The Saga of Doctor Thor

The coat of arms is composed of six elements: the shield, the helm, the mantling, the supporters, the compartment and the motto. The shield's three colours are a play on the family name: "Thor" (black for the Norse god of thunder), "lak" (blue for the waters of a lake), "son" (gold, or yellow, for the sun). The superimposed Viking broadsword with an entwined dragon (a mythical supporter of the Icelandic coat of arms) is a modified caduceus of the medical profession, and suggests a surgeon's scalpel fighting the dragon of disease.

Upon the helm (the knight's helmet) is an Icelandic falcon holding in its right claw a hammer of the mythical diety Thor, which translates into a gavel to call a meeting to order. The falcon, the official bird of Iceland, stands upon a red and silver (white) circulet and red maple leaves (the official leaf of Canada). The colours of the Icelandic flag (red, blue and white) are depicted in the mantling.

There are two supporters: a Viking with the battle ax of King Olaf, Patron Saint of Norway, to the right of the shield; and the bear (for Bjorn) to the left. (It is interesting to note that the Rynning coat of arms contains a man standing in a forest with a raised ax. Rynning is the family name of Dr. Thorlakson's Norwegian mother.)

In the compartment is the prairie grass of North Dakota, where Dr. Thorlakson was born, and also the prairie crocus, the official flower of Manitoba, where he was nurtured and spent most of his life.

The motto, "The Future is Today," is an attitude of mind which has been the basis of a life of planned achievement.

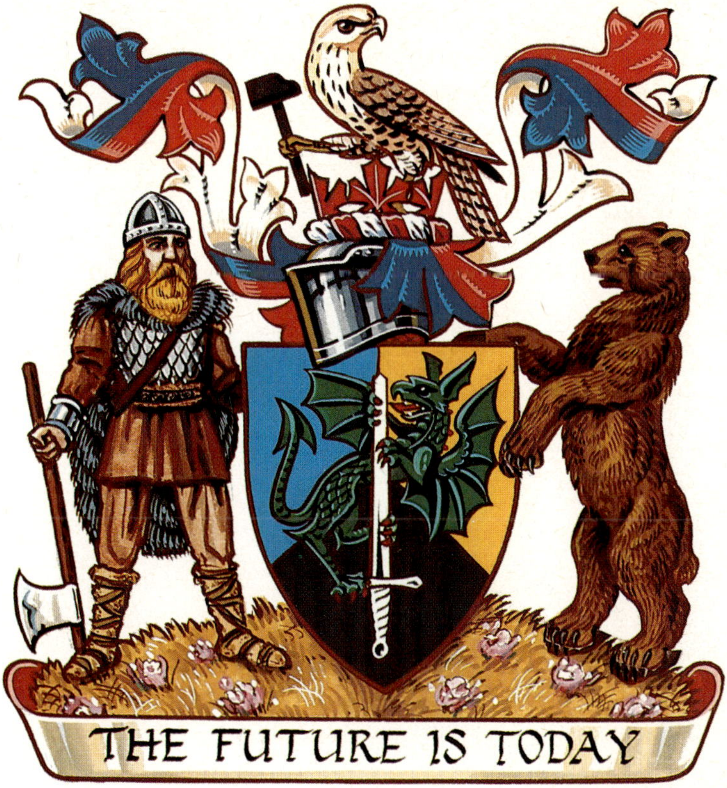

PAUL HENRIK THORBJORN THORLAKSON

CC, MD, CM (MAN), MRCS (ENG), LRCP (LON),
FRCS (CAN), FACS,

HON. LL D (MANITOBA), HON. LL D (WINNIPEG),
HON. MD (ICELAND), HON. D SC (BRANDON),
HON. FICS, HON. FACHA

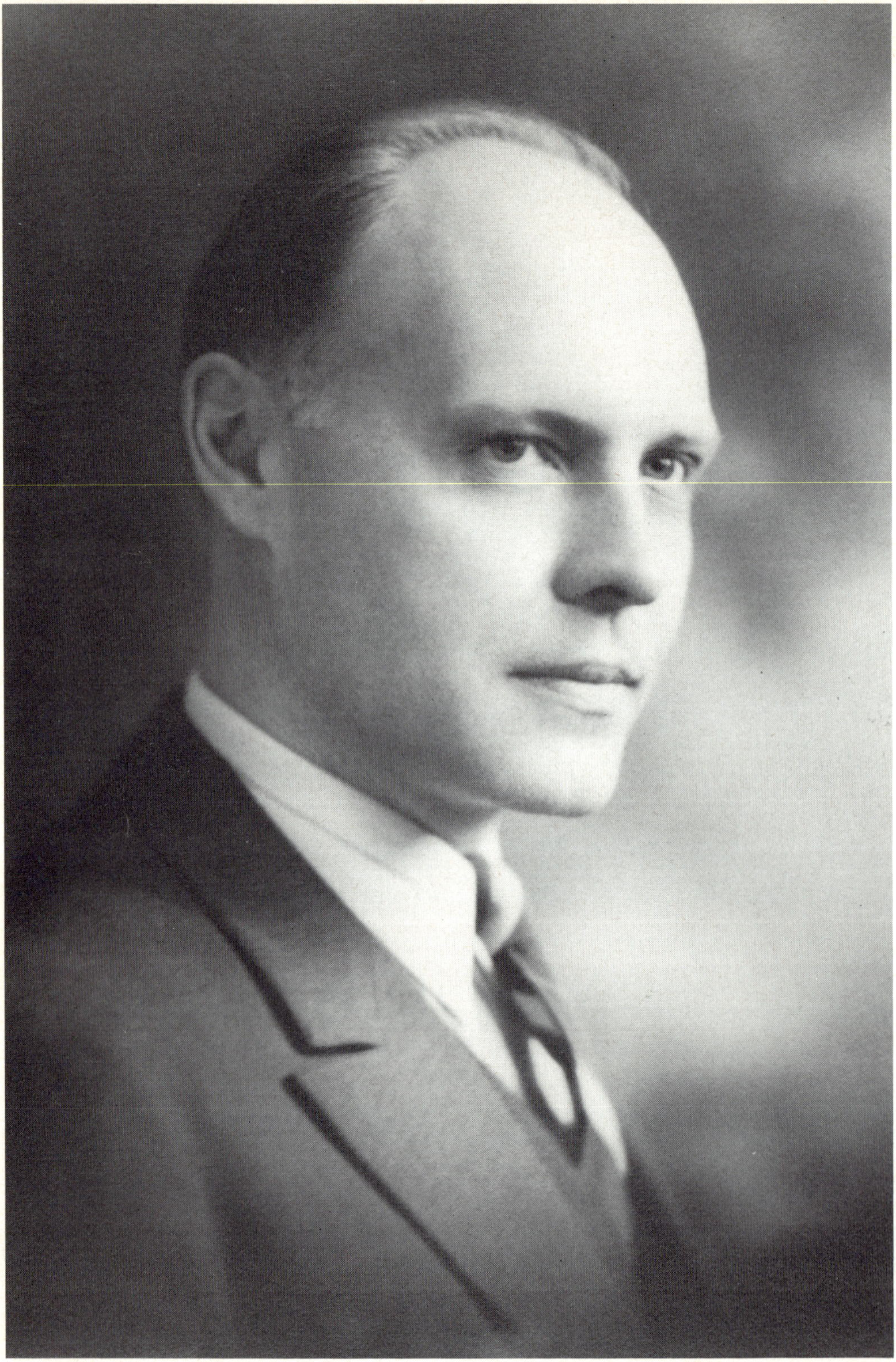

Paul Henrik Thorbjorn Thorlakson, about 1935

The Saga of Doctor Thor

Paul H T Thorlakson CC MD

A BIOGRAPHY BY T A J CUNNINGS

With the compliments
of
Paul H. T. Thorlakson
Dec 1986

The University of Manitoba

Jacket illustrations: bronze bust by Leo Mol; portrait in oils by Brenda Bury; photographs of bust and portrait by Ken McGregor, R.B.P., Medical Photography, Health Sciences Centre, Winnipeg, Manitoba; coat of arms designed by Dr. Robert H. Thorlakson; photograph of author by Bente Cunnings.

Canadian Cataloguing in Publication

Cunnings, T.A.J. (Thomas Albert John), 1908–

The saga of Doctor Thor

Bibliography: p.
Includes index.
ISBN 0-919932-25-8

1. Thorlakson, Paul H. T., 1895– 2. Physicians - Manitoba - Winnipeg - Biography. 3. Medical care - Manitoba - Winnipeg - History. I. Title.
R464.T46C85 1986 610'.92'4 C86-098093-6

TO GLADYS MAREE THORLAKSON

Many friends had urged Dr. Thorlakson to write his memoirs, but he resisted this suggestion. Subsequently Mrs. Thorlakson asked his longtime friend T.A.J. Cunnings to undertake the task of recording an account of her husband's life. For almost fifty years the fields of interest of these two men often coincided, and frequently they found themselves associated with the work of the same organizations.

This book is dedicated to Gladys Maree Thorlakson, whose devotion and constant support in her husband's family life, professional career and community involvement helped to make possible the events described in this book.

Contents

Foreword

There is perhaps no figure in the history of medicine in Manitoba whose influence has been greater than that exerted by Dr. Paul H.T. Thorlakson – "Doctor Thor" as he is affectionately known. There are of course many whose contributions in particular spheres were unsurpassed but none whose vision was broader; none whose grasp of the import of social developments for medical practice was firmer; none whose ability to transform grand designs into reality was greater. The story of the life and career of Dr. Thor, as described in the pages of this comprehensive biography, reveals much of the drive, tenacity and dynamism that animated this remarkable man; but, for each of us whose life has been touched in some special way by him, the reading of *The Saga of Doctor Thor* will bring to mind many personal recollections of the force of his personality.

I first encountered Dr. Thor when I was a medical student on the surgical wards of the Winnipeg General Hospital. It was evident, even to a novice, that here was a man of great skill and stature who commanded the respect and admiration of his peers. But equally impressive was his sensitivity to the needs and concerns of his patients and the manner in which he could, no matter how brief the interaction, establish a sense of trust and confidence in them. Dr. Thor epitomized for me what was in those days often referred to as the art of medicine.

Some years later, when I joined the Department of Physiology as a junior lecturer, I gained a fuller appreciation of the breadth of Dr. Thor's interest in the progress of medicine. My mentor, Professor Joseph Doupe, once described the key role Dr. Thor played in assisting him to establish a research unit at the Winnipeg General Hospital after World War II. Dr. Thor knew there were great advances in medical science on the horizon and he was convinced that the General Hospital could not achieve distinction as a centre for advanced health care and medical education unless its clinical staff members had available to them the stimulus of an active research program.

This appreciation on Dr. Thor's part of the importance of combining the art and the science of medicine was nothing new. His active interest in the development of a strong national program of medical research was reflected in his appointment, in 1938, as a member of the first Medical Research Committee of the National Research Council of Canada and his seminal role in the formation of the Western Regional Committee on Medical Research of the Council. Typically, Dr. Thor did not merely exhort others to support research and education. He was the founder and first president of the Manitoba Institute for the Advancement of Medical Education and Research which later became the Winnipeg Clinic Research Institute. The Institute was the vehicle through which Dr. Thor and his colleagues at the Winnipeg Clinic contributed handsomely to the financial support of many budding young medical scientists and worthy research projects.

Dr. Thor's promotion of medical research was predicated on three related beliefs. First, that an active medical research program is an essential foundation for exemplary medical care and medical education. Second, that, because of its influence on medical care and education, a strong medical research program is required in all regions of Canada. Third, that for medical research to be fostered effectively in those regions where it is underdeveloped requires the active support and sponsorship of local community leaders. His commitment to these beliefs remains undiminished to this day. How heartening it was, to those of us concerned with the erosion of federal support for research in the 1970s, that Dr. Thor, then in his ninth decade, became the founding chairman of the Manitoba Chapter of Canadians for Health Research, a coalition of lay persons and medical scientists which was instrumental in persuading the government to increase research funding.

It is not surprising in retrospect that a person with Dr. Thor's breadth of vision would inevitably concern himself with medicine not only from the perspective of the individual practitioner but also in terms of the organization of medical care. He brought his talents to bear on the problem of the efficient conduct of specialized medical practice, on the organization of medical services from a community perspective, and on the financing of medical care. Dr. Thor pioneered group medicine in Canada and became an international authority on this subject; he was an initiator of the first comprehensive scheme for insured physician services in Manitoba; he promulgated the concept of the Manitoba Medical Centre (a forerunner of what later became the Health Sciences Centre in Winnipeg and similar centres across Canada); he was an active participant in the leading Canadian and international medical societies and an important contributor to voluntary agencies such as the National Cancer Institute.

Given Dr. Thor's dedication to community service, his interest in education was not, indeed could not be, confined to medical education. He was President of the Manitoba Division of the Canadian Conference on Education and played an active part in the development of Manitoba's system of higher education. This included the establishment of the Chair in Icelandic Studies at The University of Manitoba and his election as Chancellor of The University of Winnipeg. During his nine years of distinguished service in that capacity, the University became firmly established as an independent institution with a unique mission.

It seems hardly credible that the foregoing sketch of this consummate professional man of medicine covers but a fraction of his life and work. Yet it is only that – for to encompass Dr. Thor's full measure one must also allude to his love of family, to the moving love story of Thor and his companion of more than sixty-five years – the incomparable Gladys, to his devotion to the Icelandic community both in North America and Iceland, and to his contributions to many worthy causes – in short, to his untiring effort to make the world in which he lived and worked a better place.

Dr. Thor has received many honours and awards over the years. Although these are noteworthy symbols of success, it is in the pages of this biography that one can gain a full appreciation of this outstanding man. *The Saga of Doctor Thor* is the story of an exemplar of what is best in our society – of that fusion of science and humanity to which many aspire but which few achieve; it is a story of "brave hopes fulfilled" and a vision of excellence transformed into reality.

Arnold Naimark
President
The University of Manitoba
October 1986

Preface

At the very beginning of this note of appreciation, I must record the complete cooperation of Dr. Thorlakson in the writing of this book. I was given full and unrestricted access to his personal papers, covering a period of more than half a century. They included files of correspondence, copies of speeches, published and unpublished papers on the whole range of his interests, briefs to public authorities, records of meetings, newspaper clippings, and other published records of events. As a depository of facts rather than opinions, this remarkable treasury of information was the principal source for this biography.

The material was augmented and confirmed by reference to the Department of Archives and Special Collections, University of Manitoba Libraries, the library of the Faculty of Medicine, University of Manitoba, and the reference departments in the libraries of the City of Winnipeg and the Province of Manitoba. I am grateful for the courtesy and assistance of the staff of these excellent facilities. I am grateful also to the Medical Photography and Audio-Visual Services, Health Sciences Centre, and the Communications Systems, Health Sciences Group, University of Manitoba, for their assistance with photographs.

The Thorlakson papers were acquired by the Department of Archives and Special Collections, University of Manitoba Libraries, in late 1986.

The written records were, of course, rounded out by the recollections of Dr. Thorlakson, and by discussion with those who had participated in some of the action. Some were kind enough to grant taped interviews – notably The Honourable Douglas L. Campbell, longtime Premier of Manitoba and Cabinet Minister when key parts of this story occurred; and Dr. Arthur S. Majury, for many years a member of the Winnipeg Clinic.

An account of Dr. Thorlakson's life is an important record of significant segments of Manitoba history. I have therefore quoted extensively from original documents to provide an authentic narrative of activities and events that were influential in shaping many aspects of life in this province; and indeed, in some cases, in places far away from Manitoba.

The quotations, then, express opinions and proposals from points of view held at the time. In reproducing them, no changes have been made in the text, except for necessary cutting for the sake of brevity and the avoidance of repetition. I had the privilege of having the original documents available to me, and I must take responsibility for the selection of those that have been quoted, in whole or in part.

In carrying out a work of this magnitude, one is inevitably the beneficiary of kindness and assistance from a great many people. I am grateful to them all. Numbers alone would preclude mentioning them individually, and I shall confine myself to naming Miss Edith Banks, Dr. Thorlakson's secretary from the earliest days of the Winnipeg Clinic to the present, who sorted and collated the vast store of source material into a manageable degree of topical order. Her excellent filing system (and memory) enabled her to produce with deceptive ease documents that confirmed or shed light on events associated with any aspect of Dr. Thorlakson's professional and public life. I extend to her my thanks and appreciation.

T.A.J. Cunnings
October 1986

Our Father, the Surgeon: Some Reminiscences on his Surgical Life

Father made his mark in many fields – academic, research, administrative and ethnic relationships – but he was first and foremost a surgeon. The respect and admiration he gained as an outstanding physician along with his natural abilities and remarkable energy combined to spell success in whatever field he entered. From our observation no small credit must also go to our mother, who was a force in her own right and who "held the fort" at home, raised us and our younger sister Tannis, opened her home unstintingly for meetings and gatherings, and was always available for support, encouragement and thoughtful counsel.

At an early age we were well aware of Dad's energy and capacity for work. He would leave home before dawn and often come home after midnight. Five or six hours of sleep seemed to be quite sufficient for him in any twenty-four-hour period, though he would take the occasional catnap whenever the opportunity presented itself. As we grew older we saw that his extensive knowledge of medicine and surgery was in part due to a good memory and constant reading. At home there was a large library of medical texts and journals and a well-organized filing system on surgical subjects. A surgical volume or journal was usually on his bedside table. As medical students and interns ourselves, we observed that Dad was continually on the lookout for better surgical instruments and techniques. He also encouraged his associates to develop special areas of expertise. As young surgeons we began to appreciate Dad's attention to detail in the pre- and postoperative care of patients, his manual dexterity and delicate handling of tissues, and his ability to meet and overcome unusual situations.

Even before graduation in medicine Dad took on heavy responsibilities for patient care. In his fifth and final undergraduate year he became the first full-time, and indeed the only, intern at the Children's Hospital, which was situated near the Redwood Bridge some miles from the Medical College. For nine months he was on twenty-four-hour duty during a period which coincided with the world-wide epidemic of "Spanish" flu. He assisted in the operating room almost daily and did many tonsillectomies under supervision. His commitment to the hospital's 120 patients was such that he was unable to attend many of his lectures. However, one lecture he did attend was given by Dr. Clifford R. Gilmour on gastric ulcer. It inspired him to make a special study of the disease, and it later became the subject of his Master of Surgery degree.

Although he obtained a great deal of first-hand experience in surgery during his undergraduate years under his preceptors, Dr. Neil John Maclean at the General Hospital and Dr. J.D. MacEachern at the Children's Hospital, his exposure to general medicine subjects was limited by lack of time and by the reduced availability of teachers during World War I. To rectify this, and on the advice of Dr. Maclean, Dad went to London, England, in January 1921 and spent three years in postgraduate study. His mentor in these studies was Dean (and later Sir) S. Stanley Woodwark, author of *A Manual of Medicine*. He studied neurological diseases under Sir James Purves-Stewart, and radium therapy under one of its pioneers, Mr. E. Rock Carling. During this time he passed examinations in medicine, in obstetrics and gynecology, and finally in general surgery. He spent a month in Paris studying surgical anatomy. At St. Mark's Hospital he met Mr. William Gabriel, FRCS, who later became one of the world's best-known colorectal surgeons. It is of interest that in 1951 soon after we had arrived in London to pursue our postgraduate studies in surgery, we paid a visit to Mr. Gabriel at St. Mark's. Just before we left the hospital he asked us to sign the visitor's book; then he turned the pages back to 1921 and showed us Dad's signature, penned thirty years earlier.

Dad wrote extensively on the surgical subjects in which he had a special interest and experience. The material presented in his papers was based on a study of his own cases. He maintained complete follow-up on patients with ulcerative colitis, toxic goitre and all cancer patients (thyroid, breast, stomach, colon, rectum). Most of the articles he wrote were presented at local, national and international meetings and were published later in medical and surgical journals. The first illustration of a surgical specimen ever printed in colour by the *Canadian Medical Association Journal* appeared in the February 1938 edition. Dad paid $300 (in 1930!) to the *Journal* to have this colour photograph included with the article. It was called "Carcinoma of the Rectum and Recto-Sigmoid" and was co-authored with Dr. A.W.S. Hay. When one peruses the large number of published papers and the even larger number of unpublished reports and speeches that Dad prepared, one wonders how he ever found the time to write them all. We learned his secret! He would disappear on occasion for two or three days into a small hotel across town, away from the telephone and other interruptions, until he had finished his paper. During the times he was preparing papers or speeches, a thought would often occur to him just as he awakened from sleep or while he was driving the car; he would immediately get out of bed or stop the car and jot down the wording on a scrap of paper.

In the 1920s, bacteria were thought to play an etiological role in ulcerative colitis. Dad was engaged with Dr. F.T. Cadham (Professor of Bacteriology, University of Manitoba) in a collaborative study of the disease. An autogenous serum was prepared by Dr. Cadham and used for treatment of some of their cases. Dad relates that in the surgical management of ulcerative colitis an early treatment was appendicostomy which provided a conduit for solutions needed to irrigate the affected colon. Later, defunctioning ileostomy became commonly used, "to put the colon at rest." Finally, proctocolectomy (removing all the colon and rectum) to excise all of the diseased bowel became the mainstay of surgical treatment. Dad usually did this procedure in two stages using the dictum, "It is better to do less twice than too much once" in very sick patients. Appropriate surgical intervention can be very gratifying, and on occasion spectacular, as is illustrated by the following brief 1939 case history. A healthy, physically active thirteen-year-old boy was suddenly struck by an extremely severe case of ulcerative colitis. Over a very short period he lost almost eighty pounds; (he dropped from 150 to seventy-two pounds). The ordeal with this debilitating disease kept him out of school and resulted in many complications including rheumatoid arthritis and severe ulcerations of both legs. He was in hospital for many months over the next two and a half years for observation, investigation and treatment. Finally it was decided to undertake surgery; Dad carried out an ileostomy on November 17, 1941. The operation worked "miracles." The young patient's appetite returned, his weight shot up, his leg ulcers healed, and he was able to return to school two and a half months after the operation, easily completing his school grade. Subsequently he underwent removal of the large bowel in two stages. Still later he went on to study medicine and has made substantial contributions to his chosen specialty, to the medical association and to his community.

Dad had an extensive practice in gallbladder and biliary tract surgery and an early interest and experience in dealing with liver trauma and tumour. Strictures of the common duct, always a great challenge to the surgeon, were often referred to Dad for surgical management. In the early 1930s he introduced the use of lipiodol for x-ray visualization of the biliary passages after common duct exploration. In

1927 he successfully operated upon two young patients with severe injury to the liver, one a six-year-old girl who had been injured under the wheels of a wagon, and the other a twenty-two-year-old woman who had been involved in an automobile accident. In 1960 he removed the left lobe of the liver of a patient with a solitary tumour matastatic from the colon.

In 1932 Dad sent a telegram to Dr. C. Burton Stewart, who was just completing postgraduate study in Edinburgh, requesting him to go to Germany to call on Dr. Roger Korbsh, who had recently designed a gastroscope. Dad asked Dr. Stewart to observe how Dr. Korbsh used the instrument, and to bring one home. Dad began using it in the study of stomach lesions at the Winnipeg General Hospital in February 1933. This was the introduction of the gastroscope to Canada and possibly to North America. We can remember, as ten-year-old boys, seeing the long tube in its velvet-lined case at our home before Dad took it to the hospital. We also recall seeing a picture on the front page of the *Winnipeg Free Press*, about 1935, of a patient at the Winnipeg General Hospital who had had his whole stomach removed due to cancer. The picture showed him sitting up in his hospital bed eating a normal meal. Mother explained that Father had performed the operation. It was possibly the first total gastrectomy performed in Western Canada.

In the middle third of this century, duodenal ulcer was a very common disease, and little could be done to treat it medically except diet, sedation and rest. For intractable pain and hemorrhage the surgical operation eliminated acid secretion by the stomach by removing most of an otherwise normal stomach. In January 1943, Dr. Lester R. Dragstedt, of Chicago, was the first to perform a vagotomy for duodenal ulcer. In this operation the nerves to the stomach, through which acid secretion was stimulated, were divided after reaching them through a chest incision. Dad encouraged Dr. M.B. Perrin, a thoracic surgeon, to give this operation a trial; Dr. Perrin performed a transthoracic vagotomy in some forty cases. The transabdominal route for division of the vagus nerves (supplemented by a gastroenterostomy to ensure that the partly paralyzed stomach would empty) was subsequently taken up by Dad's colleague, Dr. K.R. Trueman, who pioneered the operation in the Winnipeg area.

Because Manitoba was in the "goitre belt," operations on the thyroid were amongst the most commonly performed during the first half of this century. While on live-in duty at the hospital during the fourth year of undergraduate training, Dad had an introduction into one of this operation's postoperative complications. One afternoon he received an urgent call to East Two Ward. A patient had developed great difficulty breathing and was turning blue two hours after a large goitre had been removed. At operation it had been noted that the cartilage of the trachea (wind pipe) had been partially absorbed by the long-standing pressure of the goitre. Dad quickly opened the wound by cutting the subcutaneous wire suture with the nurse's bandage scissor. This was followed by a "large gush of blood" with immediate return of normal breathing. This quick action saved the patient's life. Years later Dad reported a series of 385 cases of goitre upon which he had operated between 1937 and 1945 (unpublished paper presented to the Regina and District Medical Society on April 20, 1945).

Before the discovery of vitamin K, uncontrollable hemorrhage was a common complication following surgery on jaundiced patients. Dad had occasion to attend a meeting of the Associate Committee on Medical Research in Ottawa where he was given samples of the newly produced vitamin K. On his return to Winnipeg he was met by Dr. Stewart McInnis, who had a jaundiced patient with uncontrolled bleeding. Dad produced some of the vials that he had in his pocket and the contents were administered to the patient. The bleeding stopped. Dr. McInnis exclaimed, "It's magic!" This was probably the first clinical use of vitamin K in western Canada.

In 1929 Dr. Alexander Fleming noted that colonies of *Penicillium notatum* mold contaminating one of his staphylococcal cultures had prevented growth of the bacteria over an area of the colonies. In 1939 a method of producing the active ingredient, penicillin, was found by Dr. Howard Florey and his colleagues at Oxford. This method was introduced to the United States during World War II where ways of mass producing the drug were developed. During the War, little penicillin was available to the civilian population. However, Dad was able to obtain a small amount to treat a young man who had developed severe subacute bacterial endocarditis, frequently a fatal infection. Administration of penicillin brought about complete recovery.

Later, Dad obtained another drug, Actinomycin D, from the National Institute of Health in Bethesda, Maryland. It was administered to a patient with cancer of the body of the pancreas who was undergoing palliative x-ray treatment at the Winnipeg General Hospital. The patient experienced relief of severe pain, was able to leave hospital and to return home, where he lived out the remaining short period of his life relatively pain-free.

Referring doctors and medical and surgical colleagues were always welcome in Dad's operating room. On many occasions he was visited during operations by surgeons from elsewhere in Canada, from the United States and abroad. One morning about 7:30, Dad had a telephone call from Dr. Arthur W. Elting, an American surgeon who had been duck hunting in Manitoba, and who was staying overnight at the Fort Garry Hotel. The visitor asked if he could watch Dad operate. As Dad was just on his way to the hospital to start the day's operating slate at 8:00, he suggested that the doctor take a taxi to the General Hospital and then go up to the operating room where a nurse would give him a gown (to wear over his street clothes!). He arrived and took his place on the observation platform and later beside Dad, where he observed the surgical procedures with great interest and from time to time offered knowledgeable comments. Since there had been little time for conversation during the morning, Dad invited the visitor to have lunch with him at the Manitoba Club. It was then that Dad learned that his guest was the President of the American Surgical Association; he had come in this capacity to see Dad operate upon the recommendation of two of Canada's leading surgeons, Dr. W.E. Gallie of Toronto and Dr. E.W. Archibald of Montreal. "If it's the last thing I do as president, it will be to see that you become a member of the Association," he said.

During the time we were doing our surgical postgraduate training in Britain, Dad was collaborator on a panel discussion on intestinal obstruction at the joint meeting of the American College of Surgeons with the Association of Surgeons of Great Britain and Ireland held in Leeds and London. He came down to Ipswich where one of us was Surgical Registrar at the Ipswich and East Suffolk General Hospital. The consultant surgeon, Mr. Arthur R. Hill, FRCS, was away on the continent at the time and had turned over the operating responsibilities to his Canadian registrar. Ken invited his Dad to "scrub up" with him for a day's surgery, which included a gastrectomy, a cholecystectomy and a thyroidectomy. It was a unique experience to have one's father operating with him in a distant land.

When we came home after our postgraduate studies in England, over a period of time we gradually assumed more annd more patients who came into the Section of General Surgery at the Winnipeg Clinic. Over the ensuing years we observed Dad's communication skills with family physicians and with patients. He had the "human touch" with patients, never seeming to be in a hurry and always taking time to listen and to explain. He never turned away a patient who asked to see him. If Dad determined that the problem was not in his field of practice, he would then and there pick up the telephone and ask one of his colleagues to see the patient, after which he would say to the patient, "You will be well looked after." Dad invariably contacted the immediate family member of every patient upon whom he had performed a major operation. Throughout his life as a doctor Dad would, whenever the occasion warranted, call at the home of a patient who was sick or who had had an operation or who was terminally ill. At Dad's side in office practice was Dr. Dallas Medd, who provided invaluable support with his concise histories and meticulous physical examinations of potential surgical patients; also with him in the office was Miss Edith

Banks, his secretary, with her infallible memory and remarkable understanding and insight.

Now, some twenty-five years after Dad has retired, hardly a day passes during which one of us does not see a patient upon whom Dad has operated during his forty-three years of busy surgical practice. The patients invariably inquire after him and usually make one of the following remarks: "Your father always had time to talk to me"; or, "When he walked into the room I knew that I could put my complete trust in him"; or, "When your father put his hand on my shoulder before I went under the anesthetic, I knew that I was in safe hands."

Dad made a point of being readily available at all times to his patients and to his colleagues. He was meticulous in communicating with others. Dad always went out of his way to insure that his patients, his staff, his colleagues, his family and others to whom he had some obligation were informed of his intentions or commitments and that he, in turn, was aware of their opinions and plans.

Dad never seemed to waste a moment. Every hour of the day was spent in purposeful activity with appropriate balance of time for work, for leisure and for rest. While completing everything that needed to be accomplished each day, he constantly looked ahead and planned for the future.

Robert H. Thorlakson, M.D.
Kenneth T. Thorlakson, M.D.
October 1986

PART ONE

Introduction

CHAPTER 1

Prologue: A Love Story

A reunion of the descendants of Niels Steingrimur Thorlaksson (1857–1943) and his wife, Erika (Rynning) Thorlaksson (1860–1947) was held in Seattle, Washington, in September 1977.

Of the 104 descendants (including wives and husbands and children of the sixty-one in direct line) eighty-five attended this family gathering. They came from the provinces of Manitoba and British Columbia, and from the states of Oregon, Washington, Colorado, Missouri and Texas.

Guests of honour were three of the six children of Niels Steingrimur and Erika Thorlaksson: Margrethe Sigmar of Kelso, Washington; Paul Hendrik Thorbjorn (Thor) Thorlakson and his wife Gladys of Winnipeg; and Erika Eastvold of Seattle. Dr. Haraldur Frederik Thorlakson of Seattle and Lorentz Halfdan Thorlakson of Vancouver, the two remaining living children, were unable to attend because of illness. The eldest son, the Reverend Steingrimur Octavius Thorlaksson, had passed away in Webster Grove, Missouri, on July 10, 1977.

The reunion festivities began in the afternoon of September 2 in the Providence Heights Conference Centre, situated in the heavily wooded hills near beautiful Lake Sammamish, several miles east of Seattle.

After the excitement and joy of first greetings and a reception resonant with the happy laughter and the exclamations of delight that signalled every new encounter, the company sat down to dinner. The Master of Ceremonies was the Reverend Eric Sigmar.

At the conclusion of the dinner, "Dr. Thor" was invited to address the assembly. His speech was entitled simply, "A Love Story":

This evening, I will tell you a love story. It was love at first sight in a romantic and beautiful setting on the occasion of a wedding which took place in the city of Horten, a naval base fifty miles south of Oslo, Norway. Visualize a spacious home surrounded by a large, beautiful garden with roses and other flowers in profusion. Here, in 1885, two young people met for the first time. The young lady was Erika Rynning from Oslo. The young man was Niels Steingrimur Thorlaksson, a theological student at the University of Christiania (now Oslo).

Here, I must first explain Father's presence in Norway. In 1873, at the age of 16, he had arrived in Wisconsin, USA, with his parents and their large family from the north of Iceland. Two years later, in 1875, he enrolled in Luther College in Decorah, Iowa, from which he graduated with honours with the degree of Bachelor of Arts in 1881. During summer vacations, he had taught school in the log cabin he had built on his quarter section of land near Mountain, North Dakota. After graduation, he spent two years in Mountain in business with his older brother, Haraldur, and was at the same time the first regular teacher and the first justice of the peace. In 1883, he travelled to Norway where he studied theology at the University of Christiania (Oslo) and from which he graduated in 1887.

While still a student in Oslo, Niels Steingrimur received a letter from one of his former teachers at Luther College, Professor O.J. Breda, who was returning to Norway during the summer holidays to marry his fiancée, Miss Emilia Braarud of Horten. Professor Breda asked his former student, Niels, to be best man at the wedding.

The bride's best friend and bridesmaid was Erika Rynning of Oslo. The day before the wedding, and unbeknown to each other, Niels Steingrimur and Erika must have travelled on the same train from Oslo to Horten. The next day was to be the most fateful day of their lives – love at first sight. How can we explain this instant, mutual attraction which occurs so often, so naturally, and so spontaneously between two complete strangers who have never seen each other before?

Mother never ceased to enjoy telling us, her children, of the excitement and thrill of that memorable and happy summer day in 1885. With a reflective smile, she would tell us of the walks in the garden that she and Father took together before and after the wedding ceremony. After sitting near Father at the wedding dinner for three hours of feasting and many speeches, and then walking with him in the cool moonlit garden, she knew that this meeting with the young student was to have an important influence on her life. That evening, she sang for the assembled guests. We can only surmise that one selection would have been the lovely Norwegian song, "Over the Lofty Mountains," a song which she would often sing for Father and the family.

We can be sure that they were no longer strangers the next day on their return journey to Oslo. Mother told us that she and the young theological student later went together to see the recent newlyweds embark for America. As the bride embraced her bridesmaid in a fond farewell, she whispered into her ear: "Erika, you will soon be engaged to Niels Thorlaksson!" What better reassurance could the young Mrs. Breda have for herself than to believe that she might be joined in that faraway land of America by her friend, Erika Rynning. And that is exactly what happened.

Mother's and Father's engagement was announced on June 6, 1886. Later that summer, when Professor and Mrs. Breda returned to Norway for a holiday, Mother and Father were on the dock to welcome them. As Mother greeted Mrs. Breda, she pressed the hand with her engagement ring into the palm of her friend and whispered: "Emilia, you prophesied correctly – we are now engaged."

When Father was about to graduate from the University of Oslo in 1887 and return with Erika to America, their plans for the wedding were well advanced. The date had been set for May 17, 1887. But here tragedy intervened. The bride's mother took critically ill and died. The wedding was postponed. Mother, as the eldest daughter in the family, stayed for a whole year to help make the necessary adjustments, which included securing the help required by a large family.

As Father had received and already accepted a call from the Icelandic congregations in and near Minneota, Minnesota, he was obliged to return to America alone. He was ordained on August 21, 1887, by the Reverend Jon Bjarnason, the president of the Icelandic Evangelical Lutheran Synod of America, in the newly built church in Mountain, North Dakota. Here his older brother, Pall Thorlaksson – known as the father of the Icelandic settlement in North Dakota – had served from 1878 until his untimely death in 1882.

At the end of another year, Erika Rynning bade her family farewell, knowing, as many others had before her, that she might never see her loved ones in Norway again. She travelled alone across the broad Atlantic. From New York, she took a train for Chicago and here again, fate intervened.

Father had left Minneota, Minnesota, and travelled the seventy miles to Minneapolis by train to await the arrival of his bride-to-be at the home of their mutual friends, Professor and Mrs. Breda, where the wedding was to take place on May 17, 1888. On the spur of the moment, Father decided to surprise Mother. He boarded a train for Chicago in the hope of travelling back with her the 400 miles to Min-

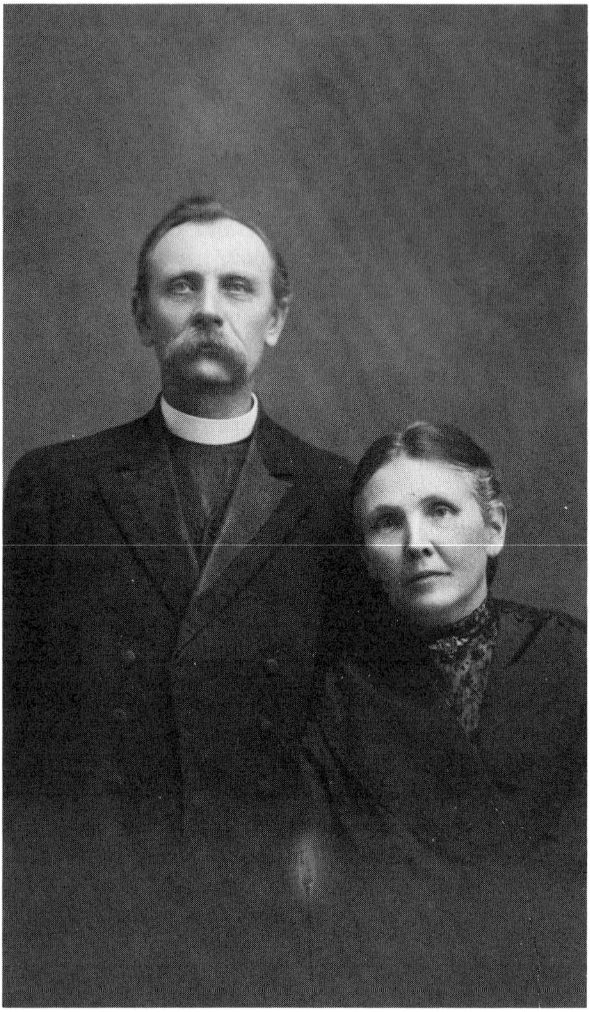

Reverend Niels Steingrimur Thorlaksson and his wife Erika (Rynning) Thorlaksson, about 1910

neapolis. The large, bustling railway station in Chicago was packed with people, some looking for friends who were to meet them, and others struggling to find the right train on which to continue their journey. Finally, Father was forced to admit to himself that either Mother had missed the train in New York or had passed through on an earlier train. When he telephoned the Bredas, he learned that the bride-to-be had already arrived in Minneapolis. Because of the mishap in Chicago, the wedding was postponed *one more* day, to May 18, 1888. We can well imagine the excitement when these four young people were finally re-united. Professor Breda, who was by then Professor of Norwegian Language and Literature at the University of Minnesota and an ordained minister, performed the ceremony.

Father's and Mother's first home in Minneota consisted of two small rooms, reached by an outside stairway, above a general store. Much of the furniture was hand-made by Father. Their good friend, Gunnar B. Bjornson, was later to recall that the accommodation was "nothing for the young bride to write home about." However, he continued by saying that "Mrs. Thorlaksson came to the Minneota Parish as a ray of sunshine. Everybody fell in love with her at first sight. She had many fine qualities: culture, geniality, beauty, charm, and music. She was accustomed to cultured society, to the gay life of a European metropolis, to comparative ease and comfort as a daughter of one of Norway's old and honoured families; and yet, cooped up in two small rooms over a dilapidated old store, she never grumbled and she never complained." Three years later, in 1891, a parsonage was built and ready for occupancy.

It was not until Gladys and I visited Norway for the first time in 1930, when Mother's brothers and sisters were still living in their comfortable homes, that I realized what Mother had sacrificed because of her great love for Father. Not only had she left the comfort and security of a gracious home and the prestige of her large family, but she had also turned down a handsome Norwegian suitor to travel alone – thousands of miles – to become the bride of a young Icelandic pastor and live in a strange and harsh new world. Only such a love could have given her both the courage to set off for America and the fortitude to surmount the hardships and heartaches which she faced in her new and vastly different environment.

Mother and Father were a happy, resourceful couple, deeply in love. And that is a fortunate combination which – when nourished and allowed to grow – never fails. They were both musical. Mother had a trained, rich soprano voice.

Mother also had a keen sense of humour and could laugh heartily at herself whenever she was the cause of some temporary embarrassment by using a wrong word in her first attempts to speak Icelandic. Some

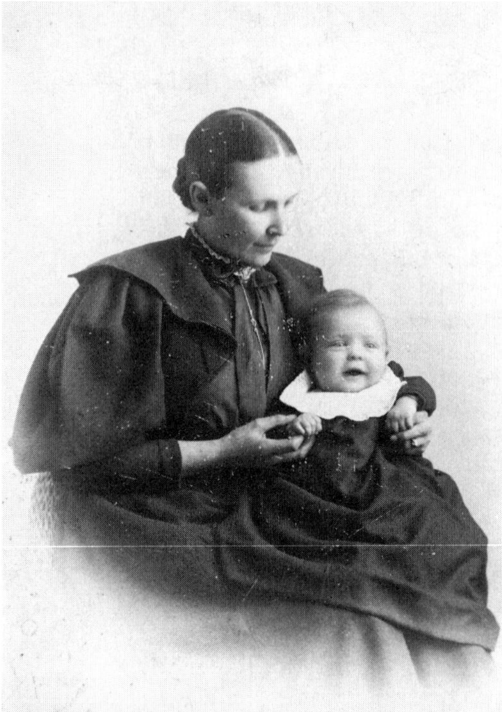

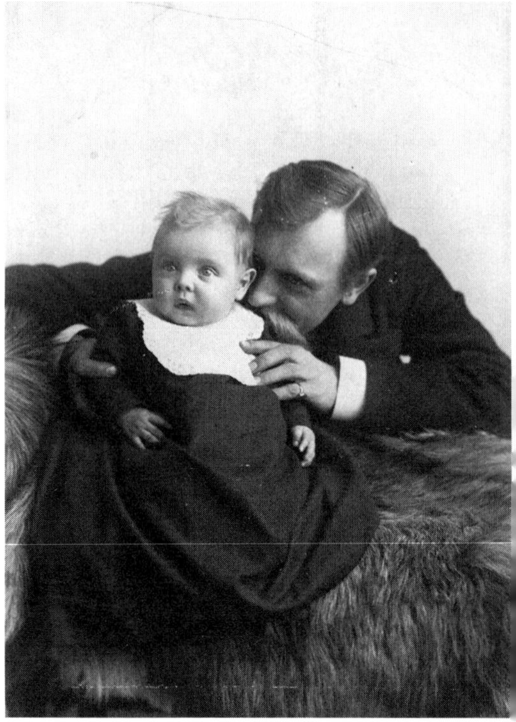

Thorbjorn, aged nine months, has his first portraits in 1896, with mother, with father

time prior to her engagement, she had followed the practice, common then for young ladies in Norway, of attending a home-making and cookery course. As all her family and many friends can attest, she was a cook "par excellence." I know that we will taste some of her favourite specialties during this family celebration, because both her culinary skills and baking artistry were passed on to many of you.

Father served four churches in Lyon and Lincoln counties in the State of Minnesota from 1887 to 1894, driving from Minneota by horse and buggy twelve miles to one church, thirteen to another and seven miles to the third.

Octavius, our eldest brother, was born in the two-room "suite" over the store in 1899 and was named after a little girl, Octavia, whom Mother and Father had adopted soon after they came to Minneota. Octavia had died the very day that Octavius was born.

Many of you must wonder how our sister, Margrethe, got the nickname Loa. Margrethe was the first child to be born in the new parsonage in Minneota. Before she was born, Mother and Father took long walks in the evenings. Passing a furniture store on one occasion, Mother spied a small corner cupboard with three shelves. She told Father that it was just what she needed for some of the things she had brought from Norway, but father replied that unfortunately they could not afford it just then.

A day or two after the birth of Anne Margrethe, Father came into the bedroom holding something behind his back. Mother was holding her new baby in her arms. Father gave her his gift – the corner shelves – and said to Mother, "This is my present to you for giving me my little Loa." Loa is the name of a little song-bird in Iceland. Fred and I were born in Park River, North Dakota, where Father and Mother served a Norwegian Lutheran church for six years. In 1900, the family moved to Selkirk, Manitoba, Canada, where Halfdan and Erika were born. We regret that Fred and Halfdan are unable, because of illness, to be with us this evening. Mother told us that when Halfdan was five or six years old, and knowing that two children had been born in each parish, he said to her, "Mamma, why don't we move again so that we can have two more in the family?"

Another anecdote that amused Mother greatly was when Harald Sigmar, as a very young boy, said to his *bestemor*, "Grandmother, you have nothing to worry about. When you take sick, you will have two doctors in the family to make you well again, and when you die, you will have two ministers in the the family to bury you. Grandmother, you have nothing to worry about."

Father and Mother had love for all people, but especially for young people. Our home in Selkirk was regularly filled with music, song and

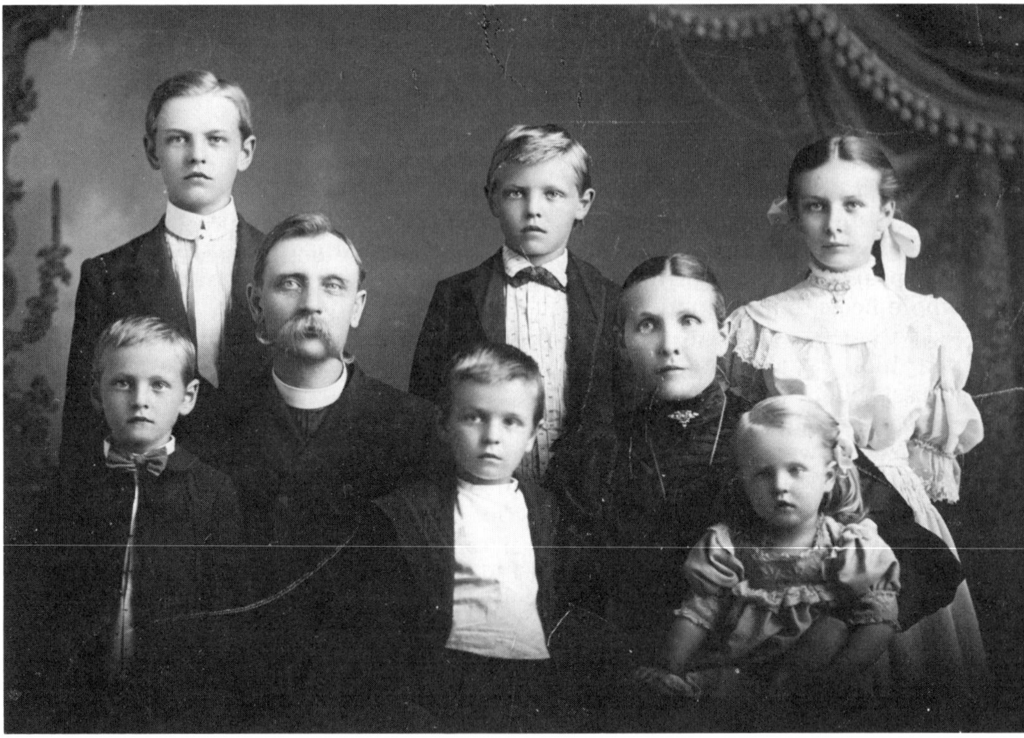

The Thorlaksson children with their parents at Selkirk: at back Octavius, Thorbjorn and Margrethe; at front Frederik, Halfdan and Erika.

laughter. There were plenty of games, both indoors and outdoors. We had a tennis and a croquet court in the garden.

I must now digress for a moment to mention *two* incidents that served to enhance our understanding and appreciation of the true love story that I have related to you. What I have said is only a fleeting glimpse – only the highlights – of the full story which would take a whole book to do it justice.

I will now transport you suddenly to a hotel room in Reykjavik in the year 1930 when Iceland was celebrating the thousandth anniversary of the establishment of representative government. Early one morning, a rap came on the door of our room. I wakened enough to call "come in" – for no doors were locked in the brand new old folks' home that had been built in time to accommodate a few of the 30,000 visitors to Reykjavik and Thingvellir on that historic occasion. The door opened and in walked a handsome young naval officer. He looked at me and then across the room at the other bed. He said to me, "I am Lorentz Holck, one of your Norwegian cousins," and then he added, "Is that Gladys, your wife, in the other bed?" I was still half asleep and, according to Gladys and Cousin Lorentz, I replied, "I hope so." After a few pleasant exchanges, he said, handing me an envelope, "I bring you this letter from our captain which contains an invitation to an afternoon reception on board our Norwegian battleship." Incidentally, I should tell you that many of the countries which sent official representatives to the thousandth anniversary celebrations sent them in war ships, which acted as hotels – very impressive hotels, I should add – for the members of the delegations. [Great Britain sent the large battleship "Rodney." Lord Stanley said in his official address to the Icelandic Nation that, "as a representative of the Mother of Parliaments, I am pleased to be here to salute the Grandmother of Parliaments."]

Exactly forty-four years later, in 1974, Gladys and I were spending a holiday in Sandefjord, Norway, situated thirty-five miles south of Horten, where Mother and Father first met. Our cousin, Lorentz Holck – now a retired officer of the Norwegian Navy – and his wife, Mary, invited us to visit them in Horten, the naval base on the Oslo Fjord. We motored the thirty-five miles from Sandefjord to Horten; it is one of the most beautiful country drives that we have had in our travels abroad.

Lorentz and Mary drove us around Horten and then took us to the former home of Mr. and Mrs. Ole Eriksen Braarud, where their daughter, Emilia, had married Professor Breda, and where Mother and Father had walked in the garden in 1885. The large house is still standing and is in a remarkable state of preservation. Evidence of its former grandeur can still be seen. As we walked in the garden, the whole story of Mother's and Father's first meeting was re-enacted in our minds. *There,* in this beautiful garden, the romance had started and *there* had begun the enduring love story that accounts for *all of us* being here today.

This evening we honour the memory of, and pay tribute to, Niels Steingrimur and Erika Rynning Thorlaksson, and also to other loved ones who are no longer with us: Octavius and Caroline (Thomas) Thorlaksson, Haraldur (Halli) Sigmar, Doris (Bousfield) Thorlakson, Harald Eastvold, and Margaret (Sigmar) Kristjanson.

I now ask you to rise and stand for a moment as we give silent thanks for the companionship, love and joy that they gave to us.

CHAPTER 2

Preparation

From early childhood, but more particularly as he worked through his high school years, Paul Thorlakson was encouraged by his parents to follow the family tradition and select one of the professions for his life work. During the family discussions of potential alternatives, it became evident that Paul himself was attracted by the challenges and the opportunities of medicine. This met with the warm support of his father and mother, and the decision was taken that Paul would become a medical doctor. It was a decision that was to have a profound impact on the practice of medicine in Manitoba and an influence on medical care in far places as well.

At that time, it was possible to enter medical school immediately after senior matriculation in high school. However, Paul's father wisely insisted that this step was premature and that Paul should spend at least two years taking courses in arts and science before turning to the study of medicine.

Thus equipped, in the spring of 1914, at the age of eighteen, the young man assembled his scholastic record and his recommendations, and sent off his application to enter medical school in the autumn of that year. It was a thrilling moment when in early summer he received his letter of acceptance; he looked forward with eager impatience to the day his professional career would be launched. The path ahead seemed clear and certain and the hindrances and impediments that lay ahead were unsuspected.

As Winston Churchill put it many years later, "It's good to

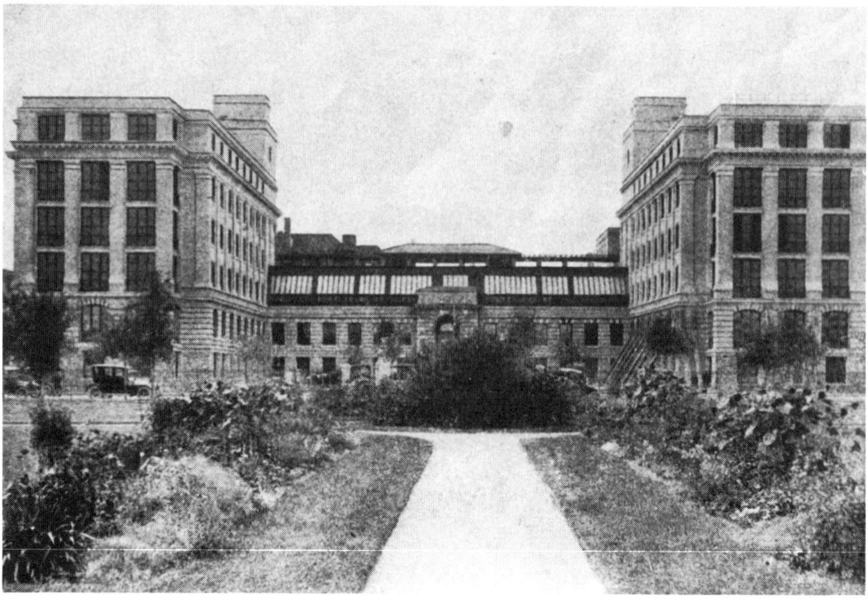

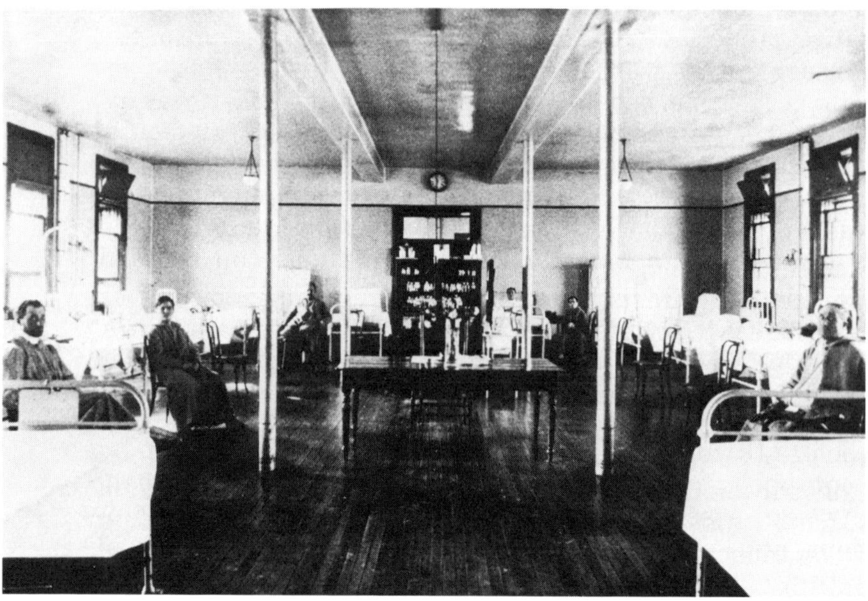

Main entrance of the Winnipeg General Hospital, about 1921

Typical ward at the Winnipeg General Hospital at the time of Dr. Thorlakson's medical training and early practice

look into the future, but it's difficult to look further than you can see." Paul Thorlakson's plans were almost overturned before his training could begin. At midnight on August 4, 1914, what had seemed until then a distant quarrel between Germany and its neighbours was transformed into the reality of World War I. The next day, young Canadians in the thousands were lining up at recruiting stations, offering themselves in the service of their country. For young men on the threshold of a career, this presented a grave dilemma. It was clear to the authorities, however, that doctors would be needed in large numbers; and students enrolled in the Faculty of Medicine were strongly urged to carry on with their studies.

Thus it was that a month later, on a September morning vibrant with the blue skies and sunshine of Manitoba, Paul Thorlakson took his place in the lecture rooms and laboratories of the Medical School of the University of Manitoba and on the wards of the Winnipeg General Hospital. It was a relationship that was to last a lifetime.

As the late Dr. Ross Mitchell[1] noted in an unpublished paper, "He was fortunate in his teachers, young and able men: Alexander Gibson in anatomy; William Boyd in pathology; E.W. Montgomery in medicine; Brandur J. Brandson, Neil John Maclean and Jasper Halpenny in surgery; H.P.H. Galloway in orthopedics; and O. Bjornson in obstetrics." To receive instruction and guidance and counsel from this distinguished group of men was a privilege which Paul (or Thor, as his friends called him) embraced with enthusiasm. Strong and healthy, diligent and keen, he took in stride the heavy demands of the lectures, the laboratories, the libraries, the things scholarly, the things practical, the long hours of concentrated study, the examinations, the demonstrations. All, due to the teaching and example of his parents, were considered as opportunities to be grasped, not as duties to be tolerated.

Continuing a pattern established during his senior high school years, he spent the summer vacation after his first year in medicine working in the commercial fishing industry, moving in harvest time to stooking and threshing on farms between Glenboro and Baldur. For two summers he was employed as a clerk at a fishing station operated on Lake Winnipeg by Captain William Robinson. The story is told that one day the cook on a

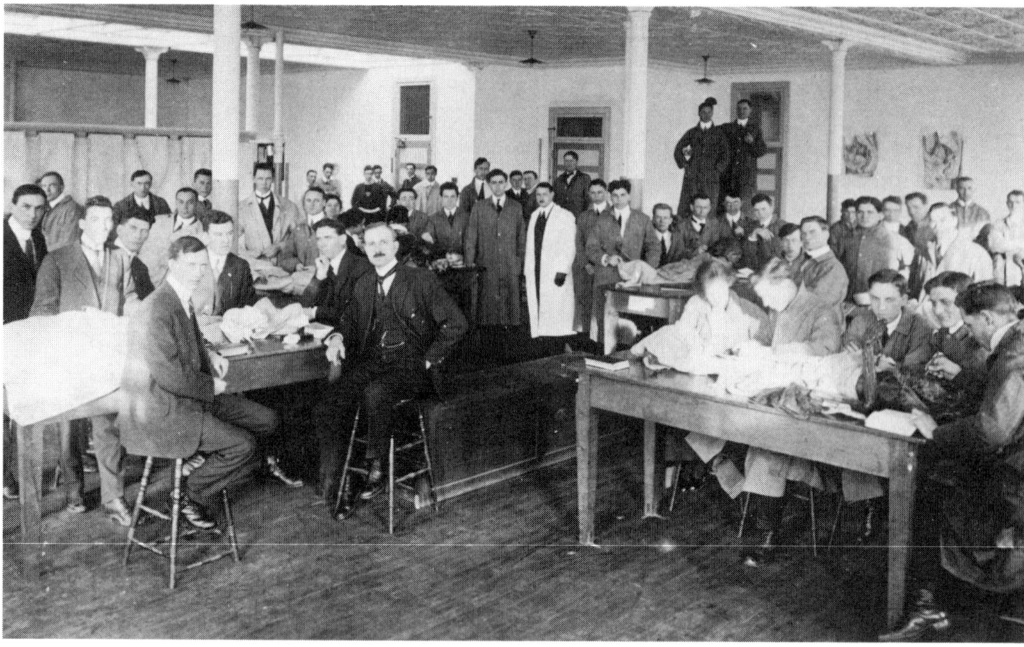

Anatomy class, Manitoba Medical College, 1914. Standing centre, in the white coat, is Dr. Alexander Gibson, professor of anatomy. Young Thor is seated at the end of the table at extreme right.

tug owned by Captain Robinson was ill, and the youthful clerk was pressed into service as a replacement. Noting a quantity of dried apples on the shelves in the tiny galley, he decided to give the men a treat by making apple pies. Following his recollection of how his mother did it, he mixed together flour, water and shortening, but the dough could not be kneaded. He tried adding more flour, then more lard, then more water; but despite his best efforts the dough remained a spongy, unmanageable mixture. In desperation, he threw the whole thing overboard, and served prunes for dessert. That evening when the nets were raised, the sticky, indigestible mass appeared, rejected even by the fish!

Dominating the life of everyone in Canada at that time were the devastating battles in Europe, which were not going well for the Allies. As the War continued, the sense of duty to their country persuaded more and more of the young men in "essential training" categories, to forsake their education and enlist. Early in 1916 Paul Thorlakson decided he must follow this course. Years later he described his initial experience:

Immediately after writing the last examination at the conclusion of my second year in medicine in the spring of 1916, I walked to the recruiting office to enlist. I was assigned to the 223rd Battalion, as a private in the medical unit. On arrival at the barracks, I discovered that Dr. Baldur Olson, who had himself graduated from our medical school just a year earlier, was the medical officer, with the rank of captain. I reported to him, and promptly received my first (and only!) promotion in the military service; I was raised from the status of a private to sergeant (medical) of the battalion.

Regularly, Dr. Olson and I would walk from the barracks on Main Street – in the wholesale area east of the City Hall – to the General Hospital to visit recruits who had been admitted to the special military ward. I learned some very important methods of clinical examination from him during these morning rounds, as well as at the daily sick parade in the barracks.

Dr. Olson gave me my first instruction in examination of the chest with a stethoscope. I gained a great deal of practice under his guidance, and he was an excellent teacher. After the War, he continued his medical practice in Winnipeg, and was recognized as one of the early specialists in respiratory disease. Together with his colleague Dr. William Lawson Mann, he performed, in the early 1930s, the first thoracoplasties in Manitoba at the Winnipeg General Hospital. These oper-

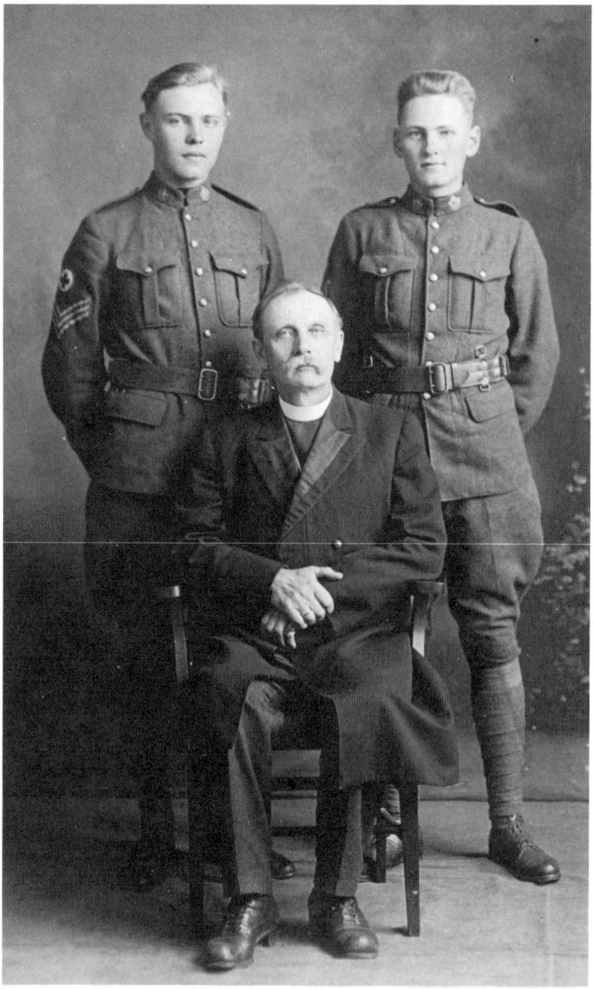

Reverend Niels Steingrimur Thorlaksson and his sons Thorbjorn and Frederik, 1916

ations were designed to close cavities in lungs which had been caused by active pulmonary tuberculosis.

Our battalion was sent to Camp Hughes for a summer of training, preparatory to going overseas. In the fall of 1916, however, instead of crossing the Atlantic, we were moved to Portage la Prairie. Shortly afterwards, Colonel Marino Hannesson, a lawyer by profession, was appointed our battalion commander, with Joseph Thorson (later to become famed in politics and the law) as his adjutant.

When Colonel Hannesson learned that I had been conducting many of the morning sick parades, but could not continue to do this daily without the direction of a qualified doctor, he suggested that the work be divided and that I should not lose the whole winter session of my medical training. He therefore arranged that I should leave on the CPR night train on Sundays to Winnipeg and return each Friday evening to Portage la Prairie to resume my medical duties. Dr. G.A. Hassard of Portage la Prairie was appointed temporary medical officer of the battalion. Under these arrangements I was allowed to register for my third year in medicine and took all my classes for that year.

One Saturday morning I was invited to assist Dr. Hassard at an operation in the hospital in Portage la Prairie. I was interested to notice, as we prepared for the operation, that he was most meticulous in scrubbing his hands and arms; but he was among the doctors, few in number at that time, who refused to use rubber gloves because they reduced the sensitivity of the fingers in dealing with human tissues. I suspect that the rubber gloves were somewhat thicker than those developed later, and they fitted poorly.

Just after I completed my third-year classes, and just before the examinations, the 223rd Battalion was ordered to proceed to Halifax, en route to England. Shortly before our departure, Dr. Frank A. MacNeil was appointed our battalion medical officer. After the War, he returned to Winnipeg to practise as a highly respected ear, nose and throat specialist. He died in October 1981.

Soon after leaving Winnipeg with the battalion, a Major Scholer suffered an attack of renal colic. He refused to leave the troop train, so I was detailed to be available to give him an injection of morphine if he had recurrent pain. On our arrival in Halifax, he and I were installed in a hotel while we waited our turn to embark on the next troop ship. Major Scholer had his meals delivered to his room, whereas I took my meals at a nearby restaurant.

One noon, after I had ordered my lunch – lobster, no less! – I was summoned immediately to the hotel. I assumed that Major Scholer needed an injection of morphine, so I took leave of my lunch and assured the restaurant keeper that I would be back to finish it shortly. However, when I reached the hotel, there was the Major sitting in a large military automobile, all ready to board ship. He had arranged for my bag to be packed and put in the car. Under these circumstances all I could do was get into the car, and off we went to England.

Many years later I happened to be in Halifax at a medical meeting. I tried to locate the restaurant, taking my bearings from the hotel, but I was unable to find it; so my mysterious disappearance remains unexplained to the proprietor.

The 223rd Battalion reached England early in May 1917, and was sent to a camp at Shorncliffe, near Folkestone, a summer resort and seaport on the southern coast of Kent. Shorncliffe had been a major centre for the advanced training of Canadian troops since 1915. The open fields near the town and the rolling Kentish countryside beyond provided almost ideal conditions for practice in musketry and training in both attack and defense in the conduct of trench warfare.

By mid-May the 223rd Battalion was well settled into the strenuous training-camp schedule, living in huts and tents, which was not unpleasant in the fine south-of-England spring.

Meanwhile, in the early months of 1917, the Germans had decided to turn from the costly and largely unsuccessful use of Zeppelin airships to carry out bombing raids on the United Kingdom, and instead use the more effective Gotha IV airplanes. The Gotha was a biplane which was forty feet long and had a wing spread of more than seventy-seven feet; it was powered by twin 260-horsepower Mercedes engines which gave it a speed of eighty miles an hour.

In daylight this machine had a ceiling of 16,000 feet, carrying 300 kilograms of bombs. For night raids, when a ceiling of 10,000 feet was sufficient, it was loaded with 500 kilograms of bombs.

On May 25, at Shorncliffe, the day was clear and sunny and the troops were hard at their training assignments. At Ghent, in Belgium, a squadron of twenty-one Gothas was preparing for takeoff in the first air attack on an English target under the new German strategy. Before them was a two-hour flight, out over the coast of Belgium and then west to their objective: the military installations and the training-camp facilities at Folkestone and Shorncliffe. Coming over the coast at 16,000 feet, the Gothas were unnoticed by the troops on the ground. Suddenly, out of the sunny Shorncliffe sky, there came a rain of bombs, causing havoc among soldiers and civilians alike. For the newly arrived young men from western Canada, this was the first trial of the devastation wrought by this new and terrifying form of warfare. They were not equipped to offer a worthwhile defence. They could only take shelter as best they could and suffer in angry helplessness. At the end of the attack there were nearly 300 casualties. Seventeen of the dead and ninety-three of the wounded were Canadian soldiers.

Foreseeing a shortage of medical officers and anticipating a prolonged war, later in 1917 the military authorities decided that medical students who had completed three years of study could be sent back to finish their training and then return to service.[2] As a result of this decision and at the urging of Dr. Frank MacNeil, his senior medical officer, Dr. Thorlakson found himself back in Winnipeg in the autumn of 1917. Here he spent a year at the Winnipeg General Hospital; he served the first three months on the emergency and "outdoor" service, which was under the capable supervision of Miss Sarah Lewis,[3] and the remaining months on the surgical service of Dr. Neil John Maclean.

Dr. Thorlakson was also attached to the service of Dr. James Wilford Good, who was the first doctor in Winnipeg to own and use radium in the treatment of superficial malignant lesions. This extra duty entailed meeting Dr. Good on J Flat at 7 a.m. to see patients with him and to receive instructions as to when the radium should be removed and safely stored. Dr. Good had come to Winnipeg in 1879 after graduating from Trinity Medical School in Toronto and doing post-graduate work in Edinburgh. He was one of the founders of the Manitoba Medical College, and became its second dean, succeeding Dr. James Kerr in 1887. (It is interesting to note that P.H.T. Thorlakson has known all of Manitoba's deans of medicine, except the first, Dr. Kerr.) His was a free and capricious spirit, uninhibited by convention. On one occasion, for example, he rented the Board of Trade Saloon on Lombard Street for a day, and there dispensed wit, wisdom and whisky to the throngs of his fellow citizens who came to see him.[4]

In 1898, Dr. Good resigned as Dean of Medicine and took advantage of the once-in-a-lifetime opportunity to participate in the stampede for gold in the Klondike. About 18,000 people rushed into this almost-unsettled area of the Yukon, with Dawson City as the main base. Dr. Good became the medical-health officer in Dawson City and won high praise from the authorities for his service. After some two years in the Yukon (apparently without finding gold) he decided to return to Winnipeg and restrict his practice to ophthalmology. In preparation, he went to Vienna for formal training and thence to India, where he had the opportunity to participate in and perform more than 200 operations for cataract. He returned to Winnipeg to practise his specialty, for most of the time in partnership with Dr. Thomas Turnbull. Dr. Thorlakson recalls that, on one occasion when the intern on the Eye, Ear, Nose and Throat Service was otherwise engaged, he was called to assist Dr. Good in performing an iridectomy.

Stories abound about Dr. Good's capacity for repartee. If he was requested by a patient to accomplish the impossible, he was wont to reply, "I still spell my name with two o's." On one occasion when he was in general practice prior to going to the Klondike, he was called to see a patient at the home of a well-to-do Winnipeg citizen. Driving by horse and buggy to the home, on arrival he was directed to the third floor to examine the maid, who was reported to be too ill to get out of bed. After a thorough examination, he could find nothing the matter with her and suggested that she get dressed and go to work. "No," she replied, "these people have not paid my wages for six months, and I'm not getting out of bed until they pay me what they owe." Dr. Good walked over and carefully closed the door. "Move over," he said, "they haven't paid me for six months either!"

By the time Dr. Thorlakson's year of surgical internship was completed in mid-summer 1918, the military situation in Europe had completely changed. The end of the War was in sight, and the need for increased numbers of medical officers overseas was alleviated. The depleted medical resources available to maintain hospital and health services for the civilian population became matters of renewed concern. Dr. Thorlakson and his medical mentors decided that he should take a further year of internship, and it became necessary to determine where this would be served. Dr. Maclean recommended a position at the Children's Hospital, which would provide an opportunity to broaden his training and experience. From October 1918 through May 1919 he became the sole intern in that busy institution. It proved to be a rewarding addition to his medical education.

Despite the demands on his time, he was able to complete a thesis on gastric ulcer, which was submitted as a basis for a master's degree in surgery. The Academic Committee found this acceptable, and he was asked to attend for the related practical examination. This consisted of an oral "quiz" by Dr. H.H. Chown, the Professor of Surgery, and Dr. Fred Jamieson, who practised at Carman.[5]

At the convocation of the University of Manitoba in May 1919 with Archbishop Matheson, Chancellor of the university conferring the degrees, Dr. P.H.T. Thorlakson finally achieved his goal and became Doctor of Medicine and Master of Surgery. At the same convocation, a charming, gracious and talented young lady, then unknown to him but destined to play a great part in his life, also graduated, with a bachelor of home economics degree.

Having earned his degrees, Dr. Thorlakson was faced with the formidable task of determining where to practise. The father of one of his classmates, Dr. Carl W.E. Seale, had a farm at Birtle, Manitoba. He reported that their local physician, Dr. Frank Smith, was leaving Birtle to become a radiologist in Winnipeg, and this might give Dr. Thorlakson an opportunity to practise there. Dr. Seale was going home for a visit after graduation. Since all postal, telegraph and telephone communication had ceased due to the Winnipeg General Strike, Dr. Thorlakson decided to accompany him to investigate the prospects in Birtle. When they arrived at their destination, almost the first person they saw on the station platform was Dr. Smith. He immediately introduced them to Dr. Philip W. Head, who was taking over his practice! This ended the possibilities at Birtle for Dr. Thorlakson.

The Seale family then suggested that there would probably be enough practice for a second doctor in the nearby town of Shoal Lake. The following day it was decided that the Seales and Dr. Thorlakson would drive to Shoal Lake to investigate. As Dr. Thorlakson tells it:

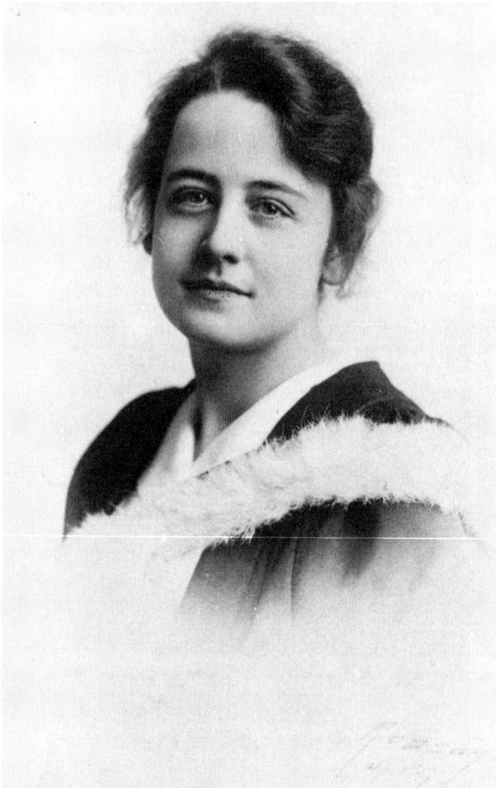

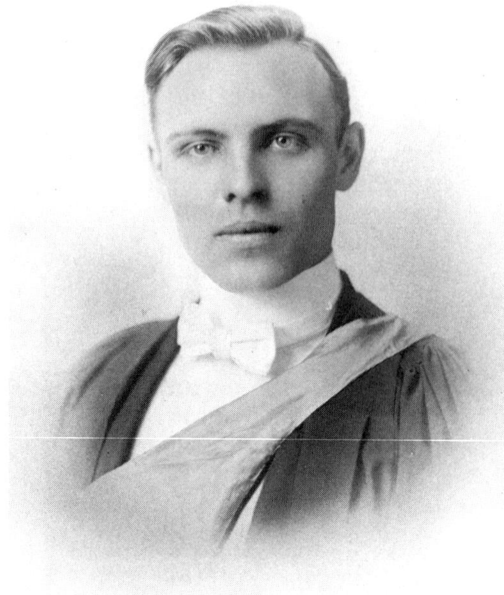

Gladys Maree Henry, Bachelor of Science in Home Economics, University of Manitoba, 1919

Paul H.T. Thorlakson, Doctor of Medicine, University of Manitoba, 1919

Shoal Lake did indeed seem to have some potential; but as a first measure I arranged to be introduced to Dr. W.H. Brothers, then the only doctor in the town. In response to my suggestion that I might like to practise there, he replied that there was not enough practice for two doctors in Shoal Lake. But I said that this was what I had been told he would say; and that I intended to try it for at least six months, partly because there was a hospital there.

I went back to Winnipeg on the train to get supplies and instruments, and then returned in a few days to Shoal Lake to find an office. While I was looking at space over a drug store, Dr. Brothers telephoned me to say that if I was determined to stay in Shoal Lake, we had better practise together. So we agreed to meet and discuss the arrangements. He suggested that we pool our income, and that his share should be sixty percent and mine forty percent – a very generous proposal on his part, which I was happy to accept.

We decided to occupy the second floor of a new building in town. We laid out offices, employed a nurse, and in a few days our joint practice was in full operation. Miss Mary Wheatley was both our nurse and our secretary. . . .

When I arrived in Shoal Lake, I had never delivered a baby. Nevertheless, as a student, I had stood in the delivery room, dressed in sterile gown, cap and mask, as a witness to the procedure. I was particularly impressed by two things: the extremely aseptic precautions taken, and the sharp slap on the behind of the newborn infant – held head down by the obstetrician – to encourage the baby to breathe.

It is worthy of note at this point that, during the first three decades of this century, ninety-five percent of all deliveries in Manitoba (including Winnipeg) were in the home. Expectant mothers were rarely seen by the doctor before childbirth; indeed, often the doctor was not notified until after the first birth pangs. Then, of course, the call was in the nature of an emergency. The doctor in the country did not have the convenience of prepared sterile sheets and towels, and no hot running water was available in the farm homes, nor in most of the houses in the town. The water had to be rapidly boiled in a kettle and brought to the bedroom in a basin.

I learned during my first few days at Shoal Lake that obstetrics was practised on an emergency basis, just as was a broken leg, a severe accident, or a sudden illness. The doctor travelled miles by horse and sleigh in winter or by car in summer to reach the home of a patient, whatever his condition of health or illness.

Dr. M. O'Brien of "Saddleback Doctor" fame was a neighbouring doctor, practising in Rossburn, a town about twenty miles northwest of Shoal Lake. He visited me shortly after my arrival and gave me many tips on practising medicine far removed from the facilities of a city hospital. He advised, for example, that one should always have a pile of unopened copies of the *Free Press* in the trunk of the car for emergencies where sterile sheets were required, such as during child-birth. He said that nothing could be more sterile than the inside pages of a large newspaper that had not been looked at, or touched by human hands.

In my Shoal-Lake experience I learned a great deal of practical "common sense" medicine from my first partner, Dr. Brothers – and woe betide the doctor who hasn't inherited or acquired a substantial degree of common sense, and the ability to extemporize in emergency situations.

On the second Sunday of the partnership, the importance of Dr. Thorlakson's experience at the Children's Hospital was demonstrated. A small baby was admitted to the fourteen-bed cottage hospital in the town, under the care of Dr. Brothers. He diagnosed an acute obstruction of the bowel, caused by the ileum (the terminal portion of the small intestine which opens into the large bowel) being telescoped into the right colon. The baby was very ill, and Dr. Brothers discussed the problem with Dr. Thorlakson. They agreed that an emergency operation was required. Dr. Brothers gave the anesthetic, and their nurse, Mary Wheatley, acted as the scrub nurse and first assistant. On opening the abdomen they found a mass on the right side, and examination revealed that several inches of the ileum had indeed telescoped into the large bowel. The complication was corrected and the abdomen was closed.

After the baby had been returned to his crib, Dr. Brothers left the hospital because his wife had invited a goodly number of people from the community to meet the new doctor, now her husband's partner. Dr. Thorlakson stayed on at the hospital another hour or so and consequently was the last to arrive at the reception. When he had been introduced to all the guests, he looked around the room for a chair. Unfortunately, the only one available turned out to be a highly cherished antique, which, when he sat down, promptly collapsed. Dr. Thorlakson found himself on his back on the floor – a most undignified and trying situation for the guest of honour!

The baby recovered. The internship at the Winnipeg General Hospital under Dr. Neil John Maclean and the year spent at the Children's Hospital, where he had assisted at operations for this extremely serious affliction of early childhood, had proved their worth.

Dr. Thorlakson stayed at the local hotel during his early days in Shoal Lake. One evening in the dining room, two weeks after his arrival, he was introduced by the proprietor to another guest, Miss Gladys Henry, who was the superintendent (and advance agent) for the Chautauqua, that famous organization which brought a combination of education and entertainment to western Canadian towns each summer for many years before radio and talking movies satisfied the need. The Chautauqua system provided for the employment of bright and personable young ladies who were university graduates; these women preceded the one-week program bookings by several months for the purpose of signing up a group of local business and professional men as guarantors of the basic costs of the performances. These guarantors then became responsible persons in the organization of the advance publicity and ticket sales. In the previous year the superintendent had failed to sign up Dr. Brothers, and this year Miss Henry had been asked to make a special effort to get the doctor on the sponsor roster. Assuming, when she was introduced to "the doctor," that this must be her special target, as Dr. Thorlakson says, "She was especially attentive to me – and has been ever since!"

Gladys Henry, of Irish and Scottish descent, the eldest daughter of Robert Alexander and Elizabeth (Anderson) Henry, was born on the family farm, ten miles southwest of Killarney, Manitoba. Her early life on the farm, and later in the town of Killarney, allowed her to develop, under the guidance and encouragement of her parents, the self-confidence and resourcefulness that are so often the gift of a free-ranging, independent rural upbringing. As a young girl she learned to ride spirited horses with skill and assurance. In due course, she studied music. She graduated in home economics from the University of Manitoba. At the University, she participated in swimming meets, was a member of the winning intramural debating team, was captain of the Snowshoe Club, and captain of the basketball team that won the inter-collegiate tournament for three consecutive years.

While still an undergraduate, she was chosen to lecture on the Better Farm Train[6] which toured Saskatchewan in 1918 to

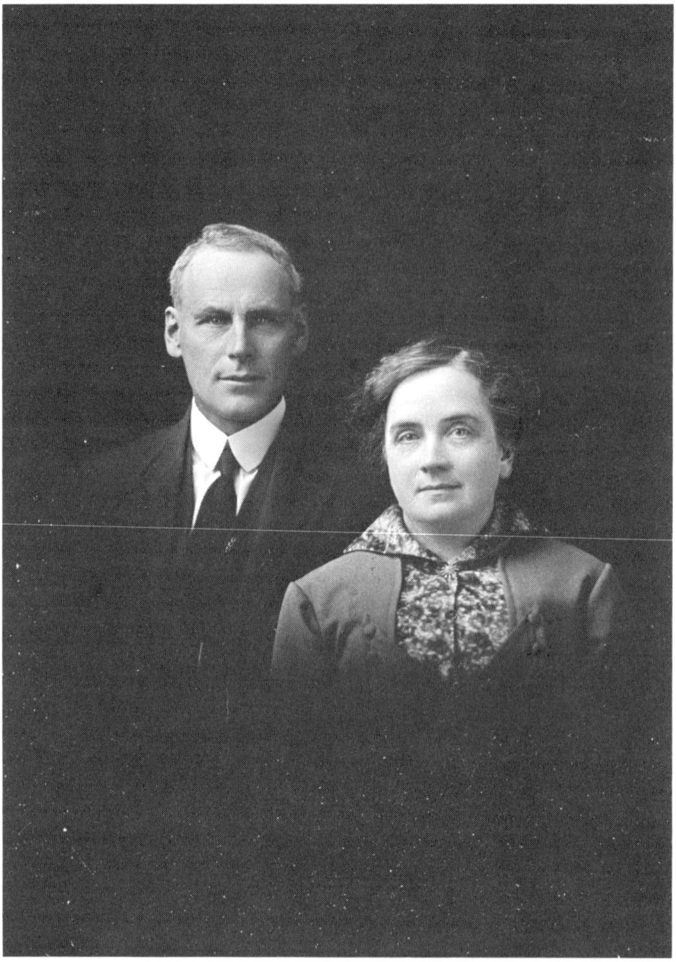

Robert and Elizabeth (Anderson) Henry

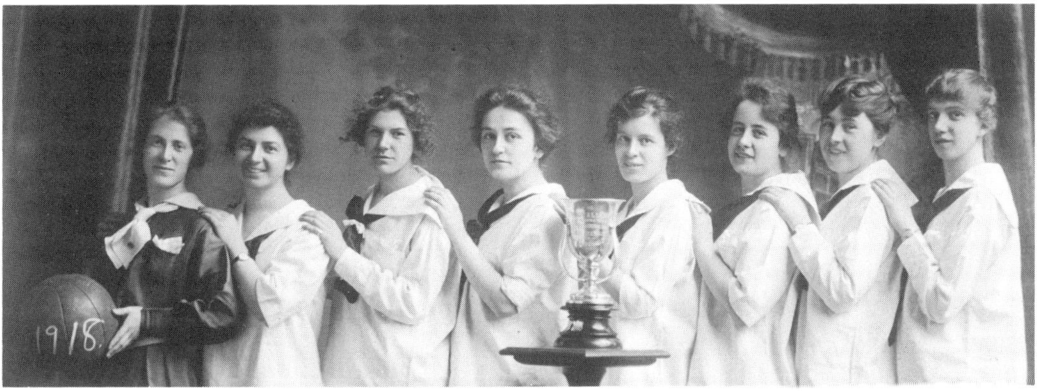

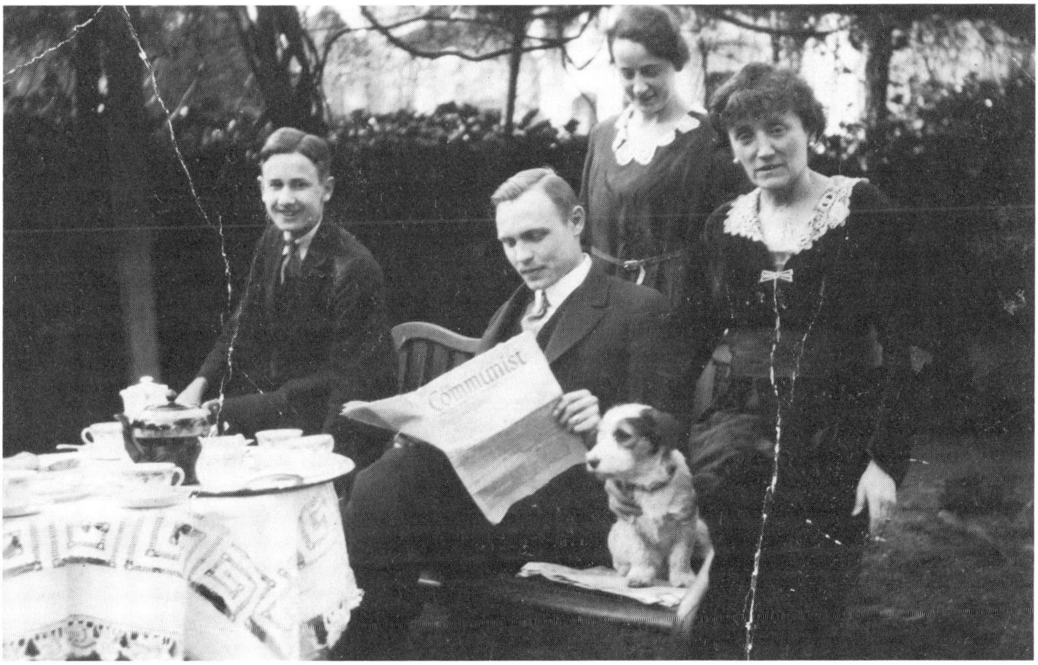

Gladys Henry was captain of the University of Manitoba basketball team that won the intercollegiate tournament for three consecutive years. The team of 1918, left to right: Anna Kennedy (instructor), Evelyn Moore, Winnie Wood, Bernice Wright, Gretta Lyon, Gladys Henry, Margaret Speechley and Evadine Judson.

For much of Dr. Thorlakson's study period in London (between 1920 and 1923), he and Gladys were paying guests at the home of Edith Brown and her son Ron at 26 Maida Vale. Here Dr. Thor has delayed Sunday tea in the garden to satisfy his curiosity about the communist view of the news as expressed in a paper handed to Ron on his way home.

teach improved methods of farm and farm home management. She also taught extension courses in rural Manitoba. And, after graduation, she joined the Dominion Chautauquas as a superintendent and organizer for the four western provinces. She found the work challenging and rewarding, and her competence was such that before she resigned in 1920 she had been given the additional responsibility of visiting the western universities to interview prospective staff for the Chautauqua.

In November 1920, Dr. Thorlakson terminated his practice at Shoal Lake and he and Gladys Maree Henry were married. His wife has been for him a constant source of strength and support throughout the strenuous days of his professional life. He and his bride left immediately for England and the Continent where they spent about two and a half years. It was a period of preparation for practice as a surgeon that had been planned for some time.

In planning his postgraduate studies in England Dr. Thorlakson had the benefit of advice from Dr. Neil John Maclean, who had studied there. This provided him with introductions to the most eminent surgeons in London. Once his schedules were established, he spent long hours daily attending clinical sessions, ward rounds, surgical operations and lectures of the teaching surgeons. This was accompanied by a heavy program of reading. He was preparing himself as a general surgeon, with special attention to surgery of the intestinal tract and surgery in gynecological conditions. He also took advantage of opportunities offered to him to study, under famed preceptors, general medicine. On occasion he journeyed outside London to gain first-hand experience of the work of surgeons of high repute in a particular field.

This whole period was a great learning experience to which he devoted his full resources of energy and intellect for two years. At its conclusion he was granted membership in the Royal College of Surgeons (England) and became a Licentiate of the Royal College of Physicians (London).

PART TWO

A Pioneer in Group Practice

CHAPTER 3

Early Experience in Group Practice

THE MACLEAN-GUNN CLINIC

Soon after his return to Winnipeg in the summer of 1923, Dr. Thorlakson was invited to visit Dr. Neil John Maclean in his office. Dr. Maclean renewed a suggestion he had made three years before, and invited Dr. Thorlakson to become associated with him in his practice in the Maclean-Gunn Clinic. The invitation was gladly accepted. "There are four people," Dr. Thorlakson says, "who have had an immense influence on my life: my parents, my wife, and Dr. Neil John Maclean." This gifted surgeon had noted young Thorlakson's energy and ability as an undergraduate student. His favourable impression was reinforced by Dr. Thorlakson's one-year experience as an intern on Dr. Maclean's surgical service at the Winnipeg General Hospital and by the reports of his work as an intern at the Children's Hospital.

Dr. Maclean's interest in his young colleague, and Dr. Thorlakson's deep respect for his professor and mentor, led inevitably to discussion of the choice of a specialty. Dr. Maclean had graduated in medicine at Manitoba Medical College in 1898. Subsequently, he took post-graduate training in surgery in Britain, and was a Member of the Royal College of Surgeons (England). He was also a Fellow of the Royal College of Surgeons (Canada) and a Fellow of the American College of Surgeons. From his own experience, he was aware of the value of training under the direction of surgeons of international reputation in Great Britain and in Europe. He encouraged Dr. Thorlakson's

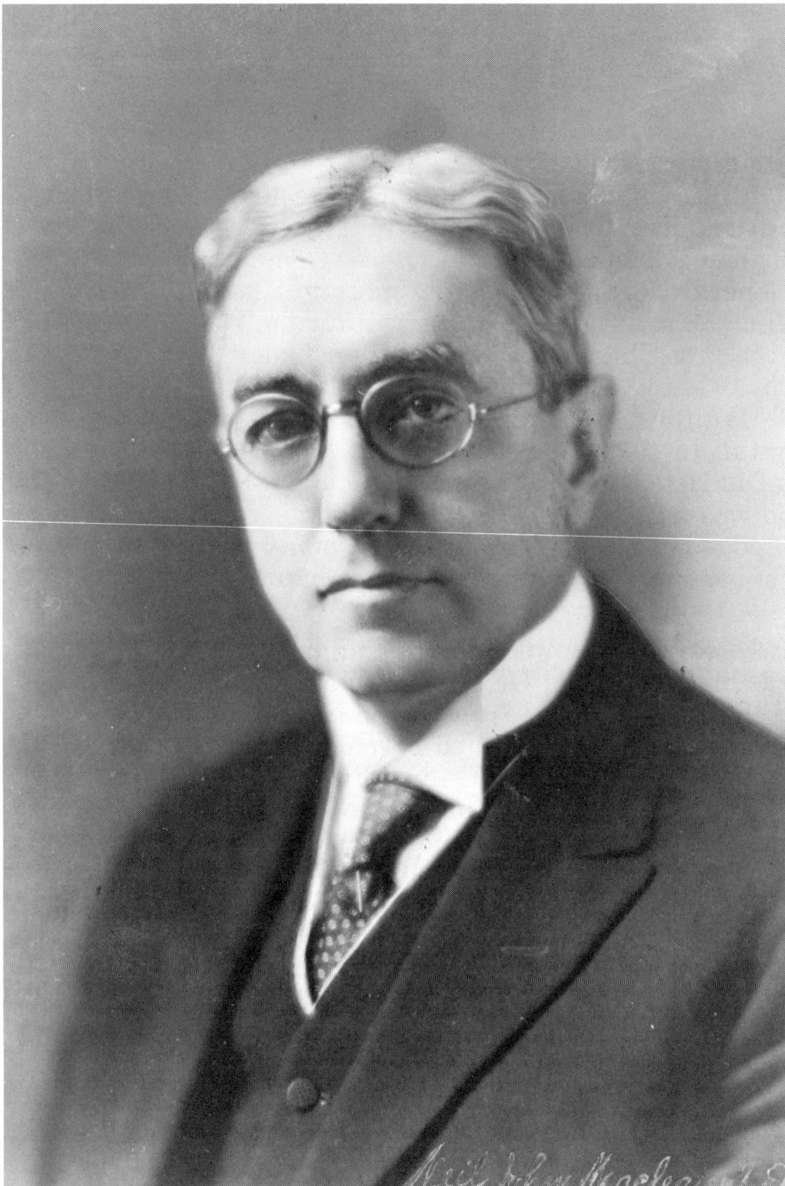

Neil John Maclean, M.D.

interest in surgery, and had strongly recommended that he obtain his British qualifications.

When Dr. Thorlakson joined the clinic, Dr. Maclean's partner was Dr. John Alexander Gunn.[1] He was a highly respected surgeon who had gone overseas in 1914 as Officer Commanding No. 1 Canadian General Hospital. He had a distinguished military career, and when he returned to Winnipeg after the War he was appointed as the first Chief of Surgery at Deer Lodge (Military) Hospital. From 1934 to 1938 he was Professor of Surgery at the University of Manitoba, and Chief of Surgery at the Winnipeg General Hospital. In 1940, he became Chief Medical Officer of the Manitoba District of the Canadian Pacific Railway. Dr. C.E. Corrigan, who was associated with him for many years on the staff at Deer Lodge Hospital, noted that "like many of the grand old surgeons of his time he was rather a dour man, who always spoke sparingly, though never in anger."

For the Thorlaksons, this period of introduction into clinic practice was a happy time. The years of preparation were finished. Temporary quarters and acquaintances overseas were replaced by life among family and friends in the city that was to be their permanent home. Dr. Thorlakson was experiencing the challenges, obligations and rewards of a busy general surgeon, who had been newly released from the ritual relationships of a graduate student to assume the self-imposed responsibilities of a consultant and teacher.

A long-time professor of surgery at Johns Hopkins University, Dr. Warfield Firor, offers this description of the general surgeon's vocation:

> The life of a general surgeon is an exceedingly strenuous one. It requires a long period of preparation, and makes great demands on one's physical, mental and emotional stamina. It is, however, an immensely satisfying vocation. This is so because the practice of general surgery provides variety, hard work, responsibility, independence, and rich rewards. The latter are not primarily monetary, but rather the satisfactions of achievement. The results of a successful operation are realized within days or weeks . . . [The surgeon meets] a steadily changing succession of people needing his help and understanding. This can be a source of interest to an enquiring mind, and gives a deep sense of gratification.[2]

Dr. Thorlakson could confirm Dr. Firor's point that the rewards were not primarily monetary. In describing his early years of practice, he said:

I mentioned a guaranteed income of $200 a month, or $2,400 a year. Today, such an amount would be derided if it were offered to an inexperienced and untrained youth, let alone a breadwinner. However, it proved adequate for us for the first year or so because Gladys was a superb manager. Actually, each month, after paying $100 for a small, furnished, third-floor, walk-up apartment and paying cash for other necessities, we had just $10 to spare. Once in a while we splurged by going out to dinner at our favourite restaurant in the Royal Alexandra Hotel. There we could dine for $2.50 each or less – without, of course, a cocktail or wine with our meal. Then we would go back to our suite by street car. On occasion, we would buy a roast and invite a couple to join us for dinner at home.

We were very happy and content with our lot because we felt optimistic about the future. We learned early how to make the most and the best of less – a lesson that stood us in good stead during the bitter days of the financial depression of the "dirty thirties," and the severe drought of the summers between 1930 and 1937. Sometimes two dozen eggs were offered by farmers in acknowledgement for a major operation; more often medical and surgical services were rendered without charge, because the patients were without means of payment.

THE MACLEAN-THORLAKSON CLINIC

Three years passed, during which the services at the Maclean-Gunn Clinic increased steadily. Dr. Maclean had been working at capacity for some time. Even when he returned to Winnipeg on the train on Sunday evenings after a weekend at his lake cottage, patients or their relatives were frequently waiting on the station platform to see him, to ask a question or make an appointment.

Dr. Thorlakson was also carrying a heavy practice, and had fully established his position in the medical community. By 1926 it was evident that both the accommodation and the medical complement of the Clinic needed to be expanded. Nevertheless, Dr. Gunn, in his position as Chief of Surgery at the Deer Lodge (Military) Hospital, was preoccupied with his commitment to the Hospital and to veteran patients. Due to this work, his substantial surgical practice at Winnipeg General Hospital and St. Boniface Hospital, as well as his community activities, he was reluctant to undertake the obligations that would be necessary in an enlarged group practice.

The Thorlakson home at this time was on Wolseley Avenue; the Macleans lived in fashionable Armstrong's Point. Not infrequently, after a busy day, Dr. Maclean and Dr. Thorlakson would walk home together. One fine spring evening in 1926, on their walk home, Dr. Maclean began to discuss the need to reach some decisions about the future. The pressure to expand the group was urgent, but Dr. Gunn had indicated continuing doubt about participation in an enlarged venture. Dr. Maclean therefore proposed that he and Dr. Thorlakson enter into a surgical partnership, to be known as the Maclean-Thorlakson Clinic, that would be located in the Medical Arts Building on Graham Avenue.[3]

In the following months, this plan was carried out. Dr. Maclean, as the senior partner, but with little interest or time for the requirements of management, asked Dr. Thorlakson to take full charge of the organization and administration of the new clinic. Dr. Thorlakson recalls the early days:

> In effect, Dr. Maclean was the president of the group and I became its general manager. This was the start of my training for long-term planning, management and recruitment. My first decision was to enlist the help and advice of people experienced in business, management and finance. By modern concepts this was a small operation; but for me, at that time, it represented a major responsibility and a serious challenge. I was convinced that I needed expert guidance.
>
> There are two ways to obtain the knowledge necessary for success in administration and finance. The modern method is to enroll in a special course of training at college or university. The alternative is to pass through the "university of hard knocks" – and this was the only way available years ago. Most successful organizers of private companies or professional groups acquired their management training in this way. They either became reasonably proficient, or they "lost their shirts" in the process. The most important lesson I learned was to consult experts in each field while preparing to make decisions.

By the fall of 1926, five rooms and a space for a small laboratory on the second floor of the Medical Arts Building were leased and furnished, staff was recruited, and the Maclean-

Thorlakson Clinic became a reality. In 1928 Dr. A.W.S. Hay became associated with the Clinic; and in 1929 Dr. C. Burton Stewart joined the group.[4]

Late in 1929 and in 1930 the great financial catastrophe that tormented the western world also struck Canada. Business failures were epidemic, thousands of jobs were lost, and deprivation and misery were widespread. "The lowest month of the depression for us was February, 1932," Dr. Thorlakson said. "In spite of seeing patients from 8 a.m. until 7:30 p.m. each day, at the end of that month only enough money had been collected to pay the rent and the salaries of the staff." Nothing was left for the medical partners.

Dr. Thorlakson tells a story that illustrates the tact and finesse, as well as the professional skill, that were required in the conduct of a private medical practice during the Depression:

In 1933 or 1934 a young couple from the far north presented themselves at the Maclean-Thorlakson Clinic. The history and physical examination revealed that the woman had delivered her first child without help other than that which her completely inexperienced husband could supply. She had suffered injury which only complex surgery could repair.

The patient was admitted to the Winnipeg General Hospital and assigned a bed in what was strangely called a semi-public ward; that is, there would be no bill to the patient for hospital care, but the physician or surgeon could attend his indigent patient on a "private" basis; either no fee was charged, or a nominal fee, depending on the circumstances.

For four days the patient was carefully prepared for the operation; the exacting surgery was successfully carried out; and by the tenth day after the operation it was apparent that complete healing, without infection, would occur. Normal function would be restored. Shortly after, the husband appeared at the clinic and asked to see me. The nurse took him to my private office where he awaited my arrival from the hospital.

As we faced each other we glowed with satisfaction – he because his wife would be so completely restored to health; and I because the surgery had been so successful and effective. He came right to the point. He said he wanted to pay me for the operation! In those hard times this was an astonishing – indeed, almost an incredible – proposal. I had heard of people in better days who walked around in overalls, the pockets of which were stuffed with bills of large denomination. Could this be . . . ?

I became a little cautious. In an off-hand way, I reached for the ultimate and said: "John, the bill should be one fifty." This was intended to be a trial balloon. To my astonishment, without a moment's hesitation he replied, "Doc, I'll pay that right now."

The situation was so unusual as to be almost unnerving, but with some hesitation and a vague unease I directed him to the office of Miss Brown, who looked after the payment of accounts for the Maclean-Thorlakson Surgical Clinic.

I went to another room to see my next patient, but I was worried; my conscience started to bother me. In his elation over his wife's recovery, perhaps he was paying me his last dollar. How would he and his wife get home? I excused myself, left my patient, and headed for Miss Brown's office, hoping to get there before she had issued the receipt for $150. But on the desk in front of Miss Brown lay a two dollar bill, and she had the appearance of one struggling with a major decision.

I quickly sized up the situation. The young man had never been in the city before, knew nothing about the cost of medical and surgical services, and to him one fifty meant only one thing. Without hesitation I picked up the two dollar bill, handed it to the young man, thanked him for his intention to pay me, but said that I had changed my mind and there would be no charge for the operation. We parted the best of friends, both of us pleased with the outcome of our relationship.

The virtue in adversity is fortitude, they say. There is no doubt that adversity tempers the mind and character of those who face it with courage, strength and perseverance, and who profit by its instruction to prepare for kindlier times. So it was in the days of the Great Depression. Little by little, economic conditions improved; epidemic unemployment was reduced; society adapted to new levels of productivity and prosperity. In western Canada, improved methods of farming and grain marketing, as well as the development of natural-resource industries, resulted in higher incomes, increased security and growing population.

The Maclean-Thorlakson Clinic shared in the general growth of the community. By 1937 the practice had expanded to such an extent that the offices that seemed so spacious in 1926 were totally inadequate and precluded any further addition to the membership in the group. Enquiries revealed that additional space could not be leased in the Medical Arts Building.

It fell to Dr. Thorlakson as general manager to find a solution to this challenge. It was not easy. Dr. Maclean, then sixty-seven, was not interested in taking an active part in developing an enlarged group practice. Other present or prospective members of the group were hesitant to take the responsibility and the risk of sharing in the investment, planning and operation of a modern clinic building and its essential equipment. Even if they had wanted to put in capital, the Depression years had left them with little chance to accumulate funds for such an investment.

Dr. Thorlakson, however, had been giving a good deal of thought to the future as the Depression years passed, and the demand for the Clinic services increased. He had accumulated, by careful management in the Thorlakson household, a modest capital. He had sufficient confidence in himself and in the future to accept some risk.

In 1938, for the sum of $14,000, Dr. Thorlakson bought the property at the corner of St. Mary Avenue and Vaughan Street. This property would eventually become the site of the Winnipeg Clinic, the city's first multi-specialty private group practice clinic.

CHAPTER 4

Founding the Winnipeg Clinic

THE EVOLUTION OF GROUP PRACTICE

The genesis of medical group practice is somewhat obscure; but by far the oldest and largest private group clinic in North America is that founded by Dr. W.W. Mayo in Rochester, Minnesota. In 1877 he entered into a partnership with his two sons, Dr. W.J. and Dr. C.H. Mayo. Drs. Judd and Graham were soon added; and when Dr. Henry F. Plummer, an internist, joined them, it became a true group practice clinic. Specialists in as many as twenty-five additional fields were added over the years, and the Mayo Clinic acquired world renown as a centre for high quality diagnosis and treatment.[1]

The prototype of medical practice has always been the independent solo practitioner. Nevertheless, numbers of doctors who had been in military service in World War I had observed the effectiveness of integrating into a well-organized system a variety of medical skills, equipment and technical support services. This combining of resources expedited and often improved the diagnosis and treatment of soldier-patients. These doctors were inclined to the view that a similar coordination would be advantageous for the treatment of civilian patients. The concept came to be known as group practice.

Medical opinion about these integrated groups of doctors was sharply divided for many years. Indeed, it was really not until 1967, when a committee appointed by the Canadian Medical Association [CMA] to study the subject issued its report, that this form of practice organization was officially recognized. The professional concerns lay generally in the potential for excessive referrals within the group, the inherent tendency to confine consultations to members of the group, and the pooling of fees (which some felt contravened the ban on "fee-splitting").

On the other hand, there is a potential for the enhancement of the quality of patient care through group practice. The CMA Committee report noted the considerable number of group practices that had become established in Canada and the United States by the time of their study. They had the following comment on the reasons for this trend, which has continued to strengthen with the passing years:

> Probably the basic underlying reason for the gradual emergence of groups, or "grouped" medicine, is a counter movement to the "division" of medicine into many specialties. At one time all medical knowledge could be encompassed within one person. Today, however, with the rapidly proliferating rate of medical knowledge in all fields and the potential development of a separate specialty for almost every organ of the body, it has become necessary to develop some form of organization which will enable all these specialties to work together. The patient, after all, remains a single person with some intangible qualities which we can attribute to the "whole." Medicine, likewise, must find some mechanism by which to remain a single entity.

The CMA Committee on Group Practice, which carried out its studies over a four-year period (1964 through 1967), recognized that there are many forms of "groups" in the practice of medicine. They may, for example, simply be solo practitioners who occupy the same building and share some services such as a common waiting room under a variety of formal or informal partnership arrangements. The CMA Committee decided on five criteria which they considered essential to define a true group-medical practice: the group must consist of three or more full-time doctors who are bound by a formal contract, share a common office and patient records, pool income and expense, and distribute the net proceeds on a pre-arranged basis. Finally, their definition states: "The multi-specialty group is the ultimate expression of the complete group practice concept, insofar as it is the one concept that attempts to bring together a range of specialties, including General Practice."[2]

It was this concept that, thirty years earlier, beginning about 1933, Dr. Thorlakson began to perceive as a means of improving both the quality of medical care and the effectiveness with which it is delivered. His first private medical practice in partnership with Dr. Brothers in Shoal Lake met the criteria for definition as a group practice, except for the number of doctors. The partners shared office accommodation, the services of the receptionist-secretary, and the patient records; and the income was pooled and divided on a pre-arranged basis. He had, therefore, an early and satisfactory introduction to group-practice principles.

Even earlier, he had noted the advantages in patient care of the easy consultation, both formal and informal, that existed on the public wards of the Winnipeg General Hospital, and in the army. He was familiar with the excellent work done at the Mayo Clinic. He had read with interest the monograph on private group clinics published by the Millbank Memorial Fund (USA) in 1931, which stated that this relatively new form of organization for the delivery of physician services was of benefit to both patients and doctors and should be encouraged.

PLANNING FOR THE CLINIC

During these years, Dr. Thorlakson visited many of the group practice clinics then operating in North America, including the famous Mayo Clinic. He spent, as he put it, "as much time with administrative groups as in the operating rooms with the surgeons." In the period from about 1935 onward, the idea of establishing a multi-specialty group practice in Winnipeg became ever more attractive to him. He gave up golf and other hobbies to devote all his spare time – evenings, weekends, holidays and any other moments he could find in the busy days – to exploring the subject, working out basic plans for a suitable building, and considering the principles under which a group practice clinic could best operate.[3] Throughout the whole period of developing, considering and reshaping of the plans, one theme was consistently maintained: provision must be made for an ongoing interest in medical education and for supporting and sharing in medical research.

The selection of a name for a private group practice clinic, which was expected to have a substantial number of participating members, was a matter of concern. Dr. Thorlakson was anxious to avoid the connotations of authority that would inevitably occur if the names of one, or a few, of the active members were included in the clinic title, perhaps to the detriment of future relationships. On the other hand, Dr. Maclean had determined that he would not take an active part in the new venture, but had agreed to be associated with it as a senior surgical consultant, in partial retirement. Dr. Thorlakson therefore suggested that the new project be called the Maclean Clinic. Dr. Maclean demurred, pointing out that he had three sons who were, or were about to be, doctors, and they might want to use the family name in a partnership practice.

After all the alternatives were considered, it was finally decided to use a geographical designation. On March 15, 1938, the Winnipeg Clinic was officially born; and with the approval of the physician associates at the Maclean-Thorlakson Clinic, the new name was inscribed above the old on the door to the offices in the Medical Arts Building.

During his travels, Dr. Thorlakson had observed an organizational and financial difficulty in a number of private group practice clinics; the problems stemmed from the question of ownership. If one member, or a few members, of the clinic owned the property and the fixed assets, their income was enhanced through recovery of capital costs from the group. But if the entire partnership owned the property, a substantial investment was required from individuals joining the group, which sometimes precluded the recruitment of new members. Even greater difficulties arose if members wished to leave the group, or if a member died, especially if property values had changed materially. All these problems left the way open to disputes that marred the professional association. In the plans for the Winnipeg Clinic, Dr. Thorlakson was determined to avoid these problems, and not to involve his professional colleagues in a personal financial obligation for which they were certainly not prepared at that time.

He therefore concluded that the members would not be asked to make a direct financial commitment for purchase of the property, building, furniture or equipment. Instead, the medical group partnership paid rent for office space, first in the Medical

Arts Building, and later as tenants in the new two-storey building that was constructed on the corner of St. Mary Avenue and Vaughan Street. Dr. Thorlakson himself undertook to raise the capital funds. In a report to Winnipeg Clinic members on February 4, 1966, he said:

> It was during these difficult years that I began to establish my credit rating on a sound basis in the business community. The assurance that obligations would be honoured and adequate protection provided for those individuals who placed their trust in my integrity and sense of personal responsibility has been advantageous during the various stages of development and expansion of the Winnipeg Clinic and the Manitoba Institute for the Advancement of Medical Education and Research. . . .
>
> During this period I was also involved in activities that brought me into close association with the members of the Board of Trustees of the Winnipeg General Hospital, the Board of Governors of the University of Manitoba, and the members of the Provincial Government, several of whom were personal friends. The contacts and friendships established then proved to be extremely helpful . . . to the Winnipeg Clinic, the Manitoba Institute for the Advancement of Medical Education and Research, and (later) in the formation of the Manitoba Medical Centre.

When it became known that he had acquired the property at St. Mary Avenue and Vaughan Street and that a building for a medical clinic would be erected on it, one of the first to offer advice and assistance was Mr. E.W. Kneeland, a Winnipeg grain merchant. Dr. Thorlakson accepted this invitation to discuss his plans, and Mr. Kneeland suggested that he review the details of his project with Cecil S. Gunn, an expert in real estate and finance.[4] "Then," said Mr. Kneeland, "I would be happy to be interested and involved in any proposition that you and Cecil Gunn think would be feasible and practical." This was an expression of confidence and encouragement; it was also a moment filled with the spontaneous sense of joy that pervades the spirit when the way is opened to realization of a long-cherished dream.

Dr. Thorlakson lost no time in consulting Mr. Gunn, who quickly put the clinic proposal into a form that would permit designers and builders to be selected. Cecil Gunn also pointed out the importance of sound legal advice. Dr. Thorlakson had already discussed his project with John A. MacAulay, K.C., a partner in the prestigious legal firm of Aikins, Loftus, Aikins and MacAulay. These preparatory actions formed the basis of an effective working partnership with Mr. MacAulay and Mr. Gunn, both highly successful in their respective fields of law and finance.

Subsequently, Dr. Thorlakson invited Dr. A.W.S. Hay, Dr. C. Burton Stewart, Dr. H.D. Morse, Dr. Lennox G. Bell, Dr. K.R. Trueman and Dr. J.E. Isaac to become members of the new clinic. He also invited Dr. C.R. Gilmour, a noted diagnostician and professor of medicine at the University of Manitoba between 1928 and 1939, who agreed to act as medical consultant. He invited Dr. Neil John Maclean as surgical consultant.[5]

The realization that a large, multi-specialty, private group practice clinic was actually coming into being in Winnipeg sent a shock wave through the medical community. It appeared to be a threat of unknown proportions to the tradition of the solo practice of medicine.

The fundamental purpose of multi-specialty group practice clinics, which by 1938 numbered about 185 in the United States and perhaps a dozen in Canada, was to provide an organization and environment for the more effective practice of medicine. The clinics offered the advantage of more efficient use of specialized staff and complex equipment. Business management was usually in the hands of lay administrators, freeing doctors to devote their time to professional activities. Joint responsibility for patient care, informal as well as formal consultation, and fully accessible patient records, gave both doctors and patients the advantage of shared service. The arrangement allowed physicians to take necessary time for continuing education, medical conferences and vacations, and avoid being continuously on call; they could leave their offices with the confidence that their patients would receive care from fully informed colleagues. The benefit to both doctors and patients was self-evident.

However, the early group practice clinics were highly suspect in the opinion of many doctors. They feared that these private groups were an economic threat to solo practitioners and smaller partnerships; that they might be centres of unethical practice; that they had an unfair advantage in attracting patients and medical referrals. On the other hand, a substantial number of doctors who themselves were solo practitioners maintained that the group practice clinics enhanced the quality of care, not only in the clinics themselves, but also in the community at large. Emotions ran high on the subject, and reactions among members of the profession ranged from approval and support to vocal and sometimes vindictive antagonism. Nevertheless, in the midst of all the debate, plans for the Winnipeg Clinic went steadily forward.

The firm of F.R. Lount and Son, Limited, was selected to prepare the plans and construct the building. It was agreed that it would consist of two storeys and a basement, and that it would provide office space and examining rooms for the invited members of the original group, along with accommodation for laboratory, x-ray, library, business office and other support services. Construction began early in 1939. It was estimated that the Winnipeg Clinic building would cost about $110,000, at that time a substantial sum for the accommodation of a private medical practice, and a considerable capital for Dr. Thorlakson to raise.

Mr. Kneeland, who had at the very beginning indicated his interest in being of financial help, died during the development of the plans.[6] In Kneeland's untimely death, Dr. Thorlakson lost both a friend and a supporter. Fortunately, he had other confident and able backers for his clinic in the persons of Mrs. James A. Richardson, Cecil S. Gunn, John A. MacAulay, K.C., and G.F. Jonasson, who joined with Dr. Thorlakson in making interest-free loans to finance the construction of the building. The land was provided by Dr. Thorlakson himself.

It was recognized that the success of the Clinic in the initial period was largely dependent on the personal efforts of Dr. Thorlakson. His large surgical practice would provide a major share of the group practice income, and his contribution as an organizer and manager was vital. As an added safeguard, therefore, an insurance policy on his life in the amount of $100,000 was purchased. Similarly, a Lloyds of London policy for $50,000 was purchased to protect against injury to his hands. Both policies were payable to a trustee for the lenders.

Throughout these exciting but often worrysome events, the steadfast and encouraging support of his wife was a source of

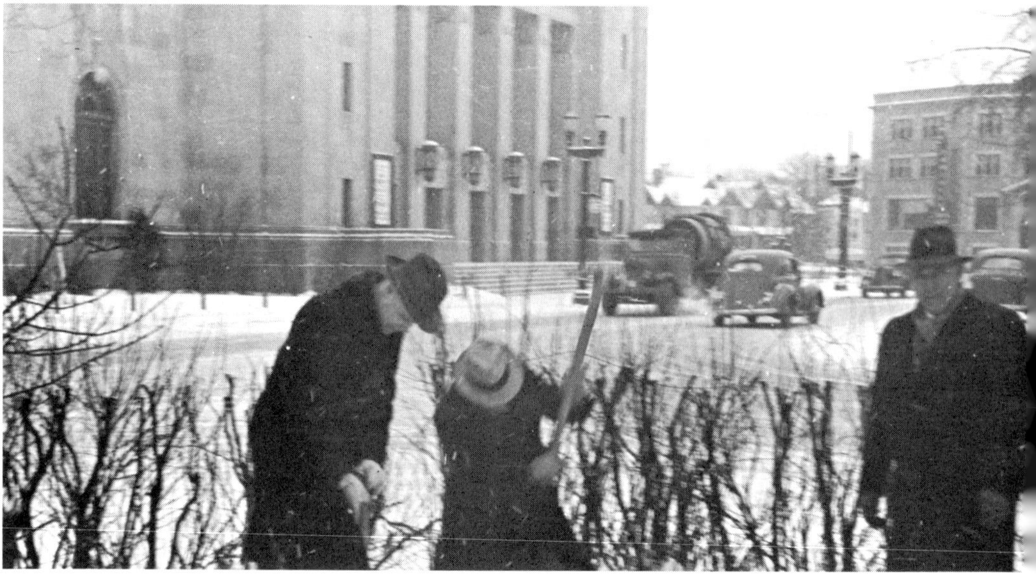

Turning the sod to launch the construction of the new Winnipeg Clinic building at Vaughan Street and St. Mary Avenue in early winter, 1941. Left to right: Dr. Thorlakson, C.S. Gunn and F.R. Lount

strength to Dr. Thorlakson: "It was vital to this whole undertaking that it had the full support and approval of Mrs. Thorlakson. Without this, in these early and difficult years, it would have been impossible to have carried on and make the personal sacrifices that were demanded."

Dr. and Mrs. Thorlakson spent many evenings discussing the plans for the new building, the property which had been purchased as its site, and the surrounding property which Dr. Thorlakson thought he should acquire, as soon as he could, for an expanded clinic of the future. They examined his personal obligations in the venture in the light of his limited financial resources. They also reviewed the names of the doctors Dr. Thorlakson had selected to interview as possible members of the Clinic. It is notable that every individual on that list subsequently accepted an invitation to join the Winnipeg Clinic, and each made a significant contribution to its continuing success.

THE FIRST STAGE REALIZED

The basement of the new Clinic building had already been excavated, and the foundation laid, when World War II broke out. For the second time in Dr. Thorlakson's life, the advent of war threatened his hopes and aspirations.

With Canada's declaration of war against Germany of September 3, 1939, the whole focus of public attention turned to the needs of the military effort. Construction resources – men, equipment and supplies – were diverted to the immediate needs for troop training camps, munitions plants and the immense industrial requirements of the war. Supplies and materials for "non-essential" projects were severely limited or cut off entirely.

Construction of the Winnipeg Clinic building was immediately in jeopardy. Controls on construction materials were swiftly enacted in Ottawa. New works requiring the use of large amounts of steel and other essential components were frozen unless they contributed directly to the war effort. From the national point of view, the building of a two-storey medical clinic was hardly a matter of pressing concern. But to Dr. Thorlakson, committed as he was both professionally and financially, the restrictions rapidly being put in place were a potential catastrophe. Nevertheless, despite small work crews and delays in material delivery, the contractor proceeded with his work and the basement walls were finally in place.

These months were marked by one depressing development after another in Europe. Poland was overrun by Russia from the east and Germany from the west; Norway and Denmark were occupied by Hitler's troops; the Baltic States of Latvia, Estonia and Lithuania were absorbed into Russia under the guise of the Mutual Assistance Pact; while the French-German border was haunted by a sense of impending disaster, although scarcely a shot was fired there during the first six months of the war.

On the morning of May 10, 1940, the German Panzers, in all their appalling might, swept into Holland, Belgium and France. Their devastating success drove home the precarious state of the Allied cause and the sacrifices that had to be made to thwart Hitler's purpose of making a national socialist Germany "lord of the earth."

The future looked very dark. The Canadian Government had established the War Supplies Board, which in turn appointed controllers to oversee the supply of essential materials such as steel, oil, timber and minerals. Priorities were instituted for their authorized use. The heavy demands on the supply of construction materials is evidenced by the 123 percent increase in the volume of building contracts during the first five months of 1941 compared with the same period in 1939.[7] In the face of the anxieties and restraints of what promised to be a long war, it seemed doubtful that the Winnipeg Clinic building could be completed. Under the circumstances, Dr. Thorlakson wrote to the Ottawa authorities and offered to discontinue the project, if they considered this to be a desirable action. Acceptance of the offer would mean that all the contracts would have to be cancelled; his personal loss would be more than $50,000 to pay off the contractors, to mothball the structure already built, and to repay the advances already made to finance the construction. But aside from the financial loss, this decision would defer indefinitely the realization of a goal for which he had worked so long and so hard and to which he had obligated himself so completely. "One evening," he recalls, "Mrs. Thorlakson and I visited the unfinished basement and were reminded (not too seriously), of the ancient proverb 'hope deferred maketh the heart sick.' "

However, amidst all the worry, relief came. After due consideration, the Ottawa authorities decided that the project should be completed, since the materials required, mainly Tyndall-stone and glass brick, were not essential to the war effort. Also, it would give employment to older men in the building trades who had not been taken into war industries. During this period of anxious waiting, representative citizens in the community and doctors not associated with the Clinic were consulted, and they agreed that no useful purpose would be served by leaving the building unfinished. With renewed zeal, therefore, construction was resumed.

The two-storey Clinic building was finally completed in the late summer of 1942. The furnishings and equipment were in place, and all other preparations completed in October; by the end of that month the Winnipeg Clinic was entirely transferred from the Medical Arts Building to the new quarters.[8]

To provide working capital, Dr. Thorlakson, from his personal funds, deposited $27,000 in the Winnipeg Clinic bank account and transferred to the current assets of the Clinic all of his collectable accounts receivable, amounting to $120,000. Thus provided with operating funds, the new Winnipeg Clinic was ready to function.

The original group of full-time doctors included: Dr. Lennox G. Bell; Dr. Arthur W.S. Hay; Dr. Jacob E. Isaac; Dr. Neil John Maclean; Dr. Harry D. Morse; Dr. C. Burton Stewart; Dr. Paul H.T. Thorlakson; Dr. Stephen B. Thorson; Dr. Kenneth R. Trueman; Dr. Clifford R. Gilmour. Part-time associates were: Dr. J. Currie McMillan (X-ray); Dr. R.A. Macpherson (X-ray); Dr. William A. Gardner (Orthopedics); Dr. George Brock (Dermatology). The Executive Committee comprised: Dr. Paul H.T. Thorlakson (Chairman); Dr. C. Burton Stewart; Dr. Harry D. Morse; Dr. Lennox G. Bell; Mrs. J. Bernice Shepherd (Clinic Manager).

The initial medical members constituted sections of general surgery, internal medicine and urology. In 1944 a section of obstetrics and gynecology, headed by Dr. Brian D. Best, was added. The ancillary services included radiology, laboratory and pharmacy. There was the nucleus of a medical library. The support staff numbered twenty.

One of the advantages of a group practice clinic, clearly seen by Dr. Thorlakson, lay in the potential for a more efficient use of the doctors' time, not only through convenient layout of the facilities and the close association of the medical members, but

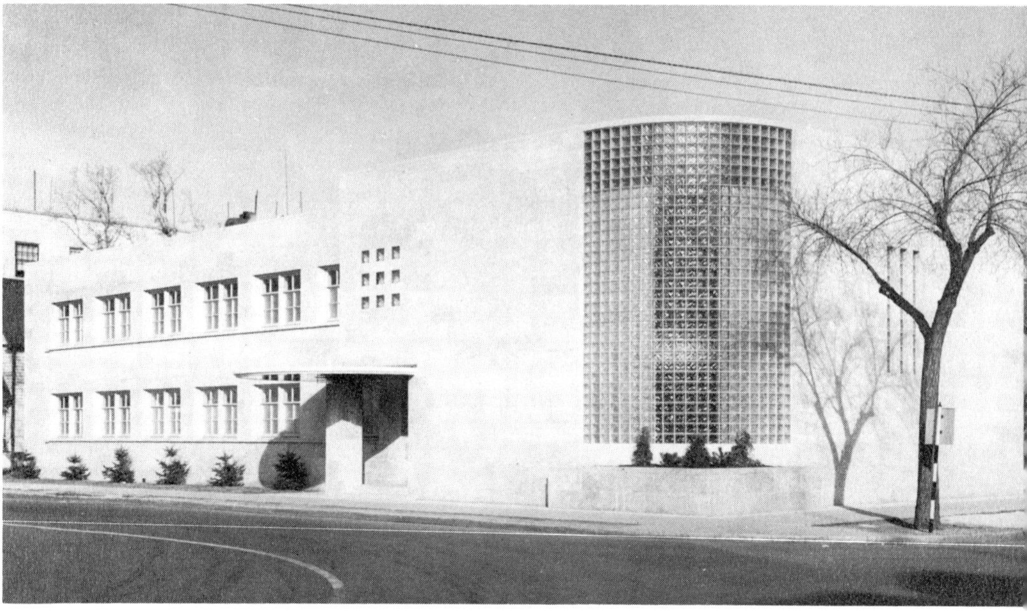

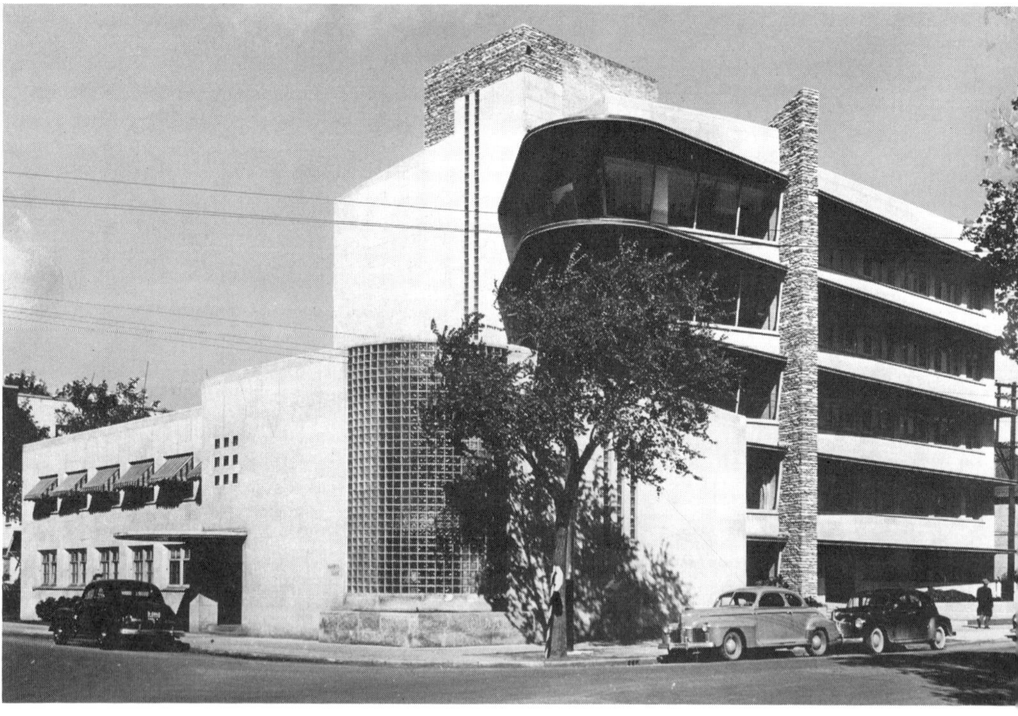

The Winnipeg Clinic, 1942

The five-storey addition, completed in 1947

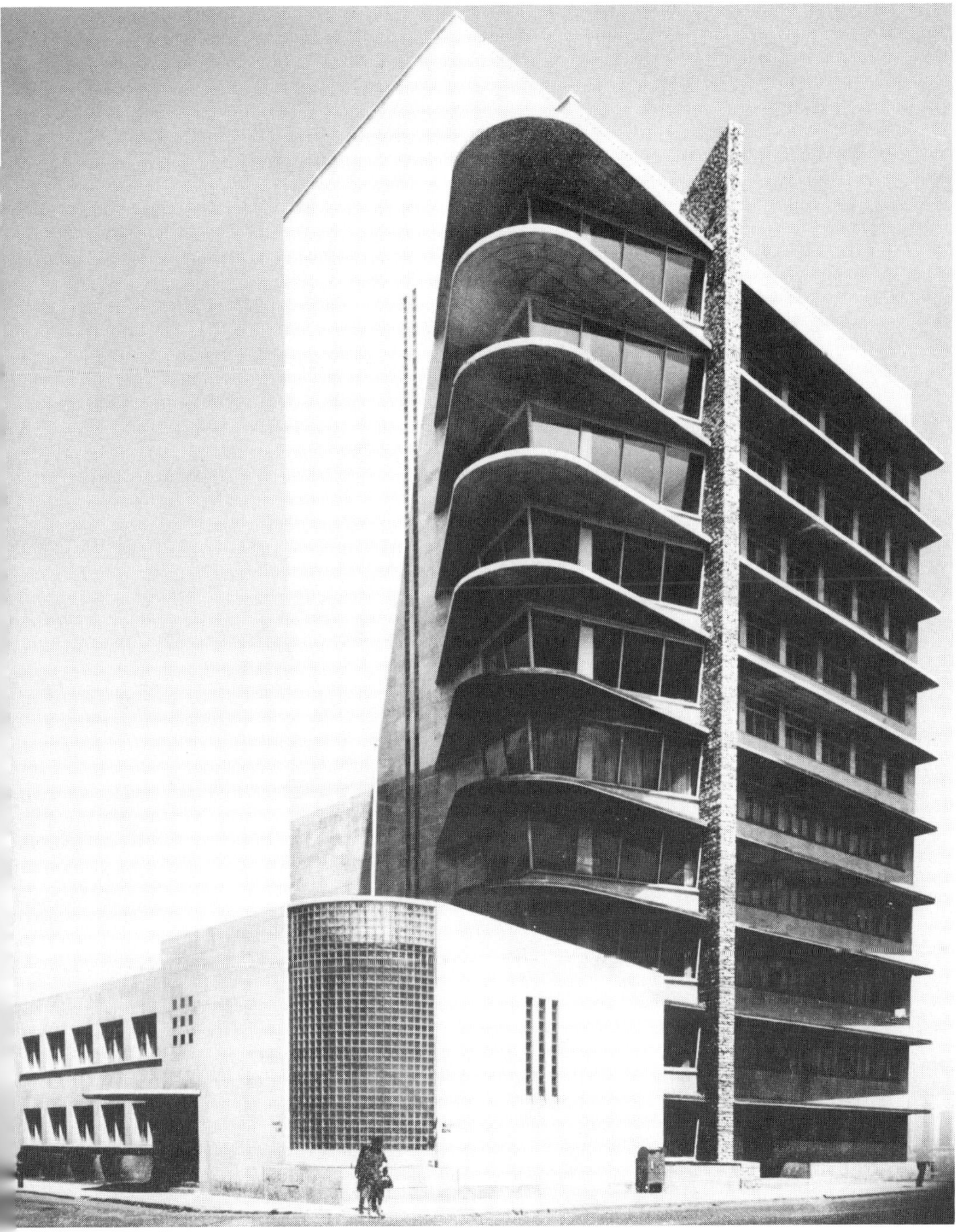

An additional seven storeys, completed in 1962

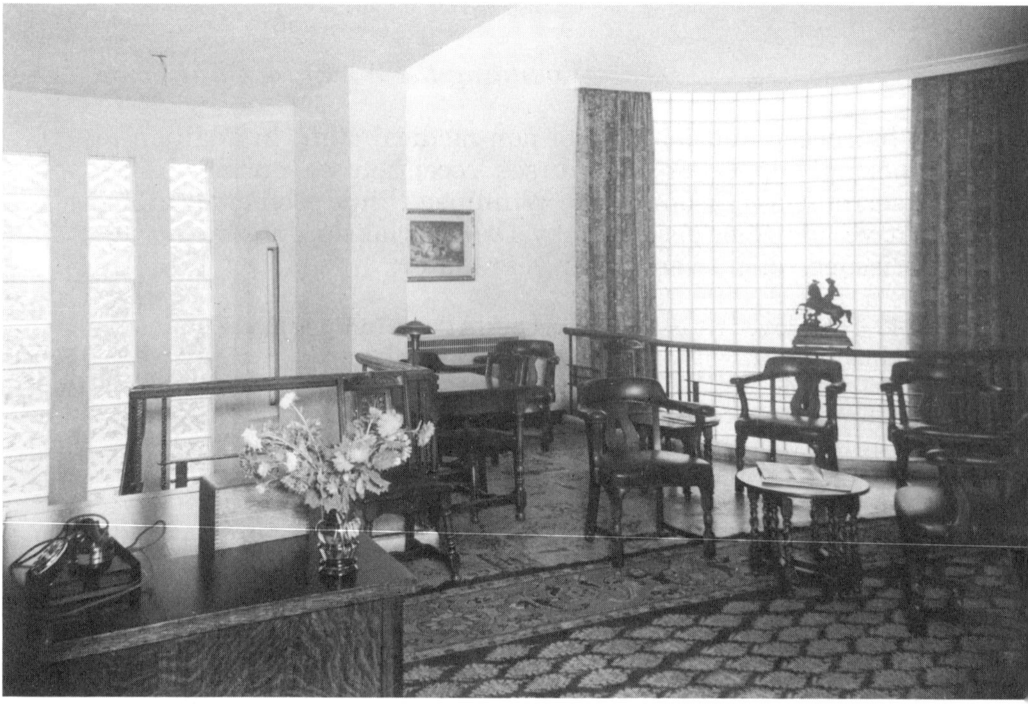

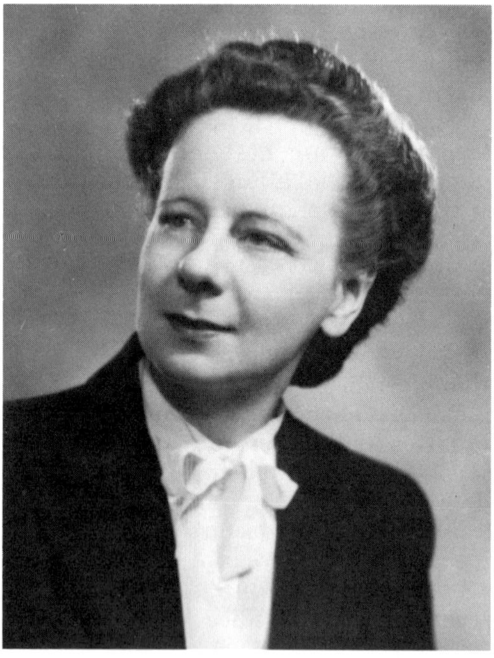

Patients' reception area, Department of Surgery, 1942

Mrs. J. Bernice Shepherd, clinic manager, 1940 to 1965. The initial patient-record and accounts system was developed by Mrs. Shepherd with the advice of Mr. R.B. Benson of the Duluth Clinic.

also by the appropriate use of non-medical staff. In addition to the normal support staff of nurses, receptionists, business office and secretarial personnel, the Winnipeg Clinic soon made an innovative addition, described by Dr. Thorlakson in a memorandum issued some twenty-four years later:

> In 1942, I employed three new members of the Winnipeg Clinic staff to assist busy doctors with their workload. I did this partly from necessity and partly by design. We were, at the time, desperately short of medical staff. We had to conserve the time of our doctors in order that they could utilize their medical knowledge and skills most effectively.
>
> One person in this category was a visiting nurse. She relieved the doctors from the considerable but, at that time thought to be necessary, follow-up of visiting patients in their homes after they were discharged from hospital. A service such as this is both good medicine and good public relations. Patients want to be remembered by their doctors. They are justifiably and noticeably hurt if their doctor does not see them every day in the hospital. Many patients wonder why they should suddenly lose touch with their doctor after they have been discharged to their homes and, in their opinion, are neglected by him. In many instances, one or two telephone calls by the doctor or his nurse will provide the patients with needed reassurance. This has a good effect on the patient. A home visit by the doctor is, of course, the most perfect way to establish the important doctor-patient and family relationship. As a profession, we all talk about the importance of the doctor-patient relationship whenever we address ourselves to governments or anyone who wants to interfere in any way with our professional affairs. It is then – and, too often, only then – that this relationship becomes a matter of vital importance and even a matter of principle. A way for the Winnipeg Clinic to partially solve this problem was to institute a home-visiting nursing service.
>
> Another person to be employed in 1942 was a dietitian who was a university graduate. Our doctors then, as now, were involved in the treatment of diabetes, peptic ulcer, flatulent dyspepsia, chronic diarrhoea, chronic constipation, obesity, etc., etc. Diet sheets were important but it was thought that careful explanation and personal advice were more important. A qualified dietitian could do this well and relieve the doctor, thereby saving a great deal of time for other professional work. This service has been available to all the doctors and patients of the Winnipeg Clinic for almost twenty-five years.
>
> The third person to be employed in 1942 was a nurse/medical secretary, who was especially assigned to the members of the medical and

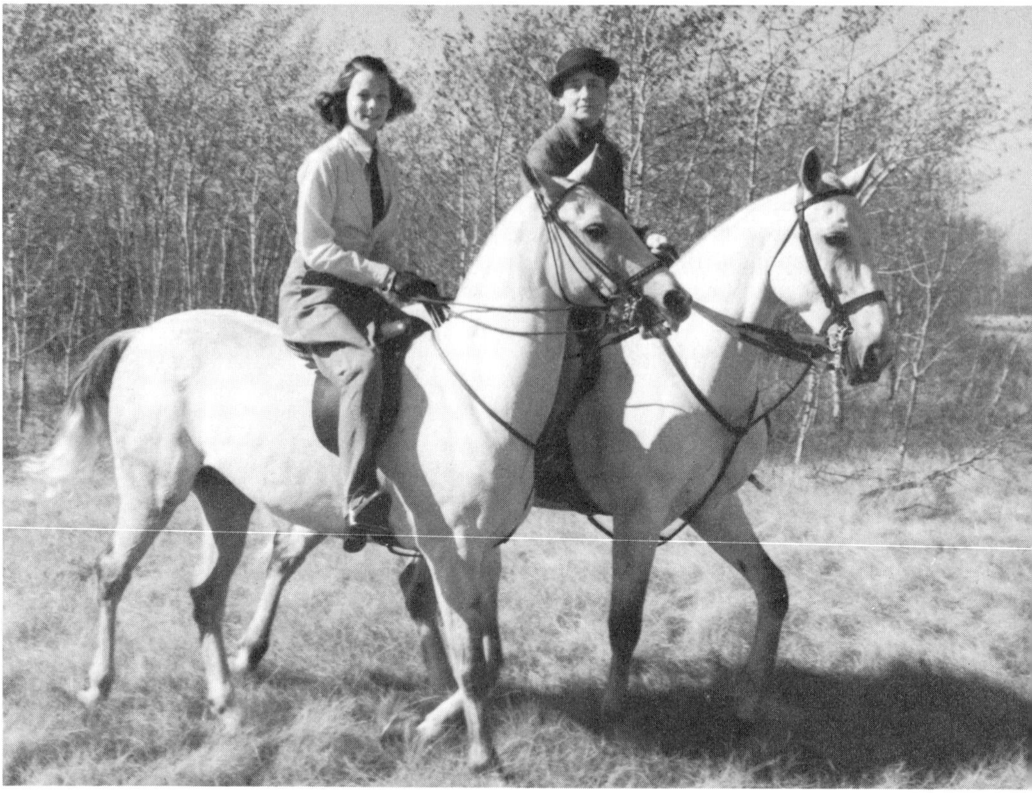

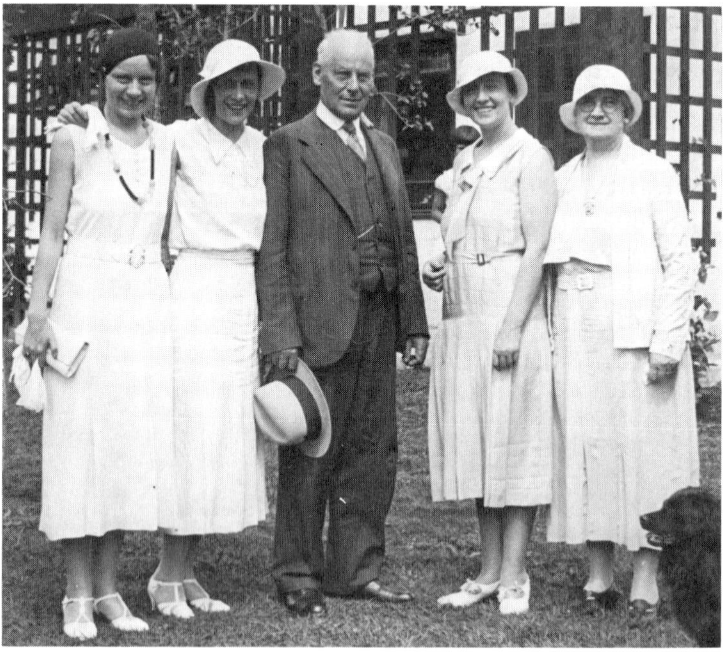

Gladys Thorlakson's love of horses and her competence in riding were shared by her daughter Tannis.

Mr. and Mrs. Henry and their three daughters, left to right: Bernice, Florence and Gladys, at the home of Thor and Gladys, 114 Grenfell Boulevard surgical staff who carried the heaviest hospital load (more than fifteen to twenty patients, on the average, in hospital). She accompanied the doctor on rounds, took down his clinical notes and instructions, transferred essential information to the Winnipeg Clinic records, and accepted the responsibility for assuring that the referring doctor was kept informed about the diagnosis, treatment and progress of the patient. This was thought to be especially important in cases of long-stay patients. The approved procedure was an initial written acknowledgement to the referring doctor which was mailed as soon after admission as possible. The second note was sent after a diagnosis was made and the course of treatment or surgery decided upon, and a final letter went immediately on discharge. We must never forget that the busy doctor in the country still appreciates this type of service. They are more impressed and pleased by these brief exchanges of information than they are by long detailed reports sent sometime after the patient has returned home.

At long last, by October 31, 1942, the Winnipeg Clinic was off to an auspicious beginning in its new premises and was breaking new ground in the delivery of medical service.[9]

ANOTHER PERSPECTIVE

Some indication of the strenuous demands on the Thorlakson family during this period was provided by Mrs. Thorlakson in an interview by the authors of *Mrs. Doctor:*[10]

Mrs. Thorlakson said that perhaps her greatest opportunity to be useful came when her husband decided to erect a clinic building on the property he had purchased at St. Mary Avenue and Vaughan Street, because in 1938 there was no more space for expansion in the Medical Arts Building. Until that time no one in Winnipeg had experience in planning a building to accommodate a multi-specialty group practice. "We needed to depend on our own initiative and to spend many evenings and weekends in making plans and trying to think of all the conveniences and facilities that would meet the needs of the patients, the doctors and the staff of the new clinic.

This was an important chapter of our lives. Many meetings, some of which were held in our home, preceded and continued after the founding of the Winnipeg Clinic and the subsequent establishment of the Winnipeg Clinic Research Institute.

In the course of his travels, Thor visited well-established medical clinics in the United States. On his return we would examine clinic building plans that he had obtained, and review his investigation into clinic organization and management. These important contacts broadened his insight into the many difficult problems which had to be resolved, including joint ownership of assets.

Over the years many difficult decisions had to be made and personal risks taken. The unique form of clinic organization that finally evolved was quite different from the accepted arrangement and had significant consequences for all members of the new clinic and for our own family.

On Sir Frederick Banting's invitation received in 1938, Thor became a member of the first Associate Committee on Medical Research of the National Research Council of Canada.

He served on the Committee until 1946. This long association could well have been one of the factors in the decision to transfer the ownership of the properties and buildings to a foundation to support medical education and research, which later became the Winnipeg Clinic Research Institute. . . .

One weekend, when Thor was in Ottawa, attending a meeting of the Associate Committee on Medical Research, Frank R. Lount – who was building the clinic – called me to say that a furniture factory was being closed but that if we could place an order at once, furniture for the clinic would be shipped to us. Mr. Lount and I spent that day with a tape measure and drawing paper to see how the furniture would fit. When we thought we had it all lined up, I called Thor in Ottawa. He was at a meeting and not available, so we just phoned in the order for the furniture!

When Thor called the next evening to check on the family, I felt a great sense of accomplishment when I told him what we had done. When he came home on Monday night, I said: "I was disappointed because you didn't seem excited about the furniture." He said: "Oh, I was impressed. But I haven't the money to pay for it." Then he added: "That furniture may be on its way but the clinic may not be finished for months. Where are we going to put it all?" I explained that I had rented an old skating rink in St. James and had arranged for it to be delivered there.

As the war progressed, hospital and clinic supplies were not easily obtained. Since the sheets we needed were not regulation size, we had to buy sheeting material and make our own. I turned the breakfast room into a cutting and sewing room and there I made fifteen hundred sheets of the required size for the examining tables. The gowns for the patients also had to be made at home. I bought material in rose, green and blue. The nurses could tell by the color what size they were. For the young patients, I bought material with Indians and cowboys. This was only the beginning – wallpaper, curtains, lamps, ash trays and even waste-paper baskets still had to be chosen. Night after night, when the children were in bed, we would go down to the clinic to make sure the painters were putting on the right colors to match the curtains and wallpaper. . . .

If I did make a contribution, it was the same as that of every other doctor's wife. We cared for our families and coped with emergencies when our husbands were at the hospital, in the office in the daytime, or out on night calls. I think it is important to remember that, in those days, acutely ill patients were always seen in their homes by their doctors before they were sent to the hospital. All doctors, in the country and in the city, were on duty twenty-four hours a day, seven days a week.

It was a good life with hardly a dull moment!

CHAPTER 5

Expanding the Clinic

PLANNING FOR GROWTH

Even before the first sod had been turned for the construction of the two-storey building which was to be occupied by the Winnipeg Clinic, Dr. Thorlakson was studying alternate ways of expanding the structure to accommodate the added professional facilities which he foresaw would be required when the war was over – if not before.

The plan provided space on the first floor for the Department of Urology, the X-Ray Department, a small laboratory, the pharmacy and the necessary examining rooms. Here too was the business office, presided over by a kind, dedicated woman, Mrs. Bernice Shepherd. The departments of Surgery and Medicine were located on the second floor, along with their examining rooms and waiting rooms. The library, which later became Dr. Thorlakson's private office, occupied the south-east corner.

Dr. George Brock and Dr. W.A. Gardner, who were part-time members of the Clinic, continued their main practice in their rooms at the Medical Arts Building on Graham Avenue.

The steady growth in the Clinic practice was making heavy demands on the space available for professional and support facilities. The pressure increased when Dr. Brian Best joined the group in 1944 to establish the Department of Obstetrics and Gynecology. It was evident by then that some structural changes would have to be made.

Only a partial basement had been provided initially, and it

was agreed that the first step must be to complete this excavation and finish the full basement for professional and support-staff services. The contractors and designers, F.R. Lount and Son, were asked to provide a plan and cost estimate and a work schedule that would permit the Clinic to operate with the least possible inconvenience during construction. At best, it would be a period of some difficulty.

The plans were finally completed, and the cost was estimated by the contractor at $15,000 to $16,000. In the fall of 1944, work began.

The clinic building, of course, was now owned by the Manitoba Institute for the Advancement of Medical Education and Research. The subject of alterations to the property was on the agenda of the Board of Directors at their meeting held on Friday, December 22, 1944, at the Manitoba Club. The President of the Institute, Dr. Thorlakson, chaired the meeting. He asked Mr. MacAulay to report on the space requirements.

Mr. MacAulay, speaking on behalf of the members of the Winnipeg Clinic (the tenants of the building) reported that the changes would consist chiefly of the complete excavation of the basement and the finishing of the space for professional, medical-record and other services. The work constituted, at least in part, an improvement to the Institute's property, and by resolution of the Board it was provided that, "out of funds of the Institute available for that purpose," the Institute would pay the contractors $10,500 as the owner's share of the cost.[1] In the end the total expenditure was about $22,000, of which the tenants paid $11,500.

At the Board meeting, Mr. MacAulay reported that even with these improvements, the building was too small to fully accommodate the Clinic needs, and it was totally inadequate to allow for the increase in the number of doctors who could be expected to join the Clinic in the near future. Consequently plans were being prepared for a further addition, and the details would probably be ready for submission to the directors at their next meeting.

For some time, Dr. Thorlakson, in consultation with members of the Clinic and with F.R. Lount and Son, had been deeply involved in estimating the needs of the Winnipeg Clinic for both the short term and the long term, considering the probable future development of the medical services the Clinic should provide. The two lots originally purchased (No. 828 on the northeast corner of St. Mary Avenue and Vaughan Street, and No. 827 next to it, facing on Vaughan), were fifty feet wide and extended 120 feet from Vaughan Street to the lane. The first Clinic building occupied only the front fifty feet of these lots, with the entrance on Vaughan Street. The expansion plan that was chosen provided for a five-storey structure to be built on the unused portion of these two lots with the main entrance on St. Mary Avenue. The design included a foundation that would carry twelve storeys, to allow for long-term needs, and it incorporated the "old" building as an integral part of the new.

In the meantime, the adjacent lot (No. 826) on Vaughan Street, became available for purchase. In case it might be needed for Clinic expansion, Dr. Thorlakson bought it, and it became part of the assets of the Winnipeg Clinic Holding Company Limited. His foresight was well-founded, for as the plans for the five-storey building progressed, it became necessary to find a place outside the main structure to build the heating plant. A location on Lot No. 826, adjacent to the lane, proved to be ideal.

It was estimated that the addition and its equipment would cost $600,000. In order to fund such an amount, it would be necessary to obtain the support of a substantial corporate lender. The logical choice was the Great-West Life Assurance Company. Founded in Winnipeg in 1891, this company had grown into one of Canada's leading corporations in the insurance field, and was a major source of funds for property development. In the mid-summer of 1945, Dr. Thorlakson made an appointment to discuss with Vice-President and Managing Director H.W. Manning an arrangement to borrow the needed capital.

As owner of the property, the primary borrower would be the Manitoba Institute for the Advancement of Medical Education and Research. The source of loan repayment would be the rent paid by the Winnipeg Clinic physicians. Mr. Manning listened with interest to Dr. Thorlakson's explanation of the expansion plans, the increase in the number of doctors in the Winnipeg Clinic that had already taken place, and the potential for adding to the group in the future. He was reminded of the steady progress in liquidating the debt on the first building.

Dr. Thorlakson then asked what the maximum amount might be that Great-West Life would lend to the institute against a first mortgage on the property. It must be assumed that Mr. Manning was not unprepared for this request. He himself had been one of the signatories to the petition to the government for legislation to incorporate the Institute. Messrs. H.E. Sellers, C.S. Riley and Joseph Harris, all directors of the Great-West Life Assurance Company, had also signed the petition for the Institute incorporation. Finally, Mr. H.E. Sellers, who was the Vice-President of the Company, had succeeded Dr. Thorlakson as President of the Institute on June 4, 1945.

Mr. Manning advised Dr. Thorlakson that his company would be prepared to lend the Institute, for the purposes of the new construction, up to $300,000, at four and a half percent, secured by a first mortgage on the property. This was encouraging.

The question remaining for Dr. Thorlakson was where to find a lender that would advance the rest of the money that was required. This question was answered when Dr. Thorlakson happened to meet Mr. W.A. Murphy and Mr. Sellers in the corridor of the Winnipeg General Hospital, where they had been attending a board meeting. They told him that they had been considering how the balance of the funding could be accomplished. They had concluded, in consultation with Mr. MacAulay, that this might be done by means of non-interest-bearing loans; and already they had arranged that, in addition to themselves, Mrs. James A. Richardson, Mr. Joseph Harris, Mr. C.S. Gunn, Mr. Harry Ashdown and other charter members of the Research Institute would each advance up to $35,000, as needed, to an aggregate total of $300,000, without interest. Mrs. E.W. Kneeland, in recognition of the deep interest of her late husband in the initial planning of the Clinic, had also offered to join this group, and advanced $25,000. Aladdin with his lamp could hardly have arranged things more satisfactorily!

With the cessation of hostilities on both the European and Asian fronts in the summer of 1945, doctors released from the armed forces became available. A number were invited by Dr. Thorlakson to join the Winnipeg Clinic, resulting in important additions to the professional staff: an allergist, Dr. C.H.A. Walton; three internists, Dr. J.M. Kilgour, Dr. H.W. Riley and Dr. Jessie McGeachy; a thoracic surgeon, Dr. M.B. (Pit) Perrin;

a neuropsychiatrist, Dr. Gilbert Adamson; and a gastroenterologist, Dr. J. Wendell Macleod. Needless to say, this expansion created a compelling urgency to gain more space. In the autumn of 1945, secure in the knowledge that the money would become available, and without waiting for completion of the legal niceties, Dr. Thorlakson launched the construction project.

THE WINNIPEG CLINIC TO 1945

From the time the Winnipeg Clinic was established, Dr. Thorlakson had made annual reports – and, where appropriate, interim reports – to the professional members of the group. With changing circumstances and the advent of a number of doctors new to the Clinic, he decided that his Report Number 24, delivered on December 29, 1945, at a dinner meeting of the doctors associated with the Clinic, would constitute a statement of the principles that had guided the Winnipeg Clinic throughout its early years; it would also be an affirmation of the spirit and ideals that should influence its affairs in the future. Following opening remarks suitable to this festive season, he turned to more serious matters:

A Summing Up

The Winnipeg Clinic has now embarked upon a programme of expansion. The enlargement of the clinic building, together with additions to the medical and surgical staffs, necessitate the re-examination of our original plans and policies.

Progress in group practice demands constant vigilance and re-organization. Re-adjustments in inter-departmental coordination, improvements in administrative methods and procedures, additions to technical equipment, and the maintenance of a high standard of proficiency in the professional personnel, is a constant responsibility to which all members of the staff must make his or her individual contribution.

The point I wish to emphasize at this time is that no plan that we agree upon today may necessarily be adequate to meet the requirements of tomorrow. The plans made for this clinic at its inception, only four years ago, are totally inadequate now.

We, as members of a profession, are standing on the threshold of new and important developments in the practice of medicine. Governments are becoming increasingly aware of their responsibility in the fields of preventive and curative medicine and in the provision of adequate facilities for the training of medical personnel.

The change in the attitude of our governments – Dominion, provincial and municipal – has been brought about largely by the demands of the people for better-organized medical care and by the fact that some members of the medical profession have kept our governments informed on the advance in medical science and advised on the possibilities for improved medical service for all people.

Another change of attitude by governments and people everywhere is the realization that scientific research in general, including medical research, is the key to all progress in any broad national plan.

The significance of the above observations and their relationship to our clinic organization becomes apparent only when we recognize the fact that the success and permanence of this group depend not only on a high standard of professional service, but also upon the contribution that we, as individuals, and as a group, make in the fields of medical education and medical research. These two concepts must actuate the policy of the Winnipeg Clinic and very largely determine changes in organization. We must, in addition, be prepared to make our plans conform with modifications in government policy and regulations and we must agree that the interest of our patients is our first and most important consideration. The prestige of the medical profession as a whole depends to a large extent upon our individual and collective attitude towards these basic considerations.

For the information of the new members of this group, it is necessary to review early steps that led to the formation of the Winnipeg Clinic. The men who originally agreed to merge their practices in order to form the Winnipeg Clinic formerly practiced in offices located in the Medical Arts Building. The Board of Directors of the Medical Arts Building found it impossible to make provision for enlarged space in spite of the fact that members of the group had repeatedly requested that adequate premises for expansion be made available. For some of us, the situation was so serious and difficult that we had to stagger our appointments from eight in the morning until seven-thirty in the evening, including the noon hour and Saturday afternoons. The shareholders had voted definitely against building expansion prior to the war. One of the officers of the Board of Directors of the Medical Arts Building notified me personally that no change in this policy could be expected and urged that new premises be secured for the new group, of which he was then a member. This was the reason for the purchase of the property and the erection of the present clinic building.

While the formation of this clinic had been discussed prior to the outset of the war, no definite action had been taken. However, accommodation for patients and staff grew rapidly more inadequate. The availability of space in other office buildings was investigated, but no suitable location could be found. It was therefore decided that a new building, situated as close as possible to the centre of the city, was necessary.

Agreement was reached early between the principals that no financial gain would accrue to any individual by reason of equities that he might establish in the building itself. . . . Having agreed that the building itself should not represent a steadily increasing asset registered in the name of any individual member of the Clinic, it was decided to deed the building and property over to an institution organized for the purpose of supporting in perpetuity postgraduate medical education and medical research in this community.

After some discussions with University officials and leading citizens, it was agreed to petition the provincial government for a charter to establish the Manitoba Institute for the Advancement of Medical Education and Research. The provisions of the Bill include no mention of the Winnipeg Clinic or its contribution to the Institute, and representation on its board gives the University and the community control over its assets and policy. Public bequests must always be supervised and controlled by a body representing the community as a whole. Inasmuch as large assets of substantial value and large sums of money might ultimately become available to carry out the aims and objects of the Institute and that a great deal of this money would be spent by the Faculty of Medicine, it was agreed that this body should be invited to examine the Bill and to have representation on the Institute Board. The donor felt that this willingness to have the Faculty of Medicine scrutinize the Bill and make such recommendations as seemed advisable from the standpoint of the University would be accepted as an evidence of good faith.

After the provisions of the Bill had been discussed at two meetings, the members of the Faculty of Medicine voted their approval of the arrangement. The understanding that I had come to with my associates, that is, that the physical assets of the Clinic as represented by the property and building would not become part of our personal holdings, was thereby completed. The deed of the property and building was immediately transferred to the Institute at less than cost.

Several other considerations were involved in arriving at this important decision. I knew from my experience as a member of the Associate Committee on Medical Research of the National Research Council in Ottawa, that no large funds would be made available for research at the University of Manitoba unless we in this community evidenced some interest in encouraging and supporting research out of local funds. It was hoped that the step that had been taken would result in wider support from the community.

In the second place, I was convinced that a permanently satisfactory solution could not be found for the equitable and satisfactory distribution of the building and property amongst the members. There would have to be constant re-adjustments. When any individual resigned, retired or died, there would always be presented to the group a difficult and at-times-embarrassing adjustment. No inflexible rules could be laid down. The building could not be sold to all the members as a stock company. Younger members could not afford to purchase shares, so this would result in the senior members taking over control and ownership at the very time when in all probability the younger group of men would have, in the passage of years, accepted increasing responsibility for the success of the Clinic. While an arrangement setting up shares in a company might be considered good and fair business, the thought had to be kept constantly in mind that we were organizing a professional group rendering a highly specialized type of individual service to the community and not a business enterprise.

In the third place, there was no particular need for paying up the mortgage on the building in order that the Clinic in twenty years' time would enjoy premises free of rent. It must be realized that property and building must always belong to someone and if it belonged to the Clinic as a whole, which was operating on a partnership basis, a retiring partner or the legal representative of a deceased partner might institute legal proceedings against the group to obtain compensation. I need not point out to you that the attitude of the individual or his legal representative might at times be quite at variance with the opinions of the Clinic group as a whole.

The arrangement that is being explained was further justified on the grounds that young men of great promise could be expected to join the Winnipeg Clinic if they knew that senior members were preparing to make substantial contributions towards post-graduate education and research. The senior members of the Winnipeg Clinic, by this act, have relinquished ownership and control of these valuable physical assets so that they in their retiring years, or their executors after their decease, could not determine or control the policy of the Clinic with regard to expansion and further development.

The above arrangement represents the most important single step that has been taken by our [Clinic associates], up to this date. I have explained the agreement that we have made with the Manitoba Research Institute in some considerable detail because I feel you should be made thoroughly familiar with all the facts and reasons leading up to this agreement. I wish to place on record our acknowledgement and appreciation of the services and assistance of Mr. John A. MacAulay, K.C., and Mr. Donald A. Thompson in the organization of the Institute.

You will be interested to know that the Institute has equities to the value of $100,000; and by reason of gifts, the Institute has approximately $15,000 in cash, a major portion of which has already been offered to and accepted by the Faculty of Medicine in the University of Manitoba.

To complete this section of my report and before dealing with recommendations that will be placed before you for your future consideration, it should be stated that, to this date, the affairs of the Clinic partnership have been managed by an agreement of partnership between Dr. H.D. Morse, Dr. C.B. Stewart, Dr. Lennox G. Bell and myself as directors. We have been assisted in the development of the Clinic, the selection of non-professional personnel and the organization of daily routine practice by Mrs. Bernice Shepherd. Furthermore, we benefited by the counsel and financial advice of the late Mr. C.S. Gunn, an enthusiastic friend of the Clinic. We have had regular visits from Mr. R.B. Benson, the manager of the Duluth [Minnesota] Clinic, who very generously gave us the benefit of his advice based on over twenty years' experience in group practice. Mr. H. Lewis, who has been associated with us as auditor and accountant for almost twenty-five years, has followed the development of the Clinic and given us much excellent advice and has worked hard and late in the interest of the Clinic organization.

Organization And Finance

The organization of a professional group presents three problems in the realm of finance:

First is the division and distribution of accumulating assets in property and building. The Clinic has already established a policy with regard to this particular problem, namely, that these assets will go to support post-graduate education and medical research in Manitoba.

Second is the ownership of diagnostic and other equipment acquired by the Clinic. Exactly the same difficulties arise in tackling this problem as those which confront us with regard to the building. Here again certain individuals had to accept the responsibility of purchase and payment. While they might feel justified in retaining ownership and control, it is felt that here again a principle is involved in which the personal financial gain of the individual must be superseded by the interests and future satisfactory relationships within the Clinic itself. At the moment, we own equipment that has a value of over $80,000. When the new building is furnished and equipped, these items will represent an investment of $150,000 to $175,000. It is therefore recommended, subject to your approval, that the Manitoba Institute be asked to act as the custodians of this valuable asset so that it will always be available to the Clinic without charge. The Institute will only come into possession of this equipment should the Clinic organization decide to disband. This arrangement serves a two-fold purpose. One benefits the Institute in that it will increase the value of assets against any outstanding loan on the building. This is added financial security which the Clinic will provide. Furthermore, it will improve the rentability of the building to another medical institution or group if it is fully equipped. In the course of years, this clinic may out-grow this building or any addition that could be made to it. Transfer to another site might become necessary. Under such circumstances an agreement can be reached with the Institute for tranfer of the equipment. We cannot determine at this date the policy of the Clinic twenty years from now. We can, however, make allowance and provision for expansion and give reason for our present decisions and agreements. This second provision [that is, transfer of ownership of the equipment in the Clinic building to the Manitoba Institute] removes another possible bone of contention and represents in a tangible way the desire of the senior members to make satisfactory provisions for the smooth functioning of this clinic organization and is a distinct advantage to you [who are] the new or younger members of the group. It places you on a parity as quickly as possible without personal financial obligation on your part to the Clinic or the senior members.

It is my firm conviction that medical men should devote their time and energy to strictly scientific and professional pursuits and not be burdened down too much with endless and often fruitless and irritating discussions on financial matters for which they have, as a rule, little aptitude. I say this with considerable feeling and emphasis. I do not regret having spent, to date, practically all my time to the exclusion of leisure and holidays on the organization of the Clinic. Nor do I regret advancing personal funds and guaranteeing substantial loans. This was done with the full approval and knowledge of my family even though, at the beginning, it jeopardized their security. However, I would not wish to burden any other individual with the same responsibility and personal risk. Money is important to the individual and to any successful organization, but what is also important is the sacrifice of time that could be made available to leisure, learning and technical training.

If this second recommendation regarding equipment is approved, then the members of this clinic can always be assured that the workshop and the tools which form such a necessary adjunct to successful medical practice are always available without involving them individually in financial responsibility or dispute with their associates over respective ownership.

Senior members may, therefore, leave the Clinic or new members may join without causing a ripple of disturbance as far as the organization as a whole is concerned. This will result in stability within the organization and security for the younger men.

Group Practice: Purposes and Principles

The advantages of group practice may be enumerated as follows:

1. To provide the individual physician with facilities that will enable him to give to his patients all the advantages of modern, scientific medicine.

2. To provide easy access to consultation with experts in special fields.

3. To provide the individual doctor with an opportunity to keep abreast with recent advances in medical knowledge and the results of medical research because of daily contacts and discussions on diagnostic and treatment problems. There is always the stimulus and challenge to do better work.

4. To provide for the division of responsibility for any important decision affecting the diagnosis and treatment of the seriously ill patient. The free expression of an honest difference of opinion should be encouraged and welcomed. It is of distinct advantage to the patient and will mean constant improvement in diagnostic accuracy and clinic efficiency.

5. The charge to the patient will be a composite fee based on the value of the services rendered and not a series of individual and other unrelated charges.

6. For the individual physician or surgeon, his time can be organized to make the fullest use of his special talents and training.

7. Regular holiday periods can be provided, during which his work will be attended to by his confreres without loss of continuity of professional service to the patient.

8. Encouragement will be given individuals to attend and participate in the meetings of medical societies and to visit other medical centres.

9. Assistance will be given to the individual so that he may study and review the results of treatment on the basis of our clinic records.

10. Security will be provided in the form of continued income during periods of illness and provision of a pension plan, to which the physician and the Clinic will contribute, to provide for his years of retirement.

Having dealt at some length with the ideas and ideals that have determined Clinic policy in the past and made certain definite recommendations in regard to the future, allow me to emphasize and epitomize the factors which I believe will, in the final analysis, determine the measure of success that can be attained by this group:

1. the highest possible standards of scientific and professional attainment;

2. a good doctor-patient relationship; a sincere interest in people and their problems;

3. professional and business integrity;

4. efficient administration;

5. good professional and public relationship;

6. hard work and perseverance;

7. confidence in the professional work of our confreres;

8. sound planning for the future;

9. effective team work;

10. the loyal co-operation of the entire staff.

I submit to you the final section of this statement as our magna carta and its very acceptance, as such, is the greatest assurance of success in providing our patients with sound, scientific, medical advice and assistance at a reasonable and fair cost.

His audience applauded this expression of enlightened leadership. But among some there were unspoken reservations about the proposal to turn over to the Research Institute, whether in trust or as a gift, the equipment in the Clinic. The subject was not considered further on this occasion.

THE SECOND STAGE

At the meeting of the Board of Directors of the Research Institute on January 26, 1946, Mr. MacAulay made a full report on the progress of the work and the financing of the five-storey addition to the Clinic building. After discussion, by resolution of the Board, "Messrs. H.E. Sellers, W.A. Murphy and Joseph Harris [were] appointed to act as members of a committee to supervise the construction and financing of the addition to the Winnipeg Clinic building now in course of construction, it being understood that Drs. P.H.T. Thorlakson, H.D. Morse and C. Burton Stewart would represent the Winnipeg Clinic on the said committee, and that the remaining members would be J.A. MacAulay, D.A. Thompson, H. Lewis [the Winnipeg Clinic's chief accountant] and William Lount, the architect in charge of construction."

The Board also designated Mr. Murphy, Mr. Sellers and Mr. Harris, on behalf of the Institute, to deal with "all matters affecting the Institute relating to the financing and construction of the addition, the purchase of the additional land required, the fixing of rent to be paid by the Winnipeg Clinic Holding Company [for both the existing building and the addition], and the disposition of donations made to the Institute by members of the Winnipeg Clinic. . . . "

On May 15, 1946, the Board of Directors of the Institute met at the Fort Garry Hotel to deal with property matters. By-law No. 2, which authorized the purchase of Lot No. 826 from the Winnipeg Clinic Holding Company Limited for the sum of $8,000 was considered and passed, thus providing a site for the heating plant. By-law No. 3, which authorized the institute to borrow $250,000 from the Great-West Life Assurance Company at an interest rate of four and a half percent was introduced and passed. It provided that the loan would be secured by a first mortgage on the Vaughan Street land and the buildings thereon, as well as an assignment to the lender of the lease from the research institute to the Winnipeg Clinic Holding Company. By-law No. 4 provided for a lease of the land and building occupied by the Winnipeg Clinic to the Winnipeg Clinic Holding Company Limited.

These actions were "ratified, sanctioned and confirmed" at the Third Annual Meeting [and the related Special General Meeting] of the members of the Institute, held on May 28, 1946.

Work on the new building went steadily forward and it was completed in about eighteen months. It was a unique structure of distinguished appearance, designed along neo-classical lines, and built largely of Tyndallstone relieved by reddish-hued fieldstone quarried at Stonewall. Functionally and artistically attractive, it was an adornment to the architectural scene in downtown Winnipeg.

The Fourth Annual Meeting of the Manitoba Institute for the Advancement of Medical Education and Research held on July 2, 1947 was an extraordinary occasion, since it was held in the library on the fifth floor of the Winnipeg Clinic building. Construction was almost completed and Mr. MacAulay reported to the meeting that the Clinic now occupied virtually all of the premises.

He informed the members of the Institute that the cost of construction was higher than had been expected, and would total $550,000. In addition, there were the usual costs for fees, interim financing and similar items. Arrangements had been made to increase the amount of the mortgage loan from the Great-West Life Assurance Company to $325,000.

Preparations for non-interest-bearing loans under the second mortgage were now almost completed. To secure the individual lenders, the second mortgage would be issued to the National Trust Company, acting on their behalf, for an amount not exceeding $300,000. Its terms provided for repayment of the principal amount without interest. When the final accounts were calculated, the amount actually borrowed under the second mortgage was $283,000. This included the balance owing on the original first and second mortgages, balance of the cost of the new construction, and other indebtedness for services related to construction and financing of the addition.

By-laws were passed at the meeting confirming and sanctioning these actions.

With the completion of these formalities, work proceeded rapidly to complete the new structure, which would provide more than five times the original space.

CHAPTER 6

Formalizing the Organization

YEARS OF GROWTH

The first expansion of the Winnipeg Clinic was completed in the latter part of 1947. As space in the enlarged building became available, more doctors accepted Dr. Thorlakson's invitation to join the Winnipeg Clinic. In 1946 and 1947, Dr. George Ryan and Dr. Bruce Loadman joined the group to establish the Section of Orthopedics; Dr. Oswald Day and Dr. Murray McLandress initiated the Section of Pediatrics. The ancillary services of electroencephalography and physiotherapy were added. A medical records librarian was appointed.

During the next three years the medical group steadily increased in number, and by the end of the decade there were thirty-one doctors associated with the Winnipeg Clinic.[1]

The postwar period was an era of unprecedented progress in medical science. Refinements in the preparation of penicillin (first used in the treatment of patients in 1940, and described as "the most spectacular single therapeutic agent in history"), along with a host of new chemotherapeutic products born in the pharmaceutical research laboratories, were not only effective in the direct treatment and prevention of disease; they also made it possible to successfully carry out surgical procedures that previously were either extremely hazardous or altogether precluded.

Regular opportunities for exchange of information between the medical specialties helped doctors keep well informed about the new resources. In December 1945, monthly medical staff meetings were inaugurated at the clinic, at which unusual cases were reviewed and papers were presented on subjects of current interest. Many of the papers were published, either in journals with general medical circulation or in the Winnipeg Clinic Quarterly, the first issue of which appeared in September 1948. The Quarterly was sent to all physicians who asked to be placed on the mailing list, and by 1962, its merit was recognized by the listing of its contents in the worldwide catalogue of published medical papers, known as Index Medicus.[2]

At that time, most of the Clinic doctors had a primary staff appointment at the Winnipeg General Hospital with a joint teaching appointment in the Faculty of Medicine. They made an important contribution to the education of both graduate and undergraduate students, and were encouraged to participate actively in the responsibilities of the medical staff organization.

Dr. Thorlakson believed that private medical groups could, and should, provide a useful and refreshing alternative to the institutionalized hospital environment for part of a doctor's postgraduate training. At his urging, supported by Dr. Lennox Bell, then Head of the Section of Medicine, in 1947 the Royal College of Physicians and Surgeons of Canada was induced to recognize the Winnipeg Clinic as a site for one year of the training requirement for specialist certification in internal medicine.

At the same time, the Clinic offered a two-year graduate course for general practitioners. The first three months of this course were spent in the Department of Pathology in one of the teaching hospitals – that is, either the Winnipeg General Hospital or St. Boniface General Hospital. The remaining twenty-one months were spent in the Clinic, generally allowing for two months in each section, with some variation to meet the interests of the graduate. Evening courses were given by Clinic doctors, and hospital rounds were provided. Throughout the two years, the trainee received a salary from the Clinic.

Between 1947 and 1951, thirty-eight doctors took this graduate training, but the Clinic reluctantly discontinued the courses in 1951. Experience indicated that it was difficult for the University to adapt to an arrangement of this kind. The work of supervision and instruction at the Clinic was an added burden to the specialists there, most of whom already had an obligation to do graduate and undergraduate teaching in the hospital and the University. The venture proved to be expensive and time-consuming for the Clinic associates directly involved with the program.

Despite this experience, Dr. Thorlakson was not shaken in his belief that the private, group-practice-specialist clinics could provide useful opportunities to broaden the base of postgraduate training in some areas; but it was evident that initiation of a plan to utilize this capability must lie with the University.[3]

REORGANIZING THE CLINIC

Meantime, Dr. Thorlakson continued to struggle with the problem of the long-term organization of the Winnipeg Clinic and the relationship between the Clinic, as a group of practicing physicians, and the Manitoba Institute for the Advancement of Medical Education and Research. The introduction of a large number of new Clinic associates, as well as the prospect of more doctors joining the group in the future, made it imperative to try to clarify and reaffirm the organizational relationships.

When new associates were invited to join the Winnipeg Clinic, they were not asked to sign any formal document acknowledging either their privileges, or their responsibilities to their colleagues. The usual practice in the operation of medical partnerships requires newcomers to spend some time in a junior capacity, and on being invited to become full partners they must make a substantial investment to acquire a "share" in the assets, including the "goodwill," of the medical group. In contrast, under the unique arrangements Dr. Thorlakson had made with respect to financial and property affairs, and his willingness to invest his own funds and give personal guarantees to lenders, no investment was asked of any of the doctors in the Winnipeg Clinic group. Indeed the group was deemed to be a partnership, but there was in fact no formal partnership agreement at that time. New associates, having been approved by the members, simply moved into the Winnipeg Clinic building and became beneficiaries of all the facilities and the operating procedures that were already in place. Similarly, if a doctor wanted to terminate his Clinic association, he could, if he wished, simply advise his colleagues and move elsewhere, taking his practice with him.

In the initial stages, when there were less than ten doctors in the Clinic, all of whom had known one another for a long time, the informality of the organization was not a problem. Dr. Thorlakson's position as founder of the specialty group practice was accepted, and his principles with respect to property ownership, pooling and division of income, support for research, and relationships with the Manitoba Institute for the Advancement of Medical Education and Research, were recognized and supported.

By the late 1940s, however, the number of doctors in the Winnipeg Clinic had more than tripled. Individual interests were more diverse. The group revenue had increased substantially. Property values had mounted. At meetings of members, questions arose about added potential benefits, such as, for example, the establishment of a pension plan. But although under the law at that time a partnership could establish a contributory pension plan for its employees, the members of the partnership itself could not participate, since they were technically owners, and not employees, of the business.

By 1947, the Winnipeg Clinic had become a specialty group practice with nearly thirty doctors in a de facto, but undocumented, medical partnership. Except for the founder, Dr. Thorlakson, none had a capital investment in the enterprise. The professional income was pooled, and after payment of costs of practice the income was distributed to members on a basis negotiated between the individual and a small committee of senior members of the group, chaired by Dr. Thorlakson. The committee was advised by the head of the section in which the member practiced, and based its decision on a number of factors, including the individual's earnings, his contribution to medical education, his published papers, and his participation in medical, clinic and community affairs.

The Manitoba Institute for the Advancement of Medical Education and Research owned the building and property where the group practised. The building and property were encumbered by mortgages to the Great-West Life Assurance Company and the National Trust Company to secure the repayment of money borrowed for construction. The Institute leased the property to the Winnipeg Clinic Holding Company Limited, at a rental that covered payment of principal and interest on the mortgages, taxes, insurance and other property costs.

The Winnipeg Clinic Holding Company Limited was wholly capitalized and owned by Dr. Thorlakson. This company managed the Clinic business, provided the building for the group practice, and had bought, and therefore owned, most of the furniture and equipment. Its revenue was derived from a charge against the professional income of the group and rent from the Winnipeg Clinic Pharmacy Limited – the latter also having been wholly capitalized by Dr. Thorlakson, and owned by him.

It was within this context that Dr. Thorlakson approached the preparation of the annual report to his professional colleagues, which he presented on December 2, 1946. His dedication to the principles that had guided him since he founded the Winnipeg Clinic in 1938 were as strong as ever. He believed that the Winnipeg Clinic should provide an exemplary standard of care, that the professional environment should be stimulating, and that the physical facilities be both functional and comfortable. He believed that it was unwise, and perhaps detrimental to the conduct of a group medical practice, for the members to be involved in ownership of property. In his opinion, it was fitting that doctors should be prepared to offer financial support for medical education and research, since this is one of the cornerstones upon which improvements in clinical practice are based.

In his report to the Clinic associates in December 1945, he had offered to turn over the furnishings and equipment, owned by the Winnipeg Clinic Holding Company Limited, to the Manitoba Institute for the Advancement of Medical Education and Research (see chapter 5). This would, in effect, fulfill his conception that no member of a professional group should own property for which other members paid rent or capital costs. Under this plan, all the fixed assets would belong to the Institute.

But this proposal had not received the full support of the group. Since Dr. Thorlakson felt a moral obligation in such matters to achieve a favourable concensus (and there may have been some legal obligation to do so), no action had been taken.

He decided to try again in his report of December 2, 1946.

The Vision Revised

In a statement presented to the members of the Winnipeg Clinic on December 29, 1945, I reviewed at some length the history of our organization and its connection and contribution to the Manitoba Institute for the Advancement of Medical Education and Research. I enumerated some unsolved problems created by the necessity for expansion and reorganization, and placed before you some matters of principle and policy which might be used as a guide to determine our attitude toward the many situations that arise to test the soundness of our plans and the stability of our Clinic organization.

In that report, I pointed out that there were three matters in the field of finance that confronted a medical clinic organization: (a) the ownership of properties and buildings occupied by the clinic; (b) the ownership and control of the equipment and furniture used by the Clinic; and (c) the fair and equitable distribution of the earnings of the Clinic, including provision for a retirement fund.

All the major nonprofessional problems and difficulties that beset a clinic organization evolve from these three sources. It need not be reemphasized here that the stability and permanency of our organization are to a considerable extent dependent upon the thought and vision and practicability of the solution that we bring to bear on these three matters. I have stated before that medical men should not be burdened down too heavily with endless discussions on financial problems to the distraction of their other more serious responsibilities.

The original plans for our organization provided for the solution of the first major problem. I am convinced that the transfer of ownership of the properties and buildings (valued presently at more than $600,000), to the Manitoba Institute is sound planning for the future. The assets and earnings of those properties will, as the Institute's major effort, support in perpetuity, medical education and research in our university. The division of these substantial assets amongst a large number of Clinic associates would not tend to provide stability for the institution or security for new and younger members of the Clinic; the senior members quite naturally would, without this provision, own the controlling interest. This is the very contingency I wish to avoid.

The Winnipeg Clinic as a medical and surgical diagnostic and treatment centre, has far outgrown the original plans, necessitating new and improved space as well as additional equipment. The Manitoba Institute, as owners of the building, were asked to provide the necessary increase in Clinic space. To assist the Institute in the financial undertaking, several personal friends agreed to provide the necessary capital, without interest, for the second mortgage. The first mortgage has been taken by Great-West Life. Actually the money in the second mortgage provides the security for the first, and it is now incumbent upon the Clinic as an organization (because individually we are no longer able to guarantee the principal) to make adequate provision to safeguard and augment the security of the second mortgage, as well as to assure the fulfillment of the aims and objects of the Manitoba Research Institute.

The only way these objectives can be accomplished is to place the supervision and management of the Clinic in charge of a board of trustees empowered to administer the affairs of the Clinic in an impartial and equitable manner, satisfactory not only to the Manitoba Institute but also to the members of the Winnipeg Clinic actively employed in medical practice. This plan envisages a situation in which no individual or small group of senior members (or their legal representatives after their demise) will be in a position to determine or interfere with the policy of the Clinic. To make the Clinic an association of free professional men, unhampered by considerations of personal financial advantages or control, it becomes necessary to divest the present owner [i.e., Dr. Thorlakson] of his legal and financial control.

The founder and his founding associates, therefore, are prepared to offer the Institute all the present financial assets of the Clinic to insure the Institute and Clinic against financial embarrassment because of involvement in personal ownership and control. This represents a major contribution and, by its very nature, establishes the fact that nothing will be left undone by the founders to insure permanency and stability in management and control. For your information, may I say that this gift from the founders represents equipment and supplies presently valued at $125,000 and accounts receivable with an estimated value of $400,000.

It is expected that the Manitoba Institute will appoint a board of trustees and a board of administration according to an agreement which is mutually acceptable. The personnel of this board of administration will be so constituted as to directly supervise and control the policies of the Clinic with regard to professional practices, financial remuneration and retirement allowances as are considered just and proper on the basis of professional ability, prestige, contribution to Clinic practice and other scientific and educational activities. On this basis only will the Winnipeg Clinic be able to attract men of outstanding ability as practising specialists and teachers, and encourage them to remain in Winnipeg to make their individual and special contribution to the medical activities of the community. It can readily be understood that a proprietorship or incorporated body with limited and personal ownership would not, in the end, accomplish the original purposes of our organization. . . .

I hope that I have made my position absolutely clear on these important matters. I am deeply interested in helping to create a sound, ethical organization, based on a high standard of professional skill and the closest collaboration between the specialists in the various fields of medicine and surgery. I am not interested in personal control and ownership. At the moment my contribution to the Clinic is substantial, and for that reason authority and control are largely vested in me; but there will come a time when others will carry the major responsibilities of the Clinic, and it would seem unwise for me to retain that ownership and control on the basis of past services and contributions, as is legitimately done in a purely commercial organization. The Clinic should not have to depend on a series of reorganizations to adjust embarrassing situations as they arise. The time to provide for the inevitable is now. Procrastinations in these matters cause both embitterment and regrets. Many difficulties cannot be foreseen, but by judicious and sound planning, many pitfalls can be avoided. The future of this clinic rests largely with the younger men of the organization. I can only assure you that, as far as it is in our competence, your organization will be built on sound, practical considerations, free, as far as possible, from selfish motives.

This statement clearly indicates that Dr. Thorlakson, who had received so much support, encouragement and advice from some of the foremost members of Winnipeg's business community, sought to preserve and even enhance this relationship in the interest of both the Clinic and the Institute. He recognized the importance of experienced and unbiased direction for these enterprises if they were to play an increasingly useful role in the medical services in Manitoba.

But another, deeper factor probably helped to shape his views on the importance of finding acceptable ways to deal with profits of the pharmacy, and with revenue or capital gains from property.

His personal philosophy had been influenced by the dedication to Christian principles and service to the community that marked the life of his father and mother. From this background, it seems evident that he had acquired a sense of the principle of stewardship, which holds that one who is given special talents or special opportunities should perceive these endowments as being held in trust, to be exercised primarily for the general good. He was prepared to rely for his personal income on his surgical practice, and to so order affairs that revenue arising outside the professional boundaries would accrue to the benefit of medical education and research, and thus contribute to the well-being of mankind.

Some of his colleagues, however, did not share this idealistic and enlightened point of view. They preferred to ask the Clinic's legal counsel to investigate, and if possible recommend, an alternate form of organization that would permit its financial affairs to come more closely under the control of the Clinic members.

A NEW LEGAL FRAMEWORK

The legal advisors to the professional group (and to the Manitoba Institute for the Advancement of Medical Education and Research) were John A. MacAulay, K.C., and Donald A. Thompson, K.C., both of whom were experienced, able and resourceful in the field of corporate law. The request to design a new legal framework for the Winnipeg Clinic became primarily the responsibility of Mr. Thompson.

It was an interesting challenge. The provisions of the Manitoba Medical Act clearly prevent a corporation from conducting a medical practice. Therefore, a simple incorporation under the Companies Act was not an available alternative.

On the other hand, in addition to the disadvantages cited earlier, the conduct of a medical practice under a partnership agreement carried with it other problems that became more serious as the number of members increased. There were already some thirty doctors in the group; and it was evident that this number would have to be increased substantially as more and more patients sought the Clinic services. With this prospect in the future, there were good reasons to seek new arrangements for the conduct of Clinic affairs.

Particularly troublesome was the legal principle that, on the death or retirement of any partner, the existing partnership would be deemed dissolved and therefore a new one established. Also in the event of the death of a partner, income tax and succession duty problems arose. The deceased member's share had to be evaluated and disposed of – normally to one or more of the remaining members. This was not only inconvenient, but it also raised the possibility of financial conflict between the partners and the estate, and indeed between one another.

To overcome these difficulties and to avoid potential problems, Mr. Thompson proposed "a novel type of corporation." The plan called for the formation "by private act of the provincial legislature, of a corporation without share capital under the name of Winnipeg Clinic, the members of which would all be duly qualified medical practitioners. These practitioners would practise their profession as individuals but would assign to the corporation their professional fees and for this would receive an agreed amount per annum, either fixed or fluctuating. The difference between the total sum agreed to be paid to the members for their services and for their professional accounts and the sum total of the professional accounts would represent the income of the corporation and would be used to offset the cost of providing the facilities [and other services]."

No membership fee would be charged to an incoming member. Membership would terminate on death, resignation or retirement of a member. The affairs of the Clinic corporation would be under the control of a council elected from amongst the members. The plan also provided that the assets of the Clinic as constituted at the time of the new incorporation would be turned over to the corporation without any consideration other than an agreement on behalf of the Winnipeg Clinic (Incorporated) to enter into contracts with the individual members of the partnership. Finally, it was proposed that the Winnipeg Clinic Holding Company Limited and the Winnipeg Clinic Pharmacy Limited would be turned over by Dr. Thorlakson to the incorporated clinic.

The reorganization plan prepared by the legal counsel was welcomed by the members of the Clinic. For his part, Dr. Thorlakson agreed to transfer the Winnipeg Clinic Pharmacy Limited and all the assets held by the Winnipeg Clinic Holding Company Limited, to the incorporated clinic for the nominal sum of one dollar. Although the value of both of these companies had increased substantially in the years since they had been established, he held to his basic principle that he would not take any personal profit either from the Pharmacy or from the capital gain that had accrued in the Holding Company. The new arrangement was not, of course, entirely in keeping with his conception of a clear and well-understood separation between the Clinic medical practitioners in their professional association, and the ownership of the pharmacy, the furniture and equipment, the business services and the property. He believed, nevertheless, that the principles he had enunciated would continue to be followed.[4]

General concurrence in the plan was gained from the parties

directly interested. The "Petition of P.H.T. Thorlakson and others for an Act to incorporate the Winnipeg Clinic" was prepared by the solicitors. It was presented in the Legislature by Lt. Col. Gordon Churchill, acting on behalf of Mr. A.J. Stringer, who was absent from the House when the bill was called for first reading, on Friday, February 25, 1949.

Passing through the customary legislative procedures almost without comment, the Act of Incorporation was duly passed, and received royal assent on Friday, March 25, 1949. The Winnipeg Clinic (Incorporated) was now a legal entity with broad powers to act.[5] This legislation was designed to be consistent with the position that the members of Winnipeg Clinic (Incorporated), each of whom had fulfilled the requirements of the Medical Act and of the College of Physicians and Surgeons of Manitoba and held a license to practise his profession in Manitoba, were in fact practising as individuals.

Nevertheless, the Act also provided for agreements between the Corporation and each of the practitioners under which they agreed to practise in association with each other and utilize the facilities and services available from the Corporation. The Corporation was to pay them a salary, the amount of which was not necessarily related to their fee earnings; provide them with other benefits such as pensions and group insurance; manage the clinic operations; and in other ways act remarkably like an employer.

What remained to be tested was the attitude of the income tax officials toward the proposal. Before actually carrying out the reorganization, the tax authorities had to be consulted to ensure that the steps being taken complied with their requirements.

The response of the income tax officials was disappointing. Despite extended correspondence and a number of discussions with senior officials at Ottawa, the tax officials insisted that since a corporation cannot conduct a medical practice, the employee-like role for the doctors was not acceptable. On the other hand, if the doctors were in fact maintaining individual practices, then their respective incomes must consist of the fees they respectively earned. Each doctor must, therefore, record his fee income in his tax return, from which the allowable expenses of conducting his practice would be deducted.

To accept this ruling would necessitate a refinement of the accounting system and a revision of a number of administrative practices. More traumatic, however, was the realization that it would preclude the establishment of corporate group pension and insurance plans.

Six months after the Act was passed, it was evident that the minds of the income tax officials would not be changed, and no further attempts at appeal would be useful. This turn of events must have vexed Mr. MacAulay and Mr. Thompson; but they were not dismayed. Alternate ways of achieving the objectives were devised and examined. By November 1949, they were prepared to recommend a modified plan to the Clinic members.

In a paper dated November 18, 1949, Mr. Thompson set out the new proposal:

> There is no objection in legal theory or from the income tax departmental point of view to the conduct of a medical practice by a partnership as distinct from a corporation and to partners engaging other practitioners. Accordingly, we propose to abandon the theory that each medical practitioner will be carrying on a medical practice individually, and substitute the theory of the conduct of the medical practice by a partnership in conjunction with the corporation providing the facilities.
>
> The incorporated Winnipeg Clinic would be organized identically as originally proposed and would acquire the capital stock of the Holding Company and Pharmacy and all facilities, equipment and supplies owned by the present partnership and would also acquire the lease of the Clinic premises. These would be turned over to the corporation by the founders [i.e., principally, Dr. Thorlakson, but two doctors who had been with him from the beginning, Dr. Stewart and Dr. Morse, were included] on the same basis as was previously discussed, namely without cash payment but an obligation on the part of the corporation to pay to each of the founders on death or retirement the stipulated sum previously discussed. The incorporation would provide all the facilities for the conduct of the practice of the Clinic as were previously contemplated.
>
> The partnership would be composed of not more than three members who in reality would be in the nature of trustees for the other members of the incorporated Winnipeg Clinic.
>
> The three partner trustees who will be designated to carry on the medical and surgical practice will enter into employment contracts with the remaining doctors. They would also enter into an agreement with the incorporated Winnipeg Clinic to use the facilities of the incorporation and to pay for such facilities a fee based on the actual cost plus

a percentage of profit, the purpose being to ensure that all surplus revenue of the partnership would go to the incorporation.

The partnership would set up a pension plan which would cover all the doctors engaged in medical practice other than the three partners. The incorporated Winnipeg Clinic would likewise set up a pension plan in which all employees of the incorporation would share. Likely the one plan could cover both the partnership and the incorporation. Some pension benefit could be secured for the three partners by appointing them officers and salaried employees of the incorporated Clinic, the extent of such benefits being necessarily dependent on the amount of their respective salaries.

In order that the partners should not be penalized by not being able to share to the same extent as the other practitioners in the pension plans, the partnership agreement could provide for supplementary pension benefits out of partnership assets to equalize such partners with the others.

The affairs of both the incorporated Clinic and the partnership would be conducted in the same manner as was previously contemplated, with the three partners simply being regarded as trustees for the larger group. The income of the partners and of the other practitioners would be determined by the Council of the incorporated Winnipeg Clinic.

A new partnership agreement would be entered into between the three partners which would provide that any partner would retire on request of the Council of the incorporated Clinic, and further that on the death or retirement of a partner the deceased or retiring partner would have no claim to any of the assets of the partnership (which would merely consist of book accounts and cash) and which would provide that in such event a new partner would be admitted into partnership to take the place of the deceased or retiring member, such new partner to be selected by the Council of the incorporated Winnipeg Clinic. The incoming partner might have to be compensated in respect of any pension rights which he might lose by ceasing to be an employee of the partnership.

The foregoing plan should accomplish the same result as was desired in the first plan and should not be objectionable in legal theory to the income tax department. The members of the incorporated Clinic would regard the three partners as trustees. The income tax department would regard them as independent partners.

Rulings on the new setup would, of course, have to be obtained, but the same delay as was experienced previously in obtaining rulings is not anticipated.

The revised form of organization was accepted by the income tax authorities.

The members of Winnipeg Clinic (Incorporated) agreed that Dr. Thorlakson, as the founder, and Drs. Stewart and Morse, as his earliest Clinic associates, should become the partners who would operate the medical practice. It was decided that the new operating structure made possible by reason of the terms of the Act of Incorporation would be brought into effect on January 1, 1950. Since it was, by this time, early December 1949, it would require a great deal of effort on the part of Mr. Thompson and his associates to determine the legal measures necessary to implement the operating plan. They proved equal to the task, and by the beginning of January all the documentation was ready.

The first document to be prepared and executed was a partnership agreement providing that Drs. Thorlakson, Stewart and Morse agreed "to become partners and associates in the practice of medicine and surgery . . . under the name 'Winnipeg Clinic' (hereinafter referred to as the 'Clinic') as of January 1, 1950." The partnership agreement was completed by the year end.[6]

On January 6, 1950, the first meeting of the Council of the Winnipeg Clinic (Incorporated) was held, with all of the eight members specified in the Act present.[7] By unanimous agreement, Dr. C.B. Stewart acted as chairman and Dr. T.A. Lebbetter was secretary. By-laws prepared by the solicitors establishing the rules and regulations under which the corporation would operate were reviewed in detail and passed.[8]

The legal transfer of all the assets of Dr. Thorlakson's Winnipeg Clinic Holding Company Limited was accomplished by means of an assignment to the Winnipeg Clinic (Incorporated) from Drs. Thorlakson, Stewart and Morse "either as a partnership or as individuals," for the nominal consideration of one dollar. There was no recognition of the fact that in the assets of the Winnipeg Clinic Holding Company Limited (wholly owned by Dr. Thorlakson), in addition to the equipment in the Winnipeg Clinic, there were four lots on the west side of Kennedy Street, across the lane from the Clinic building. Two of these valuable properties (Lots No. 771 and No. 773) had been purchased by Dr. Thorlakson in December, 1946, with his personal funds; and two (at the corner of Kennedy Street and St. Mary Avenue) with funds borrowed from the Pharmacy, which he also owned.

These properties were not necessary for the operation of the Clinic, and probably should not have been included in the assignment of the Holding Company assets which primarily consisted of the Clinic equipment and furnishings. Indeed, in his proposals to Clinic members, Dr. Thorlakson specifically named the equipment and furnishings as the assets he was prepared to turn over to the Manitoba Institute for the Advancement of Medical Education and Research, or (later) to the Winnipeg Clinic Incorporated (see pages 68, 78.)

The Assignment set out that these doctors conduct a medical and surgical practice under the name Winnipeg Clinic; that either as individuals or as partners they own certain assets; and that the Winnipeg Clinic (Incorporated) had been established for the purpose, amongst others, of furnishing them with facilities required for their practices. It was, therefore, agreed that for the nominal sum of one dollar, they would assign all properties and other assets to the Corporation, including all inventories and supplies; all equipment and fixtures; the lease of the premises from the Manitoba Institute for the Advancement of Medical Education and Research; the right to use the name Winnipeg Clinic as the corporate name, although at the same time retaining the name for use of the partnership in its practice; and all the issued capital stock (five shares) of the Winnipeg Clinic Holding Company Limited. The Winnipeg Clinic (Incorporated) assumed a debt of $61,828.43 owed by the Winnipeg Clinic Holding Company Limited to Dr. Thorlakson for money advanced by him for the purchase of equipment. He had borrowed the money from the Royal Bank of Canada, and the Winnipeg Clinic (Incorporated) paid this obligation directly to the bank.

The Assignment also transferred from Dr. Thorlakson (who held all the issued capital stock, two shares of which were loaned to others so that they could qualify as directors) all the shares of the Winnipeg Clinic Pharmacy Limited, the consideration being the same nominal sum of one dollar. The Pharmacy, however, had accumulated a reserve of between $80,000 and $100,000.

When, in 1943, Dr. Thorlakson transferred ownership of the property and building occupied by the Winnipeg Clinic to the Manitoba Institute for the Advancement of Medical Education and Research, he was, of course, fully aware that this would not immediately produce income to support the Institute objectives. It was his intention that the source of the Institute's initial cash income would be, in addition to direct donations, the profits of the Pharmacy. This would also ensure compliance with the policy of the Canadian Medical Association that doctors should not receive reimbursement from a pharmacy that filled prescriptions for their patients. As a result of this arrangement, by December 31, 1949, the Institute had received $52,058 from the Winnipeg Clinic Pharmacy Limited.

In considering the implications of transferring the ownership of the Pharmacy to the Winnipeg Clinic (Incorporated), which had been anticipated by including in the Act of Incorporation a section which authorized it to carry on the business of a pharmacy, Dr. Thorlakson sought the advice of Mr. MacAulay. There were two concerns. One was the method of dealing with the accumulated surplus; the other was the matter of future contributions to the Institute.

Mr. MacAulay suggested, and Dr. Thorlakson agreed, that in addition to the annual payment to the Institute of the maximum sum allowable as a tax deduction – then ten percent of the net profit – the Pharmacy could transfer annually a further sum of $5,000 by way of a dividend from its accumulated profits, with the Clinic Corporation acting as intermediary. This dividend could be increased as circumstances permitted.

However, the Assignment of the Pharmacy shares made no reference to this arrangement, and no special consideration was provided with respect to the transfer of ownership of the Winnipeg Clinic Pharmacy Limited. It is not clear that the new owners were aware of the dividend suggestion.

Finally, one other financial factor was recognized. At the time when a number of new associates were added to the Clinic group, Dr. Thorlakson had merged some $120,000 of his personal medical accounts receivable into the group funds, without any special consideration. It was agreed that this warranted a payment to him of $72,000 as part of the restructuring of the Clinic affairs. Dr. Morse had made a similar, but lesser, merging of his accounts, and it was agreed that this warranted a settlement with him in the amount of $12,000. Dr. Stewart had, of course, been with the original Clinic group, and his accounts had also been melded in the joint funds. On the principle of equity, Dr. Thorlakson allocated $12,000 to Dr. Stewart from the estimated value of his excess input of funds.

The Assignment, therefore, provided that the sum of $60,000 would be paid to Dr. Thorlakson, and $12,000 each to Drs. Morse and Stewart – not immediately, but on January 1, 1959, without interest.

Having put its affairs in order, the Clinic was ready to move on to a new stage.

CHAPTER 7

Director of the Clinic

MANAGING THE CLINIC

The incorporation of the Winnipeg Clinic in 1949 following its eleven-year life under what was essentially the sole control of Dr. Thorlakson opened a new era for this large specialty group practice. It was clearly established by the Act of Incorporation and the by-laws that henceforth the control of the Clinic resided in its duly qualified members, acting through its elected council and its executive officers. Each member had one vote, including the founder of the Clinic.

At the first meeting of the Council of the Winnipeg Clinic (Incorporated) on January 6, 1950, Dr. Thorlakson was appointed director. The by-laws provided that he was the chief executive officer of the Clinic; would preside at all meetings of the members and of the Council; and had authority to see that all orders and resolutions of the Council were carried out. He was authorized to make provisional appointments to the Council in case of temporary vacancies. He appointed the staff. Indeed, the by-laws provided that the director "would perform all the duties pertaining to his office [as though that office] was that of the president of a corporation."

As a result of these responsibilities, Dr. Thorlakson found himself with more demands on his time for Clinic management than there were before reorganization. Added to the conduct of his large surgical practice and other professional and community obligations, he had no relief from the weight of long and strenuous days. Dr. Thorlakson's constitution was such that he thrived on all this but, as time went on, there were some Clinic members who were troubled that the director was not always on the spot to deal with what they felt were urgent management problems.

An important event in the life of the Winnipeg Clinic occurred on August 1, 1949, when Dr. Lennox G. Bell, who was one of the original members of the group and Head of the Section of Medicine, left to take up his appointment as the first full-time Dean of the Faculty of Medicine.

At the end of the first year of operation under the new management structure, the director had bad news to report. The annual meeting of members was held on December 7, 1950. Like a surgeon describing an unpleasant reality to a patient, Dr. Thorlakson identified the condition, its cause (the great flood, which virtually closed the Clinic for three months), the immediate treatment, and measures he thought should be taken to prevent a recurrence. "After paying all professional salaries including those of the partners, and the operating expenses for the year," his report began, "there will be a deficit of approximately $80,000."

He explained that the partnership (Drs. Thorlakson, Stewart and Morse) was required to operate on a cash basis for income-tax purposes. Under the revised organization all doctors other than the partners received a salary as employees of the partnership. But the partners themselves could only be paid if there were funds available after payment of operating costs. Since there was a loss on operations in 1950 the monthly drawings of the three partners were considered to have come from a bank overdraft, and were not earned income as defined by Revenue Canada.

"This problem will have to be resolved," the report continued, "after study by the business manager and our solicitor, through liquidation of the deficit and a system of deferred payments to the partners."

Dr. Thorlakson suggested adopting a number of economies. He recommended that in future there should be quarterly business meetings of the members for the purpose of reviewing comparative statements of income and expenses. He proposed that until the financial emergency was over the members should unanimously agree that the maximum annual salary for senior surgeons should be $15,000 and for senior internists it should be $10,000.

He reminded his listeners that for every $100 placed on the books through charges for professional services, only eighty-two percent was collected.[1] From this net revenue, all the overhead costs of the clinic had first to be paid. After this had been done the sum remaining was available for payments to members.

Dr. Thorlakson concluded his discourse on the financial principles that ought to be observed with a formula for determining the amount of monthly drawings by members. "For every $100 of his basic monthly salary," he said, "an internist will provide a minimum of $160 in gross charges for professional services. Of this, on average, eighty-two percent (i.e., $131.20) is collected. Similarly, for every $100 of the basic monthly salary paid to a surgeon, he will provide a minimum of $225 in gross charges for professional services. Of this, eighty-two percent (i.e., $184) will be collected. . . . It is desirable that we have some latitude in our final adjustments, making due allowance for intangible factors. But remember that elasticity must be predicated on a surplus; not a deficit, or simply breaking even."

The clinic continued to increase the number of its members, and even by 1949 the five-storey addition had become inadequate for the growing needs for space. In 1952, a small "temporary" structure was added to the northeast corner of the main floor of the original building. This provided extra rooms for the Section of Pediatrics, and the Section of Obstetrics and Gynecology.

In 1956, a large house on two lots at the corner of Kennedy Street and St. Mary Avenue was purchased from Dr. G.W. McIntosh by the Winnipeg Clinic Holding Company Limited. The cost of $66,000 was met by a loan from the Winnipeg Clinic Pharmacy.

This house was subsequently called the Winnipeg Clinic Annex. Into it were moved the Section of Allergy, the library, the electrocardiography service, and a number of administrative offices. This released fifteen units in the main building to ease the pressure during the period of the next addition, built in 1959 and 1960.

NEW MEMBERS

Doctors who expressed an interest in joining the Winnipeg Clinic, or who were recommended by others, were always interviewed by Dr. Thorlakson himself (often accompanied by Mrs. Thorlakson) before a decision was made to issue a formal invitation to them to become associated with the group. He believed in taking immediate and direct action if a well-qualified and well-recommended candidate was available.

For example, when Dr. John M. Kilgour and his wife returned from overseas at the end of World War II, Dr. and Mrs. Thorlakson journeyed to Montreal and invited the Kilgours to meet them at their hotel. At the conclusion of a lengthy discussion about the clinic and the opportunities it offered, it was agreed that Dr. Kilgour would join the group in the Section of Internal Medicine. He remained as a valued member for the rest of his professional career.

In 1953 Dr. Thorlakson spent three weeks at the Dorchester Hotel in London, during which he interviewed twenty-seven specialists, of whom he selected four for the Winnipeg Clinic. These recruitment experiences were sometimes unconventional, but always exhilarating. Dr. Arthur S. Majury was one of the candidates on this occasion. Many years later, he described his experience.

In 1953 I was a registrar in a Belfast hospital. I had decided that there were few prospects of a consultant appointment in Britain. An advertisement had appeared in the *British Medical Journal* for a gynecologist at the Winnipeg Clinic. I responded, and soon had a letter from Tom Lebbetter[2] who then held an administrative position at the Clinic. He said that Dr. Thorlakson would be in London in March 1953, and if I could go to London at that time he would interview me for the post.

After arranging for coverage of my duties at the hospital, on the appointed weekend I crossed from Belfast by boat and boat train, arriving in London early on Saturday afternoon. I had arranged to stay with friends, and after settling in, I telephoned Dr. Thorlakson at the Dorchester, as instructed. He suggested that I come to the hotel at six o'clock, which seemed an unusual hour for our interview; but, allowing myself plenty of time, and telling my friends that I expected to be back for dinner by eight, I left for the Dorchester.

Dr. Thorlakson met me in the lobby and after the usual greeting he informed me that he had been unwell that day. He had planned to go to an evening concert in Albert Hall, but had given the tickets to his daughter-in-law and her friends. I learned later that he was referring to Lorna, the wife of Dr. T.K. Thorlakson.

We went to his room, and for the next five hours, with relatively brief interruptions when I was asked to express my thoughts, Dr. Thorlakson gave a full account of medical affairs in Winnipeg; life in that city; the services of the Winnipeg Clinic; his wishes and desires for what the Clinic should be; and information about the Winnipeg hospitals and the Faculty of Medicine. Certainly anyone accepting a position at the Winnipeg Clinic could not say that they did not know all about the situation before agreeing to go to Canada.

Suddenly the phone rang. To my surprise, it was about eleven o'clock, and Lorna and her party were back from the concert. Thor immediately ordered coffee and cakes and invited them up to his room. His disinterest in food due to his gastric upset and his absorption in our discussion had caused him to forget dinner completely. I welcomed a little food, but thought ruefully of the dinner my friends had prepared for eight o'clock. I got back to their house about one o'clock in the morning.

Working with me in Belfast was Dr. Mervin Roulston, who had also answered the advertisement and had got a similar letter asking him to come to London. We were not able to be away from the hospital at the same time, so he covered for me while I was in London and I covered for him the next weekend. His experience was very similar to mine except that he was invited for breakfast at the Dorchester at seven o'clock. Mervin hadn't been used to interviews at breakfast time, but of course he went, and had several hours with Dr. Thorlakson.

Following the interview, Thor wrote to both of us, explaining that there were going to be two positions for gynecologists at the Winnipeg Clinic, one now and one a year later. I was offered, and accepted, the first position and arrived in Winnipeg in June 1953. Mervin Roulston was offered the second position and came a year later, in June 1954.

I have never regretted the move. All the twenty-six years I spent at the Winnipeg Clinic were happy ones. I enjoyed working with Thor. I found him easy to get along with, but at the same time he was a strict director, as one would expect.

Until Dr. Majury and Dr. Roulston arrived, the Section of Obstetrics and Gynecology consisted of Dr. Brian Best (Head) and Dr. A.W. Andison.

The other two doctors selected during these interviews at the Dorchester Hotel were an ophthalmologist, Dr. Howard N.

Reed, who opened a new section in this specialty at the Winnipeg Clinic; and an ear, nose and throat specialist, Dr. Lloyd Davis. Unfortunately, after a few months in Winnipeg the wife of Dr. Davis became so homesick that eventually they returned to England.

Dr. Arthur Anhalt, a dermatologist, and Dr. Oliver S. Waugh, a neurosurgeon, joined the Clinic during this period. In January 1958, Dr. Rankin Hay became the second member of the Section of Neurosurgery.

ANOTHER EXPANSION

In 1956, continuing growth in Clinic services compelled consideration of an enlarged Winnipeg Clinic building. A Building Committee was established by the Clinic doctors to consult with the director about a suitable plan. At a meeting of the Board of Directors of the Institute on May 15, 1956, Dr. Thorlakson informed them of these developments.

Dr. Thorlakson had arranged for Ellerbe and Company, Architects, based in St. Paul, Minnesota, to study the site and make a sketch plan of the structure they would recommend. This turned out to be a five-storey eastward extension of the existing building, facing on St. Mary Avenue and continuing through to Kennedy Street.

The plan would require diversion of the lane which runs from Graham Avenue to St. Mary Avenue, at a point near the northeast corner of what was then the Winnipeg Clinic powerhouse, so that it would make a ninety-degree turn and exit on Kennedy Street. Informal enquiries indicated that this could be done at little cost by exchanging a twenty-foot strip along the north side of the Winnipeg Clinic Holding Company's Kennedy Street property for an equivalent stretch of the south end of the land which separated the Vaughan Street and the Kennedy Street holdings.

It was contemplated that construction of the new building would begin about two years later. This would allow ample time to plan and to consider alternatives. By that time, Dr. Thorlakson expected that the debt would be paid in full to the group who had made interest-free loans to help finance the 1947 addition.

Further study indicated that the proposed extension to the

east would probably be more expensive and less effective in the long run than an upward extension of the 1947 building would be. This would avoid the necessity of diverting the lane. Foundations had been designed in the 1947 structure to carry ten or twelve storeys and the plan of adding seven floors to the 1947 building was finally adopted.

The Winnipeg Clinic Research Institute, as owner of the property, had responsibility for the financing and construction of the enlarged accommodation. The Institute Board appointed the Buildings, Properties and Investments Committee, with Mr. C. Gordon Smith as Chairman, to act for the Board in these matters.[3]

At a special meeting of the members of the Winnipeg Clinic Research Institute on June 23, 1959, the addition of six floors and a penthouse (the latter to house the heating and air conditioning equipment) on top of the five-storey 1947 structure was approved, as recommended by the Smith Committee and the directors. At the same time, the Board of Directors of the Institute was authorized to negotiate a loan of $850,000 with interest at six and a half percent from the Great-West Life Assurance Company, secured by a twenty-five-year first mortgage on the property. This loan was expected to cover the cost of the new construction and liquidate the remaining balance of about $89,000 payable to Great-West Life on the borrowing for the 1947 building. The interest-free loans for the 1947 construction, secured by second mortgage, had already been repaid in full, and the second mortgage had been discharged.

At the same meeting, the terms of a new lease of the entire building to the Winnipeg Clinic (Incorporated) were approved. This lease would run for a period of twenty-five years, at a monthly rental that would cover all mortgage payments, real property taxes and insurance.

As construction proceeded, it was found that the original estimates of cost would be exceeded by about $150,000. This additional sum was borrowed from the Great-West Life Assurance Company under mortgage for a term of twenty years, with interest at seven percent.[4] A corresponding adjustment was made in the rent payable to the Institute by the Winnipeg Clinic (Incorporated), in order to cover all capital costs.

The book value of the property owned by the Winnipeg Clinic

Research Institute on completion of the building would therefore be: for the first stage, $107,550; for the second stage, $600,000; and for the third stage, $1,000,000; for a total book value a little in excess of $1,700,000. (These figures are approximate.) This is a measure of the far-sighted plan Dr. Thorlakson had in mind for providing a capital fund for the support of medical education and research when the Institute was founded in 1943.

The new construction was effectually completed by midsummer 1962. All that remained was the renovation of the first five floors, and this work was finished by the year-end. With the exception of the tenth floor, which was deliberately held open to accommodate a further increase in the clinic membership, all of the new space was occupied.

LOOKING TO THE FUTURE

By 1964, universal hospital insurance had been in effect in Canada for six years. Studies that were under way would lead to establishment of a similar plan to cover medical care. These programs brought with them uncertainties and anxieties with respect to the future organization of medical practice. University facilities for medical teaching and research in Canada were substantially expanded. This was associated with the concept that faculties of medicine should consist predominantly of full-time teachers who were also practitioners and researchers. This new outlook brought a change in the relationship between the university and physicians in private practice. At the same time the influx of relatively new members at the Clinic introduced new perceptions of the way in which it should operate.

Taking all things into account, after twenty-six years of executive responsibility for the Clinic's affairs, at the age of sixty-nine years, Dr. Thorlakson concluded that the time had come to turn over active direction of the Winnipeg Clinic to younger members. This would give them greater authority to test their ideas about policy, and to experience the exercise of responsibility and the obligation for accountability which are inherent in the mandate of the chief executive officer. In 1964, therefore, Dr. Thorlakson resigned from his position as director of the Winnipeg Clinic.

Dr. Thorlakson presented his last report as director to the annual meeting of the members of the Clinic on March 16, 1964. It is typical that the report looked more to the future than back on the past, and that it expressed some of the principles which he believed ought to permeate the practice of medicine.

Dr. Thorlakson was never overwhelmed by the size or extent of the enterprises he had shaped, nor did he ever lose sight of his original objective: to provide the means whereby patients could receive medical care of a uniformly high standard. To this end, he believed that scientific knowledge and technical skill ought to be leavened by professional integrity and dedication to the patient's needs, and the whole infused with compassion. Countless reports from his patients attest that this conviction characterized his own practice, despite the distractions of other interests and activities. It was his hope that the doctrine would always be a hallmark of patient care at the Winnipeg Clinic.

Some of this philosophy is revealed in Dr. Thorlakson's last official annual report to the members of the Winnipeg Clinic in his capacity of director, on March 16, 1964. He entitled it, "The Value of Membership in the Winnipeg Clinic."

In my previous annual reports I have dealt with such subjects as construction, renovation plans, professional organization, administration and finance. This evening I shall attempt to answer an important question which was asked at a recent administrative board meeting: What is the *real* value, the *true* value, of membership in the Winnipeg Clinic?

I shall also speak to you about two closely related subjects which should be clearly defined and understood by every member, namely, the responsibility of membership in the Winnipeg Clinic, and its corollary, our priority of loyalties. I know of no other topics that have greater significance at this particular time. Many of our acts and decisions, as well as our general attitude towards the Clinic and its patients, are determined by our individual sense of responsibility as members of this medical group and by our priority of loyalties.

In developing these topics for presentation, I chose three examples taken from the records of 1963. They illustrate very clearly how three members accepted personal responsibility for the welfare and success of their clinic.

The first example is "the relationship of doctor and patient." Mrs. F. had been a patient of the Clinic for twenty-one years. Her terminal illness began in the spring of 1963. Investigation revealed that she had a

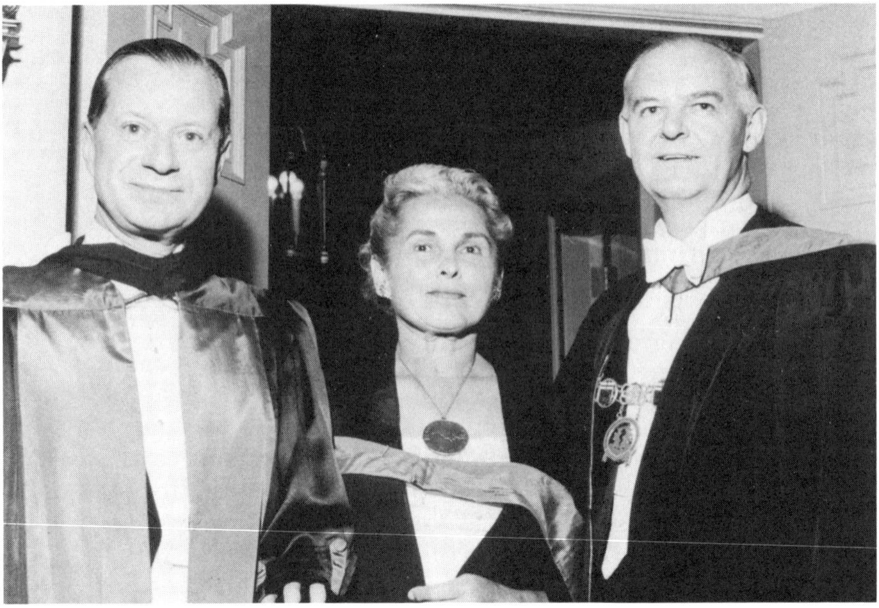

In attendance at the annual meeting of the Canadian Medical Association in Winnipeg, June 18 to 22, 1962, were: Dr. Lennox Bell, Dean of the Faculty of Medicine, University of Manitoba; Dr. Emma Adamson, President of the Federation of Medical Women in Canada; and Dr. Kenneth R. Trueman, President of the Manitoba Division of the Canadian Medical Association. All three had an association with the Winnipeg Clinic: Dr. Bell and Dr. Trueman had become members of the Clinic in 1942, and Dr. Adamson's husband was a member for some years. Dr. Bell resigned as Head of the Division of Medicine in the Clinic to accept an appointment as Dean of the Faculty of Medicine. Dr. Trueman was a distinguished member of the Clinic's Department of Surgery until his untimely death in 1977.

malignant lesion of one of the pelvic bones. She was given deep x-ray therapy to no avail. Her pain gradually became intense and, at this time, another Clinic surgeon was asked to see her. From then on, he assumed complete charge of her case. He performed a left-sided chordotomy which provided immediate relief of pain although, after a period of time, some of her discomfort returned. She died in December 1963.

On her way home to California, the patient's daughter wrote a letter of appreciation to this surgeon who had taken care of her mother during the final illness. The following is a paragraph from the letter:

". . . Most of all, let me tell you Doctor, how grateful we felt that your care of Mother was at all times the finest that we could have asked for her. There was no doubt what her future held, but our hope was that her last days would be as comfortable and as meaningful as possible. The fact that her mind remained clear and alert to the very end was a comfort to all of us near and dear to her. But most of all we are grateful that your attention was personal, sensitive and showed real warmth and care for the total needs of so sick a woman. . . . "

As the members of this family had been patients of mine for many years, her record and the letter were sent to me with the attached comment by the surgeon:

". . . There is no doubt that repeated house calls take up a lot of time, but as you see from this letter they are greatly appreciated, as a rule, by the patient. I think they are also very valuable for the doctor. I learned a great deal about this patient and her family as a result of seeing her at home. Such visits certainly help one to maintain and develop personal relationships with the patient and the family and I think more stress might well be put on such visits."

Last spring I spent a day at the Montefiore Hospital Clinic in New York City. This metropolitan group has a home care roster, on which senior specialists are glad to be included. They are beginning to realize that specialists, physicians and surgeons alike, have a social as well as a medical responsibility to their patients. Home care has an important place in the total care of the sick and it must soon be given its proper status in the minds of all the members of the medical profession.

The second example is "a proposal by a colleague who wanted to improve his own and his section's professional and administrative efficiency." He assured us that increased personal income was not his reason for trying to improve the working arrangements within his section. He suggested a plan which provided better utilization of staff and space. He was convinced that by these means his services to his patients would improve and his contribution to the Clinic increase. Good results can be achieved by individual members who try to improve their efficiency after consultation with members of their own sections and with members of the Clinic administration.

The third example is "a memorandum from a colleague requesting facts and figures to prove that the administration is both efficient and economical." This member asked for information regarding the growth of the medical and ancillary staff of the Clinic during the past few years. He also wanted to know the administration's plans for future development, a matter which I shall deal with later in this report. We welcomed this colleague's interest and enquiries and obtained the statistical information and presented it to the administrative board of which he is a member. No one would submit such a series of penetrating questions unless he had given the subject a great deal of thought, and unless he wished to use this information to improve the performance of his own section and to relate that performance to our total effort.

By quoting the three examples in some detail (and I could tell you of many other helpful suggestions by members, if time permitted), I wish to make the point that no one should underestimate the influence which each individual member can exert on the practice of medicine in his own section, and on the administrative efficiency of the entire Clinic.

In a group of sixty or more doctors there will naturally be differences of opinion and method. This is good, provided there is a basic unity of purpose and that all members adhere to the same principles of conduct and observe the usual courtesies. A member's sense of responsibility is often manifested by repeated acts of simple courtesy and by his willingness to help his colleagues and staff find solutions for their problems, be they patient care, handling of records, or articles for the *Winnipeg Clinic Quarterly.*

We all recognize that the welfare of our patients is our first consideration and first professional responsibility. Next should come loyalty to the Winnipeg Clinic. After all, each one of us chose to practice our specialty in this group.

We have also accepted a responsibility to the Medical Faculty of the University of Manitoba and to the teaching at other hospitals in which we practise. As a group, we sacrifice much valuable time and effort on the altar of medical education. In many cases the expenditure of time and effort on free medical and surgical care is substantial. All this extra work saps our strength and makes us less available to patients and to our colleagues. It lessens our capacity to earn for our families and further reduces the time we can spend with them.

I realize, however, that these separate loyalties to the Faculty of Medicine of the University, to the hospitals, and to the Winnipeg Clinic can create a problem for some individuals. Perhaps some members do not know exactly where they stand in their priority of loyalties.

Don't misunderstand me. I am not underestimating the importance and value of these other activities. My personal record proves that I believe doctors have a responsibility beyond their own practice, but let us strike a reasonable balance. Too often the Clinic is blamed for situations that develop because of non-clinic duties and responsibilities.

I know that the University and hospital boards are trying to initiate a more positive and realistic arrangement with heads of clinical departments and with the private physicians and surgeons who make up the large number of unpaid teachers of the Medical Faculty of the University and the honorary attending staff of the teaching hospitals. This is a complex and difficult problem. The government, the University and the teaching hospitals should not expect highly qualified doctors to continue to teach and give their services, even on a part-time basis, without a fair share of official recognition. The boards and these public institutions surely recognize the value of the contribution made by the Winnipeg Clinic, and other similar groups, to these essential educational and medical services.

In this connection I am constrained to say that I am aware of statements made by some senior University appointees which would suggest that there is, in some quarters at least, a deliberate attempt to bypass clinicians who are members of private groups. To deal with members of a clinic as individuals when this is convenient but treat the individual as a member of a group when this attitude would serve a particular purpose is the best way that I know of to disrupt and destroy the unity and strength on which all Clinic group effort is based.

If the situation is not soon clarified it can create disillusionment with the Medical Faculty of the University. A better climate of mutual understanding is urgently needed. Important decisions have already been delayed too long to the great detriment of our medical school. Surely one's professional fitness for a teaching position should never be assessed on whether or not he is engaged in group practice.

I should, at this juncture, remind all the members that the basis on which the Winnipeg Clinic was originally founded over twenty-five years ago was that a high quality of medical care should be provided by physicians and surgeons who also had a keen interest in undergraduate and graduate education. From the beginning, the support for medical research was also emphasized.

The Winnipeg Clinic has now come of age as an important medical institution, not only in our city and province, but also in Canada. Our relationship with other groups and institutions must be realistic and mutually advantageous. Let us continue to give liberally of our talents and our resources to strengthen and improve community effort in the University and teaching hospitals, but let us be on guard against decisions and arrangements that are unfair to the individual doctor and to the Winnipeg Clinic. Self-interest is necessary and can be good and constructive if kept within proper bounds. This type of enlightened self-interest and loyalty to the Clinic can actually form the solid base on which effective community effort can be supported and developed.

Frequently, after all other demands on our time are attended to, we are asked to see yet another patient on top of a long list of appointments. This, of course, adds to the stress and strain of our practice but we must realize that, for a few clinicians, the work week at the Clinic itself consists of only four, and on occasion only three half days a week. In every other successful private clinic in North America, every member who is not fully occupied with seeing clinic patients in hospital spends the balance of his day seeing patients at the clinic itself. . . . It is often the non-clinic work that takes many hours of time and causes delay for a few doctors in keeping their appointments and carrying their patient load over a normal number of working hours in the Clinic.

In this connection there is yet another factor which must be recognized. When a doctor earns professional income away from his clinic seeing non-clinic patients for a public institution, it always results in inefficient utilization of the space, staff, laboratory and x-ray facilities and consulting services provided in the clinic building. This type of institutional income adversely affects the ratio between net earnings and overhead for himself and for his clinic colleagues. Unfortunately the overhead remains constant for any given period, even though the trend is generally upwards.

There are many of you who accept pressures of work with equanimity and a smile, and you are most fortunate. Somehow you fit into this "push and pull" existence without blaming other people for your troubles or for your difficulties in coping with every situation. You just do your job the best way you can, and God bless you – you are a joy to this clinic and to this community! But all of us are not so constituted. Some of us, a small minority it is true, are seldom satisfied, either with what we, ourselves, are doing or what others are doing. We do not have that serene, objective discontent that begets progress; rather we blame others for our difficulties, not realizing or being willing to admit that we, ourselves, are really the authors of most of our personal feelings of frustration and discontent. Each one of us, without exception, feels this way at some time or another, but not all of us can hold our emotions and feelings under complete control at all times, and many of our personal harassments are caused by our failure to ask ourselves one vital question: In my priority of loyalties, where do my patients and the Clinic come?

I believe that we can, with considerable justification, be proud to belong to this family of physicians and surgeons and can have confidence in the integrity and professional ability of our colleagues; I believe that fairness and good business judgement have been, and are being, shown in the conduct of our corporate affairs. But let no member of the Winnipeg Clinic think for a moment that we have reached our peak of accomplishment in the fields of group practice, medical education, medical research, or administrative proficiency. As I see it, we are now only on the threshold of our potential growth. The challenge is even greater now than it was twenty-five years ago. The opportunities before us have multiplied and expanded.

The members of this organization have a satisfactory level of income, though not as high as some others in private practice. Our members have long-term financial security. We enjoy an unusual degree of freedom of action within our clinic organization. The record shows that no member of this Winnipeg Clinic has purchased any stock or paid any money to become eligible for membership. No one has obligated himself in any way financially to his senior partners who invited him to join and offered him full participating membership. The newest member has the same voting power as the original founders. The Winnipeg Clinic was probably the first professional group to provide group insurance for sickness, total disability and death and every member will benefit from our group pension and retirement program. These plans were initiated by the Winnipeg Clinic long before the federal government or the Manitoba Medical Service had formulated their plans for independent professional people. Each member owns his or her share in the Pension and Retirement Fund and nobody can take it away. Besides all these assets, we have, as advisors, a group of citizens who are among the financial leaders in Canada, and despite the many demands made upon them, they give unsparingly of their time and ability in the cause of medical education and research. They are the directors and officers of the Winnipeg Clinic Research Institute. In all these respects we are practically unique among private medical clinics in Canada. In no large group on this continent has there been more complete and equitable control of assets without a personal financial commitment to the group or to senior partners; or without some contract or other restriction on freedom of action.

Medical education and research were considered to be vitally important by the founders of the Winnipeg Clinic. They still are important to us. It is a fact, however, that we have been able to give assistance in these fields only because many Clinic members have carried a heavy patient load in the Clinic and in the hospitals. Every dollar the Clinic spends for anyone, or on anything, has to be earned by one of the doctors in the course of his professional work. There is no magic available to us in the field of finance. Personal, individual responsibility for production and economy are as essential in group medical practice as in any other type of free enterprise. In the priority of our loyalties, our patients and our clinic *must* come first because the Clinic is our professional home and our source of livelihood; without this provision, none of us could carry on part-time teaching or research. . . .

What Are the Administration's Plans for the Future?
I predict that within five years we will have a complete, self-contained Department of Nuclear Medicine. We will have a greatly expanded Department of Laboratory Medicine supervised by a full-time director. There will be three or four additional sections of internal medicine with more specialization by sections. At this juncture let me be more specific. I believe that serious consideration should be given to establishing sections of gastroenterology, cardio-vascular disease and for diseases of the respiratory tract. If we claim to be medical specialists, let us be specialists by section rather than as isolated individuals. As it is, we now have an excellent section limited to allergy diseases, another to psychiatry, another to dermatology. Some of the reasons for specialization by section in the Division of Surgery apply now to the Division of Medicine. New research resulting in greater understanding and new techniques always demands more specialized facilities and the use of new equipment to apply this new knowledge. There will always be a need for internists with broad interest and capabilities . . . but it has always been true that as a doctor becomes older and busier, both he and his patients – but particularly his patients, his colleagues, and referring doctors – contrive to restrict his work to the field in which he has special experience and a particular interest. This is the way excellent reputations have been established and real progress made in the practice of medicine. . . .

As you know, I have submitted my resignation as director, or chief executive officer of the Winnipeg Clinic, to the Executive Council and the Administrative Board, to be effective as soon as my successor is appointed. I am *not* resigning as an active member or surgeon of the Winnipeg Clinic. I can assure you that I do not come to decisions of this kind on the spur of the moment. I would have offered my resignation five years ago except for the fact that I was then responsible for the building program, which included finance and re-organization. My present decision is based on a conviction which I have always held, namely, that the hope for the future of this clinic depends on the calibre, motivation and training of the youngest third of our membership and that sound progressive clinic practice and administration should rest with those in the intermediate age group. The senior members should constantly prepare for the time when they will be available for consultation but will no longer guide the destinies of this medical organization.

In this connection, I am reminded of a recent discussion by the well-known personality and economist Professor C.N. Parkinson of England. His theme was, "How to Get Rid of the Chief Executive." He described his own plan to induce "an inclination to retirement." His plan consisted of arranging almost continuous air travel for the chief executive officer to attend meetings booked, one or two days apart, in widely separated cities such as London, New Delhi, Tel Aviv, Buenos Aires, Tokyo, etc. In this way the chief executive officer would be kept in almost constant motion. This being very tiring, he would soon decide that he was not physically up to it. Dr. Parkinson's second suggestion was to make the chief executive officer responsible for completing numerous forms every day, on all phases of his travels, including detailed accounts of his expenses. This would contribute to a rapid aging process and would soon induce "an inclination to retirement." Such a method of disposing of an executive director may be successful but, with my present state of good health, it would be time-consuming and too expensive for the Clinic. I hope it will not be necessary for you to resort to such extreme measures!

One final word – membership in the Winnipeg Clinic carries with it responsibilities as well as privileges, opportunities and values which surely can be appreciated by every member. The responsibility of membership is never to be taken lightly; it is the badge of approval that we give to every new member, entitling him to play his part in the development of an organization which represents the life work of many of us here tonight.

Let us always remember the objectives laid down for the Winnipeg Clinic and the Winnipeg Clinic Research Institute some twenty-five years ago. Surely we can look back over the years, with much satisfaction, to what we, as a group, have created together.

The future of the Winnipeg Clinic and all that it signifies has been, is now, and will always be, the personal responsibility of each member.

When Dr. Thorlakson noted in his report that he was not resigning as an active member of the Winnipeg Clinic, this was no idle statement. He continued to take a vigorous part in the management of the Clinic, and in all its affairs. Indeed, he continued for some time as the de facto director.

In the public mind, the integration of identity between the Winnipeg Clinic and Dr. Thorlakson will be an enduring mem-

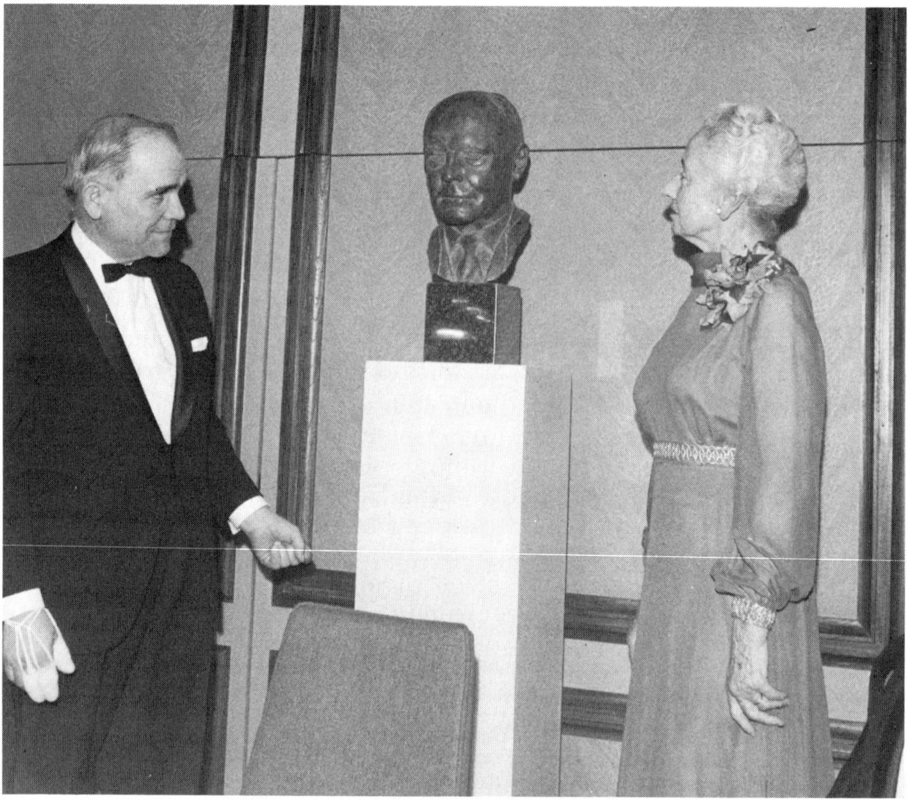

During the ceremonies related to the unveiling of the bronze bust of Dr. Thorlakson, created by the distinguished sculptor Leo Mol, the artist presented a personal gift to Mrs. Thorlakson: a sculptured head of her husband. The sculptor is seen here making his presentation.

ory. Nevertheless, the nature of that relationship changed in 1964, and the formal association was gradually terminated.

Consequently, this seems to be a fitting point at which to end our account of the Winnipeg Clinic and the crucial role it played in the life of its founder and elder statesman.

But just one last story: On December 15, 1970, at the close of Manitoba's Centennial Year, the members of the Winnipeg Clinic held a dinner to honour Thor and Gladys. Many distinguished guests were present to pay their respects.

In the course of the evening, Chairman Dr. C.H.A. Walton announced on behalf of the Clinic members and staff that a bronze bust of Dr. Thorlakson had been completed by the internationally famous Winnipeg artist, Leo Mol.[5] He invited Miss Elizabeth Clint, Chief Laboratory Technician at the Clinic since its opening, to unveil the statue.

Before calling on Dr. Thorlakson for his remarks, Dr. Walton announced that in tribute to Gladys, Mr. Mol had a surprise for her; whereupon the artist presented her with a replica of the head on the statue.

In the course of a graceful and gracious acceptance of this gift, Mrs. Thorlakson revealed the wifely insight and sense of humour that had been one of her strengths through the years. After paying tribute to the artist and his wife she said:

> Now, as Dr. Walton has told you, this bronze bust of Thor will find its permanent home in the Winnipeg Clinic. It will be transported from here to the Clinic, and then I imagine it will be put on a pedestal, or a table or something, in a very advantageous spot on the main floor of the Clinic, and there Thor will sit – doing nothing – encased in bronze.
>
> I think for the first few days, until he gets his second wind, he will probably look out of the window and see the congestion of traffic on St. Mary Avenue during the busy hours. He will see the doctors of the Winnipeg Clinic, the nurses and the staff going in and out. He will see the old patients coming in, and through the years many of them have become personal friends; and he will see the new people coming in who probably have never been in the Clinic before. And when all that is finished, I don't know quite what he will do – except sit. If, some day, the people in the Clinic hear a terrible crash and bang and fear the place has been bombed, think nothing of it. The bronze bust has simply got down off his perch and decided to organize something!

More than fifteen years passed. The Research Institute and the Clinic continued to be close to his heart and much in his mind, even though the responsibility for their affairs had fallen to others. So it was a happy occasion when, in his ninety-first year, he was able to be present at the meeting of the Board of Directors of the Winnipeg Clinic Research Institute on May 12, 1986.

On this occasion Mr. D.A. Thompson, Q.C., from the beginning legal counsel and member of the Board of the Winnipeg Clinic Research Institute, announced that the two mortgages on the Clinic property had been paid in full. He then produced the mortgages. Mr. Albert Cohen, a long-time director of the Institute and a sponsor of the Paul H.T. Thorlakson Research Foundation, commended the wisdom and foresight exercised by Dr. Thorlakson in planning the capital financing of the Clinic building, and in creating the Research Institute.

Mr. Cohen then called on Dr. Thorlakson to join him in the ceremonial burning of the mortgages. It must have been a moment of deep emotion for the founder, combined with a justifiable pride and satisfaction that the purpose to which he had devoted so much thought, energy and hard work had been fulfilled. It was a celebration of the completion of one cycle in the life of these institutions which Dr. Thorlakson had envisioned when he created them nearly half a century before; and it marked the beginning of a new era in the work of the Winnipeg Clinic Research Institute.

PART THREE

The Role of Research

CHAPTER 8

Federal Funding for Medical Research Begins

ASSOCIATE COMMITTEE ON MEDICAL RESEARCH

Dr. Thorlakson was in a position to view the field of medical research from an unusual vantage point through his appointment, in the spring of 1938, as a member of the first Associate Committee on Medical Research.[1] This committee had been appointed by the National Research Council not only to deal with grant applications in the field of medicine, but to consider how and to what extent medical research could be developed in Canada.[2] The Committee had an initial allocation of $53,000 for the support of research projects – hardly a munificent sum. Nevertheless, it was the seed from which, in 1960, the Medical Research Council of Canada evolved; and in 1982 the MRCC was allocated more than $113,000,000 by the Government of Canada for the support of medical research. By the fiscal year 1985–86, the amount was $157,700,000.

The establishment of this committee, with the famed Sir Frederick Banting as its chairman, was an historic event in the development of medical research in this country.[3]

Up to this time, almost all medical research of a substantial nature had been centred at universities in central Canada, notably the University of Toronto and McGill University. In Winnipeg, the Faculty of Medicine included a small group of trained researchers. They carried a heavy teaching load, which limited the time they could devote to research; and they were restricted

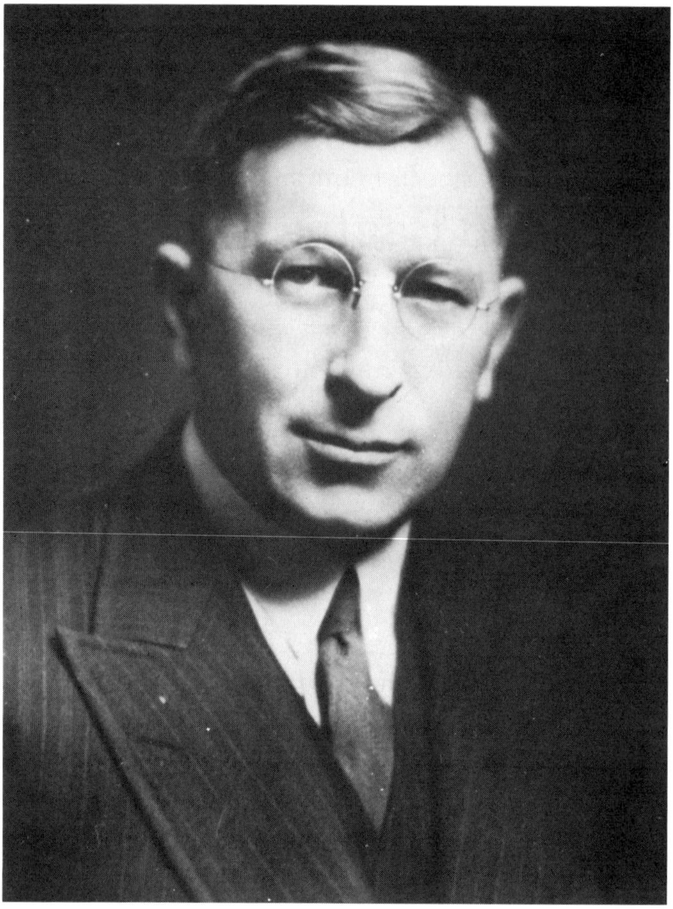

Sir Frederick Banting (1891–1941)

in what they could do by a lack of funds for the salaries of technical assistants and the purchase of special equipment.

Since he had little personal knowledge of the medical schools in western Canada and the research activities and facilities associated with them, Dr. Banting decided that he, personally, ought to visit the university centres in the West as part of a general survey of medical research facilities in Canada in order to prepare himself for his responsibilities as chairman of the newly formed committee. He spoke of this to Dr. Thorlakson, who warmly welcomed the idea. It was clear that a visit by this renowned recipient of the Nobel Prize for the discovery of insulin would be an inspiring and exciting event for faculty and students alike. The decision being taken, Dr. Banting invited Dr. Thorlakson to join him in the western survey. The invitation was gladly accepted and as the western member of the Associate Committee, Dr. Thorlakson shared the responsibility for coordination of the planning and scheduling of the journey, particularly in Manitoba.

The combination of warm informality, together with serious enquiry and discussion that were to mark this visit was intimated in a letter sent by Dr. Thorlakson to Sir Frederick on November 12, 1938:

Dear Sir Frederick:

Our information is that you arrive here the morning of the 28th and leave on the morning of the 30th. Needless to say we are looking forward to your visit with us with a great deal of anticipation.

At a recent meeting of the Faculty Council executive, at which President Smith of the University was present, I took the liberty of stating that you would like to feel that you could devote as much time as possible to your special investigation, and in view of the short time at your disposal that you would like the reception here to be as informal as possible. You have already consented to speak to the entire student body [in the Medical School]. At the Executive meeting today it was suggested that an informal luncheon be tendered you by the medical men, at which you may say as little or as much as you please. This, of course, is subject to your acceptance. Dr. Mathers[4] will be communicating with you directly in regard to these two items.

Dr. Gilmour, professor of medicine, has already invited you to a private dinner, which, I believe, you have accepted. When speaking to Dr. Gilmour in this regard he mentioned that this would likely be Monday night. This brings us to the last evening – that is, Tuesday evening. Dr. and Mrs. Mathers were over at our home last evening and we took the opportunity of discussing your visit here.

I am inviting you and Dr. Stewart to my home at 8:30 Tuesday evening to an informal fireside chat. There will be a few of our good friends there whom you will have already interviewed during the previous two days: just a handful who can conveniently sit around the fireplace. I propose to supply all with Scotch whisky and soda, and you will be at liberty to discuss anything from medicine to the situation in Europe. Dr. Mathers and I thought this would be more to your liking than another formal dinner. The important thing, of course, is that you do exactly as you would like to do, and if there is any suggestion that you have, feel absolutely free to communicate your wishes to me. I would be very happy to make any plans that you suggest.

Yours sincerely,

P.H.T. Thorlakson, M.D.

The survey began in Winnipeg with the arrival of Dr. Banting and the Assistant Secretary of the Committee, Dr. Chester B. Stewart, at 8:40 a.m. on November 28, 1938. Dr. Thorlakson met them at the railroad station, and after seeing them checked in at their hotel, he took them to the Medical College to meet Dean Mathers.

At the first meeting with Dean Mathers, an hour after their arrival in Winnipeg, Dr. Banting outlined for the benefit of the dean the purpose of the survey of medical research facilities by the Associate Committee. In turn, Dr. Mathers explained the arrangement of the various departments of the school, and discussed the facilities and the needs for medical research. He reported that there were 270 undergraduate students in the Faculty of Medicine, of whom fifty-six were in their final year. "There are practically no positions available in western Canada," he said, "for young graduates interested in research."

Following a half-hour briefing by the dean, Dr. Banting and Dr. Stewart visited Dr. A.T. Cameron, professor of biochemistry and Chairman of the Research Committee of the Faculty. Dr. Stewart noted in his report that "his department has very well-equipped laboratories with facilities for four or five additional research workers. There is at present one assistant in the Department, Dr. Frank D. White."

The visitors had an interesting and stimulating discussion with Dr. Cameron about his current projects and about the action that could be taken to expand the work. In his opinion, the immediate need was to make grants available that would allow the University to keep their best men, which the lack of funding presently restricted. "Dr. Cameron is a first-class research worker and director," noted Dr. Stewart, "and with a little additional equipment could capably manage a research staff of four or five men."

They next visited the Department of Physiology, which was under the direction of Professor V.H.K. Moorhouse. They reviewed the research work being carried on in the Department, mainly by the two full-time assistants, Dr. M.J. Ormerod and Dr. H.V. Rice. They noted that a group of clinicians was also doing research in the Department under the general supervision of Dr. A.C. Abbott, lecturer in clinical surgery.

In the Department of Pathology, headed by Dr. Daniel Nicholson, they noted that "the laboratories in the Medical College are well equipped, but the [General] Hospital department is in crowded and inconvenient quarters situated in an old section of the building." [It is of interest, and probably significant, that in Dr. Stewart's report there is never a mention of the Winnipeg General Hospital. When he is obviously referring to that institution, he invariably calls it the University Hospital!] They gained the impression that Dr. Nicholson and his two full-time assistants, Dr. J.R. Lederman and Dr. Sara Meltzer, were so busy with their regular work and their teaching that they had little time to give to research. Dr. Banting found that Dr. Ton Lung Quong, an intern in the Department who had won the gold medal in medicine in 1938, had a research project under way, and he offered encouragement to this able young man, along with suggestions on how he could deal with some of his investigative problems.

The visit with Dr. I. MacLaren Thompson, professor of anatomy, proved to be particularly stimulating.[5] He and his two assistants, Dr. D.J. Bowie and Dr. L.A. Sigurdson, had a number of research projects under way, which were reviewed in some detail. The Stewart Report comments: "Dr. Thompson is very interested in research and in progressive methods of teaching. He is carrying on some very valuable work in the correlation of anatomical, physiological and clinical facts, and doing much to stimulate interest in research. . . . Several other members of the staff at the Medical School expressed very high opinions of Dr. Thompson as a research worker and teacher."

On the second day, Dr. Banting and Dr. Stewart spent several hours at the Children's Hospital with Dr. Bruce Chown. Their report states that "Dr. Chown is carrying out some very valuable research work. The facilities available are fairly good, but he is hampered by the large amount of routine work and teaching, and lack of a graduate research assistant, for whom adequate facilities, cooperation, and direction would be available."

At St. Boniface Hospital they reviewed research work with Dr. J.D. Adamson and Dr. Digby Wheeler and reported that "there is quite an active and interested group of medical research workers at the St. Boniface Hospital, and the laboratory facilities are fairly good, although small. The lack of animal quarters prevents any animal experimental work."

Some time was spent with Dr. F.T. Cadham at the Provincial Laboratory, who, in his capacity of professor of bacteriology, had a number of research studies in progress. They observed that the laboratory was roomy and well-equipped.

Time was found to visit Dr. J.R. Davidson at his home; Dr. Davidson was a retired practitioner who claimed to have made some discoveries relating to contact with tar as a cause of cancer in mice. The experimental work was carried on in the basement of his home. The impression was that his investigative methods left something to be desired, and the results were unclear.

At the Cancer Institute the surveyors "were very favorably impressed with Dr. Pat McDonald [a physicist, and Director of the Institute] as a keen and active research worker; and with his present research project, as a fundamental investigation." They also reviewed a project being carried out at the Institute by Dr. Frank Allen, professor of physics at the University.

At a luncheon meeting arranged by the Winnipeg Medical Society, on the second day of their visit, Dr. Banting gave an address on the work of the Department of Medical Research at the University of Toronto, and Dr. Stewart spoke on the function and purpose of the Associate Committee on Medical Research of the National Research Council.

Dr. Thorlakson, losing no opportunity to capitalize on Dr.

Banting's presence in the City, arranged a brief interview with the Honourable I.B. Griffiths, the Minister of Health and Public Welfare, and a half-hour discussion with the Deputy Minister, Dr. F.W. Jackson. It was learned that the Department had a two-year morbidity survey under way in two representative rural areas of the Province, to determine the amount and nature of every kind of illness present in the population. A study of maternal and neonatal health was also being carried out. Initial reports indicated that about twenty-five percent of pregnant women in the Province had no medical care during pregnancy; and the neonatal mortality rate in this group appeared to be about seven or eight times as high as that in the rest of the newborn population. The Department was receiving financial support for these surveys from the Rockefeller Foundation and the Federal Department of Pensions and National Health.

Following the narrative account of the Winnipeg survey, Dr. Stewart concisely summarized his observations on medical research in Winnipeg in the following terms:

1. In spite of very considerable financial difficulties, over a period of years, and a heavy burden of routine work, the staffs of the Medical School and the hospitals are carrying out a substantial number of research projects.

2. There is a fine spirit of cooperation among the groups.

3. Facilities for research in the Medical School are fairly good.

4. Outstanding research workers and directors include Dr. Pat McDonald at the Cancer Institute; Dr. Bruce Chown at the Children's Hospital; Dr. A.T. Cameron, Department of Biochemistry; Dr. I.M. Thompson, Department of Anatomy; Dr. J.D. Adamson, St. Boniface Hospital; and Professor Frank Allen, Department of Physics.

There is little doubt that this concentrated two-day focus on medical research by Sir Frederick Banting and his able colleague, Dr. Chester B. Stewart, enhanced the standing of research workers in the eyes of their faculty colleagues, and provided them with much-appreciated encouragement.

It was a remarkably probing review, considering the time constraint under which it was conducted. The personal relationships that were established among the chairman of the Associate Committee, its assistant secretary and the members of the Faculty of Medicine at the University created an understanding and mutual respect that were helpful when grant submissions were being evaluated. They laid the groundwork for such special consideration as the subsequent invitation to Dr. Pat McDonald, who had applied for a grant of $4,000, to come to Toronto at the expense of the National Research Council to discuss the subject of his research with others interested in a related line of enquiry. This would enhance his insight into the intrinsic physical and chemical properties of radiation which were at the core of his studies. Dr. Banting's favourable impression was a factor in the ultimate recognition of Winnipeg as a significant medical research centre.

At 9:45 a.m. on November 30, 1938, Dr. Banting, Dr. Stewart and Dr. Thorlakson left Winnipeg by train for the West. By the time they returned on December 11, they had conducted similar surveys in Saskatoon, Edmonton, Vancouver, Calgary, Regina and Brandon.[6]

This journey of discovery did much more, of course, than identify people and review projects. Through face-to-face discussion, searching questions, specific suggestions, and addresses to doctors and students, Dr. Banting and his colleagues for the first time gave a very positive stimulus to the development of medical research in the western Universities. Researchers with a demonstrated ability to do good work were imbued with the feeling that their efforts would be recognized, and that from the limited funds available, their applications for grants in support of projects would have consideration on the same footing as those from the long-established centres in the East.

A full meeting of the Associate Committee on Medical Research was held in Ottawa on Monday, February 27, 1939. The chairman submitted a verbal report on medical research facilities in Canada, based on his survey of resources. This report indicated that there was a potential for substantially broadening the medical research base in Canada.

Since everyone on the Committee with the exception of Dr. Thorlakson and Dr. Mainland, professor of anatomy at Dalhousie University in Halifax, came from institutions in Ontario and Quebec, with well-established research departments, any suggestion that the limited funding be distributed on a Canada-wide basis was bound to be received with mixed feelings.

Among the majority of committee members there was an opinion that the planning and control of medical research in Canada, as well as the allocation of grants, should be the responsibility of the committee itself. On the other hand, Dr. Banting was of the opinion that centralization to this degree was likely to stifle independent, original and innovative research and favour support for proposals from the larger, most experienced and most influential medical centres.

Despite the chairman's views about centralization, the Committee proceeded to consider the fields of medical research that could then be supported. They concluded that immediate attention should be given to tuberculosis and rheumatic diseases. "In each of these fields," the conference press release said, "projects are to be initiated in a number of institutions throughout the country where particular investigations can be carried out with economy and advantage. The projects in these fields will be correlated by the Medical Research Committee. Attention was directed to the importance of developing research in the various institutions throughout Canada so that in due course, as the Committee extends its work, the required facilities and trained personnel may be available. To this end a number of assisted researches on a wide variety of subjects have been prepared and the various medical institutions concerned are being invited to undertake this work under the auspices of the Committee."

There is a place for directed research under contract, especially in determining clinical applications of new medical knowledge. But basic research is different. It would be hard to conceive of Einstein formulating the Theory of Relativity under a twelve-month contract drawn up by a committee, with renewal dependent on the assessment of his progress report! On the other hand, those who are truly creative – those who reveal new truths – are rare indeed.

Two letters from Sir Frederick to Dr. Thorlakson following the meeting are revealing. On April 13, 1939, Sir Frederick wrote:

My dear Thorlakson:

Your letter of April 3rd has been received.

My reaction to your suggestion of a number of the staff of your Faculty of Medicine coming for a two-day trip to Toronto is that we would be delighted. The work of the laboratory would not be interfered with and we would be very glad if your group would go about leisurely and find out everything that is being done and how it is being done. I can assure you that the other Departments of the University would welcome a visit from your group also.

I think your idea with reference to having each member of the Committee submit his personal views on the matters that have been brought up in the Committee meetings is a good one. I am not at all sure that it would be of much value, however.

The reason why the report of Dr. Stewart and myself was not tabled is because certain members of the Committee did not think it expedient or wise. I think I have already expressed to you my disappointment at the meeting. I consulted with General McNaughton several times during the meeting and he continually advised that the various members be allowed to talk themselves out.

I am glad you saw Dr. Pat McDonald on your return to Winnipeg. There are two people from whom he might get some valuable suggestions and to whom he could explain his theories. These people are Professor E.F. Burton, of the Department of Physics, University of Toronto, and Dr. Laurence, of the National Research Council. I think it would be wise, if Dr. McDonald thought of coming East, to make appointments with these two gentlemen before coming.

I have not yet received your "views on general points" that arose from the meeting, but I look forward to receiving them.

Sincerely yours,

Banting

In due course Dr. Banting did receive Dr. Thorlakson's views about matters discussed at the Committee meeting of February 27, and he replied as follows on April 26:

Dear Dr. Thorlakson:

Please pardon delay in reply to your memorandum concerning the Associate Committee on Medical Research. My reason for not replying was that there was so much to be considered in your letter that I thought it wise to discuss it with the Executive at their meeting on April 22, where it was read.

I have been requested by the Executive to ask if you would object if your letter was included in the Minutes of the Executive meeting. (The

Minutes of each Executive meeting go to all the members of the Associate Committee.)

The discussion following the reading of your letter brought out the opinion that the policy of the Associate Committee on Medical Research must evolve rather than be too definitely laid down at the beginning. It was also considered advisable that the local medical research committees should help and cooperate rather than administer the funds available for medical research through the Associate Committee.

In the discussion of the application of Dr. Pat McDonald, it was decided that he should be invited to come East at the expense of the Committee and visit Montreal, Ottawa and Toronto and discuss his problem and that following this discussion, the President of the National Research Council, Dr. Gendreau and myself would endeavour to come to some conclusion concerning his application.

May I say that I personally appreciate your memorandum and only wish that every member of the Committee were taking their responsibilities equally seriously. May I also say that I was more disappointed than you were with the outcome of the meeting of the Associate Committee the last two days of February. The only consolation is that I believe each member of the Committee had plenty of scope in the expression of his opinion, which tended to clear the atmosphere so that we can proceed. I am particularly anxious that precedents should not be too firmly established so that we may gain wisdom with time and be enabled to change policy and proceedings as necessity demands. The best we can hope to do is to make a start, be prepared to make mistakes and be prepared to learn from our mistakes, and at the same time to do the thing that seems most worthwhile at the time.

I am still of the opinion that medical research should not be centralized and on looking over the appropriations that have already been made, it will be seen from the Minutes that due consideration was given to the applications from smaller centres. As you know, the money available was far short of what was hoped for, but I am sure that if we are able to make good use of these funds, more will be forthcoming. I admit that the Committee was inconsistent in making a grant to Dr. Masson, who is a member of the Committee, when applications were not received from Ettinger, Paterson, Mainland and Gendreau. However, this inconsistency was automatically rectified in that no application was received from Dr. Masson.

The only difficulty in including your letter in the Minutes is because of the personal references which you made concerning my visit, and it may be that Dr. Stewart may only include those parts which are relevant to the activities of medical research. I wish you would drop me a note or write directly to Dr. Stewart, concerning your views and wishes in the matter.

With kind personal regards.

Yours sincerely,

F.G. Banting

By letter from Dr. Stewart on April 28, 1938, Dr. Thorlakson was advised of grants made by the Committee to Winnipeg applicants: Dr. A.T. Cameron, $1200; Dr. H.V. Rice, $300 for the purchase of special apparatus. It was confirmed that a final decision would be made on Dr. McDonald's application for $4,400 after his visit to eastern centres at committee expense. No financial support was offered for fifteen other research projects submitted: Professor I.M. Thompson (4 projects); Dr. J.D. Adamson (5); Dr. J.M. McEachern (2); Dr. C.H.A. Walton (1); Dr. Bruce Chown (1); Dr. A.C. Abbott (1); and Dr. John Hillsman (1).

With the advent of war in September 1939, the Associate Committee on Medical Research turned its attention to the needs both of members of the armed services and of civilians suffering the injuries of combat on land, sea and in the air. Burns were a major medical problem. At the beginning of World War II, the standard incendiary bomb consisted of a magnesium metal case filled with thermite, a mixture of aluminum and iron oxide. The burning of such a bomb cannot be extinguished with water. In the autumn of 1940, such bombs dropped by German aircraft gutted a large part of London. Incendiary bombs were used on both sides throughout the war, with "improvements" that made them even more devastating. Military personnel suffering from severe burn damage were being returned from overseas for long-term treatment.

Research on the medical care of burns therefore received a high priority. A sub-committee of the Associate Committee, under the chairmanship of Dr. Wilder Penfield, coordinated work on burns in a number of research laboratories in Canada.

Dr. Thorlakson reported to Dr. Penfield on May 1, 1942, that the local Regional Committee had met and recommended that the Penfield Sub-Committee on Surgery proceed to issue a set of recommendations on the treatment of burns for the guidance of those responsible for this difficult task. He also advised that the Regional Committee in Winnipeg seek approval to enlarge their membership to include a burn committee consisting of Dr. C.W. Burns, Dr. A.C. Abbott and Dr. Bruce Chown, to take charge of burn cases in the three teaching hospitals (i.e., Winnipeg General, St. Boniface General and Children's); and he suggested that Dr. Oliver S. Waugh, professor of surgery, act as chairman of the Burn Committee. The proposal got prompt approval from Dr. Penfield.

The work of the Associate Committee steadily expanded, and at the annual meeting of the National Research Council on March 16 and 17, 1944, Dr. Thorlakson submitted a paper in which he made three major recommendations on the organization of medical research in the postwar period.

First, he proposed that a western regional committee on research be established, which would periodically survey facilities in the western centres, provide encouragement and advice, and review applications for assisted research. The recommendations of this regional committee would be forwarded, along with the applications themselves, for consideration by the Associate Committee on Medical Research. He suggested that the Western Regional Committee should meet annually, perhaps in Edmonton or Saskatoon to reduce travel costs, in order to exchange information and carry out its responsibilities. The Regional Committee should have clinical representation in its membership, and its members should be appointed by the Associate Committee.

He also proposed that a systematic canvass be made of all medical officers in the armed forces to identify those who had shown special aptitude for research, so that they could be encouraged to take the necessary training to enable them to make a career in this field; and he urged the National Research Council and the Associate Committee to make strong representations to the Dominion Government to provide substantially increased financial support for medical research after the War ended.

As a consequence of this paper, the Western Regional Committee was established with the sanction of the Associate Committee and the National Research Council, and did much to maintain an interest in research in the western universities, and provide an improved flow of information about grant appli-

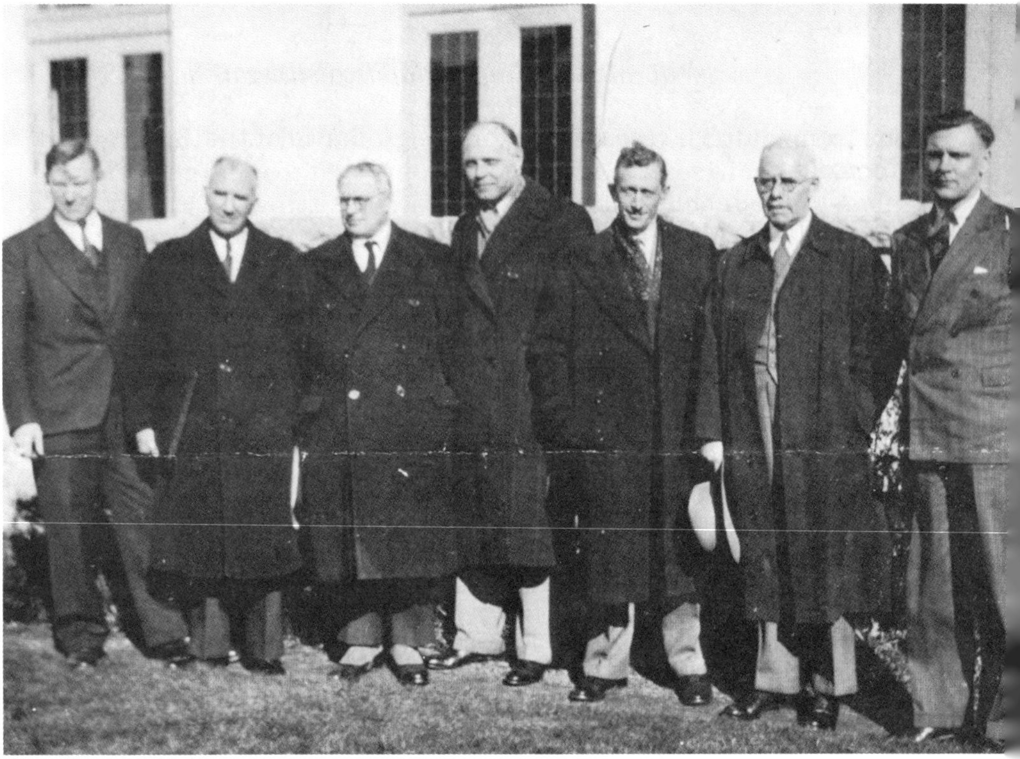

First meeting (held on February 23, 1945, in Vancouver) of the Western Regional Group, a part of the Associate Committee on Medical Research of the National Research Council. Left to right: Dr. Norman MacKenzie (President), University c British Columbia; Dr. John W. Scott, Edmonton; Dr. J.B. Collip, Montreal; Dr. Paul H.T. Thorlakson (Chairman) Winnipeg; Dr. G.H. Ettinger, Kingston; Dr. W.S. Lindsay, Saskatoon; and Dr. C.R. Dolman, Vancouver.

cations from western researchers for the guidance of the Associate Committee.

DIVISION OF MEDICAL SCIENCE

Membership on the Associate Committee was restricted to two terms, which meant that Dr. Thorlakson's direct participation terminated at the Council meeting in May 1945. He continued his relationship with its members and its work, however, as a member of the Sub-Committee on Surgery. For some time the feeling had been growing that medical research was too important to continue to be guided by an associate committee. While recognizing the many good things that it had been able to do to advance its objectives – for example, the budget considered for 1946 was $200,000 compared to the $53,000 in the committee's first year – the opinion was advanced that the Associate Committee ought to be raised to the status of a full division of the National Research Council.

To help achieve this objective, Dr. Thorlakson prepared the following brief, setting out the advantages of this new status and suggesting what its organizational structure might be. He submitted his brief to a number of people for review and criticism prior to its presentation to the National Research Council.[7] The brief was entitled, "Division of Medical Science, National Research Council":

The members of the Associate Committee on Medical Research voted unanimously, on October 30, 1945, to petition the National Research Council to alter the status of the committee to that of a division of the National Research Council. The advantages and disadvantages of establishing a separate medical council had been discussed at earlier meetings. At this last meeting, all were agreed that medical research in Canada should come under the aegis of the National Research Council and its president, Dr. McKenzie, thereby avoiding duplication of administrative organization and expense.

The change in status pre-supposes a review of the record and organization of the Associate Committee from its inception in 1938. From this study, changes in organization might be indicated.

In 1938, the Associate Committee on Medical Research was organized for the purpose of establishing a method of dealing with the applications for assisted research and to assume the responsibility of distributing a sum of money set aside for that purpose. At one of its organization meetings, the Research Committee appointed an executive to deal with matters that would come up for consideration and decision between the semi-annual meetings, and to prepare an agenda for the subsequent meetings. This was the procedure followed until the beginning of the War.

Shortly after the outbreak of hostilities, the Committee enlarged its membership and created new sub-committees to deal with the many urgent problems that were presented to it by the exigencies of war. Representation on the Associate Committee from the medical branches of the armed services was arranged, and the chairmen of the sub-committees were invited to attend its regular meetings. Associate committees on medical research were appointed for the army, navy and air force and many sub-committees, sub-sections and regional committees were created. The whole machinery of the organization was geared to the task of bringing all the resources of our laboratories and clinical facilities to assist in the solution of pressing war problems such as burns, shock, blood substitutes, wounds, gas gangrene, and a host of others. In this "second emergency phase," the work and responsibility was not limited to medical research, but included also the work of crystallizing and organizing the opinions and recommendations of scientists and clinicians from our university centres, as well as those participating in scientific investigations in the medical branches of our armed forces.

This pooling of all the scientific and clinical resources of Canadian medicine proved a most effective method in the early solution of many problems and also in the rapid transmission of information from one group to another. During this time, too, the closest liaison was maintained between Canadian, British and American research organizations. The record that has been established by the various Canadian medical organizations working under the aegis of the National Research Council is one that has brought credit to the Research Council and to Canadian medicine as a whole. However, it is obvious that the present multiplicity of committees, sub-committees and sub-sections is unnecessarily complicated, cumbersome and expensive to serve the needs of peace-time medical research. Furthermore, this organization, grown out of the needs of war, far exceeds the original plans for the Associate Committee. A consolidation of our position and another re-organization has now become necessary.

The first step in this direction was accomplished at the recent meeting of the Associate Committee when a motion abolishing all sub-committees as of a certain date was presented and carried. It was agreed that the continuity of certain committees should be assured by their immediate re-establishment; but the fact that the slate was wiped clean suggests that, in the opinion of the members of the Committee, the whole problem of medical research in Canada should be subjected to careful scrutiny and study. The motion implied that the present executive should form the clearing house for opinions and recommendations on the most effective methods for encouraging and supporting medical research in Canada. It was anticipated that the executive committee would present proposals for this re-organization at the next meeting of the Associate Committee.

In considering this problem, it is necessary to approach it from a broad national viewpoint and to make certain statements that appear to be relevant to this important question. We have arrived at a crucial moment in the scientific development of our country as far as the support from government and private agencies is concerned. Never before have the citizens of this country, the universities, the provincial governments, or the government in Ottawa been more keenly alive to the importance of supporting generously basic scientific research, for they now realize the valuable contributions that scientific discoveries can make to progress on a broad national scale. It is therefore incumbent upon us to prepare a concrete and practical plan which will coordinate the experience, the facilities and the financial resources of our National Research Council with the potential research facilities and personnel within our universities, whether they are supported by provincial governments or private endowment.

In 1938, the late Sir Frederick Banting made a tour of Canada to examine research facilities and interview research workers in the various medical centres in the Dominion. The key note of an address that he delivered on this tour was that Canada could not afford to continue to export many of its keenest young men and women, trained in our universities, to make their contributions to science elsewhere. He maintained that a part of this annual depletion was the result of a short-sighted attitude of our governments and universities in failing to provide much greater opportunities for advanced training in the fields of scientific technique; and another part was the result of the meagre rewards offered in Canada to young men and women who were determined to devote their talents and energies to the field of research, compared with the incomes and other inducements offered to these same men and women in the United States.

More recently, President McKenzie of the National Research Council has re-stated the same viewpoint and has supported his argument by an array of facts and figures.

A few weeks ago, President Trueman of the University of Manitoba took the opportunity in his inaugural address to re-emphasize the gravity of this annual exodus. He made a strong plea to government and university authorities that immediate steps be taken to rectify this situation. The burden of all these public statements is to the effect that if Canada is to rise among the nations of the earth to that eminence which its great deposits of natural wealth and the virility of its people would justify, we must offer inducements to our able young men and women that will lead them to discover by research the means to develop and conserve those resources.

The progress of medical research in Canada is an essential and integral part of the advance of scientific research. Today, one cannot separate medical research from progress in other fields such as chemistry and physics. The medical applications in the field of radio-activity, inherent in the discovery of the release of atomic energy, are the most recent evidence to show the close inter-dependence of all scientific progress. In the field of chemical synthesis lies hope for great discoveries in the field of medical therapy. It seems, therefore, that a most fortunate decision has been made, that the new organization for medical research should enjoy the closest collaboration and cooperation with other departments included under the National Research Council.

In the organization of the new Division of Medical Sciences, we must take into consideration the present general public approval of financial support for research and the need for maintaining the closest affiliation between medical research and all other research activities. We must also consider the method by which we can bring the effect of all this support and collaboration to bear on the development of active research centres in our Canadian universities. The decision that we reach in this matter now may well influence the whole future of Canadian medical research.

Judging by the opinion that has been expressed repeatedly, it seems agreed that the National Research Council should support medical research in university centres, and not in a central laboratory located in Ottawa. This decision very largely determines the form of our new organization and it is on this premise that the following recommendations are based.

While education is a provincial responsibility and the Dominion Government is loath to become involved with the provinces in this field because of certain provisions in the British North America Act, scientific research has been accepted as a Dominion responsibility through the establishment of the National Research Council and the provision of large sums of money to subsidize research.

Education and research are hand-maidens to the normal process of national development. Each depends on the other. Research men are trained in universities; university departments require the stimulus of research-minded men on their staffs. There is in this a fusion of provincial and Dominion interests. With this interdependence of interest, there should be no difficulty in devising ways and means to overcome the obstacles that stand in the way of a satisfactory arrangement.

Inasmuch as medical research is not likely to be carried on in the National Research Council buildings in Ottawa, the Director and Secretary of the Division of Medical Sciences should not be full-time employees of the Council. It would be in the interests of Canadian medical research that the director be a man with international reputation, enjoying the support and confidence of all men engaged in research. Both the director and the secretary should be on a part-time salary from the Council.

The advisory council that would be set up around these two officials should be chosen from leaders in the six sub-divisions that were suggested at the recent meeting, with the addition of dentistry as an associate committee. The executive committee would consist of representatives from medicine (1), surgery (1), pre-clinical sciences (2), industrial hygiene (1), military medicine (1), and dentistry (1).

In order that Canadian medicine as a whole be represented, the membership should include the President of the Canadian Medical Association, President of the Royal College of Physicians and Surgeons of Canada, a rotating representation from the deans of the faculties of medicine of Canadian universities and from the Association of Deputy Ministers of Health of the provinces of Canada, the President of the National Research Council, and a representative of the Dominion Department of Health.

This council and executive would function only in an advisory, supervisory and consultative capacity to discuss and determine policy and procedure regarding the manner in which the National Research Council could most effectively encourage medical research across Canada. One annual meeting would probably be sufficient for its purposes. This body as a whole would not consider and attempt to pass judgement on applications for assisted research in one day as is now done by the Associate Committee. It is suggested that as each application is submitted to the secretary, the stenographic staff of the Council should type the number of copies necessary to distribute the application to a panel of experts (two or more). The recommendations from the panel could then be returned to that member of the Council who represents the particular section concerned. The Executive Committee, with the chairman and the secretary, would meet the day preceding the annual meeting to consider the recommendations submitted by the head of each section and allocate the available funds.

To assure continuity of effort and all the year-round supervision of the work of the Council, assistant directors on full salaries from the National Research Council could be appointed and placed in research posts at key points, provided that the university concerned could arrange for proper quarters and equipment and have a number of men on the staff sufficiently interested to carry out research to justify such an appointment. This recommendation is made with the belief that the creation of such posts across Canada by the National Research Council (and there are precedents in other fields which make it possible) is not only opportune but necessary for the full and satisfactory development of any broad national plan. This recommendation is taken from a recent memorandum prepared by the Research Committee of the Faculty of Medicine of the University of Manitoba. The contacts that would be established by these key men, with men and women of the student body, with younger members on the teaching staff, and finally with the parent organization in Ottawa, could well be of inestimable value to the success of the national plan. These regional directors would be in constant communication with the parent organization, keeping it informed of the progress on research projects and recommending consideration for additional support or the withdrawal of support when justified. Having a fully paid representative in the field, the central organization would be in a better position to make provisions for work in the succeeding year.

The plan as suggested centralizes final authority and control, which is necessary for the successful management of any organization, but it serves to de-centralize the responsibility for the success of the local units and provides closer contact and supervision over work as it is being carried on.

If this plan meets with the approval of the authorities of the National Research Council, it is suggested that immediate steps be taken to develop these units in at least four centres: Dalhousie University; Laval University; the University of Manitoba; and the University of Alberta. From a geographical standpoint, the provision of two units in the East and two in the West should meet with general approval.

As this plan develops and units are established in other centres, special consideration could be given to the transfer of a research man from one centre to another in order that he might carry on his particular study with the greatest of success, realizing that certain centres will always have facilities and personnel especially capable of carrying forward any particular problem.

In addition, travelling fellowships in research should be provided so that our graduates could visit laboratories in other countries. Canadian medicine must not be allowed to develop into tight provincial compartments, each one of which educates and trains to meet little more than the immediate needs of the people of its own province. This, at the moment, seems to be the trend – according to the official opinion expressed in the four western provinces. Medical research has an opportunity to create a national attitude in the field of Canadian medicine, in opposition to a purely provincial attitude.

The provision of measures to safeguard and improve the health of the people of Canada and the advancement of medical knowledge is a national responsibility. What has been accomplished by Canadian medicine in time of war can be accomplished in time of peace, providing we carry forward into the period that lies ahead the same degree of enthusiasm, will and determination for well-directed coordinated effort on a broad national basis.

It was not to be expected that this comprehensive recommendation would be accepted in its entirety. There can be no doubt, however, that it carried weight when the final decision for change was made, and in the deliberations which culminated in the following announcement, published on June 1, 1946:

THE NATIONAL RESEARCH COUNCIL OF CANADA
announces that the
Associate Committee on Medical Research
has been re-organized as the
DIVISION OF MEDICAL RESEARCH
Director: J.B. Collip, CBE, MA, PHD, MD, DSC,
LLD FRS, FRSC, FRCP, Gilman Cheney Research
Professor of Endocrinology, and Director, Research Institute of
Endocrinology, McGill University, Montreal, Que.
Assistant Director: G.H. Ettinger, MBE, BA, MD,
FRSC, Professor of Physiology, Queen's University,
Kingston, Ont.

The final act in the evolution of a national agency to formulate policies concerning medical research and allocate funds for projects considered to be worthy of support came on November 14, 1960. The National Research Council announced the dissolution of its Division of Medical Research, and its replacement by the virtually autonomous Medical Research Council of Canada. Since that time the Council has been the administrator of almost all the funds allocated by the Government of Canada for medical research.

From October 24 to 26, 1985, the Medical Research Council of Canada celebrated its twenty-fifth anniversary by holding a symposium in Winnipeg hosted by the University of Manitoba. In response to their invitation, Dr. Thorlakson, who earlier that month had celebrated his ninetieth birthday, gave the opening address.

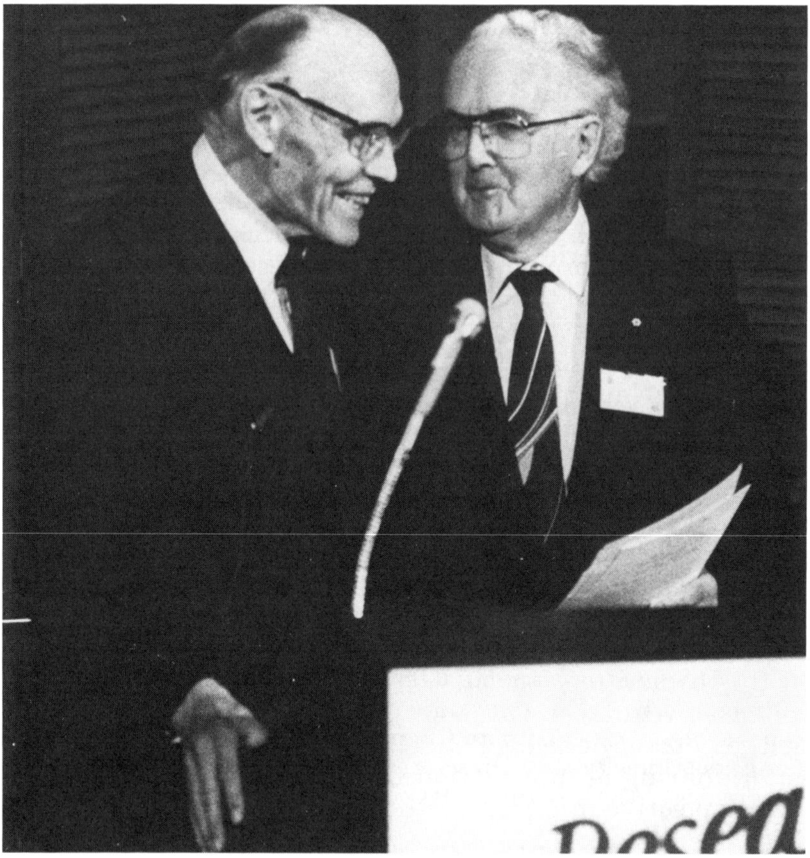

At the twenty-fifth anniversary meeting of the Medical Research Council of Canada held in Winnipeg on October 26, 1985, Dr. Thorlakson, the opening speaker, exchanges with Dr. Chester B. Stewart of Halifax happy recollections of their experiences in 1938 when they surveyed medical research resources in western Canada with Sir Frederick Banting in 1938.

His paper contributed a historical perspective to the meeting. Recalling his early experience with the development of Canadian resources for medical research, he remarked on the key role played by Sir Frederick Banting in creating the interest of the federal government in providing support for research. Banting had been urging the principle of government funding for some time before he became a member of the National Research Council in 1935. He was undoubtedly influential in shaping President A.G.L. McNaughton's decision to invite proposals from the Canadian Medical Association, the Royal College of Physicians and Surgeons of Canada and the Department of Pensions and National Health, which led to the formation of the Associate Committee on Medical Research.

Dr. Thorlakson referred to the importance of the work of the Western Regional Committee on Research which he had recommended to the Associate Committee, and which had been strongly supported by Banting. Dr. Thorlakson was the first chairman of this committee, which, after its founding in 1944 continued to meet regularly for more than twenty years. It brought together doctors engaged in research in the western universities for sharing of information, ideas and experiences, and was a strong positive influence on the recruitment or retention of medical scientists and the development of resources that resulted in centres of excellence in Western Canada of international stature.

Dr. Thorlakson had a close relationship with Banting during those years, and he closed his address with this personal note:

> During our association we had become good friends. After our last meeting in 1941 we dined together at the Chateau Laurier Hotel in Ottawa, and then walked across the street to enter the railway station. Our trains stood side by side and we had a short time to talk and plan. We agreed to meet each other again in Toronto after his return from England. By then he had established a close relationship with both English and American groups carrying out military research. This would be his second mission to England. His plane took off from Toronto the next day.
>
> I arrived back in Winnipeg thirty-six hours later. As I stepped off the train in the early morning the station master came down the train to inform me that the plane on which Sir Frederick Banting was travelling to England had crashed in Newfoundland and that Sir Frederick had been killed.

I was not able to attend the funeral but some time later I visited Lady Banting. During my visit I was shown some of the last reports he had signed. There was an account of a flight he had made one dark drab day over Toronto, checking himself on the effects of altitude on the actions of certain drugs. At the end of the report he had written, "No matter how dark it is on earth we should always remember that there is beautiful sunshine above the clouds."

CHAPTER 9

The Manitoba Institute for the Advancement of Medical Education and Research

RESEARCH SUPPORT FROM THE PRIVATE SECTOR

There was a growing conviction in the 1930s in the universities and in the medical profession generally that research programs had an important part to play in achieving standards of excellence in medical education. Students at all levels could benefit from association with medical scientists and by participation in studies under their direction. This would in turn bring about improved standards of patient care. Investment in research was seen to have value beyond adding to the bank of scientific knowledge.

In discussions during the research survey of the western provinces in 1938, described in chapter 8, Sir Frederick Banting strongly advocated the necessity to arouse among civic leaders a lively sense of the need for a well-rounded research establishment to improve the whole field of medical education and patient care. In his view, if Winnipeg was ever to become a major medical research centre, the interest and support of successful leaders in business and the professions must be sought. Concurrently, a vehicle was required in which they could personally participate as members and directors, and through which substantial contributions could be channelled. Dr. Banting did not believe in sole reliance on government funding.

It must be remembered that Dr. Thorlakson at this time was not only on the Associate Committee on Medical Research of the

National Research Council; he was also the Chairman of the Manitoba Faculty of Medicine Committee on Research, and keenly aware of the shortcomings, the needs, and the research potential in Winnipeg. It was in his nature that to see a problem was to experience a strong urge to do something about it.

In this case, in fact, he recognized two issues. One was the necessity to do something about property ownership related to the Winnipeg Clinic (which had just been established) to avoid the difficulties and disputes which he had noted elsewhere, if professional members were required to invest substantial amounts in shares. The second was the need to improve medical research resources in Winnipeg.

While he was pondering these problems, the idea gradually evolved that a single strategic plan might resolve both of them. If ownership of the Winnipeg Clinic property were turned over to a non-profit research foundation which collected rent from the medical partnership tenants, the basic income would provide a permanent source of funding for research that would increase as the capital loan was gradually reduced, and ultimately paid off in full. Such a foundation, having a board consisting of community leaders, could also become a means of attracting substantial sums for research by way of donations.[1]

Dr. Thorlakson discussed his idea with members of the Board of Governors of the University of Manitoba, with the Dean and members of the Faculty of Medicine, and with Mr. W.A. Murphy and other members of the Board of Winnipeg General Hospital. He discussed the implications of such an arrangement with his colleagues in the Clinic, pointing out the long-term benefits of keeping the members of the professional partnership out of the real estate business. At the same time, acceptance of this proposal would be a tangible demonstration that the members of the Clinic were prepared to back the profession's claims that support for education and research were essential.[2]

The very positive responses from members of the business and professional community on the University and hospital boards was an affirmation of Sir Frederick Banting's thesis that community leaders could, and should, be interested in aid to medical education and research. The Dean of the Faculty of Medicine and most of the department heads welcomed this new and potentially important source of funds. It was not surprising, however, that some who were convinced that a multidisciplinary specialty group practice clinic was inherently self-serving, raised the cry that the scheme must have been devised to save income tax for the members of the Winnipeg Clinic. It is perhaps appropriate to recall the comment on change in the scientific field made by Nobel-Prize winner Max Planck. "A new scientific truth," he said, "does not triumph by convincing its opponents and making them see the light, but rather because its opponents eventually die, and a new generation grows up that is familiar with it."[3]

THE INSTITUTE

The plan for the new foundation went forward steadily. Mr. John A. MacAulay, both as the solicitor consulted by Dr. Thorlakson and as an interested citizen, gave much study as to how it should be legally constituted. One day, Mr. Justice A. K. Dysart, then Chairman of the Board of Governors of the University of Manitoba, walked over from the Law Courts Building to the Clinic to discuss with Dr. Thorlakson the name of the proposed foundation. His choice was The Manitoba Institute for Medical Education and Research; and this, in fact, was accepted and used when applying for incorporation of the Foundation.

The Winnipeg Clinic moved into the new two-storey building in October 1942. The members of the Clinic had agreed to the Research Foundation plan. The general support expressed for the idea by members of the boards of the University and Winnipeg General Hospital and others encouraged rapid action to make the concept a reality.

On February 8, 1943, the following petition was addressed to the lieutenant governor, requesting an act of incorporation:

> To His Honour the Lieutenant Governor of the Province of Manitoba: The undersigned are desirous that they and the persons holding from time to time the following offices, namely, the Chairman of the Board of Governors of the University of Manitoba, the President of the University of Manitoba, the Dean of the Faculty of Medicine of the University of Manitoba, the Chairman of the Research Committee of the Faculty of Medicine of the University of Manitoba, and two other persons each to be appointed annually for a one-year term by the Board of Governors of the University of Manitoba, and one other person to be ap-

pointed annually by the Minister of Health and Public Welfare, together with such other persons as may from time to time become members of the corporation hereinafter referred to, may be constituted a body politic and corporate under the name of "The Manitoba Institute for Medical Education and Research" for the purposes and objects of assisting scientific, medical and surgical knowledge through research, and of assisting persons desirous of advancing their scientific, medical and surgical knowledge, subject to the proviso that no part of the income of the said Institute shall inure to the personal profit of or be paid or payable to any member of the said Institute by reason only of his membership therein, such Institute to be vested with all the powers necessary for the conduct of its affairs by a Board of Directors consisting in the first instance of Paul H.T. Thorlakson, Harry D. Morse, C. Burton Stewart, Lennox Bell, Cecil S. Gunn, Sidney E. Smith, Henry E. Sellers, William A. Murphy, and Alvin T. Mathers.

WHEREFORE your Petitioners humbly pray that your Honour may be pleased to sanction the passing of an Act for the purposes above mentioned.

As in duty bound your Petitioners will ever pray.

This petition (which is entitled to a place in history not only for its purpose and its distinguished roster of petitioners, but also for the length of its opening sentence!), bore the signatures, each duly witnessed, of thirty-two of Winnipeg's well-known and respected citizens.[4]

The Act of Incorporation of the Manitoba Institute for the Advancement of Medical Education and Research was passed in the legislature on March 15, 1943, and given royal assent on March 17, 1943. It had been referred to the Private Bills Committee to give an opportunity for any opposed to it to make representations, but none appeared. The name originally chosen was expanded to include the words "the advancement of," to alleviate the concerns of some who thought the Institute would compete in research with the University. Also, at the request of the petitioners' solicitor, Mr. MacAulay, in committee the Bill was amended to provide for eleven directors instead of nine; and the provision in the original draft that the Board would have at least four directors who were doctors associated with the Winnipeg Clinic was deleted, to meet what Mr. MacAulay described as "rumoured objections." At committee, several spoke in favour of the Bill, including Dr. Sidney E. Smith, President of the University of Manitoba. No one spoke against it.

The first meeting of the Board of Directors of the Institute was held in Salon A in the Fort Garry Hotel on June 18, 1943, with all the first directors named in the Act present. On invitation of the board, John A. MacAulay and Donald A. Thompson, the legal counsel who had guided the establishment of the Institute, were also present. With the unanimous agreement of the directors, Mr. H.E. Sellers took the chair, and Mr. D.A. Thompson was appointed secretary of the meeting. After passing a general by-law drafted by legal counsel to provide for the conduct of the affairs of the Institute, and agreeing to have it submitted for confirmation to a special general meeting of the members to be held on June 22, the chairman called for nominations for the office of president. Dr. Thorlakson was unanimously elected to this position; Mr. Murphy and Mr. Sellers were elected Vice-Presidents; and Mr. D.A. Thompson was appointed Secretary of the Institute.

On taking the chair, Dr. Thorlakson called on Mr. MacAulay, who made a statement with respect to the proposed gift to the Institute of the Winnipeg Clinic building and the property on which it stood at the north-east corner of St. Mary Avenue and Vaughan Street. Title to the property was in the name of Dr. Thorlakson, and was subject to a first mortgage to C.S. Gunn and Company Limited of $60,000, repayable with interest at three percent per annum; and to a second mortgage in favour of the same company for $47,542.84, repayable without interest. The property was leased to the Winnipeg Clinic Holding Company Limited, of which Dr. Thorlakson was the sole owner. Mr. MacAulay explained that the mortgages had been given to secure advances made to acquire the property and construct the Clinic building and that in taking the mortgages, C.S. Gunn and Company Limited was acting on behalf of the persons who had made the advances, which represented the total cost of the land and buildings.[5] He pointed out that the persons who had made the advances under the second mortgage without interest were in effect making an annual contribution to the Institute of the amount of interest that would normally have been payable. In fact, the interest on the first mortgage was also contributed to the Institute by the person who had advanced the funds, along with substantial additional gifts.

The directors were advised that the lease on the property held by the Winnipeg Clinic Holding Company Limited was for a period of ten years from August 1, 1942. The annual rental payable by the Winnipeg Clinic Professional Group to the Holding Company was $18,000 during the first three years of the lease, with taxes to be paid by the tenants. After the first three years, the amount of the rent would be determined by mutual agreement of the parties, or, in default of agreement, by a board of arbitration. Rental adjustments, if required, would be made every three years.

Mr. MacAulay stated that it was the purpose of Dr. Thorlakson and of his associates to make the revenue from the building available immediately (subject to the mortgage payments) for funding research projects through the Institute, and to provide that in due course the Institute would own, without encumbrance, a valuable revenue-bearing property. He confirmed that rentals had been accumulating since August 1, 1942, and that these would be paid over to the Institute with the transfer of title. He concluded by formally offering, on behalf of Dr. Thorlakson, to transfer the lands in question to the Manitoba Institute for the Advancement of Medical Education and Research. It was moved by Mr. Sellers, seconded by Dr. Mathers, and unanimously resolved by the directors that the gift be accepted.

On June 22, at the request of the president, Mr. H.E. Sellers acted as chairman of the special general meeting of the members of the Institute, which confirmed the actions of the directors.

At the conclusion of the regular business for which the meeting was called, Mr. Sellers announced that the first cash gifts from individuals had been received by the treasurer, amounting to $6,000.[6]

Dr. Thorlakson outlined the conception of the Institute in these terms:

I have been asked to review for you briefly the development of the idea which ultimately culminated in the formation of the Manitoba Institute for the Advancement of Medical Education and Research.

In relating the steps that were taken in reaching this objective, one might convey the impression that the idea originated with me and that I was personally responsible for its full development. Nothing is further from my mind as this was a cooperative procedure and I realize only too well that without the advice, assistance and encouragement –

as well as the criticism – of my close associates, this plan would never have reached maturity. . . .

Therefore, in this presentation, it is impossible for me to disassociate the idea of the development of a medical clinic from that of medical research. First, because the plan of establishing this institute originated with the members of the Winnipeg Clinc; and second, because the funds which go to support the activities of this new venture will come largely from the clinic itself.

Winnipeg has been one of the leading medical centres of western Canada for over half a century. Medicine, like all other sciences, has made marked advances in the last several decades with the result that the demands on a medical centre have been greatly increased. Thus, to keep Winnipeg to the front as a medical centre of the West, progress must be made in the four necessary requirements, namely:

1. A medical school with its affiliate teaching hospitals;

2. A group of medical men who have taken advanced post-graduate training to equip them to practice their specialties with distinction and to impart their knowledge and experience to medical students;

3. Facilities for laboratory and clinical research;

4. Adequate opportunities for post-graduate training in the form of extended fellowships.

There is general agreement that our local facilities are inadequate, if not entirely lacking, in post-graduate training. Thus many or most of our promising young men must go elsewhere to find opportunities for study which should be made available to them here.

It is with a desire to make some contribution towards the extension of local facilities for post graduate training and medical research that this institute, of which you are charter members, was established.

When permission was given [by the Ottawa authorities] for the erection of the Winnipeg Clinic building, the associates agreed among themselves that erecting a building at this time should not be, in itself, a financial benefit to them and that any equity established in this building, during and after the war, would ultimately be turned over to support advanced medical education in this community. It was with these ideas in view that we conceived the proposition that the property be deeded over to some charitable organization capable of administering the funds that would accumulate in trust for the purpose that has been declared.

We have, therefore, made arrangements to transfer the deed of this property to the Manitoba Institute as soon as the members of this institute are satisfied with the provisions of the agreement.

I cannot allow this opportunity to pass without acknowledging a great debt to many persons who have made it possible to complete this entire plan: first, to establish the Winnipeg Clinic; and second, to deed over the Winnipeg Clinic building to the Institute to which you have so graciously lent your patronage.

MEDICAL EDUCATION AND RESEARCH: THE INSTITUTE'S ROLE

After the Manitoba Institute for the Advancement of Medical Education and Research was incorporated in 1943, Dr. Thorlakson, as its president, lost no time in cultivating the interest and understanding that would enable it to push forward toward its objectives of aid to education and research. It was apparent that with the limited resources the institute was likely to have in the early years, care would have to be exercised to determine the most fruitful method of using its funds.

While most informed people knew something about medical education, there was less understanding about the nature of medical research and its place in the tripod of clinical practice, education and research on which progress in medical science is based. Medical research was relatively limited in the University of Manitoba at that time, and if this were to be changed it would be necessary to develop a broad interest in, and hopefully enthusiasm for, its support.

As an introductory step, it was decided t invite Dr. Charles F. Code, a brilliant young medical scientist who had graduated from the University of Manitoba and who was then on the research staff of the Mayo Foundation in Rochester, Minnesota, to come to Winnipeg and present a paper about research.[7]

On October 27, 1945, the Board and members of the Institute, together with a number of guests (thirty-five persons in all) gathered for dinner in Salon C at the Fort Garry Hotel, at which Dr. Code was the guest speaker. Entitled "The Role of Medical Research in a Medical Centre," his address was designed to be both informative and inspirational. (The title seems to reflect another of Dr. Thorlakson's major interests at the time – the Manitoba Medical Centre, an idea planted a year earlier and now becoming well-rooted in the community.)

Dr. Code proposed to discuss three questons: What is medical research? What qualities should one look for in a medical researcher? And what does medical research contribute in a medical centre?"

What is Medical Research?

In answering this question it should first be pointed out that medical research as a bona fide branch of medicine is new. In the days of man's historical beginnings, the "medicine man" was an accepted member of the tribe. The physician has had a recognized place in the community since early civilized times, but the medical research worker is a modern innovation. He is a development of the last 100 years. I believe it can be correctly predicted that the full recognition and widespread acceptance of medical research as a definite medical specialty will belong to twentieth-century medicine.

As to what medical research really is, it is the investigation of problems pertaining to people during health and during sickness. When an observation has been made, research steps in to try to answer two simple questions: why? and how? Why does it work that way? How does it work that way? As its name implies, it involves a persistent research into the phenomenon under study. It is associated with a certain stubborn unwillingness to accept existing explanations, no matter how plausible, if the slightest doubt can be cast on their validity.

The point has been amusingly and well illustrated by Dr. Alan Gregg in his book on medical research. He says, "I think of a day on the boat returning from China when one of our fellow passengers lost his wrist watch. Of course, he looked for it, as he said, "everywhere." But later the Number One Boy set his crew of relatives to work on a research whose essence was method and thoroughness. Not only did this procedure return the wristwatch, it discovered a pearl necklace, two gold rings and a stick pin!"

Research is not simply the compilation and summarization of facts. It is a more active process than that. It is a means of finding new facts. It is a means of establishing the truth. It uses the experimental method for the elucidation of its problems. By this procedure experiments are designed which show what happens, why it happens or how it happens. The master of the experimental method is the man who devises experiments, the results of which give clear-cut, decisive answers to fundamental questions. The process of research is an active one. Medical research is the active attack on a medical problem.

What Qualities Should you Look for in a Medical Researcher?

If I were asked, "What is the greatest single attribute of a good medical research worker?" my answer would be: curiosity. While necessity is the mother of invention, curiosity is the mother of research. Good research men are driven by a persistent curiosity....

The research worker must have curiosity, and originality, based on intellectual capacity. But these in themselves are not enough. He also needs the ability to get the job done, to settle down and get to work. By the very nature of their work, research people are generally left to themselves. If they are to succeed, they will have to work. All great research workers have been extraordinarily industrious people.

Such people often turn to that procedure known as cooperation. Now cooperation in research is frequently a veil behind which a person with some authority gets a research worker to carry out the investigation which he himself has not the will to do. If you get a good man in your medical research centre, don't make it necessary for him to have to "cooperate." If you obtain a man who can do good research of his own, don't make him spend his time on the research of others who are unwilling to do the work for themselves.

Alan Gregg, Director of Medical Sciences for the Rockefeller Foundation, has said, "Cooperativeness counts in this country [he is speaking of the USA] for more than it should. It is usually urged more vociferously by those who want results [such as a flow of published papers] than by those who themselves have done distinguished scientific work."

On the other hand, let your research man or any research man in your entire medical center *collaborate* with whomever he pleases. In collaborative undertakings everyone works. It is not uncommon for an investigation to carry a research worker into an unfamiliar field. It is the mark of a good man if he then recognizes his limitations and seeks collaboration. This type of undertaking in which one person brings to a problem what the other or others have not – namely, specialized experience in another field – is true collaboration and is often highly productive.

It is poor policy and it is a fallacious standard to measure a man's research worth by the number of his publications. If there is any field in which it is quality and not quantity which really counts, it is in the field of research.... In England the medical scientific group on the whole has a sounder view which is well illustrated by an experience I had while working in England.

One of the young men in the laboratory remarked one day, "You know I have not published a paper for a year, and I am a bit worried about it." Our chief, Professor C. Lovatt Evans, turned to him and remarked, "But you have been working haven't you?" "Oh yes," replied the young man. "Then don't worry – it is not the size of your bibliography which counts. Always remember this: A. Hopkins, the best biochemist in England, has a bibliography of only twelve to fourteen papers. Each is a classic."

In the biography which Eve Curie has written of her famous mother, Madame Curie, she states that from 1919 to 1934 (fifteen years), 483 scientific communications were published by the physicists and chemists of the Institute of Radium – the Institute which Professor and Madame Curie established in Paris. Among these 483 publications, Madame Curie had only thirty-one to her credit. A book by Madame Curie was published posthumously, bringing her total bibliography to thirty-two publications. Her contribution to scientific literature lay in the quality of the work inherent in every paper she submitted.

Finally, the research worker must have the precious gift of intellectual honesty. In research, if either downright fraud or simple wishful thinking is indulged in, the result is the same – fallacious, misleading conclusions to the end that the progress of science is slowed or misdirected! . . . The ability of a scientist to be completely honest, to see his experiments in their true light, is paramount to all other attributes.

WHAT DOES MEDICAL RESEARCH CONTRIBUTE IN A MEDICAL CENTRE?

If good medical research is done, contributions will be made to the better understanding of diseases, and to the lessening of human suffering. The advances made need not be dramatic, of the kind the newspapers relish, to be real contributions to medical science.

For example, I might make an important discovery in patients with that rare disease called "familial periodic paralysis," with only a few people ever hearing of me. But let me so much as mention cancer or hay fever and the press is crowded around me. A real advance anywhere in the field of medicine pushes back a little further the veil of mystery which hangs over the human in health and in disease.

If good medical research is supported by this institute, it will enhance the medical reputation of this community. It will enhance the reputation of Winnipeg. By drawing your medical group together on the common aim of progress in medicine, research assists in coordinating their efforts, in holding them together. Research is *not* the paint on the ball, if I may use a slang expression. In a medical centre, the paint is usually the buildings. Research is the strongest thread which can be woven into the stuff of which the ball is made.

Good medical research raises the standard of practice in a medical centre. It is a tangible asset which assists in attracting the best physicians to your community. . . .

[This institute should] integrate its work with the medical school, for research and education cannot be separated. Research is the process by which new truth is found. It is an investment in the future.

In a stimulating and free-wheeling question-and-answer period following his address, Dr. Code elaborated on the principles he thought should be followed in launching the work of the Institute. The light he had thrown on the nature of medical research, its methods and the characteristics of the medical scientists who devoted themselves to it, was particularly helpful at this first general meeting of the directors and members, when the Institute's course was as yet uncharted. It led to the appointment, some months later, of an advisory committee selected from appropriate members of the Faculty, to review all applications for assistance from the Institute, and to recommend to the Board the action that should be taken.[8]

POLICIES ON AWARDING GRANTS

Following its incorporation in 1943, the Manitoba Institute for the Advancement of Medical Education and Research had two quite different kinds of responsibilities. The first was to negotiate and receive the rent payable by the medical partnership for the use of the Winnipeg Clinic building, and from this income pay the mortgage obligations, taxes and other indirect capital costs related to the operation of the property. The second responsibility was to receive donations from the Pharmacy and private individuals from which grants and awards could be made in support of medical education and research. This involved determining the criteria under which such support would be offered, and applying these rules in the selection of individuals and projects that deserved recognition.

The "real estate" mandate was quite clear, and able and experienced members of the Board of Directors were available to carry it out. On the other hand, policies had not yet been determined about aid to medical education and research. As first president of the institute, Dr. Thorlakson was deeply conscious of the need to evolve a process for carrying out this mission in a manner that would not only be fair and just, and bring the best results; but that would be accepted as such by the applicants, the donors of funds, and other concerned persons.

With this in mind, he asked Dr. Bruce Chown, an experienced researcher at the Children's Hospital, to consider the subject and prepare a memorandum that would be the basis for discussion of this topic at the first meeting of members of the Institute held on June 22, 1943.

The Chown Report cited the questions that would have to be dealt with in working out a relationship between the University and the Institute with respect to grants and awards. From the beginning, Dr. Thorlakson had promoted close ties between the Institute and the University. He had confirmation of approval and cooperation from the University and the Faculty of Medicine before the Institute was incorporated. On its Board of Directors were University President Sidney Smith; Dean Mathers; Dean H.P. Armes, and Dr. F.G. McGuinness, a member of the Faculty appointed by the University. The other four doctors on the Board all had University appointments. Members of the Institute included Mr. Justice H.A. Bergman, Chairman of the University Board of Governors, and his predecessor, Mr. Justice A.K. Dysart.

An ad hoc committee appointed by the directors of the Institute (consisting of Dr. Harry Morse, Chairman; Dean H.P. Armes; and Dr. Chown) worked out a procedure that would permit a program of awards to begin. This committee recommended that, as an initial step, two undergraduate student fellowships be funded, each in the amount of $750. This proposal was discussed with the Faculty of Medicine.

On November 10, 1944, the Medical Faculty Council of the University of Manitoba adopted recommendations which were submitted to it in a Memorandum on Future Research prepared by a committee of the Faculty. One of the recommendations approved at this time was:

> Part III (2): A request to the Manitoba Institute for the Advancement of Medical Education and Research to create two fellowships of the value of $750, each to be held for one year only and to be offered to students at the end of the second, third and fourth years of medicine, of high academic standing. Recipients shall devote the year of tenure of the fellowship to the work of the B.Sc. (Med.) degree in one or two of the following subjects: anatomy, bacteriology, biochemistry, biophysics, pathology, physiology and pharmacology. . . .

To meet this request, in June 1945, the Board of Directors of the institute approved the recommendation of its Awards Committee and allocated the sum of $7,500 to be used over a five-year period to fund two scholarships annually, commencing with the 1946–47 session. In 1951 the Board of Directors approved continuance of these scholarships for a second five-year period and allocated an additional $7,500 for this purpose.

THE WINNIPEG CLINIC RESEARCH INSTITUTE

On November 5, 1953, the Board of Directors of the Manitoba Institute for the Advancement of Medical Education and Research established an ad hoc committee to review the first decade of the enterprise; and in light of experience, to consider the probable nature of its future development and the direction that should be followed in its relationships with the University of Manitoba and the Winnipeg Clinic.

Appointed Chairman of the Committee was Mr. H.W. Manning, Vice-President and General Manager of the Great-West Life Assurance Company. Members were Dr. C.B. Stewart, Dr. C.H.A. Walton, and Dr. Thomas Lebbetter, who represented the Winnipeg Clinic; and Professor I.M. Thompson, who was a full-time member of the Faculty of Medicine, a member of the board of the Institute, and a member of its Awards Committee. Dr. Thorlakson and Dean Bell also attended meetings of the Committee by invitation.

This committee presented a comprehensive report to the Board of Directors of the Institute on October 15, 1954. The most significant recommendation was that the name of the Institute be changed to identify it more closely with the Winnipeg Clinic. The Committee had considered a number of alternatives and stated its preference for The Winnipeg Clinic Research Foundation.

The directors approved the change of name in principle, subject to the approval of the income tax authorities. Even though the precise wording of a new name had not yet been settled, the members of the Winnipeg Clinic formally expressed their agreement in principle in April 1955; and in November 1955 Mr. MacAulay reported that after he had discussed the matter with the income tax authorities they had agreed that a change of name would not invalidate the status of the Institute as a philanthropic institution to which tax-exempt donations could be made.

Finally, after another year of contemplating the legal and public implications and selecting an acceptable name from among the several that had been suggested, legislation was drafted and, by an act of the Manitoba Legislature on March 30, 1957, a legal transmutation took place, through which the Manitoba Institute for the Advancement of Medical Education and Research became the Winnipeg Clinic Research Institute. The general policies of the Institute remained unchanged.

CONTINUING SUPPORT FOR RESEARCH

Commencing with the 1956–57 session, the undergraduate scholarship for work leading to the B.Sc. (Med.) was increased to $1,200 yearly, payable in two instalments of $600 each for work done in two summer sessions. The Institute allocated $6,000 to cover the awards for a five-year period. This support has continued, with the individual awards increased in 1976 to $1,500, payable in two instalments of $750 each.

At the Awards Committee meeting on November 2, 1955, Dr. Thorlakson suggested that one award be made annually to a rural general practitioner to enable him to attend short-term courses of a specialized nature that would be helpful to him in his practice. The Committee received this proposal with noticeable lack of enthusiasm and concluded that more information was necessary.

The next meeting of the Awards Committee was on November 16, 1955. By this time, the Chairman of the Committee, Dr. Lebbetter, had received a letter from the College of General Practice, Manitoba Chapter, confirming that both the local and the national organizations felt that such an award would be very helpful, and that funds for short-term training of this kind were not available from any other source. Nevertheless, the Awards Committee was loath to endorse these grants. Doubts were expressed about the quality of short courses and also their benefit to the practitioner. It was argued that the College of General Practice (which only recently had received official recognition) did not represent the general practitioners in Manitoba. The Chairman of the Education Committee of the Manitoba Medical Association (who was also a member of the Awards Committee) felt that the Association could fill the needs of general practitioners for postgraduate training, and that funds were available for this purpose. Lengthy discussion in the Awards Committee brought no concensus on the subject.

However, a new opinion seems to have been formed during the ensuing five days, and following the report of the Chairman of the Awards Committee at the meeting of the Board of Directors of the Institute on November 21, "it was resolved and carried unanimously that the sum of $400 be allocated each year for a three-year period to provide for postgraduate education for selected Manitoba general practitioners subject to mutually satisfactory arrangements between the Manitoba Chapter of the College of General Practice of Canada, and the Awards Committee."

The recipient of the award was to be determined by a special committee of the College of General Practice, Manitoba Chapter, under the chairmanship of Dean L.G. Bell.

The project was very well received, and in the period between 1955, when the first award was made to Dr. J.E. Hudson of Hamiota, and 1966, when the final award went to Dr. J. Blain Johnston of Thompson, ten physicians received grants.[9] In 1959, the amount was increased to $500.

The General Practitioner Postgraduate Awards were discontinued in 1966, because it was felt by both the Awards Committee and the Board of Directors that they had accomplished their objective, and that the funds involved should now be utilized in the support of specific research projects.

Dr. Thorlakson had established in 1947 an annual Dr. Neil John Maclean Award in the amount of $100, accompanied by a suitably engraved certificate. The amount was increased to $250 in 1957. For the first eight years, competition for this award was open to physicians on the house staff of the Winnipeg General Hospital who had graduated from the University of Manitoba not more than five years previously. The applicants were required to submit an original paper based on the observation of patients in the hospital or compiled from hospital records.

Although Dr. Thorlakson continued to fund this award personally, its administration was turned over to the Institute in 1955, and members of the house staffs of the Children's Hospital of Winnipeg, St. Boniface General Hospital and Deer Lodge (Veterans) Hospital were declared eligible.

Eighteen doctors received the Dr. Neil John Maclean Award during the nineteen years in which it was offered. Like the award for general practitioners, it was discontinued in 1966.

Special grants of from $250 to $4,000 have been made over the years by the Institute to support projects of members of the Faculty of Medicine to cover immediate needs, ranging through such items as a walk-in refrigerator for cancer research in the biochemical laboratory at St. Boniface General Hospital; a study of kidney tissue with the electron microscope; typing of a book manuscript on respiratory disease; preparation of a colour film on surgical treatment of cancer; and a variety of similar local activities.

The amounts involved were, as a rule, not large. But because they met specific needs to assist worthy projects when no other source of funds was available, they had a value much beyond the actual dollars that were spent.

It is worthy of record that outside the scope of the Institute, Dr. Thorlakson was able in a number of instances to influence the direction of other resources to the support of education and research in the health field. One such example was the James Ross Jenkins Memorial Fund. Ross Jenkins was born and educated in Winnipeg. He joined the T. Eaton Company Limited in Winnipeg in 1935, and at his retirement in 1966 he was the Executive Vice-President and Chief Executive Officer of the Company. He had many community interests, and from 1965 to 1971 was a member of the Winnipeg Clinic Research Institute. After his death in 1972, his family and friends, in consultation with Dr. Thorlakson, felt that a suitable memorial to the life and work of Mr. Jenkins would be the establishment of a fund to provide for an annual symposium on the improvement of health care in the community. The theme, "The Dynamics of the Provision of Health Care," was chosen, and the first annual session was held on September 21, 1974, in the Basic Sciences Building of the Faculty of Medicine. The general public, as well as professionals in the health services, were invited, and more than two hundred attended.

In succeeding years the James Ross Jenkins Memorial Symposia continued, covering such timely subjects as, "Health Care for the Elderly in the 1980s," and "The Provision of Health Care to Remote Communities." Internationally recognized specialists from abroad and from Manitoba have presented papers at the meetings.

Dr. Thorlakson's medical connections in many parts of the

world were helpful in selecting the international guests at the symposia. Those participating in the first three (between 1975 and 1977) included Sir George Godber, former Chief Medical Officer, Department of Health and Social Security, United Kingdom; Dr. M. Prywes, Dean, University of the Negev, Israel; Dr. A. Nody, professor of internal medicine, Tromsø, Norway; and Dr. J.A. Campbell, Chief, Department of Radiology, Martin Luther King General Hospital, Los Angeles, California.

Visiting participants from other parts of Canada have included Dr. J.F. Mustard, Dean, Faculty of Medicine, McMaster University, Hamilton, Ontario; and Dr. D.V. Bates, Dean, Faculty of Medicine, University of British Columbia.

The Winnipeg Clinic Research Institute celebrated its twenty-fifth anniversary in 1968.

In a paper prepared for members of the Institute in recognition of its first quarter century, Dr. Thorlakson noted that the Winnipeg Clinic Research Institute had contributed $188,678 in scholarships, grants and the support of other approved projects since its inception.

CHAPTER 10

A Review of Institute Policies

Meanwhile it had become apparent to Dr. Thorlakson that the sources of public funding for medical research, and the amounts available, had increased materially. This affected the need of the University for additional support from private sources such as the Winnipeg Clinic Research Institute. At the meeting of the Board of Directors of the Winnipeg Clinic Research Institute held on June 28, 1961, he voiced his concerns. He noted that eight years had passed since the Review Committee chaired by Mr. H.W. Manning had made its study of Institute policies and relationships. During this period there had been vast improvements in the funding of research, and in the resources available to medical students. New influences were also affecting the Winnipeg Clinic and the Research Institute. "Twenty years ago," he said, "there was practically no medical research done at the University of Manitoba. Fifteen years ago there were no research scholarships for undergraduate medical students. Now the picture has changed, to the extent that this year approximately $700,000 is available for medical research by the Faculty of Medicine of the University of Manitoba. . . . "

For these reasons, Dr. Thorlakson felt that the position of the Institute, and its future contribution to medical education and research, should be reviewed again. He therefore proposed a resolution, passed unanimously by the Board, that established the Ad Hoc Review Committee, consisting of President H.H. Saunderson, Dean L.G. Bell, Professor I.M. Thompson, and Mr. H.W. Manning, "to study the whole question of the relationship of the Institute, the University of Manitoba, and the Winnipeg Clinic." It was provided in the resolution that the Committee had authority to choose its own chairman, and had power to add to its membership. At its first meeting, Mr. Manning was elected Chairman, and Dr. Thorlakson and Dr. Lebbetter were added to the Committee.

During the ensuing seventeen months, the Committee held seven formal meetings, with full attendance of the members, and had frequent assistance from invited guests who could offer helpful information and advice. The Committee decided, after a searching study of the subject assigned to it, that the purpose should be to build on the accomplishments of past years. Yet it had to be recognized that the public funding of both medical education and research was quite different in 1962 from what it had been in 1943, when the Institute was founded. To utilize in an optimum way the funds then available to the Winnipeg Clinic Research Institute required a change, not in the original objectives of the Institute, but in the means by which its purposes could best be served. In an eight-page paper, the Chairman of the Committee presented its findings to the members and guests at the annual meeting of the Institute on October 11, 1962.

Following a brief reference to the development of the Institute, Mr. Manning informed his audience that the Committee had studied the organization and experience of several other foundations for medical education and research in North America; in particular, the Mayo Foundation for Medical Education and Research in Rochester, Minnesota; the Alton Ochsner Medical Foundation in New Orleans; and the Lovelace Foundation for Medical Education and Research in Albuquerque, New Mexico. His report continued:

> The most intensive study offered us was that of the Mayo Foundation for Medical Education and Research. Dr. Charles F. Code of the Mayo Clinic voluntarily and generously gave us counsel in the morning and afternoon sessions of a committee meeting held on February 17 of this year. Dr. Code is a member of the Board of Governors of the Mayo Clinic, a member of the Postgraduate Committee of the Mayo Foundation and a member of the Joint Graduate Committee between the University of Minnesota and the Mayo Foundation. Dr. Code . . . has an intimate knowledge of our own Institute, the University of Manitoba,

and the Winnipeg Clinic. . . . The following is his specific recommendation to our Institute:

"It would seem wise for the Institute to devote its funds and energies to the development of facilities for research and education within the Winnipeg Clinic; so that if and when a graduate school of medicine is established in the University of Manitoba, research would be in progress in suitable facilities, and training opportunities would be available in the Clinic of such a character that it would be appropriate for the University to use these in graduate training, and to appoint members of the staff of the Clinic to the Graduate Faculty. Simultaneously, the Institute might aid by all possible means the establishment of a graduate school of medicine in the University. . . . "

The opportunity was afforded to have Professor Ian MacLaren Thompson visit the Mayo Clinic, as well as the Tulane University in New Orleans, where he obtained information about the relationship of the Ochsner Clinic to its university. As a result, we have on file a report composed by one with keen perception of the challenges confronting this institute as it attempts [to formulate] a pattern for the next decade. . . .

[Unlike the limited support ot twenty years ago], this year approximately $940,000 is available from various granting bodies for research in the Faculty of Medicine of the University of Manitoba. It is a matter of record that during the initial phase of this tremendous development of interest in medical research and the acquisition of equipment and facilities, the Winnipeg Clinic Research Institute made a worthwhile contribution. . . .

In view of the very large sums of money from national and provincial sources and other private foundations for medical research, and on the other hand the emphasis developing in the area of graduate studies, our deliberations thus far suggest that any expanding financial support from the Winnipeg Clinic Research Institute should be directed toward a graduate program, the responsibility for which would rest with the University. Recently, the Medical Faculty of the University set up a Committee to study the graduate organization, and the Institute might play a useful role by assisting in the financing of this study. The Winnipeg Clinic has increased from seven doctors to fifty-five medical and surgical specialists, most of whom are engaged in teaching, and many of whom are interested in medical research. . . . The Clinic is now capable of providing graduate training in radiology, laboratory medicine, internal medicine, allergy and dermatology. These and other specialties could be integrated into a University graduate program. It would appear, however, that such a function must await [the establishment] of a broadly based graduate program by the University of Manitoba.

From 1945 to 1952 the Winnipeg Clinic carried on a training program for Fellows under limited approval from the Royal College of Physicians and Surgeons of Canada; but because other clinics petitioned the Royal College for similar recognition the College decided to reverse its decision. During a seven-year period, forty-eight graduate students availed themselves of this fellowship training program in the Winnipeg Clinic. . . .

From our investigation of other, similar medical foundations, closely affiliated with large medical clinics, it would appear that the Winnipeg Clinic Research Institute has a dual responsibility; on the one hand to the University of Manitoba, which in the past has received such scholarships, awards and grants as the Institute could afford,[1] and on the other hand, to the Winnipeg Clinic, its professional staff and its expanding facilities. . . .

We are impressed by the substantial contributions the Mayo Clinic, the Lahey Clinic, the Cleveland Clinic and the Ochsner Clinic have made to medical science and graduate medical education. These . . . have been made possible by the financial support these clinics have had from their research foundations. The Winnipeg Clinic should likewise have financial support from its research institute. Our institute should assist the Clinic in developing its research and in continuing to support the Faculty of Medicine in its graduate and undergraduate teaching.

The Review Committee concluded that scholarships for undergraduate students at the University of Manitoba should continue to be funded on recommendation of the Awards Committee.

With respect to future policy, the Committee agreed that the University should be the "focal organization for medical education and research in this community." However, they thought that it was important for the University to provide "leadership, advice and encouragement" for all medical education and research activities in the community, and not restrict its interest and support to institutions at present affiliated with the University. Among these additional institutions could be the private clinics that are actively engaged in supporting the University's teaching and research program.

Of special importance, the Committee proposed that in future the Institute should support graduate medical education in the

University, its affiliated hospitals, and in the Winnipeg Clinic. They also submitted that "the Institute should support research within the Winnipeg Clinic, utilizing the extensive resources that have been developed by the Clinic over the past twenty years."

The Review Committee Report was accepted in principle by resolution of the members of the Winnipeg Clinic Research Institute, and referred to the directors for detailed study and appropriate action.

This decision aroused a flurry of discussion at the Faculty of Medicine, and among the members of the Winnipeg Clinic. Dr. Thorlakson asked Dr. D.D. Gellman, an internist at the Clinic, to prepare a memorandum describing the current research being done by Clinic doctors, whether at the Clinic, the University, or a hospital. Some suggestions were to be included as to research projects that might be undertaken at the Winnipeg Clinic if funds became available. The cost of initiating such a program was to be estimated.

With the Vice-President of the Institute, Dean L.G. Bell, acting as chairman, the Board of Directors held a special meeting on December 19, 1962, to explore the new developments that should be undertaken in the spirit of the recommendations by the Review Committee.[2]

Dr. Thorlakson presented the Gellman memorandum as a basis for discussion. This included an estimate of between $31,000 and $52,000 as an initial requirement to provide a chairman of research and two associates, a full-time immunologist, and some basic equipment. Dr. Saunderson pointed out that the budget did not provide for the one and a half or two technicians that were required for every professional carrying on research. After discussion, it was concluded that probably an additional $20,000 might be necessary to pay the salaries of five technicians. Dr. Saunderson also thought that projects in immunology were expensive; work was already being done in this field by the University; and perhaps some less costly studies should be undertaken in the beginning.

Dr. Thorlakson reminded the Board that the Institute income from rent was primarily used to pay off the cost of the buildings, and it would be twenty years or more before any substantial sum could be expected from this source to support research. Any immediate funds would have to come from private donations or from development of the Winnipeg Clinic Annex property.

Mr. Manning reported on his enquiries in New York about the potential for grants from American foundations. The possibility of obtaining sponsors for research such as drug manufacturers was touched on; and it was finally concluded that Messrs. Smith and Manning would be constituted as a committee (with power to add) to examine the possibilities of raising the money necessary to carry out the Review Committee recommendations.

Almost two years passed before the next meeting of the Institute's Board of Directors. At this meeting, which was held on November 4, 1964, Dr. Thorlakson presented a report on steps taken by the Winnipeg Clinic Research Committee in the intervening period:

> The Winnipeg Clinic . . . is beginning to labour under some considerable difficulty in maintaining the high standard of medical services that were envisioned by its founder over twenty-five years ago. During this time we have been able to recruit to our staff highly trained specialists with many years of experience. Because of increasing financial inducements and other professional advantages we have lost some of these men to universities. To be specific, one of our senior associates, whom I interviewed personally in London eleven years ago, has recently accepted an appointment with the University of Manitoba at a salary of $17,000 a year. In addition, he will receive income from the Winnipeg General Hospital and will likely be permitted to participate in competitive private practice up to an amount of $25,000 a year. He is worth every dollar of this amount to his community when we take into account his long years of training, his professional qualifications, and his new responsibilities. But in private practice, because of the high overhead of thirty-five to forty-five percent to purchase and maintain expensive equipment and retain technical personnel, in order to earn this amount a doctor would have to place on his books for collection about $50,000 worth of medical services. I can tell you from personal experience that it represents a great deal of hard and difficult work, including night work and weekend work, to earn this income on the present Manitoba Medical Services fee schedule, with its thirty percent reduction from the minimum schedule of fees. [Reference is to the doctor-sponsored medical service prepayment plan, known as the Manitoba Medical Services Plan.] The doctors of the Winnipeg Clinic are all working under this financial handicap.[3]

I present this information to the Board not as a complaint but as an indication of the challenge which our two organizations have to meet if we are to continue to bring young men of great promise and ability to this community and to the Winnipeg Clinic.

My long years of active association with the Faculty of Medicine of the University of Manitoba and the public charity service of the Winnipeg General Hospital has taught me to appreciate the need for highly qualified, well-paid, properly motivated, research-minded teachers on our Faculty of Medicine. The quality of the practice of medicine in the future . . . will only be as good as the teaching of medicine today. The University of Manitoba must continually upgrade its teaching staff and improve its training and research facilities because of the rapid advances in medical science. It must also be able to hold the part-time teachers now engaged in active medical practice. No medical school in Canada could survive without the part-time teachers – private practitioners of medicine selected because of their interest in medical education. Equally important is the fact that these doctors are in constant touch with the problems of private practice outside of hospitals and the University laboratories. This is the type of practice medical students should be trained for. If these part-time teachers are not deliberately and actively encouraged, the University's Faculty of Medicine will soon lose contact with the practicing profession, and the medical students will suffer as a result.

I have in my hands two letters from highly trained specialists in medicine, one from England and one from Canada, who were interviewed recently in the hope that they would join the Winnipeg Clinic staff. Both of these men want to come to Winnipeg but declined because they did not see any immediate opportunity of pursuing their research activities either in the Winnipeg Clinic, where there are no special facilities as yet, or at the University of Manitoba because from interviews with members of the investigative units they were not encouraged to believe that they would be included as part-time workers in the research being done by the geographic full-time members of the Faculty of Medicine.

This is a practical illustration of two problems which face the Winnipeg Clinic and the Winnipeg Clinic Research Institute:

1. The opportunity for doing part-time research work is an important factor to highly skilled young doctors. It is a means of attracting such men to the staff of the Winnipeg Clinic.

2. The Faculty of Medicine of the University of Manitoba is apparently unable to include some of these doctors in the investigative units in the teaching hospitals.

For all these reasons, I submit that there is an *urgent* need to provide a new incentive which will encourage the doctors of the Winnipeg Clinic to continue to carry their share of responsibility in the field of medical education, which they now do as part-time members of the Faculty of Medicine of the University of Manitoba and as members of the honorary attending staff of the teaching hospitals. Facilities and funds must also be provided to allow some of its members to pursue their interest in medical research.

The close relationship existing between the Winnipeg Clinic Research Institute and the Winnipeg Clinic provides us with a unique opportunity to foster the academic and scientific aspects of medicine as well as its day-to-day practical application. . . .

I do not need to take your time by quoting extensively from the experience in other comparable private medical clinics on this continent and what they have said about research activities in their respective groups. However, Dr. C.E. Jackson of the Caylor-Nickel Clinic in Indiana, has summarized their experience by saying, "Our research program has improved our medical practice; . . . it has been a factor in attracting good, well-trained young physicians in our group. . . . The good records maintained by those in group practice also tend to promote long term types of study." Over twenty years ago at one of the first meetings of the Winnipeg Clinic Research Institute and earlier at one of the first meetings of the Winnipeg Clinic I emphasized that every successful medical organization (i.e., successful in providing the greatest help to its patients) should also participate in medical education and research, because these are the cornerstones of medical progress. It is recognized that the end result of all these activities is to assist in the development of the highest quality of medical care for every patient, not only in the Winnipeg Clinic but also in the whole community.

While the Winnipeg Clinic Research Committee has been actively studying ways and means of establishing medical research in the Winnipeg Clinic on an organized basis, the members of the Clinic have been considering a proposal made to them in 1963. That year I submitted a recommendation that the Winnipeg Clinic (Incorporated) transfer to the Institute the valuable property on the corner of St. Mary Avenue and Kennedy Street, which has a current value of almost a quarter of a million dollars, and also transfer to the Institute the physical assets and the accumulated financial reserves of the Winnipeg Clinic Pharmacy. The legal implications of this proposal are now being examined by Mr. John A. MacAulay and his associate, Mr. R.J. Hansell.

On December 19, 1962, I presented to the directors a proposed research budget which consisted of $10,000 to $20,000 for basic equipment, a similar amount for a specialist in medical research, and approximately $20,000 to cover loss of income by members [of the Clinic] doing part-time research. This would mean an annual expenditure for the first five years of from $30,000 to $50,000. It is my hope that the proposal I have made to the members of the Winnipeg Clinic, when approved, will go a long way towards reaching this objective.

At the meeting of the Board of Directors on December 16, 1964, it was reported that Mr. MacAulay and Mr. Hansell had discussed the property transfer with Mr. J.W. Abbott, auditor for the Winnipeg Clinic, and they had concluded that the transfer should not be made at that time. The Executive Council of the Winnipeg Clinic had agreed to donate $5,000 from the Pharmacy to the Institute by way of the Winnipeg Clinic (Incorporated), in addition to $1,900 that had already been donated in 1964. Similar amounts would be donated early in 1965, making a total of about $14,000; and this, together with an accumulated amount of about $7,000 in interest in the Dougall Trust Fund[4] and a personal donation from Dr. Thorlakson, would provide about $22,000 to provide a research capability at the Winnipeg Clinic.

Dr. Thorlakson went on to report that Dr. Samuel B. Hrushovetz had enquired about a research position at the Winnipeg Clinic. He was a graduate in medicine from the University of Manitoba, had a master's degree in biochemistry from the University of Alberta and a Ph.D. in cytogenetics and plant pathology from the University of Toronto. He was at that time engaged in research at the University of Saskatchewan on behalf of the National Research Council, with a stipend of $10,000 a year. He had made a favourable impression on those at the Winnipeg Clinic who interviewed him.

In response to an enquiry from one of the directors of the Institute, Dr. Thorlakson reported that on behalf of the Board, Mr. J. Elmer Woods (also a Board member) was investigating the use to be made of the three lots at the corner of St. Mary Avenue and Kennedy Street. These were presently held in the name of the Winnipeg Clinic (Incorporated). Mr. Woods reported that if the property were to be developed for a substantial client with whom he was negotiating, an important factor in completing the deal would be that the revenue would be used for the advancement of medical education and research in the Province of

Manitoba, and not to benefit a private corporation. He was assured that the property would be transferred to the Institute.

At this meeting, the board of directors of the Institute gave unanimous approval in principle to the expenditure of $35,000 to set up a research laboratory at the Winnipeg Clinic. It was also agreed that if qualified research staff became available, the directors would assist in developing a method of raising the necessary money to support them.

The exciting project of establishing a new research laboratory went forward rapidly. Dr. B.B. Fast was appointed Chairman of the Winnipeg Clinic Research Committee. Dr. Hrushovetz was appointed Director of the Laboratory. Special research laboratory equipment had been purchased at an approximate cost of $28,000. "And," reported Dr. Thorlakson to the Board, "we have $21,000 to pay for it!" Efforts made to obtain grants of fifteen or twenty thousand dollars from the Kellogg Foundation and the National Cancer Institute were unsuccessful. It was apparent that the most secure way to deal with the funding problem would be to turn the Kennedy Street lots into revenue-bearing property.

To this end, Mr. Woods reported that a plan was under way to construct a building on the property which could be leased to the Provincial Government for thirty years and house the Manitoba Health Services Commission. However, after a meeting with Dr. Thorlakson, Mr. Woods, and Mr. Harris, Premier Roblin remained unconvinced that the Province should enter into such an arrangement. Dr. Thorlakson pointed out that in future discussions with the Premier, it would be important to emphasize that the revenue would go to support medical education and research.

In the meantime, Dr. Bruce Chown had made an urgent appeal to the Winnipeg Clinic Research Institute for a grant to support a highly qualified research worker in the Rh Laboratory to make possible an important new facet of their work. For this he needed, almost immediately, $3,750.

This came at a time when, of course, the Institute was facing its own financial problems. However, Dr. Thorlakson described to the Board the importance of the work being done in the Rh Laboratory, its wide recognition by both medical scientists and clinicians, and the need to meet this request.

Since the Institute itself did not have the funds, it is a tribute to the sense of community responsibility on the part of the members of the Board that the minutes carry the following record: "It was moved by Mr. H.E. Sellers, seconded by Dr. Thorlakson, and unanimously resolved that the Institute would obtain $3,750 for the purpose requested by Dr. Bruce Chown." There is little doubt that the money was raised by personal contributions from a group of Board members.

A similar action was taken at the annual meeting of the Institute on October 21, 1965, when it was reported that the estimated deficit of the Winnipeg Clinic Research Laboratory for the three-year period to June 30, 1968, would be $35,000. A committee was formed to consider ways and means of raising this money, with J. Elmer Woods as Chairman, and C. Gordon Smith and Joseph Harris as members. Their solution was to write a letter to members of the Institute: " . . . In our opinion the $35,000 we are required to raise is too small a sum to approach a wide cross section of business people. In any event we feel we should first approach the forty members of the Institute. Donations can be spread over two or three years. We know that it is not necessary to try to explain the desirability of setting up this research laboratory and that you will agree that those of us who are familiar with the objective of the Research Institute should be given the first opportunity to participate in the costs." The fundraising went forward smoothly and succcessfully.

The Winnipeg Clinic Research Institute Laboratory was opened in July 1965, with Dr. Hrushovetz as its Director, and Dr. D.D. Gellman as Chairman of the Winnipeg Clinic Research Committee.

In 1968 the Executive Council of the Winnipeg Clinic formally requested that the space used by the Research Laboratory be relinquished to the Clinic for use as a clinical laboratory. By this time research facilities had been expanded at the University through the establishment of the Institute of Cell Biology. In light of these developments it was agreed that the research laboratory would be discontinued.

In 1975 the Board once more asked for a review of the aims and objectives of the Institute. The Review Committee met under the chairmanship of Mr. Robert P. Purves. Concerns had been expressed, notably by Dr. Bruce Chown, a founding member of the Board, about a possible contraction of the activities required to fulfill the original purposes of the Institute. Following the study by the Review Committee, the Board re-affirmed its acceptance of an obligation to support, as resources allowed, high-quality scientific research, both basic and applied.

CHAPTER 11

The Paul H.T. Thorlakson Research Foundation

The annual meeting of the Winnipeg Clinic Research Institute on May 18, 1978, celebrated the thirty-fifth anniversary of the Institute.

It was an occasion for recognizing the foresight of Dr. Thorlakson in conceiving the Institute as a vehicle for the support of medical education and research in Manitoba.

After paying tribute to Dr. Thorlakson's devotion to the development of the Institute throughout its existence, the Chairman of the Board, Mr. Albert Cohen, announced the creation of The Paul H.T. Thorlakson Research Foundation in his honour, to which $200,000 had already been subscribed. The objective would be to preserve the capital funds for a minimum of ten years. The earnings would be disbursed annually for approved medical research projects. It need hardly be said that this announcement was greeted by an enthusiastic ovation from the audience.

Mr. Cohen read a letter of greeting from The Honourable L.R. (Bud) Sherman, then Minister of Health and Social Development for the Province of Manitoba. Mr. Sherman said, in part:

> Because the Institute has given so much to Manitoba, it is fitting on its 35th Anniversary that the Province join others in saluting the man who made its valuable services possible, Dr. Paul H.T. Thorlakson. "Dr. Thor," as he is known by countless friends and associates, recognized an unmet need many years ago. As a private citizen with a vision, who had the wisdom and energy to work towards its fulfillment,

he laid the groundwork for an enduring and important addition to the life of Manitoba. For this achievement, Dr. Thorlakson richly deserves our honour and gratitude. I believe the creation of the new Foundation, to be named after him, that will carry on the work he saw as being beneficial to us all, is an appropriate way to show him that we know his vision was clear and we are eternally in his debt for making it a reality.

On behalf of my colleagues in the Government of Manitoba, I extend to the Institute and to Dr. Thorlakson our sincere congratulations on this milestone in the history of medical research and education, and our very best wishes for the future.

Greetings from the University of Manitoba were expressed by Dr. D. Ralph Campbell:

I am delighted to bring greetings from the University of Manitoba. . . . Members of the University of Manitoba have participated over the years in the activities of the Institute, both as supporters and as beneficiaries. Many of the current members of the Faculty, including Dean Naimark and one of the most recently elected Fellows of the Royal Society of Canada, Dr. Henry G. Friesen, have been supported by this Institute.

I am particularly pleased to pay tribute to Dr. Thorlakson, the motivating genius behind the Winnipeg Clinic Research Institute from the beginning and an outstanding citizen of this Province. Dr. Thorlakson's contributions to medical science, medical services, and the welfare of the Province generally, are quite outstanding.

Dr. Arnold Naimark, Dean of the Faculty of Medicine of the University of Manitoba, presented Dr. Thorlakson with a plaque inscribed as follows:

Dr. Paul Thorlakson will be remembered by future generations for his role in establishing Winnipeg as a leading medical centre. He recognized from the outset that modern medical care depends on the advancement of medical science and he was instrumental in the development of young scientists as part of the fabric of the medical profession in Manitoba.

The existence of the Winnipeg Clinic Research Institute is a continuing manifestation at the local level of Dr. Thorlakson's high ideals and dedication to the pursuit of excellence. Beyond Manitoba, as a member of the first Committee on Medical Research of the National Research Council, with Sir Frederick Banting, he promoted active programs of medical research in the western provinces and continues to champion the cause of medical research to this day.

In his acknowledgement of these tributes, Dr. Thorlakson spoke in part as follows:

> This evening I find myself the recipient of a most unique honour – an honour which I consider to be also a tribute to my family, to my friends, and to my professional associates who have helped me along the way. One person, in particular, deserves equal credit for anything I may have achieved and that is my wife Gladys. . . .
>
> [The] early contact and association with Sir Frederick [Banting] forty years ago, prompted me to enter into discussions concerning medical research with the University of Manitoba and its Faculty of Medicine, as well as with doctors and leading citizens in Winnipeg. These discussions persuaded me to divest myself of ownership of the Winnipeg Clinic building, and the property on which it stands, in order to create the nucleus of a foundation around which local financial support could be generated. . . .
>
> For me, there could be no happier way of marking the thirty-fifth anniversary of the Winnipeg Clinic Research Institute than to have my early efforts in supporting medical research culminated by the establishment of this new foundation, which will also support medical education and research in my Alma Mater, the University of Manitoba.

Two and a half years later another memorable event was organized by the members of the Foundation Board. On Monday, October 20, 1980, more than three hundred friends of Dr. and Mrs. Thorlakson gathered for dinner at the Fort Garry Hotel to (as the invitation read) "recognize the contribution to our community of Dr. Paul H.T. Thorlakson, C.C."

Hosts for the occasion were The Honourable Douglas D. Everett, President, The Honourable W. John McKeag, Vice-President, and the Board of Directors of the Winnipeg Clinic Research Institute and the Paul H.T. Thorlakson Research Foundation. The date was chosen to mark Dr. Thorlakson's eighty-fifth birthday, which had occurred on October 5, 1980; and the sixtieth wedding anniversary which he and Gladys would celebrate on November 20.

Dr. Charles F. Code, who had been involved at times of special importance in the life of the Clinic and the Institute in times past, came from California to address the guests. Representatives of government and the community paid tribute to Dr. Thorlakson, and a group of his friends chose the occasion to

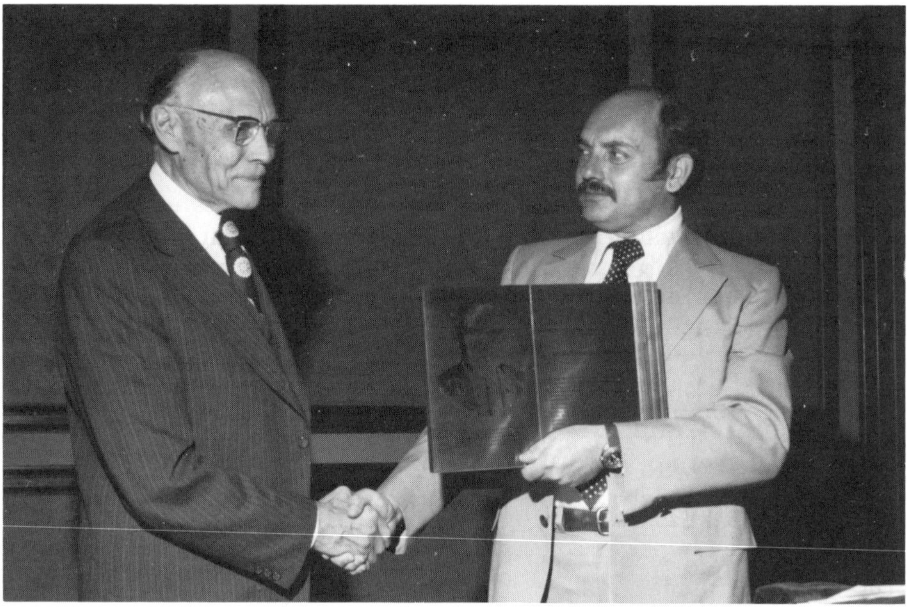

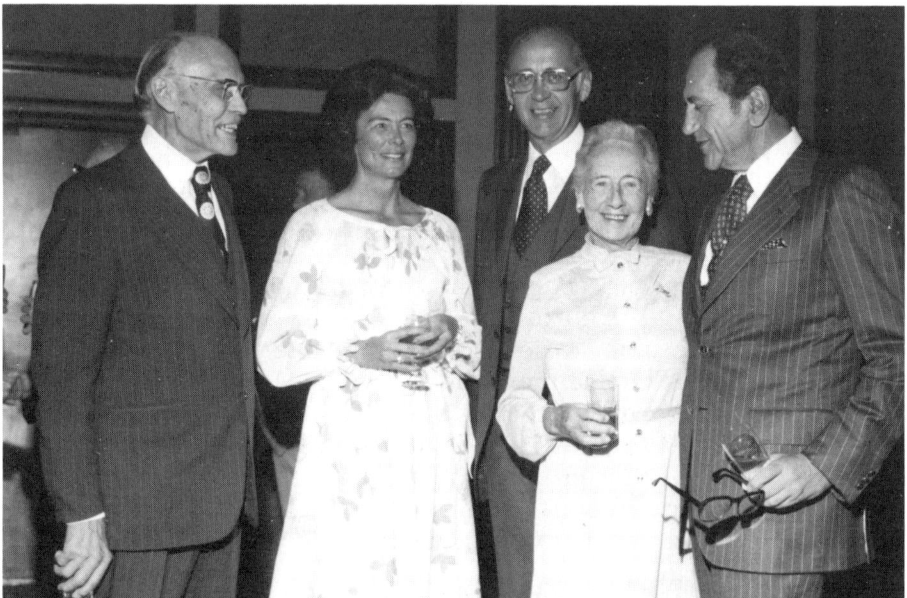

At the thirty-fifth anniversary meeting of the Winnipeg Clinic Research Institute on May 18, 1978, Dr. Arnold Naimark, then Dean of the Faculty of Medicine and later President of the University of Manitoba, presented Dr. Thorlakson with a bronze plaque paying tribute to his lifelong support for medical research.

Mr. Albert Cohen, Chairman of the Board of the Winnipeg Clinic Research Institute, at the thirty-fifth anniversary meeting on May 18, 1978, announced the founding of the Paul H.T. Thorlakson Research Foundation Inc., to which $200,000 had already been subscribed. Conversing after the meeting are Dr. Thorlakson, George and Tannis Richardson, Mrs. Thorlakson and Mr. Cohen.

make a gift of $100,000 to the Paul H.T. Thorlakson Foundation.

Among the distinguished guests at the head table was Manitoba's Chief Justice Samuel Freedman, a man highly esteemed for his qualities of mind and person, for his wisdom in the administration of justice, and for his eloquence as a speaker on occasions of ceremony and celebration.

As the events of the evening moved to a conclusion, the chairman called upon Chief Justice Freedman to introduce the guest of honour. He did so with these words:

I am pleased to have been asked to perform this very pleasant assignment. In my day I have had some very interesting experiences with regard to being asked to perform certain functions.

Some years ago a ladies' organization was planning to have a bazaar, and for this bazaar they needed a master of ceremonies. The ladies met in executive session for the purpose of selecting a master of ceremonies. Someone proposed the name of Sam Freedman. One of the other ladies said, "Oh, he would never accept. It's not in his line." The proposer said, "I'm not sure. I think he would accept it." That started a merry debate, some saying he would accept, some saying he would not accept, until the chairman, who knew her rules of order, said, "Girls, what are we arguing about? Let's put it to a vote. How many think he would accept? How many think he would not accept?" The question was solemnly and formally put. The majority decided that I would not accept, and I was not asked.

Because our guest of honour is a distinguished surgeon, I may perhaps be permitted a quick story or two about surgeons and surgery.

What is the difference between surgery and legal advocacy? I suggest one clear difference. When the lawyer in court is about to conclude his presentation, he turns to his assistant and asks, "Have I left anything out?" [Laughter in the audience.] I see that I do not have to complete this story.

Then there was the surgeon who, when called upon to operate on Lucius Beebe, the famous connoisseur of wine, postponed the incision for two hours so that Beebe could be opened at room temperature.

History is the biography of great men, Carlyle tells us; and in the history of our country, the life, career and accomplishments of Dr. Paul H.T. Thorlakson stand forth in shining splendour. Many have been the areas he has entered, and wherever he has gone he has served with conspicuous distinction. His eminence in the field of medicine is universally recognized and acknowledged. But that is only one part of this man. Surely another part is his contribution to the field of education, whether it be as the organizer and leader of several conferences of education – both at the provincial and the Canadian level – or as an outstanding chancellor of a distinguished university. In an age when the academic debate continues on the so-called two cultures of science and the humanities and of the lack of effective communication between them, Dr. Thorlakson walks with sure foot in both fields, being at once an illustrious man of science as well as a true lover of the humanities. Truly this is a man whose life has been starred with greatness, whose career at so many points has touched the superlative. I do not intend this evening to recite to you the many and varied activities which illuminate the curriculum vitae of Dr. Thorlakson. They are far too numerous for a short introduction, especially when the hour is late and when, like an Egyptian mummy, we are pressed for time. Rather, let me touch on just a few aspects of Thor's remarkable career.

I will divide my treatment in two – the doctor, and the man.

1. The Doctor: It was the year 1919 when our guest of honour received his medical degree from the University of Manitoba. That was sixty-one years ago – and truly they have been crowded, tumultuous, creative years. The problem I face is this: what to select, and what to omit?

A. Let me go back to 1938, when Thor became a member of the first Medical Research Committee of the National Research Council of Canada, under the chairmanship of Sir Frederick Banting, an office which he held over the next seven years.

B. In 1954–55, we see him as Surgeon-in-Chief, Winnipeg General Hospital, followed by his appointment as Professor of Surgery, University of Manitoba Medical Faculty.

C. I move back a bit to 1938, the year when Thor founded the Winnipeg Clinic; and to 1943 when he became the first President of the Winnipeg Clinic Research Institute. That incidentally (1943) was when Dr. Thorlakson transferred to the Research Institute – as an outright gift – his ownership of the properties and buildings of the Winnipeg Clinic.

D. In 1951 we see Thor as President of the National Cancer Institute of Canada.

E. In 1970 he was the President and General Chairman of the First International Congress on Group Medicine. He started this, and I am glad to say that this International Congress has been continued triennially ever since. The list of Thor's accomplishments in his profession is virtually endless. As doctor, author, medical trailblazer, Thor's record possesses a radiance of its own.

2. The Man: Let me say a few words about Thor, the man, the exemplar of the good citizen. Many centuries ago a great Rabbi said, "If I am only for myself, what am I?" Dr. Thorlakson has never been only for himself. The effort of his life has consistently been directed outwards – towards making the world about him a little better, a little happier, a little more civilized. That the effort was crowned with success is attested to by an unending series of great honours that others have bestowed upon him. Here are some of them:

A. Commander of the Order of the Falcon, conferred by the Government of Iceland.

B. National Human Relations Award, conferred by the Canadian Council of Christians and Jews.

C. Honourary Degrees bestowed upon him by the University of Manitoba, the University of Iceland, Brandon University, the University of Winnipeg.

D. Chairman of the Campaign Committee which founded the chair of Icelandic Language and Literature at the University of Manitoba.

E. Companion of the Order of Canada, a distinction limited at any one time to fifty Canadians. (This was perhaps the highest of all honours, conferred in 1970.)

So tonight we salute a great doctor and a great human being. Others have already mentioned two things: that Dr. Thor has just had his eighty-fifth birthday; and that he and his wife stand on the threshold of their sixtieth wedding anniversary. Let me add that we honour Thor not for the quantity of his years but for the quality of his daily life. But as he looks back on those years the events of tonight must surely be one of sanctified memories, of glorious reminiscences, of brave hopes fulfilled.

From the depths of a full heart, Dr. Thorlakson expressed his gratitude, and that of Gladys and their family, for the kind and generous words and messages, and the honour, that had been his portion on this memorable evening; and he extended his appreciation in the warmest terms to those who had created the Paul H.T. Thorlakson Research Foundation.

* * *

Presidents
of the
Manitoba Institute for the Advancement of Medical Education and Research,
Winnipeg Clinic Research Institute
and (since 1978)
The Paul H.T. Thorlakson Research Foundation

Dr. Paul H.T. Thorlakson, 1943 to 1945
Mr. H.E. Sellers, 1946 to 1950
Mr. W.A. Murphy, 1951 to 1956
Mr. Victor Sifton, 1957 to 1960
Mr. Joseph Harris, 1961 to 1968
Mr. C. Gordon Smith, 1969 to 1974
Mr. Albert Cohen, 1975 to 1980
Senator Douglas D. Everett, 1981 to 1983
Hon. W. John McKeag, 1984
Mr. William E. Shields, 1985 to –

PART FOUR

A Medical Centre for Manitoba

CHAPTER 12

Manitoba Medical Centre: A Glimpse of History

The Manitoba-Medical-Centre concept evolved from an idea born in the mind of Dr. Thorlakson in 1942 about the time the Winnipeg Clinic began its operation in the new two-storey building on Vaughan Street. Dr. Thorlakson thus became the moving spirit in a whole series of events that brought about a new approach to the delivery of hospital services in Manitoba. Three institutions in the health field also played important parts: the Faculty of Medicine of the University of Manitoba, the Winnipeg General Hospital and the Children's Hospital of Winnipeg. Several other health facilities had lesser roles. A brief note on the history of these institutions provides the necessary perspective for understanding how some of the changes occurred.

THE MEDICAL COLLEGE

In 1882, serious discussion began in Winnipeg about the need for a school of medicine in Manitoba. At that time, young men wishing to enter the medical profession had to go to Toronto or Montreal (or the United States) for their education – a long and arduous journey and a burdensome expense to their parents for the three or four years this training required. A number of local doctors were keenly interested in changing this situation.[1] As a consequence, in the summer of 1883, thirteen Manitoba physicians applied to the Manitoba Legislature for a charter that would enable them to establish a medical college in Winnipeg. This was granted on April 20, 1884.

It was typical of the pioneering spirit of Manitobans that the founders of the College did not feel it necessary to await the final word from the legislature to get their project under way. The College actually began its teaching program on November 15, 1883, when the newly appointed Dean, Dr. James Kerr, gave an introductory address to the first student class, the members of the faculty, and interested members of the profession. With the cooperation of the Winnipeg School Board, the first lectures were given in the Central School Building, at 567 Bannatyne Avenue, where the Hugh John Macdonald school now stands; and the first classes in anatomy were given in a cottage on Isabel Street. The following year, with funds almost entirely furnished by members of the faculty, a building was erected at the corner of McDermot Avenue and Kate Street which was ready in time to accommodate the second session of the College. The College (unlike many of its counterparts elsewhere) was affiliated with the University of Manitoba from the very beginning.[2] The first graduating class of six students received their degrees from the University Chancellor, Archbishop Robert Machray, in May 1886.

The number of registrants in the Medical College increased steadily, and the original building was soon too small to accommodate the teaching requirements. The members of the faculty subscribed funds to provide a new building at the corner of Bannatyne Avenue and Emily Street, the first section of which opened in 1906.[3] With substantial additions, alterations and renovations, the College has remained on this site to the present time.

With the 1918–19 session the Manitoba Medical College as a separate institution ceased to exist. Its trustees made a gift of its property and equipment to the University of Manitoba "on condition that the University establish a Faculty of Medicine and carry on the work of medical education in an efficient manner."[4]

THE WINNIPEG GENERAL HOSPITAL

From the time of the founding of the Medical College, the primary centre for clinical teaching had been the Winnipeg General Hospital. Opened in 1870, the Hospital had moved to its present site in 1883–84, occupying a new building, part of which was still in operation in 1942 as Wards A and B.[5] In 1953, Dr. Thorlakson wrote:

> From its very beginning, [the Hospital] has supported medical teaching and research beyond the limit of its financial ability. During this long period, one-third to one-half (actually seventy-six percent in 1931) of its beds have been under the control of the heads of departments of the Medical Faculty, for the treatment of indigent patients from Winnipeg and the Province. In fact, the men who created and those who have developed the Medical College over the past eight decades have, very largely, been the same individuals who have contributed to the development of the General Hospital. These two institutions have, therefore, been very closely associated and have complemented each other in supplying the people of the Province of Manitoba, and a great part of western Canada, with medical education facilities as well as specialized diagnostic and medical care. It is usual for the heads of departments of the University Faculty to be chiefs of their respective departments in the Winnipeg General Hospital.

Although the Faculty of Medicine and the Winnipeg General Hospital had been successful in attracting a medical staff of high quality – many with national and international reputations in their specialties – the Hospital had suffered in its financial and administrative affairs. Particularly during the Depression decade of the 1930s, a major portion of its beds had been devoted to the care of indigent patients for whom the municipal and provincial payments did not cover the cost of the service. Because so many people could not afford to pay for medical care, the Out-Patient Department was crowded with patients, and the Hospital's cost for this service was not included in the per diem rate paid by government agencies for indigent in-patients. The doctors served in the Department without charging fees.

The Hospital was constantly plagued by income deficiencies for both operating and capital expense at a time when advances in medical knowledge required sophisticated equipment and skilled technical staff. By 1942 the need for major renovation and rebuilding was a matter of pressing concern.

THE CHILDREN'S HOSPITAL OF WINNIPEG

At the same time, the Children's Hospital of Winnipeg, which had occupied its three-storey building on Aberdeen Avenue in North Winnipeg since 1912, had an urgent need to renovate and expand its facilities, or to replace them entirely. They had insufficient space to accommodate patient needs. The Out-Patient Clinic and waiting room areas were seriously overcrowded. Heating, laundry, elevator and other service equipment was rapidly becoming obsolete. New program requirements could not be provided because of lack of space.[6]

OTHER FACILITIES

The Grace General Hospital, operated by the Salvation Army, also was faced in 1942 with the problem of inadequate facilities to meet demands. This hospital was located on Arlington Street just south of Portage Avenue, in a solidly built-up residential area, on a relatively small and closely circumscribed site. Their requirement for expansion presented a particularly difficult problem. Should they try to deal with it within the constraints of their present site, or look for a more suitable location?

Similarly, on the near north side of the city, the Sisters who operated the St. Joseph's Hospital on an even more cramped site on Salter Street found themselves faced with a need for modernization and expansion which would be impossible to accomplish on their small property. To continue their highly respected hospital service, they would have to relocate.

Finally, the student enrolment in the Faculty of Medicine had grown steadily, and in 1942 there were 279 in the undergraduate classes. This created pressure for additional accommodation not only in the Medical College, but in the hospitals in which the clinical training was provided.

CHAPTER 13

A New Concept is Born

"Where there is no vision the people perish," says the ancient proverb. But if a man's vision is to shape the course of human events, it must be matched by his conviction that the vision is worthy of becoming a reality; by a steadfast confidence in the persuasive power of his purpose; and by a resolve to dedicate his integrity, perseverance and enthusiasm to its accomplishment. He must be prepared to risk being misunderstood; and to patiently nurture the insight and support of others who are willing to become partners in the enterprise. All these qualities were evoked in full measure in the evolution of the Manitoba Medical Centre.

During the summer of 1942 all the present and future difficulties that were perceived to be threatening Manitoba's medical services were the subject of countless discussions in hospital boardrooms, at medical gatherings and in government offices. In the course of his busy days, Dr. Thorlakson listened to widely varying assessments of the problems, and opinions and counter-opinions as to their solutions. As one deeply involved in the standards, organization and supply of private practice medical care, and at the same time fully cognizant of the importance of adequate teaching facilities, he pondered the disparate views. To him, there seemed to be a common thread running through the discussions, a thread that might lead to a collective solution. On the one hand, several hospitals had a pressing need to renovate and expand their facilities, but in three instances there were difficulties in doing this at their present locations.

On the other hand, the Medical College needed to expand its clinical teaching base and improve its potential for graduate and undergraduate education. From both points of view, shortages of funds made it imperative to spend money in the most advantageous manner, and this might be accomplished by the sharing of special diagnostic and support services.

From this point, it was a short step to the idea that several needs could be fulfilled and many difficulties could be resolved by grouping the Children's, Grace and St. Joseph's hospitals, along with other health care facilities not yet identified, around the Medical College and adjacent to the Winnipeg General Hospital. Each hospital would retain its full autonomy and responsibility for its own management, finance and service programs. The medical staff organization of each would be preserved. Specialized diagnostic services and common support facilities, such as the heating plant and laundry, could be shared. Opportunities for graduate and continuing education would be enhanced. The availability and the convenience of specialist consultations in the group of institutions might improve the quality of patient care.

To Dr. Thorlakson, these ideas were exciting and challenging. He recognized that they would be disturbing to some; that they would, if implemented, engender arguments about priorities and powers; that very large capital sums would have to be raised and expended according to a master plan over a lengthy time period; and that an immense effort would have to be made to bring about a broad interest in cooperating in this complex endeavour. Dr. Thorlakson recalls:

> During the early autumn of 1942, I met Mr. W.A. Murphy, Chairman of the Board of Trustees of the Winnipeg General Hospital, in one of the hospital corridors. I told him that I had been developing an idea, and wished to discuss it with him.
>
> We met at his home during the next weekend and I presented him with an outline of my ideas. I suggested that we should deal with the current problems of the Winnipeg General Hospital in the light of a new concept, specifically, that of developing a Manitoba medical centre as a postwar project. At that first meeting I said that the Medical College, the Winnipeg General Hospital, the Central Tuberculosis Clinic, the Cancer Foundation and the Provincial Laboratory could form the nucleus of a future Manitoba Medical Centre.

Mr. Murphy presented the plan to the Board of Trustees of the Winnipeg General Hospital at its next meeting, which I was invited to attend. The Board authorized me to make some preliminary enquiries, particularly about the possibility that the Children's Hospital might move to the centre, since it was thought that this should be our first step.

During the thirty years since the Children's Hospital had moved into its Aberdeen Avenue buildings there had been a substantial change in space and design requirements for hospitals. There were good arguments to be made for constructing an entirely new building to meet their expanding role as a treatment centre for the special needs of children, not only in Manitoba, but also for large parts of Saskatchewan and western Ontario.

Dr. Thorlakson's plan saw this development taking place in a new hospital to be built in the proposed medical centre. Here, instead of being nearly three miles from the Medical College and its major teaching hospital, they would be an integral part of the larger medical activity, fulfilling their role as the specialized facility for the care and treatment of children, and also be the focus of education and research in pediatrics. The Winnipeg General Hospital would close its sixty-bed pediatric ward and gain space to accommodate other services. The Children's Hospital would enlarge its bed complement and its support services to admit the children who had been cared for at the General. Opportunities for research and the development and application of the most modern programs of treatment would be enhanced by concentration of pediatric patients in a single hospital adjacent to the Medical College.

About this time throughout North America, concern was being expressed about the incidence of infection in women admitted to obstetrical services in general hospitals. There was a substantial body of medical opinion that favoured separate buildings for obstetrical services. In Winnipeg, a view was evolving among obstetricians that a 200-bed women's pavilion was required – a detached hospital that would remove the obstetrical and gynecological services from the central structure of the Winnipeg General Hospital. If this idea were carried out, it would be advantageous to locate the major pediatric facilities in close proximity, in order to expedite neo-natal care.

With the approval of the Winnipeg General Hospital Board, all these grounds for favouring a medical centre site for a new Children's Hospital were placed before its board and medical staff by Dr. Thorlakson early in 1943. The presentation was favourably received and a provisional joint committee was appointed to explore the project more fully. Dr. Thorlakson was the committee chairman; Dr. Bruce Chown, representing the Children's Hospital, was the vice-chairman; and Dr. Harry Coppinger, Superintendent of the Winnipeg General, was the secretary. This committee of three eventually acted as the Executive Committee of the Medical Centre Co-ordinating Committee.

Having gained the interest of the Children's Hospital with what might be termed ecumenical zeal, Dr. Thorlakson opened discussions with the Salvation Army and the Sisters of St. Joseph to interest them in moving Grace General Hospital and St. Joseph's General Hospital respectively to the medical centre site. Again, his presentations were met with a positive response and the boards and medical staff members of these hospitals agreed to examine the proposition more fully.

Concurrently, since the Medical College was the axis of the medical centre design, Dr. Thorlakson discussed his plan with Dean Mathers; and after hospital responses indicated their interest, he discussed it with President Sidney F. Smith of the University of Manitoba. Both gave assurance of their support.

CHAPTER 14

The Road to Incorporation

The initial reaction to the medical-centre plan had been remarkably encouraging. Those who had been approached by Dr. Thorlakson had been impressed with the idea, and were prepared to consider it sympathetically as an answer to their own and public needs. A few members of the medical staffs of the community hospitals did express some reservations. These doctors felt that if their hospital were built in the shadow of the Medical College and the Winnipeg General Hospital, difficulties might arise due to the domination of their large and powerful institutional and professional neighbours. To others, however, these objections seemed to be outweighed by larger considerations.

It was apparent that the next step was to bring together the representatives of all the immediately concerned institutions and agencies and establish a body that could formulate and guide subsequent planning. Consequently, at the invitation of Mr. W.A. Murphy, an historic meeting was convened in the Winnipeg General Hospital boardroom at noon on Friday, May 7, 1943. Those present were representatives of the institutions immediately concerned. They included, from the Winnipeg General Hospital: Mr. Murphy, Dr. Harry Coppinger and Dr. Thorlakson (the latter representing the medical staff); from the Children's Hospital of Winnipeg, Mrs. Ralph Baker (Chairman of the Board), and Dr. Bruce Chown; from the Sanatorium Board of Manitoba, C.E. Stockdill (Chairman of the Board) and Dr. D.L. (Tony) Scott (Superintendent of the Central Tuberculosis

Clinic); from the Cancer Relief and Research Institute, Dr. Pat McDonald (physicist); from the Faculty of Medicine, Dean A.T. Mathers; and from the City of Winnipeg Health Department, Dr. Morley Lougheed.

Mr. Murphy opened the meeting by explaining that he was simply acting as the host to bring together a concerned group to consider a medical-centre development that had been proposed. He then asked Dr. Thorlakson to outline the medical-centre concept and report on his initial discussions of the subject with University and hospital representatives.

Following Dr. Thorlakson's description of the plan and his account of the positive responses in his first meetings with the University and the hospitals, there were general expressions of support from the guests. It was suggested that there ought to be at least an informal organization to provide a forum for communication and advice. Discussion brought agreement that, as an immediate measure, those present should constitute themselves the Medical Centre Coordinating Committee, "to keep alive and active the movement for the organization of a medical centre in the neighbourhood of the Medical College and to encourage the institutions represented to carry their own individual plans steadily forward to completion."

A committee having been established, the first item of business was to consider its expansion! It was agreed that the following should be invited to become members: President Sidney E. Smith of the University of Manitoba; Dr. H.D. Kitchen of the Winnipeg General Hospital medical staff; R.G. Persse, Chairman of the Board of the Cancer Relief and Research Institute; Arthur Chipman, Chairman of Board of the Shriners Hospital; and an undesignated additional representative from the medical staff of the Children's Hospital.

The first committee officers were named, and it was agreed they would also act as an executive committee. Dr. P.H.T. Thorlakson was elected Chairman; Dr. Bruce Chown, Vice-Chairman; and Dr. Harry Coppinger, Acting Secretary.

The Executive Committee was forthwith instructed to discuss with Professor John Russell (Faculty of Architecture) a number of details relating to the site, and the probable relationships between the institutions now in the Medical-College area and the potential newcomers. This was a constructive note on which to end the meeting.

This lunch-time gathering on May 7, 1943, was a milestone in the evolution of medical care in Manitoba. The medical-centre idea, conceived nine months earlier by Dr. Thorlakson and nurtured through its period of gestation by its parent, now was born, complete with an important roster of godparents who would foster and encourage its future growth and development. A memorable day!

CONSIDERATIONS

In 1943 the concern that occupied the hearts and minds of everyone in Manitoba was the progress of World War II. Local matters had, as a rule, a lesser priority. Dr. Thorlakson was heavily engrossed with his surgical practice and the organization and management of the expanding Winnipeg Clinic, then entering the second year of its life in the new building on Vaughan Street. Discussion of the medical centre continued from time to time in medical and hospital circles, but there was a feeling among many that nothing in a major way could be undertaken until the war was settled. A number of people (conscious of the devastation of the air raids on European cities) were of the opinion that it would be foolish to put Winnipeg's major hospital facilities in such close proximity to one another, since one or two well-placed bombs could obliterate them all.

It was six months, therefore, before the next meeting of the Medical Centre Coordinating Committee was called. On November 17, 1943, the Committee met in a private dining room at the Hudson's Bay Company store. Invited guests were Ralph M. Pearson, Deputy Provincial Treasurer; Professor John Russell and Eric Thrift of the Faculty of Architecture; and F.W. Crawford, Comptroller of the University of Manitoba.

Dr. Thorlakson, as chairman, reviewed the advantages of a medical centre, stressing the potential for improved medical care in the province, and its important pre-requisite, an opportunity for enriched medical education and research. He suggested that there might be economies in administration, equipment and support services. He noted the difficulties faced by hospitals in raising the capital funds that would be required to enable them to build in the medical centre. There was a pressing need to determine a method for acquiring the property necessary to create the space for medical centre development. A careful study was necessary to determine the medical relationships that should exist between the staffs of the participating institutions.

The problem of property acquisition was particularly apparent when Eric Thrift presented a set of line drawings on which were indicated the present ownership of the land around the Winnipeg General Hospital and the Medical College. In the main it was built-up residential property, with some light industrial and commercial penetration. The General Hospital had acquired a substantial property holding in the vicinity of the Hospital. They gave no indication that this might be sold to other hospitals which decided to locate in the new centre. In any event, much more land would be required if the centre were developed. Realtors predicted that, on the announcement of a centre, land values in the surrounding area would rise, partly due to purchases by speculators. They recommended that any property in the neighbourhood which came on the market should be purchased by some agency on behalf of the centre and banked for future development. But the agency and the source of capital were never determined.

Dr. Thorlakson recommended that the Committee establish three sub-committees to study three areas of concern: property, finance and medical affairs. The recommendation was accepted; although it was subsequently agreed that the Winnipeg General and the Children's Hospital were faced with pressing immediate problems in these matters, and that they would individually and jointly study their own needs, particularly with respect to property and funding.

There is no indication that the sub-committees on medical relationships and property were ever activated. The Finance Committee was established under the chairmanship of F.W. Crawford, and in due course it was concluded that it should not take any direct responsibility for fundraising; that it should confine itself to advice and consultation with the Coordinating Committee and the institutions; that it should consist of two representatives from each major participating facility; and that each individual unit within the Medical Centre should be responsible for its own financial arrangements, subject to discussion with and approval of the Finance Committee. Four sources of funds were suggested: the City, the Province or the University – or perhaps from all three, and from the public.

APPROACH TO BUSINESS COMMUNITY

So far, discussions about a medical centre had largely been confined to those with special interest in the project: doctors, hospital trustees and health officials. Opposition began to be expressed by those who thought a medical centre would detract from the much-needed improvement of rural health facilities and the necessary upgrading of other hospitals and health services in the city. But Dr. Thorlakson was well aware that "new opinions are always suspected, and usually opposed." He possessed in full measure that quality in a physician or surgeon which the great Osler counted so important: imperturbability, which Osler defined as "coolness and presence of mind under all circumstances, and calmness and clearness of judgement in times of difficulty." It was plain to him that the medical-centre message must be put before a larger audience of those in the community who shaped public opinion.

The first opportunity came in the form of an invitation to address the Civics Bureau of the Winnipeg Board of Trade on April 14, 1944. Dr. Thorlakson readily accepted. He found a large and interested audience. At the meeting, he said:

> The plan for the project which your Executive has asked me to present today is one which I trust will commend itself to you and will ultimately receive the approval and support of the citizens of Winnipeg.
>
> It is proposed to establish in Winnipeg a medical centre which will serve this city and province with the most modern and complete facilities for the diagnosis and treatment of disease. It is an ambitious program involving the cooperative effort of several hospitals, institutions and public health agencies. The estimated cost of this project is at least one and a half million dollars.
>
> The Committee which has been charged with the responsibility of preparing plans and estimates for this project is known as the Medical Centre Coordinating Committee and is composed of representatives from the University of Manitoba, the Board of Governors and medical staff of the Winnipeg General Hospital, the Medical Faculty of the University of Manitoba, the Board of Directors and medical staff of the Children's Hospital, the Manitoba Sanatorium Board, the Department of Health of the Province of Manitoba, and the Department of Health of the City of Winnipeg.
>
> Prior to the formation of this committee, there had been a number of informal discussions and interviews between representatives of these various organizations. Some of the representatives have been officially

appointed by their organizations while the attendance of others at the meetings has been an indication of their interest in the possibilities of this venture.

The necessity for this medical centre has become obvious with the increasing demand by the public for hospital accommodation and specialized treatment. The indications are that this demand will continue to increase to the point where this community will be forced to provide an additional accommodation of one thousand treatment and convalescent beds.

The reasons for the present increased demands are obvious: the public has become convinced that the safest place to be sick is in a hospital. This is in marked contrast to the attitude of thirty years ago when patients went to hospitals only as a last resort. One might almost say that the fear of entering a hospital has been replaced by a feeling of confidence and hope. It might interest you to know that twenty years ago, eighty percent of maternity cases in this province were attended in the home; now over eighty percent are hospitalized.

The second factor which has accelerated this change is the improvement in transportation. Patients are brought in now by car, ambulance, train and often by airplane. In the postwar period, airplane ambulances will become, I am sure, a common means of conveying patients to hospital centres.

The third factor, undoubtedly, is the Manitoba Hospital Service Association plan whereby facilities for pre-paid hospitalization are being extended to increasing numbers of citizens of this province.

The fourth factor is the tremendous strides of medical progress during the last three decades, leading to a realization by the average doctor that the simple methods of investigation possible in the home are totally inadequate in the diagnosis and treatment of seriously ill patients. Twenty years ago, intravenous therapy, including blood transfusions, were used only on extremely ill patients, and even then by only a few members of the medical profession. Now it is a daily hospital routine used to prevent and relieve shock in cases of injury, burns or major surgical operations. The dramatic control of hemorrhage by the intravenous injection of vitamin K in jaundiced patients is something that can only be fully appreciated by the surgeon who was confronted with this fatal complication before vitamin K for intravenous use was available less than ten years ago. There are a host of other diagnostic and treatment procedures that have resulted in a great increase in accuracy and in proficiency. It is impossible to overemphasize the great advantages of these improvements to the patient. Many of these things can only be done under close supervision and control aided by facilities which the well-staffed laboratory and x-ray departments can provide. Another factor at the moment is the difficulty of securing help in the home and the fact that most adult members of the family are employed.

It is my conviction that home treatment of disease with its attendant inconvenience and inefficiency is definitely a thing of the past. The factors that have operated to segregate sick people in hospital will continue. Any form of national health insurance will place a terrific load on the already hard-pressed hospitals.

Up to this moment I have attempted to familiarize you with some of the facts which confront any group that is giving serious consideration to future requirements for adequate hospital and medical services to this community.

The Medical Centre

It is recognized that no medical institution can attain a high standard of proficiency and skill unless it takes an active interest in medical education and medical research. These two activities are the cornerstones upon which all medical progress is built.

It is, therefore, obvious that a medical centre in Winnipeg should be in close proximity to the Medical School. The Manitoba Medical College is the pioneer institution in medical education in western Canada. The establishment of the Medical Centre would be an appropriate way to mark sixty years of medical progress in this community.

Already, in close proximity to the Medical College, we have a group of medical institutions which are operating in close cooperation. The Winnipeg General Hospital at present provides bed accommodation for 600 patients, private, semi-private and public. In connection with the hospital there is a large and well-equipped laboratory under the direction of Dr. Daniel Nicholson, professor of pathology at the University of Manitoba. In addition to his regular duties and apart from the Red Cross Blood Donor Clinic, Dr. Nicholson has been able to develop a large blood bank in his department that not only serves the Winnipeg General Hospital and its closely associated institutions, but also supplies whole blood and blood plasma to other hospitals in Winnipeg. The facilities of the Provincial Laboratory with its emphasis on bacteriology, under Dr. Fred Cadham, professor of bacteriology, are also available. Recently there has been installed electro-encephalography equipment for the study of lesions of the brain. This has been built and is operated by Dr. H.V. Rice of the Department of Physiology.[1] Additional laboratory facilities are provided by the Department of Biochemistry under the supervision of Dr. A.T. Cameron.

The departments I have mentioned have carried on medical research for many years. The stimulus that is being derived from investigative work cannot be over-emphasized. There are other activities and services which could be enumerated but I have mentioned sufficient to indicate to you the value to a medical centre of having experts in special fields associated with it.

Dr. H. Coppinger, the Superintendent, and the Board of Governors propose to continue the renovation that has been proceeding for a number of years, until the older part of the General Hospital is completely modern in its convenience and arrangement. At the present time the public teaching wards are scattered throughout the hospital. The building of a 350-bed University Unit, facing upon McDermot Avenue, will increase the private and semi-private accommodation by about 250 beds. In arranging for this building, the present A and B wards, which now accommodate fifty to sixty patients, will be demolished. The plans for the teaching unit have for some time been receiving the consideration of Dr. A.T. Mathers and the Faculty of Medicine.

One of the most important features of the project is the transference of the Children's Hospital from its present site to a new building in the area designated. Dr. Bruce Chown of the Children's Hospital has recently returned from an extended tour of eastern Canada and the United States. This was undertaken to familiarize him with recent developments in hospital planning and construction. He has just placed his report and recommendations before the Board and medical staff of the Children's Hospital.

Many of the services which are now duplicated by the two larger institutions of the project would be merged in the proposed plan, thereby making a substantial reduction in the cost of services such as heating, laundry and power. The advantages to the Children's Hospital in having consulting services available and interchangeable need hardly be mentioned.

Within the past year the Manitoba Cancer Relief Institute has taken over the operation of the Forlong Memorial[2] which is equipped with high-voltage x-ray machines for the treatment of cancer.

The Psychiatry Department, under the superintendency of Dr. T.A. Pincock, provides facilities for consultation and treatment of various mental and nervous disorders.

The Manitoba Sanatorium, at the instigation of the late Dr. D.A. Stewart, established the Central Tuberculosis Clinic on the corner of Bannatyne Avenue and Olivia Street, which is situated within the limits of the proposed medical centre. From this clinic, Dr. Scott and his staff provide expert consulting service in the early diagnosis of tuberculosis, a service which would be extended to include the new, enlarged medical centre.

To reduce the cost of hospitalization, it has been proposed by the provincial government that a 300-bed convalescent hospital be built within this area. The Department of Health of the City of Winnipeg would probably place one of its district health units in or near the centre. The situation of the present buildings and possible sites for the new structures are indicated on the plan which has been drawn at the request of the Committee.

Gentlemen, this is the project. It may seem to some that these plans are too ambitious or premature. On the contrary, I would urge that the development of this plan be proceeded with, if possible, without delay, not necessarily as a post-war project, but just as soon as men are released from war industry and skilled labour is returned from overseas. Thus, we may establish in Winnipeg a medical centre which will provide the citizens of this city and province with the most modern facilities for the prevention, diagnosis and treatment of disease. The well coordinated medical and laboratory services of the various institutions mentioned will be a guarantee that this organization will mark a forward step in maintaining the reputation of this city as the recognized medical centre of western Canada.

The speech was warmly received by the audience, and was a major factor in enlisting the interest and support of the business community in the medical-centre project.

A SEARCH FOR CAPITAL

No one understood more clearly than Dr. Thorlakson did that in the final analysis the development of the medical centre would stand or fall on the ability to raise large amounts of capital. Government funds would certainly be needed; but in the 1940s senior governments did not have the responsibility (later assigned to them by the hospital insurance legislation of 1958) for the immense task of financing hospital construction. It was expected that hospital boards would raise through their own efforts all, or a substantial part, of the money needed to build and equip new institutions.

One of the initial needs for the medical centre was perceived to be an institute of pathology, in order to modernize the resources for teaching, research and specialized service. A well-earned reputation in laboratory medicine had been achieved in Manitoba. To maintain this standing, attract well-qualified specialists, and continue to expand and strengthen the medical sciences in both education and service, improved accommodation and equipment were clearly desirable.

Mr. Samuel Bronfman, who headed the great multinational

operations of the Seagram companies, began his career in Manitoba and Saskatchewan. In view of his western roots, it was suggested that he might be prepared to make a substantial contribution toward the cost of building an institute of pathology as part of the University facilities in the new Medical Centre. In the early spring of 1943, to explore this possibility, the University Board of Governors appointed a representative group to interview Mr. Bronfman in Montreal. Named to stimulate Mr. Bronfman's interest and extend the invitation for support were Mr. Justice Dysart, Chairman of the University Board; President Sidney E. Smith; Mr. A.J. Andrews, K.C.; and Dr. Thorlakson, representing the Medical Centre Coordinating Committee.

With an appointment duly made for the group to meet Mr. Bronfman, Dr. Thorlakson arranged to attend a meeting of the Associate Committee on Medical Research, scheduled in Ottawa for the day before the Bronfman appointment. The Ottawa meeting completed, he took the evening train to Montreal and settled in comfortably to await his colleagues at the Mount Royal Hotel, directly across Peel Street from the executive offices in the House of Seagram.

The next morning, however, he found to his dismay that a heavy snowstorm had interfered with the train schedules and the rest of the interviewing party was still in Winnipeg! Thus he found himself the lone emissary from the West as he crossed the street to fulfill the eleven o'clock engagement with Mr. Bronfman. Dr. Thorlakson reported:

> I found Mr. Bronfman to be a very affable person, and most friendly. A number of members of his Board of Directors had arrived from New York and elsewhere and were meeting in the Company boardroom adjacent to his office. In view of this, I suggested that I could come back at a more convenient time; but he said, "No, I have set this time aside for you and in any case they (the members of his Board) are enjoying themselves smoking my cigars and drinking my whisky."
>
> He listened politely to my request for a donation toward the cost of building a free-standing institute of pathology as a unit of the University in the medical centre, to provide improved facilities for the work already being carried out; but also to allow for expanded programs of research and teaching, and an advanced pathology service not only for the institutions expected to participate in the medical centre, but for all of Manitoba. The institute could act as a referral centre for doctors

and hospitals outside the major towns which did not, and could not, individually attract the services of a pathologist.

Mr. Bronfman considered my proposal. Finally, he commended the objectives but expressed the opinion that Montreal charities should be supported by people of Montreal; that Toronto charities should be supported by the people of Toronto; and similarly, the people of Winnipeg should support Winnipeg projects. Nevertheless, when I suggested that Manitoba charities might have some claim on his generosity he seemed to be ready to re-examine his position.

As I was leaving he put his hand on my shoulder and wished me luck. He concluded by giving me a sound piece of advice. "Dr. Thorlakson," he said, "you can sell anything provided you package it properly." Coming from one of Canada's most successful merchandisers, I could hardly disagree with him.

Dr. Thorlakson made one more attempt to interest Samuel Bronfman in supporting a medical-centre project. On April 5, 1944, he addressed a letter to Mr. Bronfman at his home in Westmount, Quebec.

The letter began by referring to the earlier discussions about support for medical teaching facilities at the University of Manitoba. It continued:

In the intervening time, our committee plans have developed much further and we now have in mind a substantially enlarged program which I am sure will be of great interest to you.

We propose to set up a medical centre in Winnipeg involving an aggregate outlay of about $1,500,000. It is badly needed . . . and would be of incalculable service to western Canada.

This humanitarian project would involve several undertakings, the major one being the erection of a 350-bed hospital entirely devoted to medical teaching. It would cost at least $600,000. . . .

Alas, Mr. Bronfman stuck to the philosophy he had expressed earlier, and left support of the medical centre to the generosity of local benefactors and the government.[3]

PLANNING FOR POSTWAR RECONSTRUCTION

At the next meeting of the Medical Centre Coordinating Committee, on May 15, 1944, the first specific estimate of cost was introduced.

It had been agreed from the beginning that the most important immediate step was to ensure the establishment of a new Children's Hospital on the medical-centre site. At this meeting Dr. Bruce Chown reported that preliminary studies indicated a requirement of $1,000,000 for construction and equipment. Unfortunately, no one on the Committee had any idea how such a sum could be raised, so the matter was disposed of by a resolution directing that Dr. Chown's report "be filed as part of the permanent record."

However, Mr. G.W. Northwood, a widely experienced Winnipeg architect, had recently been elected Chairman of the Sanatorium Board of Manitoba, and as a consequence had become the Board's representative on the Coordinating Committee. During the War most building had been done under government contract and he was sensitive to the potential for government support.

Mr. Northwood pointed out that in addition to the funding required for the Children's Hospital, the City of Winnipeg had already listed as a postwar reconstruction project a $600,000 expenditure for building and renovation at Winnipeg General Hospital. He held the opinion that hospitals would have a high priority in postwar reconstruction, and that an immediate approach to Ottawa was essential, backed up by the approval and support of the City of Winnipeg Council and the provincial government.

The Committee agreed with this proposal. Dr. Thorlakson was authorized to appoint a sub-committee to present the needs of the medical centre to the municipal, provincial and federal authorities, after gaining the endorsement for this action from the governing boards of the Winnipeg General Hospital, the Children's Hospital and the University of Manitoba and its Faculty of Medicine.

It will be recalled that when this meeting was held, the bombing of German rail and production centres had reached a peak; "operation overlord" (the invasion of France) was in final preparation; Allied troops were advancing up the waist of Italy toward Rome; the Japanese armies had been thrown back from the very threshold of India by the victory of British and Indian troops at Imphal; and American forces were rapidly regaining control in the Pacific.

There was a consensus that the War would soon be over and

that governments at all levels would be anxious to support worthy projects to provide employment for the members of the Armed Forces returning to civilian life. This might provide motivation for substantial government funding for the medical centre. An air of optimism pervaded this meeting in May 1944.

Nevertheless, no one expected that all the necessary capital funds would be supplied by government. Since the institutions would almost certainly have to borrow, the Committee members were reminded of a recent amendment to the Bank Act that provided for low-interest loans to farmers with a federal government guarantee to the lenders. The Committee felt that hospitals should be similarly assisted, and by resolution instructed the secretary to request the Manitoba Hospital Association to recommend to its national counterpart the opening of negotiations with the federal government to this end.

The recommendation was quickly acted upon by the Canadian Hospital Council. They found however, that "a view had been expressed in Cabinet and . . . seems to have influenced the Ministers most concerned to the effect that hospital construction is not as urgent as had been stated and that the program of hospital construction in Canada might well wait until the housing program and other phases of the reconstruction program had been completed."[4]

Nevertheless, this initiative was not without ultimate value. Although the low-interest arrangement was not accepted, a system of federal grants toward the cost of hospital construction was eventually established which was even more advantageous. The Committee initiative helped to focus attention of the Canadian Hospital Council and the federal government on the need for aid in meeting hospital construction costs.

CITY COUNCIL

Although Dr. Thorlakson tried to carry out his mandate from the Coordinating Committee to formally approach the Winnipeg City Council for support, a meeting could not be arranged during the summer months. It was particularly important to have all the members of the Council's Postwar Reconstruction Committee, of which Alderman H.B. Scott was the Chairman, in attendance when the Council hearing took place. Eventually,

Mayor Garnet Coulter accepted an invitation to meet with some members of the Coordinating Committee in the Winnipeg General Hospital boardroom on September 1, 1944. The Mayor brought with him Aldermen H.B. Scott, L.C. Stinson and J. St. John; and the Chairman of the City's Planning Commission, C.E. Joslyn.

Dr. Thorlakson outlined the medical-centre proposal; initial site plans were shown; and the impact on city planning and zoning was discussed. The City representatives were keenly interested, and Mayor Coulter suggested that a delegation from the Committee formally present the plan to City Council at a special session which he would call for that purpose. In the meantime he asked that the Thorlakson address to the Civics Bureau of the Board of Trade be circulated to all Council members.

In preparation for the presentation to City Council, and in anticipation of the public discussion that would follow, Dr. Thorlakson called two important meetings.

The first, held on Sunday, September 10, 1944, was attended by thirty-two members of the honourary attending (medical) staff of the Winnipeg General Hospital. Following a detailed and searching discussion, they endorsed the medical-centre plan and its presentation to City Council.[5]

The second, held on October 12, 1944, in the General Hospital boardroom, was attended by an invited group of fifteen influential professional- and businessmen. The reaction to Dr. Thorlakson's discussion of the medical centre was friendly and favourable, and remained so after a period of clear and candid interrogation by his audience. It was apparent that, if and when a larger committee was appointed, many of those present would be prepared to render assistance if called upon.

The delegation from the Coordinating Committee duly appeared before City Council on October 23, 1944. Dr. Thorlakson's formal statement consisted of four concise paragraphs:

Your Worship and Members of the Council:

We, the members of this delegation, have the honour to present to you the plan of a community enterprise which, we are convinced, is a necessary and desirable development for this community.

We envisage a medical centre that will provide this city and the Province with the highest type of medical service obtainable. It will give to the patients of this area the advantages of medical science which, as you realize, has made remarkable strides in the past two or three decades. If the authorities and the public wish to assure the people of this community the benefits of medical science, then we require the utmost in cooperation between the hospitals, the doctors, the Medical Faculty of the University of Manitoba, the City Council, the provincial government, and the public.

The efficiency and adequacy of medical services to the people of this country depends in part on the quality of medical training. The plan which we present to you this evening goes a long way in providing facilities and opportunities for such training.

The purpose of the whole plan is to give the patient the best care possible, and this can only be done by full utilization of the medical and surgical consultant services available in the community, organized so that this specialized service is readily available.

The preliminary site plans were presented, and an animated discussion followed. Expressions of support for the project were general.

Before the delegation withdrew, Dr. Thorlakson emphasized that its purpose was to inform Council and hopefully gain their approval, so that they would be willing to support the Coordinating Committee in an appearance before the provincial cabinet.

The climate of the meeting had been sunny and warm. Only one very small shadow was cast: one alderman mentioned that he could not support St. Joseph's Hospital leaving its north-Winnipeg location.

CHAPTER 15

Broadening the Participation

"Getting up early in the morning is like gaining an extra day," quotes Lin Yutang in *The Importance of Understanding*. The marshalling of events that culminated in formally establishing the Manitoba Medical Centre by an act of the Manitoba Legislature proceeded at an accelerated pace during the next six months. To plan, direct and participate in these activities while maintaining his practice and fulfilling his other professional obligations meant that Dr. Thorlakson had to rise early and retire late. Fortunately his constitution was such that he could function with a minimum of sleep.

The meeting with Winnipeg City Council and the newspaper publicity which followed set off a surge of discussion throughout the Province. The tone of editorial comment in the *Winnipeg Free Press* and the *Winnipeg Tribune* was favourable and indeed at times highly laudatory. On the other hand, the rural view was more reserved and was perhaps typified by the following somewhat waspish note that appeared in the *Killarney Guide* in December 1944:

A RURAL VIEW
The movement among leading doctors in Winnipeg to spend over a million dollars in creating a large medical centre in that city is premature. The Province is asked to subscribe $600,000 of this huge amount.

While the idea is good it is altogether too costly at the present time. Not until the Department of Health and the Hospital Council have finished their work of supplying adequate hospitalization for the rest of

Manitoba should the Winnipeg idea receive consideration by the Government.

Despite occasional dissent, the balance of opinion publicly expressed was in favour of the medical centre concept. However, it was becoming clear to the Coordinating Committee that positive action required authoritative decisions, which could not be reached and carried out effectively by a voluntary, unofficial group of representatives from organizations having different points of view, and sometimes conflicting interests. A legally constituted body was necessary to make binding decisions about site planning, land acquisitions, zoning applications and finance; to communicate officially on behalf of the Centre with government; and to enter into agreements with full authority to act on behalf of the Centre.

On the other hand, a move to establish the Manitoba Medical Centre as a legal entity could be expected to arouse apprehension among present and potential Centre facilities. They feared that their autonomy would be eroded. A bigger and more broadly based voluntary board would be a useful interim measure to ensure that a wide spectrum of opinion could have a voice in the design of an appropriate organizational structure.

A crucial beginning was made at the meeting of the Medical Centre Coordinating Committee on November 15, 1944, at 8 p.m., held in the Winnipeg General Hospital boardroom.

A number of additional people had been named to the Committee since its meeting on May 10, so that twenty-two members were present when the November meeting was called to order.

Of most significance, however, were the invited guests who were in attendance: Dr. A.C. Abbott, surgeon, medical staff, St. Joseph's Hospital; Dr. A.C. Aikenhead, Chief Anaesthetist, Winnipeg General Hospital; Mr. Justice H.A. Bergman, K.C., Chairman of the Board of Governors, University of Manitoba; Mr. F.W. Crawford, Comptroller, University of Manitoba; Mr. A.L. Crossin, Director, Manitoba Hospital Service Association; Mr. Philip Dawson, Associate Director, Manitoba Hospital Service Association; Mr. C.E. Fillmore, President, Manitoba Hospital Council; Mr. Justice J.M. George (Morden), Vice-President, Manitoba Hospital Association; Dr. Alexander Gibson, orthopedic surgeon, Winnipeg General Hospital; Dr. E.S. Moorehead, Manitoba Hospital Service Association (later known as Manitoba Blue Cross); Dr. P.H. McNulty, Vice-President, Manitoba Medical Association; Dr. T.A. Pincock, Provincial Psychiatrist; Mr. Ralph Pearson, Deputy Provincial Treasurer; The Honourable Ivan Schultz, Minister of Health and Public Welfare; Mr. H.E. Sellers, Vice-Chairman, Winnipeg General Hospital Board; Mr. John Spalding, Secretary, Union of Manitoba Municipalities; Dr. O.C. Trainor, President, Manitoba Hospital Association, and pathologist, Misericordia General Hospital; Dr. O.S. Waugh, Chairman, Faculty of Medicine Committee on Postwar Reconstruction.

These carefully selected guests constituted, both in person and through the organizations and interests which they represented, a group which would exercise an enormous influence on the perception of the Manitoba Medical Centre held by government, the University, the professions, the hospital authorities, and the public, both urban and rural.

It must be borne in mind that the provincial government had recently set in motion a number of measures designed to improve medical and hospital services in rural Manitoba. However, reports about the Medical Centre development continued to arouse fears in some people's minds – they feared that the plans for health services outside Winnipeg would suffer.

The prospect of locating community hospitals adjacent to the Winnipeg General Hospital in the core of the City of Winnipeg did not commend itself to a number of the councillors in the suburban municipalities. They felt that hospitals would serve the suburban population best if they were dispersed into the several regions of the metropolitan area. Furthermore, they had reservations about this multi-million-dollar expenditure of public funds in one centre within the City of Winnipeg, resulting in taxation and employment benefits for the city. Satellite business would inevitably be attracted to the area. The dissident council members argued that such an enterprise would have detrimental economic and social effects on the suburban municipalities.

Again questions were raised about the wisdom of concentrating such a high proportion of the Province's health facilities in one location, which could be closed down by a single misfortune or destroyed by an isolated major disaster. As World War II moved into its final stage, there was a growing sensitivity to the devasting effects of concentrated bombing raids!

The people present at this meeting of the Coordinating Committee were opinion-makers; they were leaders who, if they were well-informed and convinced of the advantages of a medical centre, could contribute effectively to creating the favourable attitudes essential for realization of the medical-centre plan.

Dr. Thorlakson was conscious of the need and the opportunity to inform, to reassure, and to convince his audience of the potential of a medical centre. He spoke to the issues with clarity and sensitivity:

> Representatives of various organizations have, up to this point, accepted responsibility for developing an idea and soliciting public support for a community project which has been called the Manitoba Medical Centre. The development of this idea has now reached the stage at which most of the organizations concerned have expressed approval and enthusiasm for the plan. Other groups have indicated their interest in the project and have agreed to support it. One important group met here in this room recently and, after the plan had been presented to them, they expressed themselves individually as being wholeheartedly behind the medical-centre idea. They are prepared to support the project with substantial financial donations. Both daily papers of this city have given the plan wide publicity and have supported the scheme in their editorial columns.
>
> This project is going forward with increasing public support and is planned to meet the demands for adequate and complete medical service to the people of this province and to the West. It is conceived in such a way as to enlarge and improve the teaching facilities so necessary to ensure an adequate supply of well-trained medical personnel to the rural parts of Manitoba and to western Canada.
>
> Sixty years ago, when Winnipeg was little more than a frontier town, a group of doctors and other citizens conceived the idea of erecting a medical college in this city. That was a momentous decision for western Canada. There is no way of accurately computing the value of this step to the people of western Canada but we who are sitting in this room must acknowledge the fact that a large proportion of subsequent developments in medical and surgical care to the people of this western country have been influenced by those who have held important positions on the teaching faculty of that institution. The citizens of this

country should realize that the foundation of the Manitoba Medical College was a milestone in the history of the West. Many important things have transpired in the years since 1883 when the College was first opened.

I believe it is the conviction of a very large and important section of this province that now is the time to carry forward the work of the pioneers by the development of a medical centre, using the Medical College as the cornerstone of the project. The Medical School provides facilities for medical teaching and medical research, two activities that are vital, and upon which depends the future standard and adequacy of medical care to the people of this province.

Wide as our contacts have been, we have yet to approach the most important and, provincially speaking, the most influential section of our community, that is, the section that will ultimately receive many of the benefits of this plan. I refer to the residents of the rural parts of the province. This is not a Winnipeg medical centre; this is a Manitoba medical centre. The representatives of rural Manitoba, both in our legislature and in the various committees of the Union of Manitoba Municipalities, must be made fully aware of the significance of this development in relation to their own plans for improved medical care for their constituents. There must be no conflict here between the city and the country. In the future, the provision of medical and hospital care must be based on a spirit of cooperation and a recognition of the fact that specialized care can only be given by men and women who are specially trained. There is a great volume of preventive and curative medicine that can be properly attended to within the rural districts themselves, providing the doctor is given the opportunity to train himself for the special job that is expected of him and if he is given proper facilities and assistants to permit him to discharge his responsibilities in an efficient and scientific manner. On the other hand, there is still a considerable amount of medical care that requires the teamwork of specialists. Further, I would say without fear of contradiction, that it is cheaper and more sensible to bring the patient to the specialist for care, whether it is to the Manitoba Tuberculosis Sanatorium at Ninette or the the Cancer Relief Institute in Winnipeg, than it is to take the specialist to the patient.

A most significant and far-reaching decision will be made in the next few months with regard to the relationship of the Manitoba Hospital Service Association, which sells hospital care to the people of this province, and the rural municipalities of Manitoba. I have been given to understand that representatives of the rural municipalities have approached the Manitoba Hospital Service Association with the request that the citizens of their municipalities be covered through this association and that the cost would be charged against the rate payers of each municipality. Some legal technicality stood in the way of an agreement. To circumvent that difficulty, an amendment to the Act has been recommended and will undoubtedly come before the provincial legislature in the near future, authorizing the municipalities to enter into [an agreement for] some such hospital coverage for their residents. If this movement becomes widespread (and I earnestly hope it does), it will mean that all citizens of this province are provided with hospital care on an insurance and contributory basis which is not only reasonable to the individual but is also fair to the hospitals. Such a plan has been devised and the people responsible for the Manitoba Hospital Service Association are to be congratulated for doing a magnificent job.

However, this raises a most urgent problem. If the plan is extended to include the people of Manitoba in increasing numbers, then the present acute shortage of beds – at the moment there are 160 patients waiting to enter this hospital besides many others who have gone back to Saskatchewan and western Ontario because they could not get accommodation – will increase, and the waiting list will probably exceed 300 in the space of a year. Those of us who are interested in providing hospital care will then be forced to say that the Manitoba Hospital Service Association has over-sold the available accommodation unless construction plans go forward now.

It therefore becomes apparent that a project which was originally planned as a post-war development has actually become one of immediate urgency. The only solution to this challenge is new hospital construction, which must commence and go forward not later than early next spring. The intervening months must be utilized to complete details of construction, to obtain the necessary approval and support for this development from the citizens of the Province and to accumulate the funds that are necessary.

Superficially, this tendency toward complete coverage of the citizens of this province by hospital insurance will eliminate that large class of people who present themselves at our doors as indigents. They are inadequately provided for, because the present rate of provincial and municipal support does not pay hospitals for the services that they are rendering. These people are a direct charge upon the authorities and therefore come into the public wards where they get hospital care at less than cost, and all medical and surgical care without cost, because they are a charge upon the charity of the medical profession. With improved economic conditions and better organization of the care of the sick, we hope that these people will be taken care of through such agencies as the Manitoba Hospital Service Association. This trend can only mean one thing, unless serious consideration is given to the subject, namely, it will mean the closing down of our medical school because the medical school cannot survive and can serve no useful purpose unless it has clinical material in abundance and in great variety. If these facilities are not provided by our governments through the Board of Governors of the University of Manitoba and its medical faculty and supported by organized medicine, then our future doctors will not be sufficiently trained to look after the citizens of this province in a capable and efficient manner. That is the cold fact that you and I as citizens of this province must face.

I must confess, however, that these prospects do not worry me very much provided responsible people can familiarize themselves with the facts of the case and tackle the problem in a fair and straightforward manner. The people of rural Manitoba and the people of the City of Winnipeg must accept the fact that, medically speaking, what is of advantage to one group cannot help but be of advantage to the other, provided there is a spirit of cooperation and intelligent planning.

I submit to you the thought that the Manitoba Medical Centre is a project that deserves the support of every citizen of this province.

Dr. Thorlakson followed his address with two specific proposals. Since interest in the project was developing favourably, it would now be appropriate to broaden the membership in the Coordinating Committee to include spokesmen for a wide variety of community organizations and for business and the professions. Secondly, the present committee, consisting primarily of persons named by institutions having an established interest in the site, should be replaced by a permanent board and a full-time secretary. He estimated that the operating cost of this office would be $15,000 a year.

An animated discussion followed. It commenced with an enquiry from Mr. Justice Bergman about how the centre would acquire the property necessary to carry out the plan. This was a question, as yet unanswered, that had troubled members of the Coordinating Committee, as well as others with an interest in the project.

In response to Judge Bergman's enquiry, an experienced and respected realtor who was a member of the Coordinating Committee, J.P. Nutter, stated that it was hoped to purchase the needed property, consisting mainly of older homes and apartments but including some commercial and light industrial premises; but in some instances it might be necessary to gain legislative authority to expropriate. He offered no comment on how it was expected to find capital for the land acquisition program.

On behalf of the Manitoba Hospital Service Association, Mr. A.L. Crossin reported that there were about 160,000 Manitobans presently enrolled in this prepaid hospital plan. He confirmed that negotiations had commenced with rural municipal councils, negotiations which were intended to lead to universal prepayment of hospital care for their residents. Municipalities would pay the premiums and recover the costs through the tax collection system. Taking into account the requirement for special legislation to authorize municipalities to enter the scheme and the subsequent requirement for a referendum to gain approval of the premium assessment plan from local taxpayers, it seemed unlikely that full coverage of rural residents could be achieved before 1946.

Mr. Crossin was followed by John Spalding, a highly respected, informed and articulate spokesman for the rural community. He had been secretary-treasurer of the rural Municipality of Miniota since 1927, postmaster at Miniota for sixteen years, and secretary-treasurer of the Union of Manitoba Municipalities since 1931. He had listened carefully to the chairman's address, and to the discussion. Now, clearly and concisely, he stated the needs for an improved health service for Manitobans living outside Winnipeg. He said that he could appreciate the merits of the medical-centre plan. Nevertheless, he felt it was his duty to point out that the municipalities would have a sufficiently difficult time establishing their local hospitals, which they believed were essential; and in his opinion the medical centre sponsors should not expect substantial financial support from the rural municipal councils.

These remarks led to a consideration of the effect of improved hospital services in rural Manitoba on the need for referrals to Winnipeg. It was agreed that difficult and specialized medical services would still have to be provided through the admission of patients requiring this care to Winnipeg hospitals – and in particular the teaching hospitals.

The chairman reiterated his view that there was no conflict in the need for a first-class medical teaching centre with the government's plans for improved medical and hospital services throughout the Province; indeed, the two proposals were complementary to one another. He pointed out that excellent hospital buildings only become excellent hospitals if they have excellent doctors to treat the patients. "People in the country," he said, "are vitally interested in medical teaching because they are vitally concerned about the type of doctor who gives service in their own community; but the responsibility for providing adequate clinical teaching facilities is primarily the obligation of the Government of Manitoba."

The Honourable Ivan Schultz, who had a reputation for frugality in committing provincial funds, remained prudently silent in response to this gambit from the chairman.

Mr. C.E. Fillmore, President of the Manitoba Council, discussed the need for comprehensive plans for the future, noting that "there is a strong feeling throughout the country that state medicine is coming, and the municipalities expect that in due time the government will take over the management of the rural hospitals."

Dr. E.S. Moorehead, a member of the Board of the Manitoba Hospital Service Association, wondered how, if only specialized cases were going to be referred to the major teaching hospitals, the undergraduate and graduate students were going to receive sufficient training in the care of ordinary ailments, which would constitute the principal part of their practice.

At the conclusion of the meeting, it was agreed that every effort should be made to inform people throughout Manitoba about the principles underlying the medical-centre plan. No time was lost in launching this operation. Within the next two weeks, Dr. Thorlakson had addressed the annual meeting of the influential Manitoba Federation of Agriculture; and he had given a detailed account of the medical-centre proposal to the newly elected Executive Committee of the Union of Manitoba Municipalities.

Continuing the effort to reach a larger section of the public, at the next meeting of the Coordinating Committee on December 1, 1944, Dr. Thorlakson proposed that many of the leading public organizations in Manitoba be invited to name representatives to the Committee. He suggested that invitations be sent to (among others): the Federated Budget Board (the forerunner of the United Way); the Winnipeg Foundation; the Winnipeg Suburban Municipal Association; the Union of Manitoba Municipalities; the Winnipeg Board of Trade; the Trades and Labour Congress; the Winnipeg City Council; a number of women's organizations; selected business and professional groups and the major service clubs.

To lend further strength and status to the work and decisions of the Coordinating Committee, it was suggested that all members of the Committee, including those now serving, should have their appointments ratified by the body they were representing.

Also, it was now evident that a new maternity pavilion would be an early objective of the Winnipeg General Hospital, and it seemed advisable to add two prominent specialists in obstetrics and gynecology, Dr. J.D. McQueen and Dr. F.G. McGuiness, to the Committee.

The Committee agreed with these recommendations and authorized the chairman to carry them out.

STRUCTURE

Following the meeting, Dr. Thorlakson must have been deep in thought as he drove along the quiet, snow-bordered streets to his home in suburban Tuxedo. The Coordinating Committee had unanimously supported the broad expansion of its membership. To do this, however, brought up questions of power, authority and responsibility with which the Committee had not dealt.

In his view, an underlying principle must be maintained; even though a group of hospitals might be brought together in the medical-centre area, their individual boards of directors should continue to have full responsibility for their administration, finances and day-to-day operations.

Institutions, like people, manifest unique attributes of character and personality, shaped by their purpose and their history, and moulded by the minds and hearts of those who guide and direct them. Their achievements rest on the competence and loyalty of every member of the staff, each of whom in his own way makes a contribution to the whole.

Dr. Thorlakson firmly believed that these qualities needed to be retained. In his mind, coordination and cooperation, with the sharing of appropriate support services, did not mean an indiscriminate fusion of established, effective and disparate health organizations.

On the other hand, something more than membership on an informal coordinating committee was needed to attract the interest and utilize the talent of the representatives from the organizations now about to be approached. A legal entity seemed to be needed, one that would give a measure of jurisdiction in the centre without infringing unduly on the essential authority and responsibility of the boards of the individual participating institutions.

By next morning Dr. Thorlakson had come to a conclusion. It was Saturday, December 2, 1944, and as usual he arrived at the hospital early. He had only one case slated for surgery. After this, he would see his hospital patients, spend an hour with the surgical residents in his teaching schedule, and by noon he could turn his attention to the medical centre. He left word with his secretary, the incomparable Miss Edith Banks, to arrange for Dr. Bruce Chown and Dr. Harry Coppinger to have lunch with him.

At this meeting of the Executive of the Coordinating Committee, Dr. Thorlakson quickly sketched his concerns about achieving the objectives agreed upon the previous evening. He proposed a solution: since the Coordinating Committee had originally been designed as an informal interim measure to explore the medical centre idea, it should now be terminated. It should then be replaced by a new representative body, broadly based in the Province, to be known as the Manitoba Medical Centre Advisory Council. This large group would deal with matters of general policy; its more detailed responsibilities would be delegated to appropriate sub-committees. This arrangement would not only provide extensive community participation in policy making, but would also facilitate dealing with the details of medical-centre business. How it would affect the autonomy of the participating hospitals and health agencies seems not to have been considered.

Dr. Chown and Dr. Coppinger endorsed this proposal, and it was decided to proceed. Invitations to appoint representatives were extended to forty or fifty organizations in the Province.

THE UNIVERSITY OF MANITOBA

The Comptroller of the University of Manitoba, F.W. Crawford, was a strong supporter of the medical-centre concept. He was also secretary of the Board of Governors of the University, and he pointed out to Dr. Thorlakson that although President Sidney Smith had been invited to attend meetings of the Coordinating Committee, it had been on a personal basis. He suggested that it would now be desirable to apprise the University officially of the medical-centre plans and prospects.

Discussing the request with his colleagues on the Executive Committee, Dr. Thorlakson suggested that Dr. Coppinger or Dr. Chown might undertake this task; but they quickly produced reasons why the chairman was most appropriate to carry out this important responsibility. It was subsequently agreed that the presentation would take the form of a letter sent to Mr. Crawford for submission to the Board of Governors at an early meeting. At the same time, a copy would be sent to Dean Mathers for presentation to the Faculty Council.

The letter went forward to Mr. Crawford and Dean Mathers on December 5, 1944. It summarized the situation as it then stood, and invited the active support and participation of the University.

Dear Mr. Crawford:

Over two years ago a group of men and women, representing various hospitals and other educational and welfare agencies, met to discuss the desirability of creating a Medical Centre in close proximity to the Medical College buildings. A central coordinating committee was set up which included direct representation from various groups. Others, at the request of the organizers, associated themselves individually with the work of the committee because they felt that the Medical Centre idea would ultimately influence the position and attitude of the particular body in which they held an official position. Dr. Sidney E. Smith, then President of the University of Manitoba, belonged to this second group.

I believe that I am correct in stating that no previous communication has been sent to the Board and that Dr. Smith made no request to the Board of Governors for any definite action.

It is envisioned that the Medical Centre will include at least the following:

1. Medical Faculty of the University of Manitoba
2. Winnipeg General Hospital
3. Children's Hospital of Winnipeg
4. Cancer Relief and Research Institute
5. Central Tuberculosis Clinic
6. Convalescent Hospital
7. Psychiatric Hospital
8. Provincial Department of Health Laboratories

It is hoped that in addition, the following will develop in the Centre:

1. St. Joseph's Hospital
2. An obstetrical unit, either as a separate unit or as part of the General Hospital
3. A neuro-psychiatric unit
4. A unit of the City Department of Health in association with the Children's Hospital
5. A convalescent and observation unit
6. An infectious disease hospital
7. A research unit
8. A social welfare unit
9. Shriners Hospital for Crippled Children

It is not intended that the units of the Centre will be directed by one central authority; they will remain autonomous, with such cooperation and coordination of services as meets the needs of efficiency and economy.

The development of such a Centre, while of obvious advantage to the citizens of Winnipeg and Manitoba as a diagnostic and treatment centre, is of even greater importance to the Province and to the Middle West as a centre of medical education. The Manitoba Medical College is the key institution of the Centre. In the Centre all the pre-clinical, and the major portion of the clinical, teaching of the medical undergraduate will be done.

St. Boniface Hospital, St. Boniface Sanatorium, Ninette Sanatorium, and the King George Hospital will continue as teaching units, unless in the last case a new infectious disease hospital is built in the Centre.

Equally important, the Centre will serve as a focus for graduate medical education; and for continuation courses for both urban and rural practitioners, that they may be kept fully conversant with the steady advances in medical knowledge.

The value to teachers and students, both undergraduate and graduate, of the closest association with clinical and pre-clinical teachers cannot be over-emphasized. Basic new scientific knowledge must be continually tested and applied to clinical practice. The clinician must be kept fully conversant with this new knowledge, so that his patients may receive full benefit from it. Equally, the laboratory worker must be in a position to see and appreciate the problems of the clinician so that he may direct his efforts towards aiding in the solution of those problems. The value of this two-way stimulation is beyond estimate. *It is essential to the best in medical progress.* The provincial government has plans for improving the care of the rural population. Small modern hospitals will be built in selected towns. The diagnostic and treatment facilities in the Dauphin and Brandon Hospitals will probably be made more complete. Both these steps seem to be most desirable but, if first-class medical care is to be provided for all the citizens of Manitoba, it is an absolute essential that the medical personnel receive, and continue to receive, the best medical education possible. The finest hospital building staffed with third-rate personnel becomes a third-rate hospital. Here is where the Medical Centre will serve the whole Province; it will serve to raise and hold medical education and training at the peak.

The Centre then becomes of direct and immediate interest to the University as the teaching authority at this level. The present Coordinating Committee earnestly requests that the Board of Governors appoint one or more representatives to the Committee. It seems to the Committee that the development of the Centre will require that the University, in consultation with the Department of Health and Public Welfare, consider a plan for the provision of patients and patient accommodation for clinical teaching and a decision as to how the costs, both capital and operating, shall be met. We have been informed by the Deputy Minister of Health and Public Welfare (Dr. F.W. Jackson) that there is need in Winnipeg for five hundred beds for patients requiring active treatment. It is the opinion of the Committee that a teaching unit of about 350 beds, which would go far to meet the need for five hundred active treatment beds, should be included in the Centre; most economically as a wing of the Winnipeg General Hospital.

The Committee has, of late, given wide publicity to the plan for a Medical Centre. One or more members of the Committee have placed the plan in outline before the City Council, the Manitoba Federation of Agriculture, the Reeves and Councillors of the Suburban Municipalities, a committee of the Board of Trade, a group of Jewish business men, the Sister Superior and representatives of the medical staff of St. Joseph's Hospital and other groups.

The Committee now feels justified in approaching the Government of Manitoba for endorsation of its plans and for financial support. Before taking this step they desire to place the matter before the Board of Governors of the University to obtain from them their opinion of the plan as it would affect future medical teaching and training, and to have representation from the Board on the Committee. We believe that the Board of Governors will be interested in the facilities that the Medical Centre will provide for the education and training of medical personnel and in the raising of the standard and efficiency of medical care in this Province. We trust that they will see their way to appointing representatives to the Committee at the earliest possible date.

Yours respectfully,

P.H.T. Thorlakson, M.D.

CHAPTER 16

A Reception Hospital for Psychiatric Patients

Three months earlier, quite unexpectedly the medical-centre concept was reinforced from a new quarter.

During the first week of September 1944, Dr. R.E. Wodehouse, the Deputy Minister of Pensions and National Health in Ottawa, telephoned Dean A.T. Mathers to make an extraordinary proposal. The responsible federal officials had been receiving reports that raised concern about the effectiveness of the diagnosis and treatment of members of the armed services who suffered from psychiatric and neurological conditions. Generally in Canada such cases were treated in the psychiatric hospitals and clinics operated by the provincial departments of health. This was the system followed in Manitoba. Dean Mathers was himself chief psychiatrist for the Province. He was also neuropsychiatrist at Deer Lodge (Veterans) Hospital, where he was seeing 150 to 200 patients a month.

Dr. Wodehouse proposed an entirely new building for the diagnosis and basic treatment of military patients. The federal government, he said, would be prepared to build, in Winnipeg, a 150-bed "reception hospital" for patients from the armed services who had psychiatric and neurological symptoms. The federal authorities wanted it built on a site near the Medical College; they wanted it to be used as a teaching facility for undergraduate and graduate students; and they suggested that it be operated by the University. Quite unprepared to deal with this proposal on the telephone, the dean could only express his interest, and it was agreed that the proposal would be made in writing. A letter from Dr. Wodehouse dated September 11, 1944, formalizing the offer, arrived on the dean's desk in due course. At the same time a similar letter was sent to the Honourable Ivan Schultz, Minister of Health and Public Welfare.

The inherent attribute of resistance to change promptly revealed itself in the reaction to the federal proposal. The plan would remove part of the diagnosis and treatment of neurological and psychiatric patients from the established provincial service which operated in the Psychiatric Institute in Winnipeg, and the mental hospitals at Brandon and Selkirk. The purpose of the proposal was to seek innovative methods of diagnosis and treatment in the vigorous climate of the Faculty of Medicine, with its orientation toward research and evaluation, and subject to the enquiring minds of the faculty, and the questioning of graduate and undergraduate students.

From the standpoint of Dr. Thorlakson and the Coordinating Committee, the establishment of this new institution in the medical centre would be a tangible stimulus to the project; and giving it even greater attraction, it would be totally funded by Ottawa. But it was not to be.

On October 5, 1944, Dean Mathers transmitted the proposal to President Armes for presentation to the Board of Governors of the University in the following memorandum:

> Thinking that the Board of Governors would desire to have some expression of opinion from this Faculty, I have discussed it [i.e., the Federal proposal] with the Faculty Council Executive, and the Executive is entirely in favor of the proposal. . . .
>
> On receipt of Dr. Wodehouse's phone message, I undertook to ascertain unofficially the attitude of the Deputy Minister of Health of the Province. He stated that while he could not give very much more than his personal opinion, he was favorably disposed towards the proposal. I have since heard some information that suggests that it might be in the mind of the Provincial Government to make an attempt to divert the funds for the proposed hospital to the enlargement of the Mental Hospital at Selkirk.
>
> This of course would be ruinous to any plan to utilize the new hospital for teaching purposes. As I have said, this information is not official.

When the Minister of Health received his letter of September 11 from Dr. Wodehouse, it was natural for him to turn to his departmental authorities on psychiatric matters: his brother, Dr. Stuart Schultz, longtime superintendent of the Brandon Mental Hospital; Dr. T.A. Pincock, respected head of the Psychiatric Institute in Winnipeg; and Dr. Edward Johnson, the experienced superintendent of the Selkirk Mental Hospital, for which expansion plans had been under consideration for some time.

On October 10, Dr. Pincock set out his views in a lengthy letter to the Deputy Minister of Health, Dr. F.W. Jackson:

Since the first intimation of the Dominion Government's proposal to build a unit for neuropsychiatric patients, I have not only had certain conversations with you, but also with the Minister of Health and Public Welfare, the Honourable Ivan Schultz, and Dean Mathers. I am exceedingly anxious that the decision reached by all concerned in the proposal be one which in the long run would best serve the psychiatric needs of the Province, and fit in with the future programs which we have planned.

The terms in which Dr. Wodehouse couched his letter offering to build such a hospital unit were perhaps unfortunate, but I do not think we could expect Dr. Wodehouse to understand our particular provincial needs and make a final proposal which was to be accepted or rejected without modification. I presume that was not Dr. Wodehouse's intention.

If one interprets the letter literally, the proposal is impractical on more than one score:

1. The 150-bed unit proposed is unnecessarily large for present, or anticipated early, future needs.

2. The operation of the unit by the Faculty of Medicine of the University of Manitoba is impractical under existing legislation for the control of mentally diseased persons in this province.

3. The asked-for guarantee that accommodation be provided for all soldier patients and that civilian patients be admitted, provided beds are available, is in need of clarification and definition.

In my opinion we would be very short-sighted should we assume that these proposals are not subject to modification, and such modification as would result in a mutually beneficial arrangement for the Dominion Government, the University and our Department. . . .

May I also set down what in my opinion would serve our psychiatric needs:

1. Two wards of thirty beds each, a total of sixty beds, equally divided between men and women, which would provide single room segregation and protection for the acutely disturbed, together with adequately furnished day sitting-rooms for both disturbed and the better socially behaved patients. . . .

7. This portion of the proposed unit to be under the control of the provincial government, Department of Health and Public Welfare, and all the clinical facilities made available to the Faculty of Medicine of the University and the Winnipeg General Hospital School of Nursing, as at present.

8. The additional beds – as many as considered advisable, probably forty – could be devoted to patients suffering from neurological disease and the psychoneuroses or borderline states. Patients admitted to these beds would be under the control of the staff of the Winnipeg General Hospital and would be eligible for hospital privileges under the Manitoba Hospital Service Association.

9. Provision would be made for the reception of soldier patients referred from the Department of Pensions and National Health, on the understanding that they would be given care during the acute phase of their illness only, and that they would be, if the staff considered it in the interest of the patients themselves, or in the interest of the other inmates, transferred to the Provincial Mental Hospitals, as has been the practice in the past . . .

In the meantime, a committee[1] named to consider a reply to Dr. Wodehouse's letter to Dr. Mathers reported the following conclusions of their deliberations:

1. The University is not in a position to undertake the operation and financial responsibility of the hospital. . . .

2. The University has no property suitable as the site for the proposed hospital . . . in the vicinity of the Medical College.

3. As the treatment of all mental cases in the Province is administered by a department of the provincial government, the offer of the hospital by the Dominion government should be directed to the Department of Health and Public Welfare of Manitoba.

4. In the event of the erection and equipping of the proposed hospital, it would be most desirable that the facilities should be made available for teaching purposes for the students of the University.

5. The most suitable location of the building, if facilities for the students of the University are to be secured, would be in the vicinity of the Winnipeg General Hospital; and the proposed hospital might form a unit of the Winnipeg [sic] Medical Centre.

The committee report was endorsed by Cabinet, and the Minister so advised Dr. Wodehouse by letter on November 6, 1944; in his letter he also took the opportunity to strongly recommend Dr. Pincock's view that sixty psychiatric beds were all that were needed in Winnipeg, and that these should be operated by his department, but that forty neurology beds should be included in the plan to be operated by the Winnipeg General Hospital. This would take care of patients requiring active treatment, and others would be "institutionalized" at Selkirk.

The response came, not from Dr. Wodehouse, but from W.A. Woods, Deputy Minister of Veterans Affairs. He was agreeable to most of the Manitoba proposals, including the reduction in the number of beds; but he also pointed out that the Department already had decided to put a neurosurgical unit in Deer Lodge Hospital and it also had property directly across the street from it on which the psychiatric unit could be built. The inclusion of neurosurgical beds in the new unit was not acceptable. He professed not to understand the allusion to using federal money saved on the Winnipeg unit (from the reduction in size) for additional accommodation at Selkirk.

Negotiations proceeded actively during the succeeding weeks. Preliminary plans were submitted by the Department of Veterans Affairs for review by Dr. Pincock and Dean Mathers. Dr. Jackson visited the federal authorities early in January, and on January 9, 1945 after his return, he expressed his pleasure that Ottawa and the provincial government were now "in agreement on all points with the exception of doing neurosurgical work at the proposed new unit; but it was agreed that this would be given consideration at a later date."

Matters went briskly forward for another three months. Plans for the new building were prepared in Ottawa, and line drawings were forwarded to the provincial authorities for their critical review. Then, unaccountably, all activity with respect to the new building ceased. Apparently, Treasury Board in Ottawa decided that the expenditure was not really necessary – it became apparent that the War would be over before the end of the year, and military and veteran needs could be accommodated at Deer Lodge and in civilian institutions. The hope, aroused by the federal government's unexpected proposal, that the first new unit in the Manitoba Medical Centre would be almost immediately put in place, was ended. It was disappointing.

CHAPTER 17

Approval and Support

The closing months of 1944 brought a wide surge of interest in the medical-centre concept. Largely as a result of personal presentations by Dr. Thorlakson, formal endorsement of the Manitoba Medical Centre came from many quarters.

MANITOBA MEDICAL ASSOCIATION

Although some doctors in the community had private reservations about the heavy concentration of medical facilities around the Medical College and the potential effect this might have on their practice, the Manitoba Medical Association, at its meeting in September 1944, passed a carefully worded resolution supporting the expansion of hospital resources and the increase in teaching beds that were inherent in the medical-centre plan:

1. Whereas the maintenance of the present high standards of medical practice or any future modifications which may develop to improve the medical services to the people of Canada depends upon the high standards of teaching and training;

2. Whereas this training depends primarily on an adequate supply of clinical material (since) only in this way may the young doctor receive an opportunity to observe and become familiar with the many, varied problems of disease before he is ready to practice medicine in the community;

3. Whereas the responsibility for supplying clinical facilities and material does rest on the State primarily;

4. Whereas the present source of patients in our public wards, available for teaching purposes, is gradually becoming less; and that by virtue of plans now being developed by our Governments, both Dominion and Provincial, by industry, and by labour and other bodies, the group of indigents will continue to diminish;

BE IT RESOLVED that the Manitoba Division of the Canadian Medical Association, now assembled in Winnipeg, places itself on record that it will assume a measure of responsibility in devising and supporting a plan which will assure an adequate number of cases suitable for both undergraduate and postgraduate instruction.

This agreement is reached with the understanding that in the final analysis the solution of the problem of proper training of medical students rests with the Provincial Government and its Department of Health, and with the University of Manitoba with its Medical Faculty, and with organized medicine as represented in this Province by the Manitoba Medical Association.

THE ASSOCIATED BOARDS OF TRADE

The representatives of the Winnipeg Board of Trade who were guests at the Coordinating Committee meeting on November 7, 1944, as well as the members of the Civics Bureau who had been present at Dr. Thorlakson's address to that body, were much impressed by arguments in favour of a medical centre. Consequently, the Winnipeg Board of Trade sponsored a resolution at the Annual Meeting of the Associated Boards of Trade of Manitoba on December 7, 1944, which was duly passed in the following terms:

WHEREAS it is in the interest of the people of Manitoba, as a whole, that proper and adequate clinical and educational facilities be made available for the training of medical personnel for the Province, and also for facilities for the care of the more serious types of illness and for patients requiring the use of expensive x-ray and other equipment which could not be available in the smaller hospitals; and
WHEREAS the most suitable place for these facilities to be provided is in close proximity to the Manitoba Medical College where study and research are in progress at all times;
THEREFORE BE IT RESOLVED that the Manitoba Associated Boards of Trade hereby endorse the proposed plan for a Medical Health Centre in the City of Winnipeg, and urge that the Manitoba Government and all the Municipalities give it their support, provided that the

whole plan be co-ordinated with the plans of the Manitoba Hospital Council.

THE WELFARE SUPERVISION BOARD

Early in 1944, the provincial government commissioned the Welfare Supervision Board of Manitoba to examine all aspects of the system of hospital care in the Province, and bring in a report and recommendations to guide government planning. They reported in September 1944, making two important references to medical and paramedical education:

> A special study should be made of the hospital needs of Greater Winnipeg. A modern medical centre, planned as the teaching unit of the University of Manitoba's Faculty of Medicine and for the instruction and training of other technical personnel in the health field, should be planned for the future; and no further hospital construction in Greater Winnipeg should be authorized until this special study has been made and the future programme mapped out. . . .
>
> It should be said that any expenses incidental to the teaching of medical students and technical personnel at the teaching hospitals in Winnipeg connected with the Medical School should be excluded from the cost of operating the hospitals.

These recommendations were of special significance since they were made by an independent body appointed by the provincial government, after they had studied the need for hospital facilities throughout Manitoba. They added an important dimension to the function of the Medical Centre in the teaching of nurses, health scientists and technical personnel, as well as doctors. At that time, there was no adequate training program in place for meeting the growing need for skilled technicians to operate advanced equipment for diagnosis and treatment.

THE DEPUTY MINISTER

The Deputy Minister of Health and Public Welfare, Dr. F.W. Jackson, was one of the guests at the meeting of the Coordinating Committee on November 15, 1944. He expressed his views in a letter to Dr. Thorlakson two days later:

Dear Dr. Thorlakson:

I thought, while it was fresh in my mind, it would be a good idea to set down my impressions of the meeting on Wednesday evening, which, by the way, served a very useful purpose. . . .

I have gone over the recommendations that I have made to Government in respect to the hospital requirements for the province and I am still of the same opinion, . . . that we do need 1,000 additional general hospital beds, and probably 750 beds for convalescent or chronic patients; and that this distribution should be 500 for Greater Winnipeg and 250 for the remainder of the Province.

I still think that if one takes the whole field of the general practitioner's service and the surgical work that will be allowed to be done in the smaller hospitals, that ninety percent of the medical care of people can be provided in their own localities, but that the other ten percent will have to come to a [hospital centre], such as Winnipeg.

Under the Manitoba Hospital Council, in our division of the Province into Hospital Districts, we show an area around Winnipeg as tributary to the hospitals of Greater Winnipeg, for all types of cases, of approximately seventy miles east and west, and sixty miles north and south. This area, together with Greater Winnipeg, would have a population of about 325,000 persons [requiring] all types of medical care. The hospitals in Greater Winnipeg will be directly responsible for most cases of elective surgery from the area extending from Winnipeg east to the boundary of the Province; eight miles west from Winnipeg; south to the boundary of the Province; and north as far as there is any settlement. Besides these, . . . there will be the special cases which were referred to at our meeting which would have to come from all over the province to the Medical Centre.

I do not think that one needs to worry very much about whether or not an additional 300 beds are justified at the Medical Centre site, because I think this number is probably the minimum that will be required. This . . . would be exclusive of anything the St. Joseph's Hospital group might have in mind. . . .

I am sure that you know that we will be only too glad to do anything we can to further this project, as in our opinion it is something that is long overdue.

Dr. Thorlakson lost no time in replying to Dr. Jackson's letter. After acknowledging the Deputy Minister's courtesy in commenting favourably on the meeting of November 15 and expressing warm appreciation for Dr. Jackson's interest and support, Dr. Thorlakson tackled the controversial issue of the extent to which rural Manitobans would benefit from the development of the Medical Centre:

> I am interested in your estimate that ninety percent of all medical care can be provided in a small local hospital. In your estimate, you must include a large measure of public health and preventive medicine which is not now being provided. That will, of course, increase the total value of medical care to the community. This will again modify the percentage of the total that has to be sent out to special centres. Are you thinking in terms of the future? If you are, I would be inclined to agree with you; but if you are thinking in terms of the present set-up, then I cannot believe . . . that the average doctor in the country has reached the stage of efficiency in which he can give the community ninety percent coverage of medical services.
>
> However, whether it is seventy-five, eighty, or ninety percent, it does not really matter. The objective is to make the local hospital and the local doctor so efficient that they can accept increasing responsibility consistent with safety for the patient. That is your objective and my objective, and there can be little disagreement between us as to the methods necessary to accomplish our end. Whether you think in terms of hospital services or medical services, the Manitoba Medical Centre, situated in close proximity to the Medical School, is one of the strongest factors in the fulfillment of your plans.

THE UNIVERSITY OF MANITOBA

The full support of the University of Manitoba was expressed in a letter from the secretary of the Board of Governors dated December 16, 1944:

> Dear Dr. Thorlakson:
>
> . . . The following resolution was unanimously passed by the Board of Governors at the meeting held on December 14.
>
> That the Board approves in principle the project of the Medical Centre as outlined in a letter from Dr. P.H.T. Thorlakson, Chairman of the Medical Centre Coordinating Committee to the secretary of the Board dated December 5, 1944, and that a committee of six members, three of whom shall be members of the Faculty of Medicine, to be named by the Chairman of the Board, [shall] be appointed to represent the University at all meetings held in connection therewith, but without power to give official approval of plans or to commit the university to the expenditure of any money.

The Committee will be appointed by the Chairman of the Board after he has had an opportunity to consult with Dr. Mathers and others interested. I believe that I may say to you that every member of the Board is in favour of the project. In fact, I heard two or three members say that they could not understand anyone being opposed to it in principle. I believe, therefore, that you can count on the active cooperation of the University Board of Governors.

THE SISTERS OF ST. JOSEPH

The interest of the Sisters of St. Joseph in establishing their new hospital in the Manitoba Medical Centre was expressed in a letter from the Mother General in Toronto dated November 27, 1944:

Dear Dr. Thorlakson:

After carefully considering the possibility of having a hospital in the proposed Medical Centre of Winnipeg, we are interested to the extent of accepting the invitation of Dean Mathers and your Committee for St. Joseph's Hospital to become a unit of the Centre, under conditions which will be satisfactory to all concerned.

Our community appreciates the consideration you have already shown in this matter and we thank you.

Yours respectfully,

The Sisters of St. Joseph
Sister M. St. Bridgid, Mother General

WINNIPEG SUBURBAN MUNICIPALITIES

Prior to the creation of a metropolitan government for the Greater Winnipeg area, the municipalities surrounding the core city were members of the Winnipeg Suburban Municipal Association, which formulated policy and coordinated action to be taken respecting matters of mutual concern. Following a presentation at their meeting of December 21, 1944, by Dr. Thorlakson and Dr. Coppinger, Mr. Ernest Gagnon reported that their full support was recorded in the following resolution: "... This Association recommend(s) to its member Councils the approval of the principle involved in the proposed Medical

Centre, as outlined at this meeting by Dr. Thorlakson and Dr. Coppinger, Chairman and acting Secretary respectively of the Medical Centre Coordinating Committee, the setup of which (is) outlined in the memorandum annexed hereto."

WINNIPEG TOWN PLANNING COMMISSION

At a planning meeting organized by the executive of the Medical Centre Coordinating Committee and held on January 6, 1945, Mr. C.E. Joslyn was present in his capacity as chairman of the newly established Winnipeg Town Planning Commission. He reported that although there had been no formal request for the official approval of the Commission, he could assure the chairman that "every member of the Commission approved individually of the aims of the Medical Centre Coordinating Committee."

ST. BONIFACE GENERAL HOSPITAL

There had been an uneasy feeling at St. Boniface General Hospital that the development of the Medical Centre might affect them adversely, particularly with respect to their affiliation agreement with the University for participation in medical teaching. This arrangement had been somewhat tenuous in the past, and it was feared that if all the proposed facilities were built in the Medical Centre, the University might be tempted to terminate the St. Boniface affiliation.

To explore and hopefully allay these anxieties, Dr. Thorlakson and Dean Mathers, along with Dr. Bruce Chown and Dr. Coppinger, were invited to a dinner hosted by Father D'Eschambault at the St. Boniface Hospital. Representing the Hospital were Sister Superior A. Boisvert and three of the senior sisters on the hospital staff, four members of the medical staff, and Senator Davis and Mr. Lees from the Advisory Board of the Hospital.

After an excellent dinner, Dr. Thorlakson described the aims and proposed organizational structure of the Medical Centre; he and his colleagues answered a number of questions, and Dean Mathers gave assurance that the relationship with the Medical College would not be impaired. After a thorough discussion in response to a direct question from Father D'Eschambault, each of the hospital representatives present expressed satisfaction with the explanations given, and indicated the support of the St. Boniface Hospital for the medical-centre project.

CHAPTER 18

Incorporation Achieved

All who knew Dr. Thorlakson in this period were aware that, once launched on a project, difficulties became challenges, not deterrents, for him. Possessed with the instinct for leadership and the stamina to undertake prodigious effort, he had been able, in the short span of two years, to guide his medical-centre concept from the status of a novel idea to a potential reality that would have far-reaching effects on the nature, organization and cost of medical services in Manitoba.

However, it had become apparent that this project could not continue to develop satisfactorily without a legally constituted body to conduct its affairs. Staff and resources were needed in order to develop specific plans, prepare informational material and briefs, and formulate proposals for determining the relationships between a medical-centre authority and its participating institutions. A corporate entity was required to employ staff, receive and disburse funds, acquire land, make contracts and generally pursue the objectives of the enterprise on a formal and consistent basis. The speed with which events were moving during the last quarter of 1944, as well as the growing intensity of the demands on the time of the chairman of the Coordinating Committee, dictated a need for early action. Indeed, an immediate decision was required if an act of incorporation was to be drafted in time to be introduced in the 1945 session of the Legislature.

On December 30, 1944, a meeting of the Coordinating Committee Executive was called. In addition to the three Executive

Committee members, (Drs. Thorlakson, Chown and Coppinger), three invited guests attended the meeting in the Winnipeg General Hospital boardroom: A.E. Johnston, K.C., the Hospital Board Vice-Chairman; F.W.L. Judge, the Business Manager; and P.W. Dawson, the Executive Director of the Manitoba Hospital Service Association.

Dr. Thorlakson explained that the meeting was called in order to consider the advisability of seeking incorporation and to determine methods of organizing a public relations program.

As the minutes of this meeting record: "There was a rather exhausted [sic] discussion as to the final set-up of the organization." Invitations had already been extended to a large number of Manitoba organizations to appoint members to the Manitoba Medical Centre Advisory Council. Many had responded and named their appointees. Many were not health agencies and had no direct involvement or interest in hospital or medical affairs. If this advisory council were now incorporated as the Medical Centre Authority, it was evident that control might be exercised by those without any proprietary interest in the project. It seemed unlikely that this would be acceptable to the medical and hospital people who would be affected, or to the Medical College.

It was eventually decided that the Advisory Council could remain as planned, but that legislation must provide that a majority of the Medical Centre Board would be selected from among Council members who represented institutions located in the Centre (at that time primarily the Winnipeg General Hospital and the Medical College). At this Executive Committee meeting it was decided to invite Mr. D.G. McKenzie to act as Chairman of a Public Relations Committee.[1]

Meetings of the Coordinating Committee or its executive, with special guests invited to consider special problems, were now scheduled every Saturday afternoon. The boundaries of the Medical Centre, which were originally considered to lie between Notre Dame Avenue and William Avenue on the north-south axis, and between the lane east of the Central Tuberculosis Clinic and the lane west of the Medical College on the east-west axis, were now extended for planning purposes east to Sherbrook Street and west to Tecumseh Street. The effect of zoning by-laws was studied; the potential for expropriating property, if necessary, and the closing of streets was examined, and it became obvious that the cooperation and support of city and provincial governments would be necessary in these matters. Alternatives in property allocation, traffic flows and access routes were investigated by the planners, headed by Professor Milton Osborne of the University's Department of Architecture. Among other innovative ideas, Professor Osborne recommended that underground parking for staff only would eliminate the problem of a "parking yard"; this idea was considered to be such an intemperate surrender to comfort and convenience that it was received without comment.

At a meeting on Saturday, January 13, 1945, when the Executive Committee met with Sister Superior Girarda and other representatives of St. Joseph's Hospital, it was reported that St. Joseph's and Grace Hospitals would require nurses' residences of 150 beds each to accommodate their staffs. This space had not been allowed for in any of the tentative site allocations that had been made up to this time. It was also disclosed that the Mother General of the Sisters of St. Joseph had written to R.H. Avent, the city surveyor, enquiring about the possibility of securing Lots 128 to 131 facing on Notre Dame Avenue and bordered by Pearl and Emily Streets; and she had advised the chairman to this effect.

Although this meeting had been designated as a "meeting of the Executive Committee of the Medical Centre Coordinating Committee with representatives of St. Joseph's Hospital and Others," in fact all of the eighteen persons present could reasonably be considered Coordinating Committee members, either because of formal designation by participating institutions or because they had special interests in the project and had been co-opted by the chairman for their ability to make useful contributions to the discussions and planning. Consequently the proposal to incorporate the Medical Centre was raised at this meeting, and some of those present had enquiries about the terms that were being considered for the incorporating document. Mr. Johnston replied that it was not intended that an act of incorporation would require participating institutions to acquire share holdings in the Centre; rather, a not-for-profit incorporation would be sought, "along very broad lines." In response to requests for further detail, he agreed to have some material on the subject available for presentation "at the next meeting." However, it appears that this was the only reference to the subject at a meeting with substantial Coordinating Committee representation present, before the passing of the incorporating legislation.

In the meantime, it was decided to call the first meeting of the newly formed Manitoba Medical Centre Advisory Council for February 2, 1945. Plans were made, notices were sent out, and invitations were issued to an additional group of interested people who were not formal members. As a consequence, more than 100 people gathered in the Law Amendments Committee Room in the Legislative Building on that Friday evening to hear the presentations.

As chairman, Dr. Thorlakson kept his opening statement brief, to allow plenty of time for the featured speakers. He was followed by Dr. Bruce Chown and Professor Milton Osborne, who spoke to the question, "What is the Medical Centre Plan?" Next came University President H.P. Armes and Dean A.T. Mathers on the topic, "What Relationship Does the Plan Bear to Medical Teaching and Research?" Finally, the issue, "What Does the Plan Offer to the Public?" was discussed by D.G. McKenzie, chief of the Board of Grain Commissioners (now a member of the Coordinating Committee); and by Mr. Justice J.M. George of Morden, a distinguished and well-informed hospital trustee who was then Vice-Chairman of the Manitoba Hospital Association.

Both Winnipeg newspapers published lengthy reports of the meeting in their next editions, and both had major editorial comments a day or two later.

The *Winnipeg Free Press* editorial on February 6 under the headline, "New Medical Centre," is typical:

> Definite improvement in the medical service available, not only to the people of Winnipeg but to all Manitoba, is promised through the development of a medical centre about the Winnipeg General Hospital, and there is every reason to believe that this exceedingly desirable purpose will be achieved. A great variety of medical institutions and services would be grouped in that area. Cooperation and coordination of effort would bring greater efficiency and economy.
>
> The centre would have a distinct value for the instruction of practising physicians, medical students and nurses. The advantages of the

knowledge and training received there would spread over the province through raising the qualifications of medical personnel and improving the standard of service in the local hospitals.

The plan which was placed before a meeting of an advisory council last Friday night included in the Centre the General Hospital, Medical College, Children's Hospital, Cancer Relief and Research Institute, Tuberculosis Clinic, Convalescent Hospital (which would relieve the demand on accommodation in the General Hospital), the Psychiatric Hospital, provincial laboratories and St. Joseph's Hospital. St. Boniface Hospital would cooperate in the plan. These institutions would all be self-governing but they would work closely together.

Additional medical services would be provided, including an obstetrical unit, a neuropsychiatric unit, a research unit, a dental unit, and others.

The creation of the medical centre would not mean any centralization of medical services in the province. The local hospitals throughout Manitoba would continue and the only effect on them would be to raise their standard of service. Hon. Ivan Schultz, Minister of Health and Public Welfare, in announcing recently the new program of health services for the province, said that local hospitals would be placed within reach of all the people of Manitoba. The medical centre would be in line with the Government's programme of improved health services, and would give it effective support.

It is because the benefits flowing from the Medical Centre will be so widely diffused that the advisory council has been made representative of all parts and all the varied interests of the province – the University, the Provincial Health Department, Union of Manitoba Municipalities, Manitoba Hospital Association, the Medical Association, Winnipeg Board of Trade, the two Labour Councils, the Federation of Agriculture and other organizations.

In similar vein, under the by-line of A.W. Hanks, the respected Managing Secretary of the Manitoba Division of the Canadian Weekly Newspapers Association, a press release was circulated to all the rural newspapers in the Province, with the promise that other articles would follow as development of the Centre proceeded. Most of the weeklies published the release without comment. The *Killarney Guide,* however, was not to be easily dissuaded from its earlier position of resistance to the plan. Its editor, Tom Wilkins, stated his views in three terse paragraphs in the issue of March 12, 1945:

MEDICAL CENTRE
The Guide has been asked to lend its support to the proposed Medical Health Centre in Winnipeg. Readers have probably read a brief resume of meetings which have been held in connection with the organization. What we really want to know is how this grandiose scheme can be put into operation without detriment to the plans of the Manitoba Department of Health and Public Welfare which outline better country hospital facilities.

In the first place, no matter how desirable the scheme may appear, it will cost the Province $600,000 and the Province has only a limited amount of money to spend. This cannot help but detract from the country hospital and health scheme.

However desirable the Winnipeg Medical Health Centre may appear, *The Guide* cannot lend its support until the medical and hospital requirements of the country are fully met. In this instance rural Manitoba must stand firmly on its rights of priority of service. We have suffered patiently too long.

Heedless of all the meetings, discussions and publicity, steady progress was being made, under the guidance of Mr. A.E. Johnston, K.C. (Vice-Chairman of the Winnipeg General Hospital Board), in drafting a bill to incorporate the Manitoba Medical Centre. Dr. Thorlakson had followed a developmental principle which he felt was essential in carrying an idea to fruition; that is, to test the proposal with all the interested publics (in this case the medical profession, civic and provincial governments, the university authorities, urban and rural leaders, and the press); and having done this, to press forward toward the goal. The balance of opinion weighed heavily in favour of the medical centre concept. It seemed eminently desirable, therefore, to take advantage of the generally favourable climate and proceed without delay to get the bill of incorporation through the Legislature at the session that was slated to commence on February 6, 1945.

At a meeting of a group of interested people arranged by Dr. Thorlakson in the boardroom of the Winnipeg General Hospital on February 10, 1945, the subject of information releases to the public through the press was uppermost in the discussions. Mr. D.G. McKenzie, who had agreed to act as a chairman of a public relations committee, pointed out that some costs were involved. Simply to prepare a mat of the isometric plan of the Centre to accompany a release to the weekly newspapers would cost $30 – and the postage would be another $10!

To answer this problem, Mr. H.E. Sellers and Mr. W.A. Murphy, both of whom were present at the meeting, "agreed to accept responsibility for raising $1,500 for the immediate needs" of Mr. McKenzie's committee on public relations; and authority was given to spend $50 on preparing copies of a plan for distribution. However, there seems to be no evidence that Mr. Sellers and Mr. Murphy ever needed to be asked to fulfill this responsibility, since no costs beyond the initial $30 were ever incurred for "public relations."

Of significant consequence to the development of the Medical Centre, however, was the second item introduced at this meeting. It was in the form of a letter addressed to the secretary of the Coordinating Committee from the obstetricians and gynecologists practising at the Winnipeg General Hospital and was presented by Dr. F.G. McGuinnes. It read:

Dear Sir:

In considering the immediate plans for increased accommodation to the Winnipeg General Hospital or the Medical Centre, I [we] would like to draw your attention to the necessity of a separate maternity pavilion. A maternity department in a general hospital is a source of ever-present worry on account of the increased possibility of infection. All authorities are agreed that best results can only be obtained in a separate building.

The Welfare Supervision Board in its report on the study of hospitals in Manitoba makes the following observation with regard to obstetrical practice: "During 1941, 73.6% of all live births in Manitoba occurred in hospitals. From 1930 to 1941 the volume of this work nearly doubled. Ideally all these cases should be cared for in a completely separate department of the hospital. The rapid increase in volume and the layout of most of the older hospitals have, however, handicapped efforts towards segregation. It is suggested that standards governing maternity and nursing care should be developed to encourage modernization and ensure adequate provisions in future hospitals."

Our present maternity department, which is the oldest in the City, has not kept pace in accommodation with similar departments in other local hospitals.

We now have a department with only fifty beds, two labour rooms and three nurseries; yet in the department last year, 1,399 mothers were confined: public patients, 232; semi-public 287; semi-private, 713; and private, 167. . . .

The department has been overcrowded for the past fifteen years and in spite of the increased accommodation added two years ago, many times even the members of the Honourary Attending Staff are unable to get patients into this department.

In spite of these physical handicaps this department's statistics are unsurpassed in Canada. . . .

The present physical layout is not ideal for an obstetrical department. The accommodation for the teaching of nurses and medical students is hopelessly inadequate, as 75% of the clinical teaching in obstetrics in the University of Manitoba is carried on in this department without any suitable facilities. There is no premature unit, and many other defects. . . .

The erection of a new maternity pavilion would release ideal accommodation for approximately 60 patients, . . . providing fifty-five to sixty beds for surgery and medicine with very little alteration expense.

The letter went on to urge the construction of a maternity pavilion of at least 100 beds, with the potential for later increase to 200 beds, with complete facilities for ante-natal, natal and post-natal care; and with space for teaching requirements. The request was signed by five members of the Department of Obstetrics and Gynecology: Dr. Brian D. Best; Dr. Ross Mitchell; Dr. J.D. McQueen; Dr. Elinor F.E. Black; and Dr. F.G. McGuinness.

The proposal for a women's pavilion was accepted as information by the chairman, and Dr. McGuinness was advised that it would be taken into consideration in the planning by the Coordinating Committee.

In the meantime, in the offices of Johnston and Finlayson, Barristers and Solicitors, then located at 910-911 Electric Railway Chambers, work was accelerated on the preparation of the final draft of a bill to incorporate the Manitoba Medical Centre. This was difficult because of the imprecise understanding of the objectives of the endeavour, and the nature of the powers that should be granted to it.

In the process of informing the medical profession, the hospitals, governments and the public, scores of people had been drawn into deliberations about the Centre. While the chairman consistently propounded his view that the participating institutions should retain their individual authority and responsibility, it was inevitable that those who privately and publicly discussed the concept from a particular personal or institutional bias tended to interpret the function and purpose of the Medical Centre in their own way. This tended to cloud a number of issues.

The concerns are illustrated in a letter addressed to Dr. Thorlakson on March 7, 1945, by D.G. McKenzie in his capacity as Chairman of the Public Relations Committee:

Dear Dr. Thorlakson:

During the last two or three weeks, in conversation with several people whom I thought might be of assistance to us in promoting publicity for the Manitoba Health Centre, some matters have arisen which I think are sufficiently important to warrant early consideration.

You will recall that at our last Committee meeting I was requested to find someone to promote publicity through the press and radio. Accordingly I approached Mr. Tom Green of the Tribune, whose name was recommended, Mr. F.J. O'Malley[2] and one or two others. In every case these individuals felt that before any aggressive publicity should be undertaken, a number of questions must be answered and more detailed information made available. Among others, the following are suggestive of the type of information required:

1. What will be the corporate set-up of the Health Centre?

2. What will be its principal functions in relationship with the various units making up this Centre?

3. While it is generally understood that each of the units will be completely autonomous, what will be the special functions of the Health Centre?

4. Will it own any property in its own right?

5. What will be the specific character of the services it will render to the units making up the Centre?

6. If any appeal is to be made for public financial support, will it be made in the name of the Health Centre, and (or) in the interests of the Centre related to the respective units financed?

7. In any building program undertaken, which unit or units will

have priority position; and in respect of a public appeal for funds, will the monies raised be used exclusively for the promotion of the program of the units; and what proportion, if any, will be devoted to the work of the Health Centre as such?

8. Again, what is the real significance of the term "Manitoba Health Centre" Does it mean anything more than a convenient descriptive title of a community in which several hospital facilities may be located, or has it any additional corporate rights and special functions?

The above is illustrative of the queries that are in the minds of many people and effective publicity seems difficult until there are a little more specific definitions. . . .

When Mr. McKenzie's letter was written, the Bill of Incorporation must already have been in the hands of the Legislative Counsel, who is required to review the form and content of all bills prior to their presentation in the Legislature. It was just twelve days before its first reading in the House.

The Journals of the Legislative Assembly of Manitoba record that at the sitting of the House on Monday, March 19, 1945, at 8 p.m., Mr. C. Rhodes Smith[3] introduced Bill 89, which he presented in response to "the Petition of Garnet Coulter, and others, praying for the passing of an Act to incorporate the Manitoba Medical Centre."

The Rules, Orders and Forms of Proceedings of the Legislative Assembly require that every petitioner for a private act shall publish (prior to consideration of the petition) in the Manitoba Gazette and in two issues of a Manitoba newspaper a notice "clearly and distinctly specifying the nature and object of the application, signed by or on behalf of the applicants." In the case of Bill 89, the required publication had not been made. To deal with this difficulty, on March 23 a motion was passed in the House "ordering that the Rules of the House regarding publication of Notices be suspended in relation to the Petition of Garnet Coulter and others, praying for the passing of an Act to incorporate the Manitoba Medical Centre."

Six days later, on March 29, the Bill was read a second time. In speaking to the Bill at second reading, Mr. Rhodes Smith said that "the scheme envisaged acquisition of the land bounded by Notre Dame Avenue on the south, Tecumseh Street on the west,

William Avenue on the north and Sherbrook Street on the east." He also said that "within the Centre itself the separate institutions will be autonomous and not subject to control of the Medical Centre."[4]

A considerable effort had been made to ensure the support of St. Boniface Hospital for the medical-centre idea. Although at the meeting of January 24, 1945, their representatives had signified St. Boniface support, this had not been confirmed in writing; and even though the Bill of Incorporation had now passed second reading in the Legislature, some uneasiness remained. This was resolved, however, by a letter dated March 31, 1945, addressed to the secretary of the Manitoba Medical Centre by Sister Superior A. Boisvert and her assistant, Sister N. Dron on behalf of the trustees of St. Boniface Hospital, which offered a number of recommendations:

Following the joint meetings held on January 24, 1945, between your provisional committee and the representatives of St. Boniface Hospital, we felt that in view of the possible implications and repercussions of the new undertaking, it would be wise for us to clarify and fully define our relationship with the University authorities before giving our final decision.

The St. Boniface Hospital authorities have gone on record as approving the general plan as outlined by your representatives at the joint meeting of January 24, 1945. As one of the two main teaching units in this Province, we now agree to participate in the undertaking and cooperate with the other institutions and agencies. We feel the plan is very promising, capable of great possibilities and that your Committee is to be commended for having conceived a measure so beneficial to the welfare of the people of this Province and conducive to the advancement of medical science.

In establishing our connection with the proposed plan, we submit the following recommendations:

1. That the term, *Manitoba Medical Centre,* be not construed as a physical unit but as a group of autonomous institutions and agencies, acting for the purpose of medical, educational, research and health service for the Province.

2. That the St. Boniface Hospital be granted equal representation to that of other teaching hospitals on the Board of the Manitoba Medical Centre.

3. That the City of St. Boniface be represented on the Board by two members.

4. That the Manitoba Medical Association be represented on the Board by three members.

5. Pending the regular appointment of the Board, the Trustees of St. Boniface Hospital submit the name of Reverend Father A. D'Eschambault, D.D., D.C.L., as their representative on the Provisional Board.

6. It would be appreciated if the name of Mayor George C. McLean of the City of St. Boniface be also included on the Provisional Board.

We thank you for the consideration you have given our institution in your project and know you will realize that our suggestions are made in a spirit of cooperation.

After debate on second reading, the Bill was referred to the Law Amendments Committee for further study, and to provide an opportunity for the public or other interested parties to express their views. This procedure was significant, since ordinarily private members' bills were referred for study to the Private Bills Committee; only government legislation was considered by the Law Amendments Committee. At that time no official record was kept of the proceedings at Law Amendments Committee; but on April 3, 1945, the Honourable James McLenaghan, then the Attorney General, reported to the House: "Your Committee [on Law Amendments] . . . considered Bill 89, an Act to Incorporate Manitoba Medical Centre . . . and has agreed to report the same with certain amendments. . . . "[5]

Later that day, the House sat as Committee of the Whole and considered Bill 89, along with other measures. It then reconvened in formal session, and among others the Bill to Incorporate the Manitoba Medical Centre was reported back from Committee of the Whole, read a third time, and passed.

The terms of the Act gave the Manitoba Medical Centre broad powers, with full authority for its actions vested in a board of governors. The preamble states: "Whereas it is desirable and in the interest of the public welfare to create a voluntary corporation for the purpose of establishing a medical and educational and research and health centre for the Province of Manitoba, . . .

there is hereby created a corporation which shall be a body corporate and politic under the name Manitoba Medical Centre."

The corporation was composed of members of the Board of Governors and the members of the Advisory Council. The powers vested in the corporation were "to establish and assist, by grant or otherwise, maintain and operate clinical, scientific, chemical, pathological, medical and surgical, and research, institutions and hospitals and institutions of all kinds, and laundries, heating and power plants, and services of all kinds, in connection therewith; and in addition it has the usual corporate authority to acquire, own and control property of all kinds; and to borrow or to invest funds in accordance with corporate needs."

The Board of Governors had full and unlimited authority to carry on the affairs of the Centre, including the making of bylaws, rules and regulations concerning the number, election and appointment of its own members and those of the Advisory Council. The Board, as constituted in the Act, was composed of appointments from: Winnipeg City Council, 3; University of Manitoba, 6; Winnipeg General Hospital, 3; Union of Manitoba Municipalities, 2; Manitoba Hospital Association, 2; Minister of Health and Welfare, 1; St. Joseph's Hospital, 3; Children's Hospital of Winnipeg, 3; Sanatorium Board of Manitoba, 2; St. Boniface Hospital, 3; Cancer Relief and Research Institute, 2; Manitoba Medical Association, 1; The Advisory Council, 4; City of St. Boniface Council, 1. The Total board membership was 36.

It was provided, however, that the Board of Governors, upon an affirmative vote of two-thirds of the members present at any regular meeting could delete from the list the name of any corporation or organization having authority to appoint Board members, whereupon its right of appointment would cease.[6]

Similarly, the Board could add the names of "suitable corporations or organizations" and give them the right to appoint one or more members to the Board. The Board was also given power to appoint to its membership any person resident in Manitoba, as long as the number so appointed did not exceed one-third of those representing corporations or institutions.

It was prescribed that the advisory council was to consist of representatives of corporations and organizations as determined by the Board of Governors, together with such other persons as the Board appointed;[7] and the Board might refer to the Advisory

Council from time to time such matters as the Board might determine "for the information of the Advisory Council and its advice thereon."[8]

The Provisional Board, named in the Act, was composed of the following: Garnet Coulter, Mayor of the City of Winnipeg; Hon. H.A. Bergman, Chairman of the Board of Governors, University of Manitoba; H.P. Armes, President, University of Manitoba; Hugh McIntyre, President, Union of Manitoba Municipalities; Russell Barrett, Vice-President, Union of Manitoba Municipalities; His Honour J.M. George, Vice-President, Manitoba Hospital Association; C.C. Miller, President, Associated Boards of Trade, Manitoba; Violet C. Fillmore, President, Children's Hospital of Winnipeg; George O. Vale, member of the Board, St. Joseph's Hospital; W.A. Murphy, President, Winnipeg General Hospital; R.G. Persse, President, Cancer Relief and Research Institute; George W. Northwood, Chairman, Sanatorium Board of Manitoba; Dr. O.C. Trainor, President, Manitoba Hospital Association; Dr. A.T. Mathers, Dean, Faculty of Medicine; W.J. Parker, President, Manitoba Pool Elevators; H.E. Sellers, member of the Board, Winnipeg General Hospital, and Manitoba Institute for the Advancement of Medical Education and Research; Dr. P.H.T. Thorlakson; Rev. A. D'Eschambault, member of the Advisory Board, St. Boniface Hospital; George C. McLean, Mayor, City of St. Boniface.

On April 7, 1945, – the last day of the 1945 session of the Legislature – the Bill was assented to by the Lieutenant Governor. The Manitoba Medical Centre, despite unanswered questions as to its purpose, its operating structure, and its cost, was now a corporate entity, with broad power and authority, and a fully autonomous board of governors. It could now speak and act with authority, and dispense with the practice of depending upon concensus in carrying the plan forward.

CHAPTER 19

The Manitoba Medical Centre (Incorporated)

The medical-centre idea had been conceived by Dr. Thorlakson, and its incorporation was the culmination of more than three years of persistent organizational effort on his part. It was a remarkable demonstration of the capacity of one man of imagination and influence to marshal divergent forces in support of an idea. It was also a tribute to the wide respect accorded to Dr. Thorlakson by community leaders that, despite uneasiness and even expressed reservations among some doctors and hospital board members and some members of government as well, no-one opposed statutory recognition of the concept. In an interview many years later, the Honourable Douglas L. Campbell, a member of Cabinet at the time and later Premier of the Province of Manitoba, was asked the reason for the government's acquiescence. He replied that there was a hopeful feeling among his colleagues that the new arrangement might somehow alleviate the strain of their periodic confrontations with the Winnipeg General Hospital Board about money.

The Medical Centre was now, in the closing months of the War, a corporate entity, with a provisional board of nineteen influential community leaders and hospital Board members. Ottawa was seeking proposals for projects that could be undertaken as a postwar means of providing employment for the thousands of men and women soon to be discharged from the armed services. It was a time for action.

In the view of Dr. Thorlakson, the Faculty of Medicine and the Board of the Winnipeg General Hospital, the most urgent need was to upgrade the quality and increase the number of beds at that institution. They believed that both teaching and patient care could be improved most expeditiously and effectively by constructing a 300-bed "teaching" wing at the Winnipeg General Hospital to accommodate patients receiving their care as part of the medical education program. Some or all of the old wards in the Hospital would be renovated, providing on balance a substantial increase in the Hospital's capacity to admit private patients.

Although the plans for the new wing were in a very preliminary stage, the cost was estimated at $1,200,000. The effect on operating costs seems not to have been considered as a problem. The plans had been submitted to the Manitoba Hospital Council, and to the Minister of Health and Public Welfare, and both had approved the concept in principle. The proposal had to go next to the City Council, and with these approvals it could then be submitted to the Ottawa authorities for inclusion on the postwar project list. Sketch plans and firm financial estimates were urgently needed for this purpose.

Eleven days after the Bill of Incorporation was passed, Dr. Thorlakson arranged a meeting at the Manitoba Club between representatives of the Manitoba Medical Centre Coordinating Council [the Provisional Board of the Centre had not met as yet], some members of the Board of Governors of the University, and representatives of the Faculty of Medicine.

As chairman, Dr. Thorlakson, in order to decide what to do next, posed a question that needed an unequivocal response: "Assuming that the University and the Faculty of Medicine have the responsibility (including the financial obligation) for clinical teaching, which can only be done in hospitals, the Manitoba Medical Centre would like to know how far the University is prepared to go in backing the Centre in an appeal for financial support for the construction of a teaching wing at the Winnipeg General Hospital."

After a short pause, President H.P. Armes, on behalf of the University, responded that the University Board of Governors had approved the Manitoba Medical Centre idea in principle and would undoubtedly support any request by the Centre for a capital contribution from the provincial government. Dean Mathers observed that the very existence of the Medical School depends on having adequate teaching facilities in hospitals.

D.G. McKenzie, a member of both the University Board of Governors and the Centre's Coordinating Committee, was not satisfied with these statements. "More is needed at this time," he said, "than the bare acceptance of a principle. University of Manitoba has been criticized for a lack of clinical resources for medical teaching. The whole success of the Government's plan for rural hospitals . . . depends on the quality of medical teaching and other types of training."

He suggested that the Faculty of Medicine and a committee of the Board of Governors of the University jointly design a program and policy that would meet educational needs; and that when this had been done a written proposal in appropriate detail should be submitted to the Manitoba Medical Centre for an estimate of costs.

After discussion, this plan was agreed upon, and Mr. Justice Bergman, Chairman of the University Board of Govenors, gave assurance that the work would begin without delay. There seems to be no record, however, that such a program and policy were ever prepared.

The first meeting of the Provisional Board of the Medical Centre was held on the evening of Tuesday, May 8, 1945, in the boardroom at the Winnipeg General Hospital.

By motion put to the meeting, Dr. Thorlakson was elected Chairman of the Board and Dr. H. Coppinger was elected Secretary.

After dealing with a number of organizational items, including the establishment of an ad hoc committee to review the draft of the by-laws with the honorary solicitor, Dr. Thorlakson read a letter that it was proposed to present to the Board of Governors of the University on behalf of the Winnipeg General Hospital. In brief, the letter stated that the Winnipeg General Hospital offered to make available to the University a new wing of 300 beds. This would be a specially designed teaching unit, with patients under the care of the teaching staff of the Faculty of Medicine. Diagnostic services would be provided by the x-ray and laboratory facilities of the Hospital. The Hospital estimated that one third of the construction cost ($400,000) would be allocated to "teaching" – which implied University funding to this extent. A resolution was passed approving the dispatch of this letter.

Some reservations had been expressed, however, about the

validity of the proportion of the cost allocated to teaching. Consequently, by resolution, the chairman was authorized to appoint a committee to study hospital costs and establish the percentage cost differential between teaching and non-teaching hospitals.

The task assigned to the Committee was, of course, very difficult to carry out with any degree of validity. Important variations occurred due to hospital size, capital debt costs, personnel costs, the nature of the case load, the complexity of medical services, the extent of the diagnostic services, the out-patient services, the composition of the medical staff, and the effectiveness of the management.

Presumably the question for which both the Government and the University wanted an answer was: What is the extra cost in the major teaching hospitals attributable to medical education and research, over and above the cost of patient care? This would have required a carefully designed cost accounting study, based on reliable management and accounting data.

In any event, the Committee appointed to carry out the study consisted of Dr. Bruce Chown, Chairman; Dr. A.C. Abbott, representing St. Joseph's Hospital; Dr. G.S. Williams, representing Children's Hospital; Dr. Harry Coppinger, representing Winnipeg General Hospital, and Dr. D.S. McEwan, representing St. Boniface General Hospital.

Shortly after incorporation, Dr. Thorlakson asked, on behalf of the Centre, for an interview with Premier Garson. Unexpectedly, on Thursday, June 22, 1945, a message came from the Premier's office that he could meet a delegation from the Medical Centre the next morning at 10:30 a.m. Incredibly, no less than forty-three representatives of the Board, the Advisory Committee, the University, and the participating hospitals assembled to meet the Premier, who was accompanied by the Minister of Health and Public Welfare and his Deputy, and the Minister of Education.

During his opening presentation, Dr. Thorlakson urged the Government to associate itself with the objectives of the Manitoba Medical Centre. He also asked that the Government appoint two members to a committee on which each of the City of Winnipeg and the University of Manitoba would also be asked to appoint two members, to make a study of the financial needs of the Manitoba Medical Centre program. He asked that the Government make available immediately $15,000 to fund this study.

Dean Mathers and President Armes spoke in support of Dr. Thorlakson's proposals. Dr. Bruce Chown outlined the needs of the Children's Hospital for a closer relationship with the Faculty of Medicine and other hospitals. He took the position that in view of the development of Greater Winnipeg to the south and west, the Children's Hospital, located in the north, was not well placed to serve the needs of the City's children.

In response, Premier Garson said that formation of the Medical Centre was a worthwhile project but that the Government could not make any financial commitment to it until the affairs of the Province had been "stabilized." [It is perhaps proper to note that all governments were deeply involved at this time in trying to plan for the unknown social and economic demands of the transition from war to peace.]

The Government did agree to the appointment of a committee to examine Medical Centre program costs as requested by Dr. Thorlakson. Later this was established, with R.M. Pearson (Deputy Provincial Treasurer) and Dr. F.W. Jackson (Deputy Minister of Health and Public Welfare) representing the Province; Alderman C.E. Simonite and W.B. Brown, Commissioner of Finance, representing the City of Winnipeg; and F.W. Crawford and Dean A.T. Mathers representing the University.

The Committee met on September 21, 1945, in the boardroom of the Winnipeg General Hospital. Dr. Thorlakson and Dr. Bruce Chown also attended the meeting, at which Dr. J.D. Adamson replaced Dr. Mathers, who was unable to attend.

After recapitulating the plans and needs of the Manitoba Medical Centre, Dr. Thorlakson quoted from his statement to the Premier to show that he had asked for the committee "to determine a fair and just proportion of financial responsibility for providing the hospital facilities for teaching and the care of the sick. . . . The Province makes no special contribution to these hospitals for the special teaching facilities of our University."

Following the election of F.W. Crawford as Chairman of the Committee, a lengthy discussion on the scope of its work ensued. It had been designated as the Committee on Hospital Costs which seemed to indicate a different task from that envisioned in Dr. Thorlakson's proposal. It was ultimately agreed that the terms of reference should be provided by the Medical Centre. Dr. Thorlakson agreed to prepare them in consultation with others, in the course of which the name became The Special Committee on the Costs of Hospital Construction and Maintenance.

The Committee decided that they would need professional help in their work, and agreed to invite Mr. Donald M. Cox, Administrator of the Winnipeg Municipal Hospitals, to act in this capacity on secondment by the City for a period of three months.[1] Mr. Simonite agreed to make this arrangement, if Mr. Cox were willing. It was agreed to ask the Province and the City to provide $2,000 each to fund the Committee's expenses.

The money was granted as requested; and Mr. Cox was given leave from Municipal Hospitals to assist the Committee.

The Provisional Board of the Manitoba Medical Centre met again on October 10, 1945. They approved the revised name of the Crawford Committee; they changed its terms of reference and instructed that they be set out in a letter to Mr. Crawford, with copies to the Premier and the Minister of Health and Public Welfare, and to the Minister of Education. The meeting was advised that the Committee members and the executive officers of the Board would meet the Premier and the ministers at 2:30 p.m. on October 19, 1945.[2]

Dr. Thorlakson reported to the Provisional Board that, after a private meeting with the Minister of Health and Public Welfare, he had been left with the impression that the Government would provide nothing in the way of special financial assistance for the Medical Centre at this time.

He also informed the Board that the construction of a new wing at the General Hospital would require the demolition of some wards then in use, and that in the face of a waiting list of 372 patients, the Hospital Board had decided that constructing a new wing would not be practical. Instead, they would proceed with the building of a new maternity pavilion on the Notre Dame site earlier allocated for the Children's Hospital. The construction would be funded by gifts from members of the Hospital Board and a bond issue for $800,000 guaranteed by the City of Winnipeg.

At this meeting, the Provisional Board received the report of the Medical Committee, under the chairmanship of Dr. Bruce Chown, which was to determine the differential costs of teaching hospitals. The Committee had decided that there were two elements to the problem: capital costs and operating costs. They chose to deal only with capital costs.

The Committee recommended the following formulae for determining the portion of capital costs to be allocated to teaching:

1. For a wing such as that contemplated by the Winnipeg General Hospital and the St. Boniface General Hospital: one third of the [construction] cost. [For the first time it appeared that St. Boniface was going to have a new "teaching" wing.]

2. For x-ray and laboratory departments: one half the cost.

3. For a complete new hospital such as that contemplated by the Children's Hospital "in which a large proportion of the patients will be teaching patients": one third of forty percent of [construction] cost, plus one half of laboratory costs.

4. For a hospital such as contemplated by St. Joseph's "in which a smaller proportion of patients will be teaching patients": one third of twenty-five percent of [construction] cost plus one half of laboratory costs.

The Provisional Board received this report as information and asked that it be forwarded to the Crawford Committee.

These were interesting formulae, but no evidence was given to support their validity. Nevertheless, since the Medical Centre authorities had been urging the principle that medical teaching costs were the responsibility of the provincial government by way of the University, the Cabinet must have been alarmed to find themselves being assigned an obligation for several million dollars of capital costs, which would not only impinge heavily on the modest provincial budget but could also arouse political controversy.

This was the last meeting of the Provisional Board of the Manitoba Medical Centre.

It was followed, on April 16, 1946, by the first and only formal meeting of the Board of Governors of the Manitoba Medical Centre Incorporated.

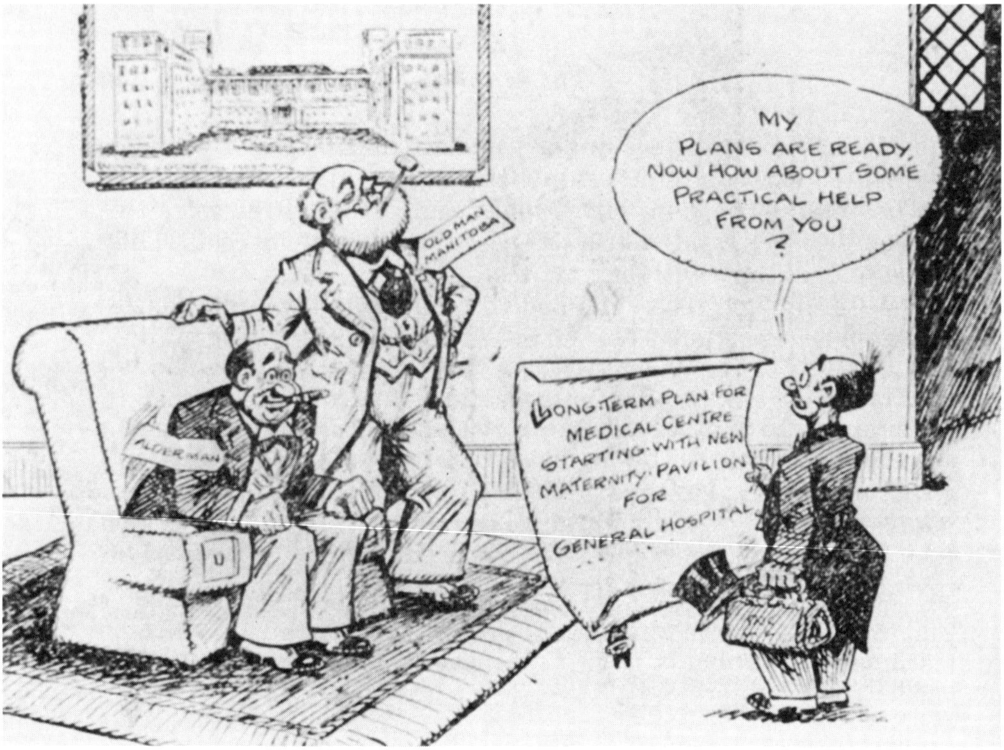
MY PLANS ARE READY, NOW HOW ABOUT SOME PRACTICAL HELP FROM YOU ?
OLD MAN MANITOBA
ALDERMAN
U
LONG-TERM PLAN FOR MEDICAL CENTRE STARTING WITH NEW MATERNITY PAVILION FOR GENERAL HOSPITAL . . .

Free Press cartoonist Arch Dale depicts Dr. Thorlakson's plea for support from th City of Winnipeg and "Old Man Manitoba" for the Manitoba Medical Centre (January 22, 1946).

At this meeting, Dr. Thorlakson was elected President of the Board. Dr. Bruce Chown was elected Vice-President, and Dr. Harry Coppinger was elected Secretary. It was agreed that these officers would act as the Executive Committee of the Centre.

During the meeting, the president reported that Grace Hospital had decided to proceed with plans to expand their hospital on Arlington Street, and would not be moving to the Medical Centre.

For a number of years, the Shriners had been operating a twenty-seven-bed unit for the care of crippled children in a structure attached to the Children's Hospital. They had now announced that they would build a new hospital on property which they had acquired on Wellington Crescent. They had refused an invitation to build in the Manitoba Medical Centre on the grounds that it would be too costly; because the site was less attractive for the care and rehabilitation of children than was the property they already owned on the Crescent; and because they were concerned that they might lose their identity if they were located in the shadow of much larger institutions.

Despite these setbacks, Dr. Thorlakson continued to work vigorously to advance plans for the Medical Centre. He accepted a number of invitations to give public addresses on the subject, an indication of the extent to which the idea had caught the interest of the community. His audiences included a variety of organizations, such as The Young Men's Section of the Board of Trade and the Annual Meeting of the Manitoba Music Teacher's Association. In these addresses, he stressed the principle that institutions moving to the proposed centre "will remain free to decide their own policies" and that there would not be "a mammoth campaign for funds to include simultaneously all the various participants. The public," he said, "will have an opportunity to examine each appeal on its own merits."

After a time, St. Joseph's Hospital changed its position. Following a visit by Dr. Thorlakson to the Mother General of the Order in Toronto, where the Sisters of St. Joseph operate the highly-respected St. Michael's Hospital, he received a letter from Sister M. St. Bridgid (the Mother General) accepting the invitation to build a replacement for their Salter Street Hospital in the Manitoba Medical Centre.

Be Sure to Hear DR. P. H. T. THORLAKSON, Speaking on a Subject of Vital Interest to Every Section Member

THE PROPOSED MANITOBA MEDICAL CENTRE

HUDSON'S BAY DINING ROOM, MONDAY, MARCH 11th, at 6 p.m. - Tickets 85c

The Scheme . . .

The scheme calls for the centralization — around the present General Hospital site — of virtually all the city's and province's principal medical services. Present medical departments in and around this site would remain where they are while others would be transferred to the area. Where necessary, new facilities would be added. It is estimated the complete centre would cost in the neighborhood of $1,500,000 and would be designed to serve both the city and province. It would be equipped with the most complete and modern facilties for diagnosis and treatment of diseases.

Get your tickets from a ticket seller at the Board Office—85c.

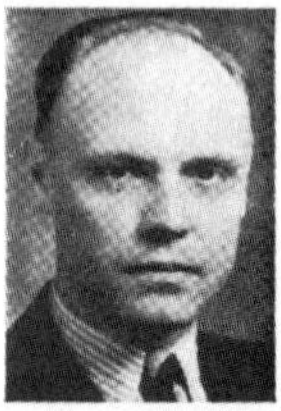

DR. P. H. T. THORLAKSON

who, as chairman of the Provisional Board, Manitoba Medical Centre, is well qualified to enlighten the members of the Section on this important proposal. He enjoys an excellent reputation as a forceful speaker.

Highlights . . .

WHAT CENTRE WOULD INCLUDE

1. Manitoba Medical College.
2. Winnipeg General Hospital (with its 600 beds).
3. Large, well-equipped laboratory under the direction of Dr. Daniel Nicholson, pathology professor at the university.
4. Large blood bank, apart from the Red Cross clinic, already established in the medical college.
5. Erection of a 350-bed university unit.
6. Transference of the Children's Hospital to a new building in this area.
7. Building of a 300-bed convalescent hospital, to reduce the cost of hospitalization.
8. Possibly a dental clinic. And many other units.

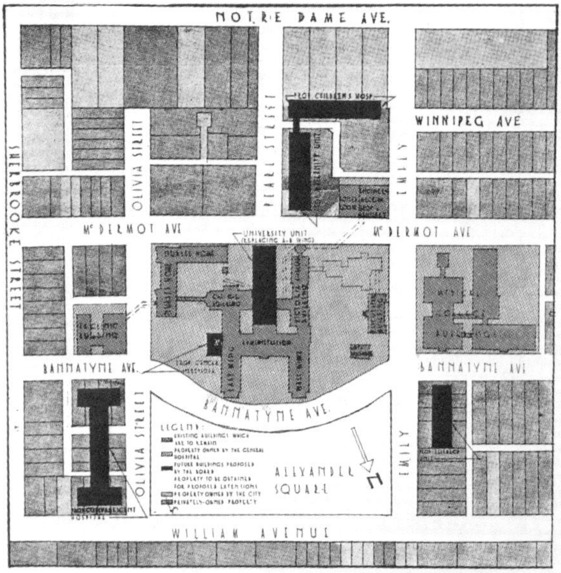

The community medical centre planned by the Medical Centre Co-Ordinating Committee is shown in the above diagram. The new buildings would be conveniently placed in proximity to the Winnipeg General Hospital and the Manitoba Medical College. The diagram also shows what land is city-owned, what land is owned by the General Hospital and the land which would have to be acquired from private owners.

A poster announcing a speech by Dr. Thorlakson about the Manitoba Medical Centre delivered to the Young Men's Section of the Winnipeg Board of Trade on March 11, 1946

However, after further consideration of how best to fulfill their mission in Winnipeg, the Sisters of St. Joseph decided against continuing their hospital operation. Instead, they converted their building to a personal care home. Here the sisters provided a warm-hearted, kindly and effective service to the people in the community which they had served for so many years.

The Children's Hospital had expressed interest in moving to the Medical Centre from the time of Dr. Thorlakson's first meeting with their Board in 1942. Dr. Bruce Chown, who had been a member of the Medical Centre executive from the beginning, had been appointed the Acting Medical Superintendent of the Children's Hospital when the incumbent, Dr. G.S. Williams, joined the armed forces. Dr. Chown never wavered in his view that the Children's Hospital ought to move to the Centre and become more closely related to the Faculty of Medicine. However, some of his colleagues and some of the Board members continued to have reservations about the ability of the Hospital to maintain its identity and its prestige as the major pediatric hospital in Western Canada if they moved into the orbit of the University and the Winnipeg General Hospital. Some felt their autonomy would be threatened.

Finally, to settle the matter, in 1945 the Board of the Children's Hospital asked for a specific recommendation from their medical staff with respect to building a new hospital in the Manitoba Medical Centre. The medical staff opted in favour of moving to the Centre. On the strength of this recommendation, the Board authorized planning for the new 200-bed Children's Hospital.

After some negotiations, it was agreed that the building could be located to the northeast of the General, provided Olivia Street could be closed between Bannatyne and William Avenues, and permission could be obtained to encroach on Alexandra Park. This property had been bequeathed to the Winnipeg General Hospital many years earlier to enhance the appearance of the approach to its main entrance and serve as a restful outdoor area for amubulant patients.

These requirements were finally met, but almost ten years elapsed before construction of the new Children's Hospital began. The sod-turning took place on October 15, 1954. Construction took two years, and the heavy responsibility of moving the patients from the old hospital to the new took place during the first real blizzard of winter on December 11, 1956.

The cost of the Children's Hospital was about $4 million. The first $1 million was raised in 1948 through a public fund-raising drive.

Five years later, in 1953, under the chairmanship of Mr. H.E. Sellers, the Joint Building Fund campaign was launched to complete funding for construction of the Children's Hospital, and for major additions and reconstruction at the Winnipeg General Hospital. It was estimated that a total of $8 million was required.

The Children's had on hand the $1 million it had raised in 1948, together with $200,000 offered by the Red Cross for a Red Cross Wing in their hospital. The General Hospital had accumulated for building purposes $1,200,000, mostly from the estate of Mrs. Ethel Shea, supplemented by other gifts and bequests.

The Joint Building Fund appeal was expected to raise $3 million, of which $1 million would be allocated to the Children's Hospital and $2 million to the General Hospital. Thus a total of $5.4 million would be provided from private sources for construction in the Medical Centre, with the balance of $2.6 million coming from statutory and special grants from federal and provincial governments.

Dr. Thorlakson was Chairman of the Doctors' Committee of the Joint Building Fund project, and shortly after the appeal began he was able to announce that members of the medical staff of the two hospitals had contributed $185,000 to the Fund.

The campaign was highly organized, with strong teams directing the appeal to corporations, employees and private givers. Mrs. Harold J. Riley, Chairman of the Women's Division, and Mrs. L.J. Orlikow, Chairman of the Residential Canvass Committee, rallied 2,000 women to solicit the support of women's groups and stage a "blitz" residential drive.

The Joint Building Fund appeal reached its goal, enabling the Children's Hospital to build in the Medical Centre, and the General Hospital to commence its much-needed additions and renovations.

CHAPTER 20

From Manitoba Medical Centre to the Health Sciences Centre

In 1957 the federal Hospital Insurance and Diagnostic Services Act came into effect. This provided for Federal-Provincial sharing of the cost of most hospital services, including diagnostic procedures such as laboratory and x-ray and their necessary medical interpretations.

The choice of method of financing and administering a provincial plan was the responsibility of the provincial government.

The Manitoba Government, then headed by Premier Douglas L. Campbell, immediately set about formulating a program, in consultation with the Manitoba Hospital Association, the Manitoba College of Physicians and Surgeons, the Manitoba Medical Association, and other concerned groups. They established an implementation target of July 1, 1958. To achieve this would require an intense effort on the part of the Minister of Health, the Honourable R.W. Bend, and his senior officials.[1]

However, in the spring of 1958, Premier Campbell called an election for June 16, 1958. The unexpected happened: the Liberals were defeated and the Honourable Duff Roblin was asked to form a new ministry.

He appointed as his Minister of Health and Public Welfare the Honourable Dr. George Johnson, the newly elected member for Gimli.[2] He found himself responsible for implementing, at the end of his first week in office, the most complex and far-reaching health service legislation that had ever been enacted in Manitoba.

In designing the plan to provide insured hospital care in Manitoba, attention was paid primarily to general hospital services, in which average length of stay was ten to twelve days. Those studying demand for hospital beds under the new scheme as against the supply apparently failed to take into account the fact that five percent of the patients admitted had long-term illness requiring thirty days or more of care.[3] Studies showed that these patients utilized about one-third of the patient days in general hospitals. It was known that there were many people with long-term illness who would be eligible for hospital admission under the new plan, who had been denied access for economic reasons, and who might now be seeking care. It follows that if the proportion of long-term patients increased even from five percent to six percent of admissions, they would utilize forty percent of acute-care hospital-bed capacity. This would result in long waiting lists of people needing hospital services.

Within two months of the inception of tax-supported hospital care, complaints began to reach the new Minister's office about the "blocking of beds" by patients needing lengthy periods of hospital care, which impeded the admission of acute-care short-term patients. It was evident that something needed to be done.

In this situation, the Government, through the Minister of Health and Public Welfare, turned to the Sanatorium Board of Manitoba, which was winning its half-century campaign against tuberculosis. It had experience in caring for long-term patients of all ages in the five hospitals it operated for the treatment of tuberculosis and chronic respiratory disease. The Board had pioneered in a rehabilitation approach to patient care.

As part of a comprehensive plan to develop alternatives to general hospital care for long-term patients, the Sanatorium Board initiated arrangements to allocate sixty beds in its Clearwater Lake Hospital at the Pas, as well as the whole of its 200-bed Assiniboine Hospital at Brandon, for "extended treatment,"[4] that is, essentially for the care of patients who needed thirty days or more of hospital care.

Within a relatively short time, this arrangement provided, in the northern and western part of the Province, regional centres with a strong rehabilitation component for the care of the elderly sick. Physicians practising in The Pas and Brandon were accorded admitting privileges in these hospitals to enable them to continue to treat their patients. Nurses were given special training. Physiotherapy and occupational therapy services were introduced for the first time in these regions. These arrangements produced 260 beds for long-term patients. They were quickly filled by transfers from general hospitals or by direct admission, and helped to relieve the demands on the acute care facilities.

An initial long-term plan proposed that the Sisters of Charity (Grey Nuns) should build an extended treatment hospital adjacent to St. Boniface General Hospital (which was ultimately done); and recommended that an extended treatment hospital and an active treatment rehabilitation hospital be built in the vicinity of the Winnipeg General Hospital. The Rehabilitation Hospital would act as a provincial centre for patients needing relatively short-term specialized rehabilitation care, to speed their restoration to the highest level of activity possible within their physical capacities.

The Minister of Health, the Honourable George Johnson, invited a representative committee of the Manitoba Medical Association to review these proposals. With their concurrence, he proceeded to implement this plan to provide improved facilities designed to meet the needs of patients with major disabling conditions.

The Sanatorium Board of Manitoba was asked to proceed immediately with the design and construction of the Rehabilitation Hospital in the block on Sherbrook Street between McDermot Avenue and Bannatyne Avenue, where it had operated the Central Tuberculosis Clinic for nearly thirty years.

The Manitoba Rehabilitation Hospital was opened in 1962. It incorporated a wing known as the D.A. Stewart Centre for Respiratory Diseases, which replaced the old Central Tuberculosis Clinic.[5]

As an organization, the Manitoba Medical Centre Incorporated had been dormant since 1946. With the announcement of the plans for the Manitoba Rehabilitation Hospital, there were suggestions that it ought to be revived.

On Saturday, January 31, 1959, Dr. Thorlakson invited to an informal luncheon meeting at the Manitoba Club representative members of the Boards of the Winnipeg General Hospital, the Children's Hospital, the Sanatorium Board of Manitoba, and the Cancer Treatment and Research Foundation, Dean L.G.

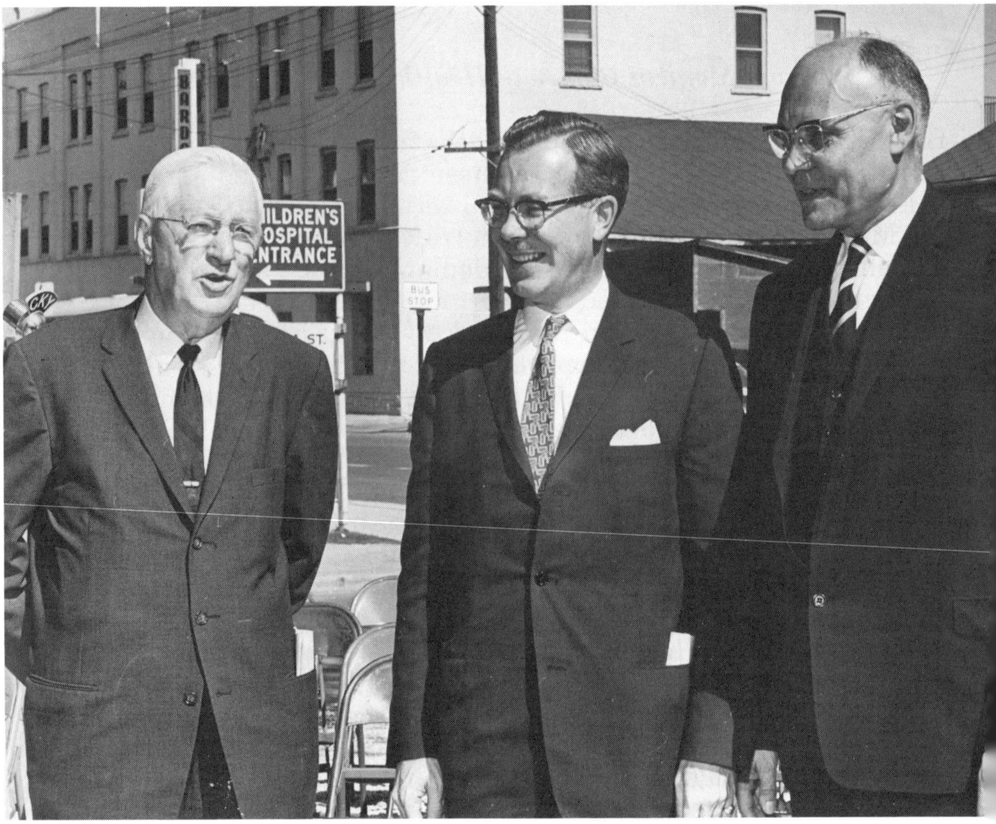

Dr. Thorlakson was the guest speaker at the laying of the cornerstone of the Manitoba Rehabilitation Hospital by Premier Duff Roblin on August 31, 1961. With Dr. Thorlakson are Premier Roblin and Mr. J.W. Speirs, Chairman of the Sanatorium Board of Manitoba, which built the Hospital and operated it until 1973. (Photo by David Portigal.)

Bell, and the Honourable George Johnson – a total of fifteen guests.

Following a pleasant lunch, the host gave a short history of the Manitoba Medical Centre about which at least some of those present knew very little. He reviewed briefly the authority with respect to the area bounded by Sherbrook and Tecumseh Streets between Notre Dame and William Avenues, granted to the Medical Centre under its act of incorporation. He outlined the substantial development that had taken place in this area since 1945, mentioning in particular the expansion and renovation of the Winnipeg General Hospital, construction of the Children's Hospital, the Women's Pavilion, the Dental College, the Medical Centre Apartments, and the enlarged Medical College. Now the Sanatorium Board had plans under way for a rehabilitation hospital and there was a possibility that an extended treatment hospital would also be built in this vicinity. The purpose of the gathering, he said, was to see if there was a concensus about whether it would be appropriate to reactivate the Manitoba Medical Centre Board or an equivalent coordinating body.

Agreement was expressed that it would be desirable to revitalize the Manitoba Medical Centre Corporation, perhaps with necessary amendments to the Act of 1945 to alter the membership, authority and responsibility in the light of current circumstances. It was decided to hold a formal meeting of Medical Centre representatives in the boardroom of the Winnipeg General Hospital on the following Saturday, February 7.

This meeting, chaired by Dr. Thorlakson, was attended by two Board members and two senior executive officers of the Winnipeg General Hospital and the Dean of the Faculty of Medicine, Dr. Bell.

The chairman presented a draft resolution that provided for the formation of the Manitoba Medical Centre Council. Among other powers, it would be authorized to engage legal counsel to prepare an act of incorporation for this new body. It was expected that this would replace the Manitoba Medical Centre Corporation.

A.E. Johnston, Q.C., Winnipeg General Hospital Solicitor and a member of its Board, pointed out that no active measures had been taken under the Medical Centre Act of 1945. He advised that in considering the membership and objects of a new planning body in the Centre the old Act should be disregarded and a new start be made. On motion of Mr. Johnston and his colleague from the General Hospital Board, C. Gordon Smith, it was agreed to organize the Medical Centre Planning Committee, which was composed of representatives of the five institutions then located there.

There were conflicting views about the terms of reference of the Committee. Some held that its work should focus primarily on the coordination of ancillary services such as joint laundry and power facilities; zoning matters, and traffic routes in and around the Centre; and an exchange of information with respect to new developments by individual institutions. But Gordon Smith stated bluntly that as he understood it, the institutions would submit their individual plans for development to the Committee for approval, which would be required before proposals were made to official agencies. Others pointed out that the public interest was already protected, since the Government had ruled that any plan for hospital structural change or development had to be first submitted to the newly formed Metropolitan Hospital Advisory Committee, which would in turn make recommendations to the Manitoba Hospital Commission and the Minister. From this point of view, requirement for prior approval by the Medical Centre Council, the members of which all had vested interests of one kind or another, would simply act as a block to getting anything done.

One of the basic principles, repeatedly stated, in Dr. Thorlakson's plan to assemble a number of hospitals in the Medical Centre area provided that although they would consult on matters of mutual concern to achieve cost efficiency, they would retain their operational autonomy. It was evident that this principle was now about to be abrogated.

The ensuing months brought a great flurry of activity in Medical Centre planning. The "Committee" became known as the Manitoba Medical Centre Council. A sub-committee composed of the chief executive officers of the several institutions was established, which met regularly under the chairmanship of Dr. Thorlakson to examine needs in the Centre and to consider solutions. The Medical Centre area was extended to reach from Sherbrook Street west to Arlington Street, and from Notre Dame Avenue north to the Midland Railway tracks, beyond Elgin Avenue. Indeed, when the plans were discussed with Mayor Juba, he was so enthusiastic that he advocated extending the Medical Centre area west as far as McPhillips Street. An informal arrangement was made with City zoning authorities which provided that zoning variations (which might be requested to allow new commercial or industrial enterprises to locate in the area) would not be granted without prior consultation with the Medical Centre Council.

Mr. Eric Thrift of the Faculty of Architecture had been acting as the primary planning consultant to the Council. At his suggestion, enquiries were launched to identify a planning and architectural design firm with the resources and experience to prepare a master plan for development. World-famous architects I.M. Pei and Associates of New York, and Jack Meltzer and Associates of Chicago, submitted proposals for the work, and sent representatives to Winnipeg to look at the site and gain first-hand views about what was intended.[6]

The legal firm of Johnston, Jessiman and Gardner was appointed by Council to draft appropriate amendments to the Medical Centre Act of 1945. Mr. Johnston's earlier opinion that the Medical Centre Act should be disregarded, and a new medical centre council incorporated, had apparently been overruled or forgotten.

A proposal was made to build a hotel, either in or on the perimeter of the Medical Centre. It was ultimately built on the south side of Notre Dame Avenue and is known as the Maryland Hotel. There were lengthy meetings with parking and traffic authorities. A Toronto investment group showed interest in building a parking facility and a motor hotel in the Centre. The Cancer Treatment and Research building was started. City Hydro offered to put all the electrical distribution lines underground for a cost of $31,000. Jack Meltzer submitted a new proposal to do a master plan for $37,000, which was accepted by the Medical Centre Council, provided the money could be raised. (The Chairman and the Secretary tried to get a grant from the Winnipeg Foundation, but were unsuccessful.) The Evangelical Church of the Cross enquired about obtaining a site for a church, in or adjacent to the Centre. Proposals were considered for structural improvements at the Children's Hospital and the General Hospital. Brochures were published, and an elabo-

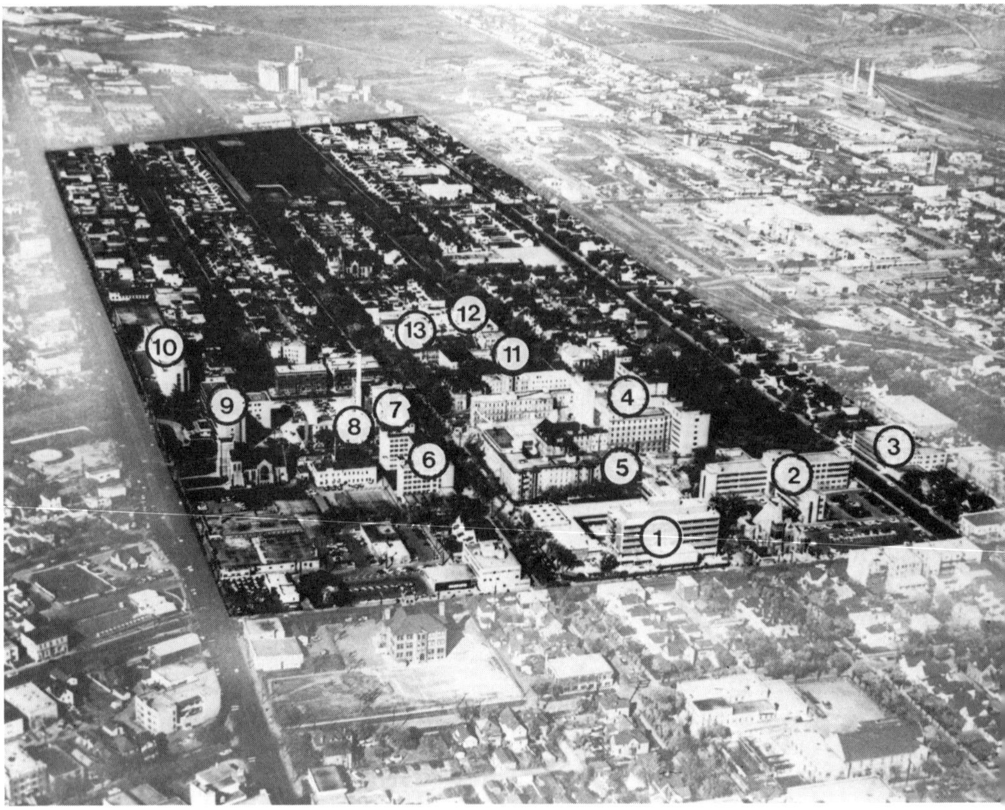

This aerial photograph shows the area for which zoning control was exercised by the City of Winnipeg for potential Manitoba Medical Centre development (1961). The numbers identify: 1) Manitoba Rehabilitation Hospital; 2) Children's Hospi of Winnipeg; 3) Children's Hospital Nurses' Residence and School; 4) Winnipeg General Hospital; 5) Manitoba Cancer Treatment and Research Foundation; 6) Winnipeg General Hospital Nurses' Residence; 7) Interns' Residence; 8) Married Interns' Residence; 9) Women's Pavilion; 10) Medical Centre Apartments; 11) Medical College; 12) Dental College; 13) Medical Library. (Photo by David Portigal.)

rate model of what the Manitoba Medical Centre might look like in the future was built. In many respects this was the most exciting period in the history of the Medical Centre.

However, in 1960 the Government appointed a committee to survey the hospital resources of the Province and make recommendations to guide the planning for future needs. Since no new capital projects for hospitals would be considered by the Manitoba Hospital Commission pending the report of the Hospital Survey Committee, any immediate developments of facilities in the Medical Centre were effectively blocked. The momentum and the enthusiasm that had been generated in the previous two or three years were lost.

Dr. Thorlakson was appointed a member of the Manitoba Hospital Commission in 1962, so he resigned as Chairman of the Manitoba Medical Centre Council; however he stayed on as a member. He was succeeded by Mr. C. Gordon Smith. The Medical Centre Council continued to meet periodically, but at lengthening intervals, until 1967.

In July 1965 the Minister of Health returned from a federal-provincial conference with news that as a supplement to the medicare program which was soon to be brought into effect, the federal government would establish a fund of $500,000,000 called the Health Resources Fund. It would be spent over the next fifteen years in Canada "to support the construction and equipment of facilities for health research and training." To the University (in particular its Faculty of Medicine) and the primary teaching hospital, the Winnipeg General, this was heady news indeed. It was scarcely believable that all this largesse was suddenly to be poured out on professional and technical health training facilities – primarily those requested by faculties of medicine.

But two more federal-provincial conferences on the details confirmed that funds would be made available to the provinces generally on a per capita basis, after first allocating $25 million to the maritime provinces. The federal funding would cover fifty percent of the construction and equipment costs for approved projects.

The Minister of Health (the Honourable C.H. Witney, who had succeeded Dr. George Johnson) asked the University to coordinate proposals from its department heads and the teaching institutions for expenditure of the Health Resources Fund money that would be allocated to Manitoba. The Hospital Commission supplied such assistance as was requested. The University appointed a Minneapolis firm of hospital consultants, represented by Mr. James Stephan, to act as their professional planning advisor.

By the beginning of May 1966, these efforts produced a plan which would require expenditure of $60 million, one half of which would come from the federal Health Resources Fund. These plans were submitted to the Minister and the Manitoba Hospital Commission on May 6, 1966. Subsequently, under the chairmanship of Mr. R.G. Goodman, Director of Research and Planning for the Manitoba Hospital Commission, a technical committee was appointed to examine the proposals and verify estimated costs. This committee reported in October, confirming that $60.8 million would be required for the submitted proposals. They also estimated that another $6.8 million might be added for other capital proposals. The additional operating costs that would be incurred were estimated at $10 million annually.

Apparently no-one thought of involving the Manitoba Medical Centre Council in all this activity. Dr. Thorlakson was aware of the planning through his position on the Manitoba Hospital Commission. At the meeting of the Medical Centre Council on June 17, 1966, he asked Dean Fyles if the University was carrying out a study of the Medical Centre in connection with the funds which were to become available from the Health Resources Fund. Dean Fyles confirmed that a study was under way which would develop a broad plan to meet the University's requirements in the Medical Centre for the next fifteen years.

In the light of the direct relation of the Faculty of Medicine with the Government in the proposals for the expenditure of $60 million (which proved to be much more than this in the long run) it was almost inevitable that any authority the Medical Centre might have had in planning would be swept aside.

The last meeting of the Medical Centre Council was held on October 16, 1967. By 1968 there was talk of bringing all the health facilities in the Centre into the direct orbit of the Faculty of Medicine and the primary teaching hospital, the Winnipeg General Hospital.[7]

Plans went forward vigorously, and as ideas expanded the

projected costs increased. The estimated cost grew from $60 million plus extras to $97 million, and an announcement was released by Premier Roblin on October 30, 1967, indicating that $97 million would be spent.[8]

Some suggestions were made indicating that perhaps some of the proposals would bear re-examination in view of the capital and operating costs that were anticipated. It became evident that debate would be avoided and progress would be easier if a consolidation were arranged.

In the meantime, Ed Schreyer was elected as Premier, and his administration was concerned about the projected costs. They were convinced that a single management for all the facilities would be more efficient and would save substantial sums of money through economy of scale. Unfortunately, economies of scale are rarely realized in industrial firms beyond a certain size. In the Canadian hospital system they are virtually impossible to achieve in large institutions.

In 1972 an act of the Legislature did away with the independent status of the several institutions and melded them into a new corporate body known as the Health Sciences Centre. This legislation came into effect on January 31, 1973. It marked the end of an important era in the development of health services in Manitoba during which its people had been well-served.

CHAPTER 21

The Paul H.T. Thorlakson Building

Recognizing that the Manitoba Medical Centre conceived by Dr. Thorlakson in 1943 and incorporated in 1945 was the precursor of what in 1973 became the Health Sciences Centre, the Board of Directors of the Centre determined to create a permanent testimonial to him by naming one of the splendid new buildings in his honour. There may be some symbolic significance in the fact that the ground-floor level of the structure they selected for this purpose encompasses the glass faced main entrance to the Centre, and the spacious entrance mall leading to all the sections into which the Centre is divided.

At a ceremony on Wednesday, June 26, 1985, presided over by Board Chairman W. John A. Bulman in the yet unfinished medical services building it was formally designated as the Paul H.T. Thorlakson Building. This would be affirmed by a suitably inscribed bronze plaque, which the chairman announced had already been commissioned, and which would be inset into the wall of the entrance mall. Several hundred guests and friends were in attendance.

The chairman then invited the President of the Health Sciences Centre, Mr. Peter Swerhone, to address the gathering. He sketched the half-century relationship of Dr. Thorlakson with the Medical School and the Winnipeg General Hospital, and his activities as the driving force behind the creation of the Manitoba Medical Centre in 1945. He went on to describe the building which was being named in his honour:

As we look around us at this impressive building – the newest on our campus – I think that we can say without a doubt that Thor's dream has truly been a vision fulfilled. Unfortunately, however, a sneak preview is all that we will be able to give you today. The upper floors of the building are still under construction. We are looking forward to the official opening . . . in about January 1986.

Most of you have entered the building today through the attractive two-storey glass mall and waiting area fronting on Sherbrook Street. This is more than just a doorway into a building. For the first time in the history of the Health Sciences Centre, we will have a central, visible main entrance. From this point the visitors, patients and staff will have access to every facility in the entire complex.

The seven-storey main portion of the building will serve as a key connection to the major patient care facilities. . . . It will have direct connection to the Rehabilitation/Respiratory Hospital, the Children's Hospital, the Manitoba Cancer Treatment and Research Foundation, the Sherbrook Parkade, and all levels of the General Hospital. The lower level will house our mailroom, micrographics, medical transcription, records, and pharmacy storage. It will also give access to the rest of the Health Sciences Complex.

Level 1, as you can see, is for admitting, pharmacy, medical records, social service, chaplaincy, cashier and information, as well as the attractive new gift shop for the White Cross Guild, and the CNIB canteen.

Level 2 will house adult physiotherapy, security, medical photography, beauty and barber shop, and the new home of the Bank of Montreal.

Level 3 will provide our not-for-admission-surgery patient facilities. Levels 4, 5 and 6 will have laboratory space devoted to clinical chemistry, pathology, hematology and urinalysis. It will house state-of-the-art equipment and technology, making it one of the most scientifically advanced laboratory facilities of its kind in Manitoba and in Canada. This integration of clinical laboratories will greatly benefit the delivery of clinical services in all areas of the Centre.

Last but not least, we are pleased to have space for the Health Sciences Centre Research Foundation on the seventh floor. When this building was originally planned, it called for six floors only. The Research Foundation, recognizing the critical need for research space, seized the opportunity to take on the responsibility of constructing and furnishing the seventh floor of the building. Thanks to the commitment of many citizens, businesses and organizations in Canada and Manitoba, the Research Foundation has raised over two million dollars toward the $3 million goal, for which we are very appreciative. . . .

Through all his hard work and varied activities, Dr. Thor's wife and family have gladly supported him and it is a pleasure to see here today

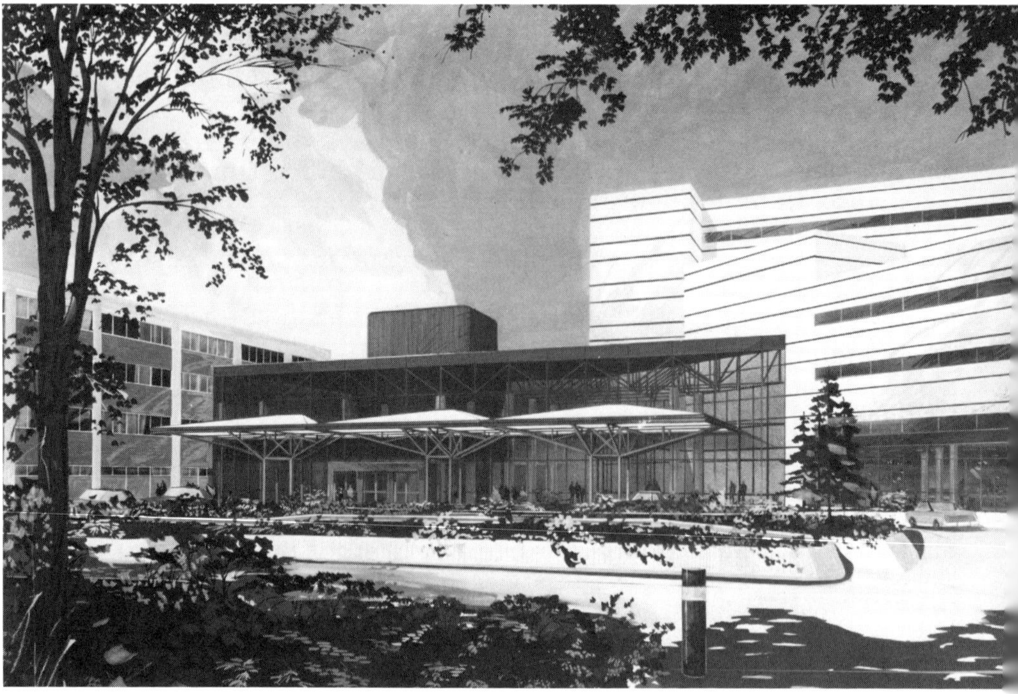

Entrance to the Paul H.T. Thorlakson Building, Health Sciences Centre. The building houses a variety of medical support services including clinical laboratories, the Physiotherapy Department, facilities for pediatric and adult day surgery, medical photography, and other essential services. The seventh floor is occupied by the headquarters and laboratories of the Health Sciences Centre Research Foundation.

Mrs. Gladys Thorlakson, along with their daughter, Tannis Richardson, and their two sons, Dr. Ken and Dr. Bob, and their families.

It is, indeed, an auspicious occasion for all of us today and I am very proud to have been associated with it.

Mr. Swerhone then introduced Her Honour Pearl McGonigal, Lieutenant Governor of Manitoba. She expressed in sincere, warm and informal terms her friendship with the guest of honour, and her respect for "his wisdom, his intelligence, and particularly his sense of humour." She said:

I think the fact that Dr. Thorlakson's family has been so supportive of his work is indicative of the fine image that he projects to his family and to all of us. And so, as the Queen's representative in the Province of Manitoba, I am particularly proud and pleased to be here as your friend too, as you are honoured with the opening of this splendid building.

My good friend, I'd like to present this scroll to you, and I'd like to read it, for the words are very important and very special. They say what we all feel about this great Canadian and fine Manitoban who is standing next to me.

THE BOARD OF DIRECTORS
OF THE
HEALTH SCIENCES CENTRE
presents this Scroll to
Dr. Paul H.T. "Thor" Thorlakson
CC, MD, CM (Man), MRCS (Eng), LRCP (Lond),
FRCS (Can), FACS
Hon LLD (Man), Hon MD (Iceland), Hon DSC (Brandon),
Hon LLD (Winnipeg), Hon FACHA, Hon FICS
At a special ceremony, which recognizes his unique part in shaping the origins of the Health Sciences Centre. A testimonial is mounted in the approach to what, with pride we have named the

PAUL H.T. THORLAKSON BUILDING

His was the vision, in 1942, of a community of hospitals centered around the Medical College. Together, they would be a place where excellence in learning, associated with challenging research, would provide for new achievements in the effective and efficient delivery of patient care. For thirty years he sustained the concept of a Centre,

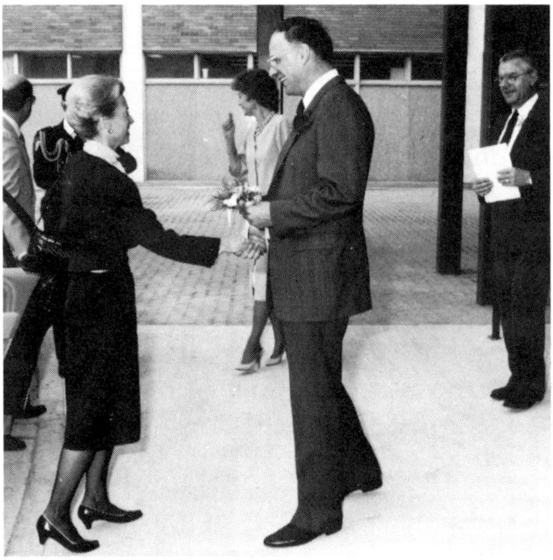

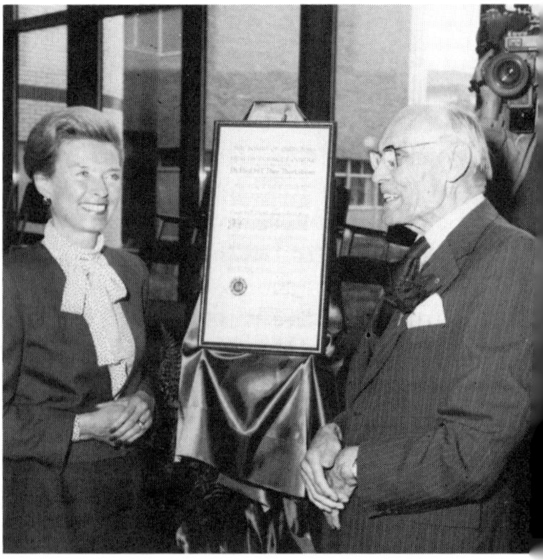

Her Honour Lieutenant-Governor Pearl McGonigal is welcomed by Chairman of the Board John Bulman and President Peter Swerhone when she arrives at the Health Sciences Centre to participate in the dedication of the Paul H.T. Thorlakson Building. (Photo by Photography Department, Health Sciences Centre.)

Her Honour Lieutenant-Governor Pearl McGonigal and Dr. Thorlakson beside the scroll she presented to him on behalf of the Board of Governors o the Health Sciences Centre. The event officially linked his name to the Medical Services Building. (Photo by Photography Department, Health Sciences Centre.)

both before and after its incorporation in 1945 as the Manitoba Medical Centre. Idea became reality by the incorporation of the Health Sciences Centre in 1973.

We honour Dr. Thorlakson's outstanding accomplishments in surgery, his pioneering introduction of Group Practice through the founding of the Winnipeg Clinic, and his international acclaim when he organized the First International Congress on Group Medicine, held in Winnipeg in Manitoba's Centennial Year.

We laud his consistent support of medical research, affirmed as a member of the First Associate Committee on Medical Research (the forerunner of the Medical Research Council of Canada); as President of the National Cancer Institute; and as the founder of the Manitoba Institute for the Advancement of Medical Education and Research.

We pay tribute to his contributions to the betterment of society in countless ways. They are exemplified by his interests in multiculturism, particularly his leadership in projects of special concern to the Icelandic community. His life long involvement in education extended beyond the medical field as evidenced by his term as Chairman of the Manitoba Council on Education, and his nine years as Chancellor of the University of Winnipeg.

Dr. Thorlakson's life has been distinguished by a sense of mission, nourished by his extraordinary physical stamina, self-discipline, patience, perseverance, and "the capacity to command events." He has been a sterling example of the intrinsic merit of Sir William Osler's dictum that "the Master Word in Medicine is Work."

W. John A. Bulman
Chairman of the Board
P.E. Swerhone
President

The chairman then called on Dr. Thorlakson, who responded with the following remarks:

Mr. Chairman, your Honour, a long-standing friend and co-worker and the President, Mr. Swerhone, ladies and gentlemen: You have accorded me an extraordinary honour today. Not only Gladys and I, but all of our family are grateful for the generous thoughts you have expressed and for the testimonial recorded on this elegant scroll.

It is a rare and exciting gift to be allowed to experience the fruition of an idea that one planted more than forty years before. In the year 1942 I suggested to the Board of Governors of the Winnipeg General Hospital the advantages of joining the Children's and other hospitals, and with the University, to develop a comprehensive Manitoba Medical Centre. This led to much discussion and tentative planning in hospital, medical, business and government circles.

As time passed it became evident that the broader community wanted to be informed about the nature and the purpose of these studies. An opportunity came when on April 14, 1944, I was invited to address a large meeting of the Civic Bureau of the Winnipeg Board of Trade. That dinner was held at the large dining room in the Hudson's Bay Store and I am going to shock you right now – we had a full-course dinner, a good dinner, and it cost 85¢. . . .

A few words from that address would indicate our intentions at that time in 1944 and I quote: "It is proposed to establish in Winnipeg a medical centre which will serve the city and the province with the most modern and complete facilities for the diagnosis and treatment of disease. It is an ambitious program involving the cooperative effort of several hospitals, institutions and public agencies."

The objective of the original proposal was the creation of a composite centre made up of individual self-regulated units sharing some physical resources, cooperating in teaching and dedicated to patient care and medical research.

Throughout my medical career I was actively involved in reporting my research on topics related to my surgical practice and, therefore, I am particulary pleased to know that through the efforts of the Health Sciences Centre Foundation, the seventh floor of this new building was added for clinical research. For the immense progress that has been made, I congratulate the Health Sciences Centre Board and its staff, the medical staff, the Government of the Province of Manitoba, and the Manitoba Health Services Commission, who together have created the splendid facilities which are in the course of completion here.

I would be remiss on this memorable occasion if I did not refer to the numerous persons in the health services and in public and private who supported the Manitoba Medical Centre and its successor, the Health Sciences Centre, throughout the past forty-three years.

Without their initial and continuing support the concept may not have survived. I cannot help but feel that in accepting this honour today, in a sense I am their representative; therefore, for all those countless others who caught the vision as well as for myself and my family, I say sincerely, very sincerely, "thank you."

Before closing the ceremonies, the chairman read letters of congratulation from Mayor Bill Norrie and from the Minister of Health, the Honourable Larry L. Desjardins, neither of whom was able to be present. As the formal proceedings ended, scores of friends pressed forward to offer their congratulations and best wishes to Dr. and Mrs. Thorlakson.

PART FIVE

Faculty of Medicine, University of Manitoba

CHAPTER 22

Early Association with the University

Dr. Thorlakson's parents were imbued with the pleasure and satisfaction that came from learning, and they were active in educational affairs in the community. Through their example, and by the encouragement of intellectual curiosity in their children, they passed on this love of learning for its own sake. At the same time they instilled in them a sense of obligation to share knowledge, and introduced them to the exhilaration that can be found in the interaction between teacher and student. It was a natural evolution of the family tradition that, not long after his own graduate training was completed, Dr. Thorlakson became a teacher in his profession, and in due course was invited to participate in the planning and development of medical education.

His first University of Manitoba appointment came in 1926, when Dr. Thorlakson was appointed as a demonstrator in the Department of Surgery. In 1928, he was appointed Lecturer in Clinical Surgery in the Faculty of Medicine. In 1934, on the recommendation of the Faculty Council, he became Chairman of the Committee on Graduate Studies,[1] constituted to recommend improvements in this essential component of medical education. In due course a comprehensive plan was submitted to Dean Mathers:

PRELIMINARY REPORT OF THE
COMMITTEE ON POSTGRADUATE EDUCATION (1934)

On August 11, 1934, I was notified of my appointment as Chairman of the Committee on Postgraduate Study. In presenting this preliminary report, I wish to emphasize the fact that I am seeking to approach the problem of postgraduate teaching from a broad perspective. Some of the proposals to be submitted cannot be implemented at once; others do not come directly within the scope of a postgraduate programme. These latter, however, in my opinion, will have an important bearing on the future working of the plans of this Committee.

Objective

The purpose of organizing a department is to acquaint the profession with the fact that we have excellent facilities for postgraduate study in our medical school and teaching hospitals. In other words, we hope to establish a recognized medical postgraduate centre in Winnipeg, especially adapted to the requirements of the profession in Manitoba and the other western provinces.[2]

Name of the Department

It has been suggested that the phrase *postgraduate work* be replaced by *continuation studies*. The idea behind the latter phrase, I understand, is to create in the minds of the profession the thought that postgraduate study begins immediately on graduation and continues throughout an individual's professional career. Furthermore, periodic organized guidance is an essential stimulus to continued study and clinical research by men in individual practice.

If this idea could be more adequately conveyed by designating this department The Department of Continuation Studies, I would recommend the adoption of such a name. However, after careful consideration, I feel we have more to gain by adhering to a name which has definite connotations in the minds of our fellow practitioners. I would, therefore, suggest that this department be named The Department of Postgraduate Studies of the Faculty of Medicine.

Organization

It is recommended that the personnel of the Department be as follows:

1. Director – appointed annually by the Faculty of Medicine.

2. Directorate – four members chosen from the Faculty of Medicine. Duties of the Directorate: to map out policies, decide on courses, appoint lecturers, plan publicity, and control finances.

3. Advisory Committee – to consist of: (a) the Registrar of the College of Physicians and Surgeons; (b) the Secretary of each of the rural Medical Societies; (c) the Secretary of the Winnipeg Medical Society

and the Manitoba Medical Association; (d) the Chairman of the Provincial Board of Health; (e) the Editor of the Manitoba Medical Review.

The reason for suggesting such an advisory committee is to keep the department in immediate touch with the needs of every section of the profession; and to enlist the personal cooperation of the above mentioned officials who, through their personal contacts, should be able to link up this department with their respective societies.

Full-Time Secretary
The duties of the full-time secretary will be to keep records, attend to correspondence, notify lecturers of their appointments, answer calls regarding courses, gather information concerning other postgraduate institutions, be able to direct casual visitors to work or clinics in which they may be interested. She should be a wide-awake, ambitious and intelligent girl who will grow into the large possibilities which will open up as the functions of this department enlarge. Preferably, she should have secretarial training and some familiarity with medical terminology. We would suggest a salary of $75 a month to begin with. This department should, as soon as possible, be provided with a private office in the College.

Finances
The initial outlay for the minimum office equipment, stationery, etc., would probably come to about $150. The monthly expense of the department would amount to approximately $100. I am informed that this department cannot expect a University grant; but I have reason to believe, because of previous associations with the College of Physicians and Surgeons, that the formation of a department of postgraduate study will meet with their sympathetic consideration. I would, therefore, recommend that the Council give us authority to approach the College of Physicians and Surgeons with the object of enlisting their support. Ultimately, the plan should become self-supporting – funds being secured from registration and tuition fees.

Courses of Instruction

1. We must first make arrangements for the doctor in the country and provide him with intensive short courses in general medicine, surgery, etc. Further, we must prepare short courses in individual subjects such as neurology, gastroenterology, paediatrics, etc.

2. Then, a more extended programme could be mapped out for doctors

in the city, consisting of weekly or semi-weekly lectures and practical demonstrations lasting two to four months, depending on the subject.

3. For doctors preparing for higher degrees, such as the FRCS or MRCP of Canada, England or Edinburgh, the Department would arrange courses as desired.

4. Special arrangements could be made for individual instruction to doctors who may be in the city for a few days only. The task of directing such visitors would be part of the duties of the secretary, who would make the necessary arrangements with the clinicians for individual instruction.

It has been suggested by the dean that this committee assume the responsibility for providing the Review with short practical articles similar to those that have been appearing.

Although this concludes the report proper, there is a related proposal in which I have been interested for some time and which I should like to place on record for consideration and discussion.

Proposal Regarding Pre-Internships

The average final-year student thinks largely in terms of the disabling types of disease presented by hospital patients. His experience is limited to this class of patient. The average intern has not been taught to meet the public and to deal with many of the common ailments that he will encounter from day to day in practice. Those limitations could be, to some extent, overcome by making arrangements for our undergraduate students – following the completion of their fourth year and before entering hospital for a year's internship – to be attached to a general practitioner, preferably in a rural district, for a period of six to nine months. This arrangement would bring the student into intimate contact with the every-day problems, professional and social, of general practice before the completion of his undergraduate studies and would enable him to better prepare himself during his final year for private practice.

This would benefit the practitioner in whose care such a student might be placed by bringing the former into closer touch with the medical educators. The stimulus that he would derive from discussing his problems with a student would undoubtedly raise the standard of his practice and would encourage him to read and keep abreast of recent advances in medical science. Every member of the faculty realizes what a stimulus he derives from his associations with keen, inquiring students. The benefits that would accrue to our school as a result of such arrangements might be striking. The experience of such apprentice students would enable us to discover the needs of rural practitioners and to make such changes in our curriculum as seem desirable as the result of such contacts.

The student might be able to attend the office; take calls for appointments; attend to accounts; and perform blood counts, urinalyses and other minor laboratory procedures which a busy country practitioner has little time to carry out. The student would receive his board and room and, in some cases, he might receive a small remuneration for any such period of *locum tenens* during the final weeks of the apprenticeship that the senior practitioner wishes to leave to his junior; allowing the rural doctor an opportunity to do postgraduate studies or to enjoy a necessary and long-planned vacation.[3]

By changing our present system to this extent, we should be carrying out the primary duty of a medical school, viz., to train general practitioners. In doing so, we should eliminate the common criticism that we are training specialists and not general practitioners. This plan has been in my mind for seven or eight years. I have discussed it with many country practitioners who seem to approve of the suggestion.

The plan would make regular postgraduate studies possible for a larger number of our rural practitioners.

The recommendation to give senior students the opportunity to take part of their training in "real-life" situations, directly under the tutelage of experienced medical practitioners in rural Manitoba, was fully supported by a number of prominent doctors practising in the country. They had themselves experienced the problems faced by newly qualified physicians who go directly after their basic training and a year of hospital internship into rural practice, where many of the support services in the teaching hospitals are not available. Among those who were supportive of the idea and ready to participate were it implemented were Dr. G.D. Shortreed at Grandview; Dr. George Clingan at Virden; and Dr. E.D. Hudson at Hamiota.

Dr. Thorlakson had himself experienced the potential advantage of such training. When the doctor at Neche, North Dakota (across the border from Altona, Manitoba) wanted a few weeks away from his practice for his marriage and honeymoon, he wrote to the Dean of Medicine to see if he could recommend a senior student who could temporarily look after his practice. Dr. Thorlakson was recommended for the post, and successfully acted as a *locum tenens* until the resident doctor returned.

The work of the Committee on Postgraduate Education led to a substantial development of training opportunities for doctors seeking additional training, whether in formal classes, or in short-term association with specific specialists.

However, nothing was accomplished regarding the recommendation that students be involved for a certain period of their training in the office practice of private physicians. Three years after the first report, Dr. Thorlakson and his Committee tried again:

A REPORT OF THE COMMITTEE ON POSTGRADUATE EDUCATION (1937)

The Dean has outlined to you the activities of the Postgraduate Committee over the three-year period since it was first organized. The teaching done during this period is the outcome of a programme drafted by the Committee and submitted to, and approved by, the Faculty Executive Council. The Committee invites your frank criticism of its past activities, but the time has now come when we must plan for the future. It is our hope that, as a result of the discussion which will take place tonight, the next three years' effort may definitely constitute a forward step in the field of postgraduate instruction.

In planning further courses we have to answer four main questions:

1. Why should this school interest itself in postgraduate training?

A. We know there is a genuine demand on the part of prairie practitioners for postgraduate courses.

B. The time will come, probably in the near future, when every doctor will be required periodically to attend special courses in order to retain his license to practise.

C. Any further expansion of our school must be through the medium of postgraduate teaching rather than an increase in undergraduate facilities. Not until the population of the prairie provinces has increased very considerably will there be any demand for additional undergraduate facilities above what we now have available. The Faculty must be organized for postgraduate teaching as thoroughly as it is organized for undergraduate work. Haphazard and undirected efforts will lead us nowhere.

2. What can this faculty do to create a reputation for Winnipeg as a postgraduate centre? There are three things necessary to attract men

to any medical centre: (a) the presence of outstanding teachers; (b) the stimulus of new leads in the shape of original research; (c) the abundance of clinical material.

In order to attract men from the country, we must establish Winnipeg in the minds of the profession at large as a centre where original research work and thinking is being done. I refer especially to the possibility of additional clinical research being attempted in this school.

At the present time, we recognize the valuable work that is being done by Dr. Cameron (professor of biochemistry) and Dr. Cadham (professor of bacteriology) in their fields, and we know that good work has been done by men on Gordon Bell and Banting fellowships. This work, however, could be extended. Any clinical research that is now done is limited to the sporadic efforts of individuals who gather together some hospital records and compile data for a clinical paper from them. We could, and should, do more than we are doing in the realm of clinical research.

Fundamental contributions to our medical and surgical knowledge have been made and will still be made by clinical research. That all modern research work must begin in a laboratory is a notion that should be discouraged. One does not imply that we do not recognize the progress that has been made in biochemical and physiological researches, etc., in the last twenty-five years, just as these had been preceded by numerous fundamental contributions in the clinical field during the previous fifty years. In the future, progress will depend more and more upon the closest cooperation between these branches of medical research and clinical research.

3. What form should the instruction take? We must arrange our courses so that they will be as useful as possible considering the constraints under which the men to whom we are lecturing are obliged to work. There is no use trying to teach them the use of complicated apparatus and so-called instruments of precision, because they will not have available many of these instruments. Our teaching will have to be practical and always thought out from the point of view of the man in the country.

During these courses, we have an opportunity – by talking to these men – of obtaining their viewpoints and seeing practice the way they see it, and of understanding some of their peculiar problems.

4. What can we do, as a postgraduate faculty, to make it possible for busy country practitioners to find the necessary time to avail themselves of the opportunities presented? We come now to a proposal which is somewhat revolutionary but which is, in our opinion, quite feasible and should have a distinct value in linking up the country

with the city in providing better opportunities for students to see some of the less serious diseases and infections, which they do not now see until after they have graduated. This proposal should be a source of stimulus to the country practitioner, to the student, to the teaching faculty and to the Postgraduate Committee.

[Here Dr. Thorlakson restated his 1934 proposal that arrangements should be made for undergraduate medical students who had completed their fourth year of study to serve as assistants to selected physicians in their offices – preferably in rural Manitoba.]

It would be a great advantage to the student to obtain some first-hand knowledge of the problems confronting the practitioners in urban or rural communities. It would be an advantage to the School to have such students return with questions relating to common diseases and their management in the home environment or in a small cottage hospital devoid of the laboratory equipment on which we are sometimes inclined to rely rather too much. Such a period of training would be of much more use to a student than serving as a handmaiden to the charge nurse by ordering laxatives and cough sedatives, or holding forceps by the hour while a surgeon performs some major operation, too intent on his work and too much occupied by the details of technique to give satisfactory instruction to the weary neophyte.

It would be a source of great stimulus to the general practitioner – who, for years may have been isolated and too busy to do a great deal of reading and to keep up with recent developments – to have with him a keen student inquiring earnestly into the causes of disease and the reason for certain lines of treatment.

Finally, such an arrangement would provide the practitioner with a *locum tenens* at a reasonable cost, which could be arranged between him and the student, so that the former could get away for post-graduate instruction or for a well-earned holiday. Arrangements could be made to legalize such a procedure, because most of the work done by such an assistant practitioner would be done under the supervision of his senior. Writing histories, doing routine physical examination, blood counts, urinalyses and routing calls – all could be taken care of by a fourth-year student in return for his board and room and possibly a little pocket money. A certificate of competency from the University of Manitoba would, we believe, satisfy the authorities for a period of six months and thus legalize the work that an undergraduate student might do.

By changing our present system to this extent, we would be carrying out the primary duty of a medical school, namely, to train general practitioners. By doing so, we should eliminate the common criticism that we are producing specialists and not general practitioners.

Before throwing the meeting open for criticisms and suggestions, I would like to point out the opportunity that presents itself: We are strategically situated in a centre of a field extending from the head of the lakes to Alberta, a field containing some 2,000 medical men as a potential student body.

MEDICAL RESEARCH

In 1938 Dr. Thorlakson was elected a member of the Executive Committee of the Medical Faculty Council. This active participation in the affairs of the Medical College and in the requirements for professional education and research reinforced his view that good medical teaching must be founded on a broad spectrum of excellence in medical practice. He believed that doctors who held the respect of their peers, however busy they were with their practice, had a duty to share in the training of their younger and less experienced colleagues. This sharing would have a double benefit. Those receiving the training would profit by the exposure to the discriminating judgment and the acumen harvested from years of professional practice. At the same time, for the practitioners, the requirements for teaching and the association with bright and enquiring minds would provide a continuing exposure to new ideas and encourage high standards of performance.

Concurrently, at the request of Dean Mathers, Dr. Thorlakson undertook the chairmanship of The Faculty Committee on Medical Research. It was the beginning of a lifelong support of the search for new knowledge, and a concern for the advancement of science in medicine.

Dr. Thorlakson's approach to medical problems, as was his approach to all situations and circumstances in which he was involved, was essentially practical and direct; so it was natural that he rather favoured clinical research, from which there seemed to be a more immediate benefit to medical practice. His own first effort in this direction was a study of ulcerative colitis, undertaken in association with Dr. Fred Cadham, which was reported to the American Association of Proctology in 1928.

Nevertheless, he was thoroughly aware of the essential nature of basic research and gave full support to finding and organizing the resources necessary for its support, both nationally and locally.

In specific instances of need that came to his attention, it is characteristic, however, that he bypassed the institutional structures and used more expeditious measures. An instance or two will illustrate.

Dr. J.D. Adamson, the Professor of Medicine, reported one day at a Faculty Council meeting that he had been approached by a resident who wanted to devote himself to medical research. Dr. Adamson was impressed with the young man's ability but, to finance a first-year position for him in a suitable research laboratory, $3,500 was needed. Neither University nor research funds were available. After the meeting, thinking about the loss to the research field if Dr. Adamson's young man were denied his dream, Dr. Thorlakson recalled that Mr. E.W. Kneeland, a prominent member of the Winnipeg business community, had offered financial help if an appropriate occasion arose. The next evening he went to see Mr. Kneeland, described the young man's desires and the need for supporting this ambition, and suggested that, if he (Dr. Thorlakson) put up $1,750, Mr. Kneeland might invest the other $1,750 necessary to launch this research career. Mr. Kneeland was glad to oblige, and proffered his cheque.

About a week passed before Dr. Thorlakson was able to arrange to meet Dr. Adamson, at which time he announced the good news: the one-year funding for Dr. Adamson's research protege was in hand. "Oh, it's too late," Dr. Adamson replied, "he's decided to get married and go into practice!"

On a later occasion, Dr. Joe Doupe, who was directing a research project having to do with the effect of cold on circulation in the body extremities, wanted to build a cold room in his laboratory. For this he needed $1,000, which was not available from the University or his research grant.

When Dr. Thorlakson heard of the dilemma, there was a patient on the private ward of the General Hospital who had offered to contribute to the support of any worthy medical project Dr. Thorlakson might suggest. On his next visit, Dr. Thorlakson explained Dr. Doupe's difficulty, and suggested that his patient might donate $1,000 to the University to finance the cold room. The patient (Mr. R.A. [Alex] Purves) was happy to do this, and Dr. Doupe was happy to find that the obstacle to his research plans had disappeared.

CHAPTER 23

A Department of Research

Banting's visit in 1938, the subsequent work of the Associate Committee on Medical Research, and some planned wartime research requested by the military authorities (the treatment of burns, wound infections, shock and the effects of mustard gas were some of the problems investigated in Manitoba) had resulted in a growing interest in improving the resources for research in the Manitoba Medical College and the teaching hospitals. The incorporation of the Manitoba Institute for the Advancement of Medical Education and Research in 1943 directly involved members of the University Board. The discussions surrounding the Institute brought about an improved understanding among the members of the University Board of Governors of the place of research in the program of medical education. The Institute's request to the University for an indication of specific ways in which support would strengthen medical research in the University compelled the Faculty of Medicine itself to seriously consider its position with respect to research.

Among Faculty of Medicine members there were mixed feelings on the subject. Virtually everyone was eloquent in support of the importance of research until it came to considering the allocation of Faculty resources. Then the needs of the clinicians, the surgeons, the laboratory specialists and the academics devoted primarily to undergraduate education, each group with their special priorities, seemed to become paramount.

The Faculty Executive Committee decided to ask Dr. A.T. Cameron, Chairman of the Research Committee, along with his colleagues Dr. Bruce Chown and Dr. Ian MacLaren Thompson, to prepare a comprehensive statement on principles and policies that should be adopted as a guide for research activities, which then, "as presented or as subsequently modified by the Faculty Council, would be transmitted to the Board of Governors of the University, and to such other bodies as the Council might direct."

In response to this request, Dr. Cameron prepared a discerning and candid statement of the basic conditions that are essential to successful research programs, and then discussed their application specifically to the Winnipeg scene. He wrote:

> Research may be defined as an orderly attempt, by observation or experiment, or both, to solve a problem, or to confirm or disprove a theory about a problem, or to check the conclusions of others about it. It may be carried out by an individual, with or without assistants working under his direction, or by two or more individuals working as a team . . . with assistants as required.
>
> Such assistants may be technicians . . . each adequately trained in one or more of the techniques involved in carrying out [the project]. Alternatively, assistants may be persons with partial training in the requisite background, who will gain more of such training through the experience gained while giving the assistance. Research Fellows are typical examples of the latter; they are not considered competent to undertake independent research.
>
> The above statements apply, whatever the nature of the research; for example, literary research, archaeological research or research in the pure or applied sciences. . . .
>
> Research always involves money. At a minimum, an investigator invests some of his time in it, and that time has a money value. It frequently involves much money in paying for the needed accommodation, the apparatus (frequently very expensive) and the salaries of the investigators and their assistants.
>
> Where research is carried on in Universities and similar institutions, the salaries . . . are partly in recognition of their duties as research workers, as well as their duties as teachers.
>
> The majority of scientific researches involve experiment. Some, such as astronomical research, chiefly involve observation, and in them experiment is confined to development of the tools for research. Some medical research is chiefly observational, . . . but experiment is seldom wholly absent.
>
> Anyone can attempt to do research, but successful research is very rarely accomplished except by persons trained in research methods.

Such training invariably involves drudgery, as it does in all disciplines.

With very rare exceptions, only those who themselves have been trained in research methods are competent to direct the research work of others.

The majority of people, including members of the medical profession, today are in favor of research being done. Few of them, unless they have been trained as research workers, realize what is required to usefully undertake it. Fewer still are willing to undertake true research work themselves, with the invariable routine and drudgery which cannot be completely dissociated from it.

They are very willing that research work should be done by somebody else. They consider that if they make monetary provision for it, and pass resolutions in favor of it, their part is accomplished. But you cannot order research as you can a roast of beef, or, in normal times, a new automobile.

However research is conducted, whether by individuals or groups, and even if it is adequately or perhaps lavishly financed, positive results can never be guaranteed; nor can the time needed to get results be calculated in advance – and this includes results sufficiently negative to indicate that a particular research should be stopped. However, the more money available, the greater the chance of obtaining results of consequence; although often a particular research may require several years, and it may be useless to commence it unless adequate support for a number of years is assured. . . .

University teachers ought to carry on research as part of their regular duties, which ought to include the training of others in research methods; but the subjects of their investigation should be decided by them. Any other arrangement will tend to lessen that atmosphere of freedom of thought, without which no University can [achieve greatness]. . . .

It is probable that no persons over forty years of age are (with rare exceptions) capable of being trained to do research work. The age limit for such capability is much lower. It follows that (since most of the clinical teachers in a University are above that age), unless they have earlier received the requisite training in research methods, they are incapable of directing research properly; with, of course, rare exceptions. . . .

In faculties of medicine . . . true research has too often been the work of the few, and not of the many. One essential for proper research work which has too often been neglected in the training of potential research workers in medicine is instruction in the proper appreciation of the literature bearing upon the subject under study, and in the presentation of the results of the research in a form fit for publication. The writing of scientific papers is an art, and the few (if any!) essays which a medical student has to write in the course of his studies afford completely inadequate preparation for it. Inability to practise this art is probably the reason that so many valuable observations made in any large hospital are not recorded in the literature.

When there is any real research activity in a medical faculty (as contrasted with the sporadic activity of a few individuals), a system of sharing common facilities, such as animal accommodation, special technicians, and special equipment, will prove inadequate. Each department must be itself almost completely equipped for its own researches. . . .

[With regard to our own needs], the quickest way of developing this University as a first-class medical research centre would be the establishment of research professorships, such as, for example, a professorship in experimental medicine. But this method is the most expensive one of all. To achieve any results of real value a relatively young man of proven ability as a research worker and as a director of the research work of others must be appointed as professor and director of an independent department. . . .

His salary, if he is any good, will be in the order of $7,000 to $10,000 a year, and this salary is only part of the expenditure needed. His department would need adequate accommodation, several full-time research fellows, technical assistants, equipment. Moreover, no really capable person would accept such an appointment unless this machinery for efficient work were guaranteed him. . . .

Present sources of monetary assistance include: the National Research Council; the Banting Foundation; the College of Physicians and Surgeons of Manitoba; the Manitoba Institute for the Advancement of Medical Education and Research; and the University itself. Of these only the Manitoba Institute is at present a potential source of any fairly large amount of money. It is the best potential source of funding fellowships, although its policy concerning them has not yet been completely made known. . . .

The paper inspired a lively discussion at the next meeting of the Faculty Council.

Quite unexpectedly, in the midst of the discussions about research in the Faculty of Medicine, Dean Mathers received a letter from India. The writer, well-known to the Dean, was Major Joseph Doupe, then stationed at the headquarters of the 33rd Corps, South East Asia Command, Doges Bank, New Delhi.

Joseph Doupe was born in Winnipeg, the son of C. Somerville Doupe, an official with the CPR. He graduated in medicine from the University of Manitoba in 1934, and went to England to take graduate work at the London Hospital; and later, at the National Hospital for Nervous Diseases. He obtained his membership in the Royal College of Physicians, London, in 1936. In 1938 he went to the University of Pennsylvania for further training in research methods with Professor H.C. Bazett.

With the outbreak of World War II, he returned to Canada and, after a period at the Banting Institute in Toronto, he joined the Royal Canadian Army Medical Corps. He served in France and went through the evacuation from Dunkirk. He resumed research work in Britain and established his scientific reputation as an outstanding clinical physiologist with his work on peripheral nerve injuries. He then returned to service in uniform in the Middle East, India and Burma. Now, four months before the war in Europe ended, but with victory assured, Dr. Doupe was a member of an Operational Research Unit in New Delhi. With the end in sight, he longed for early return to the peace and freedom of civilian life, and to professional work that would offer challenge and a sense of self-fulfillment. His training, his varied experience and his special gifts of intellect and character, opened the door to appointments of many kinds, in many places. But he had a special interest in returning to his home city and his alma mater.

On February 1, 1945, sitting in his rooms in New Delhi, his mind filled with concerns about the direction his personal and professional life should take in the postwar years, he made the decision to write to Dr. Mathers.

Dear Dr. Mathers.

I have many times considered writing you about the prospects of a job in Winnipeg after the war. However I have never really decided on the kind of work I would like to do. Recently I have been forced to do this because I have been offered a chance to start a clinical research unit at Toronto. My reply was non-committal but I was stimulated to formulate some views on the organization of clinical research. I propose to outline them to you as a means of indicating the sort of Utopia for which I am seeking.

I have had several opportunities of watching the evolution of clinical research units and in fact built one for the MRC in 1941. This experience convinces me that such units have three main defects. The job of

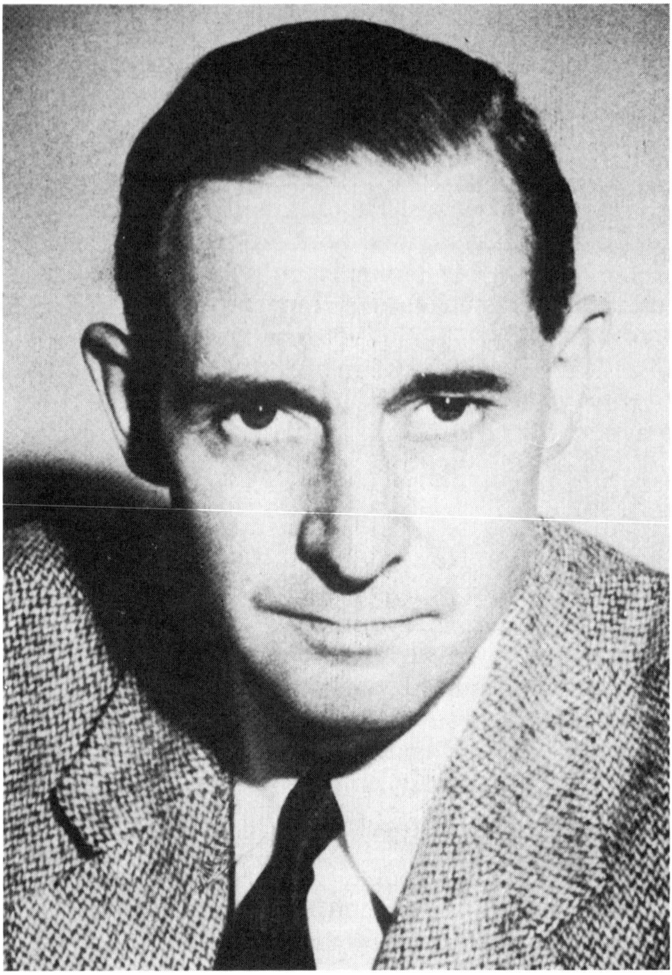

Dr. Joseph Doupe, 1910–1966, brilliant scholar and teacher, was appointed Director of the Department of Medical Research at the University of Manitoba in 1946, and Professor and Head of the Department of Physiology and Medical Research in 1948. He achieved national recognition for his role in medical research and was a member of the Medical Research Council of Canada.

director looks grand to a young man but in truth is apt to be a blind alley. It offers little opportunity for either pecuniary or academic advancement. Moreover having a research unit in a medical department tends to discourage rather than encourage research by the clinical staff. I believe it removes the onus of making progress from those best qualified to bear the burden. My third and perhaps most important criticism is that research workers in such units become segregated from the rest of the community and particularly from the coming generation. This does not happen to those working in other departments such as physiology. In this way they cannot exercise their proper educational function – a loss both to themselves and to others. To themselves because they can still feel that they are serving a useful function when, as is inevitable, experiments go wrong. A loss to others because it must be advantageous for students to come into contact with those whose profession is based on critical and individualistic thinking.

Were I asked to formulate an alternative scheme to promote clinical research I would propose the appointment of an "advisor in clinical research" to the staffs of medical schools and of large teaching hospitals. His work would be to actively stimulate enquiry by others, provide special facilities for the work, help with unusual techniques, give counsel about the general approach to the problem and advise regarding preparation for publication. He would also be required to conduct informal discussion groups such as journal clubs and perhaps to give or arrange lectures on the relation of science to medicine, the fundamentals of statistical analysis, etc. In return he would expect a living wage and facilities to carry on research. Such facilities would be one of the most valuable perquisites of the job and would include access to patients and a laboratory in the hospital.

I believe this scheme would give ample opportunities for the "advisor" to advance in the faculty; he could teach, he could research and when his ideas ran out he would not be left high and dry.

I don't know if this idea is sound but I think it would be an interesting experiment and I think that the Medical College because of its size and the composition of its faculty would be an ideal trial ground. Should you react at all favourably to this proposal I would be extremely delighted.

Yours very sincerely,

Joe Doupe

P.S. For important personal reasons I would like very much to return to Winnipeg as soon after the war as possible. Therefore if you could suggest any other way of employing me I would be grateful. J.D.

Dean Mathers discussed Dr. Doupe's letter with members of the Faculty Executive Committee and other senior Department Heads. They may have had mixed feelings about the suggested appointment of an "advisor in clinical research." In any event, the dean had no funds in his budget to support the position proposed by Dr. Doupe. Consequently, Dr. Mathers, in his response, welcomed Dr. Doupe's interest in joining the Faculty, but pointed out the lack of money, and some of the problems that might be presented in establishment of a position of the kind described in his letter.

The correspondence continued from time to time without apparent progress, and in December 1945 Dr. Doupe sought the advice and assistance of his friend Dr. Charles Code, who was now well established in research at the Mayo Clinic. Dr. Code promptly telephoned Dr. E.W. Montgomery, one of Manitoba's most respected physicians. For some years Dr. Montgomery had been Professor of Medicine, and both Dr. Doupe and Dr. Code had been among his students. He had been President of the Canadian Medical Association in 1927, and was appointed Manitoba's first Minister of Health in 1928; but by 1946 he had returned to his practice at 308 Medical Arts Building. In the telephone discussion Dr. Montgomery expressed his interest in finding a place for Dr. Doupe in Winnipeg after his discharge from the military service and invited Dr. Code to write to him on the subject. On January 11, 1946, Dr. Code wrote:

Dear Dr. Montgomery:

This letter is written to follow up our recent telephone conversation in regard to Joe Doupe. As you know, Joe has been a friend of mine ever since we were in school. He is one of my oldest and best friends. We have always worked in similar or allied fields and this has probably sustained our friendship during the last eight years when our activities have been in widely separated areas of the world. I feel I have a sound appraisal of Joe's accomplishments, and I thought you might be interested in some of these.

Joe has always been and always will be a good doctor. This interest in the sick and his strong sense of responsibility towards the sick person have kept his studies close to the bedside. He has elected a career in research and investigation. He has always and I imagine he should always combine this with medicine – either by practicing medicine or certainly by having access to clinical material for study.

Joe had an excellent record at the Winnipeg General Hospital where his unstinting energy in the interests of the patients, his keen insight, active mind, and his generosity won for him the respect and friendship of all.

After leaving the Winnipeg General Hospital Joe went to England where he took his MRCP and it was there [that he and] I renewed our friendship and shared so many happy, lively and stimulating experiences.

Joe was studying hard and obtained an appointment under Dr. E.A. Carmichael, Director of Research at the National Hospital, Queen's Square, England. Dr. Carmichael is one of the outstanding medical neurologists and clinical neurologic investigators in Europe today. I know if he could write to you that he would recommend Joe most highly. In his final year with Carmichael, Joe was his right-hand man and, besides conducting many investigations himself, he provided ideas and carried the major burden of Dr. Carmichael's own investigations during that year. I understand Dr. Carmichael has invited Joe to take an appointment with the Medical Research Council of England. It is my feeling that Joe would prefer to live in Canada.

Joe has many excellent research publications. He has been kind enough from time to time to send me reprints. His papers belong in the top category of medical research. He has been productive in the past and I am sure he will continue to be so in the future. He could, I am sure, provide you with reprints if these were necessary.

Dr. Robert W. Wilkins at the Massachusetts Memorial Hospitals, Boston, Massachusetts, is Chester Keefer's right-hand man in that hospital. Bob is a great mutual friend of Joe's and mine. He has invited Joe to join him at the Massachusetts Memorial Hospitals in an appointment that would combine neurologic research and medical practice with a service on the medical wards. Joe, I know, has considered the appointment, but once again I believe he is anxious to return to Canada. I hope the Medical School in Winnipeg will be able to take care of Joe. He is one of the most productive graduates we have had from the School. If he were to join the staff now, he would come at a time when the development of modern clinical research is much needed. I hope that every effort will be made to arrange an appointment which will enable him to teach, do research and see patients. I believe you would find his presence a stimulating and important factor in the further development of our Medical School. Anything that I can do to be of assistance in making such an appointment possible will be undertaken vigorously and with pleasure.

Yours sincerely,

Charles F. Code, M.D.

In the meantime, Dr. Doupe was about to receive his discharge from the military service, return to Winnipeg to visit family and friends, and renew in person his endeavours to gain an appointment on the University staff.

Dr. Montgomery was convinced that Dr. Doupe could make an important contribution to medical education and research in Winnipeg. He confirmed with the Dean that if funds could be raised for its support, the Faculty of Medicine would like to establish a new department of medical research, with Dr. Doupe as its director.

Dr. Montgomery decided to test the possibility of a grant from The Winnipeg Foundation. He put the case to Peter Lowe, the long-time, highly respected Secretary of the Foundation. The reply from Mr. Lowe came on January 31, 1946:

Dear Dr. Montgomery:

In discussing or considering the promotion of medical education and research, the members of our Board have always put forth the opinion that when any effort of this nature is undertaken it should be done through the University of Manitoba and its Medical Faculty, and should include support from all the medical or surgical associations within the Province. While there have been a number of discussions and meetings with representatives of the medical and surgical groups on the subject, on no occasion have they ventured to suggest what financial assistance they would provide to make a start towards the objective. It has long been felt that the sum of $10,000 would only be a beginning, and that such a department [i.e., Research] of the University would need increasing funds from year to year to meet new requirements in personnel and equipment.

It is the writer's opinion that our Advisory Board is not likely to show any further interest in the subject until such time as the medical and surgical associations of Manitoba are able to come forward with a concrete plan for reaching the objective and an undertaking in respect of the financial support they will give. . . .

On the strength of Mr. Lowe's statement, Dr. Montgomery wrote to the president of each of the medical associations and societies in Manitoba, and appealed for financial contributions from the doctors that would form the basis for a matching grant from the Winnipeg Foundation. Sadly, the request for seed money fell on stony ground.

It was on a stormy night in mid-February that the climax to these events was reached. The University of Toronto was pressing Dr. Doupe (who had returned to Winnipeg) to give a firm answer to their offer of a position as director of a research unit. It appeared that all efforts to achieve an acceptable appointment in Winnipeg had failed. Very reluctantly, Dr. Doupe agreed to go to Toronto and complete arrangements with the University there.

He was spending the evening before his departure with, among others, Dr. Lennox Bell. Dr. Bell was one of the original members of the Winnipeg Clinic, and was now full-time Dean of the Faculty of Medicine. Dr. Bell suggested that even at this "eleventh hour," they should lay the problem directly before Dr. Thorlakson. After confirming by telephone that he was at home, they drove out to Grenfell Boulevard to see him.

Dr. Thorlakson was, of course, generally familiar with the story, but now he heard it directly from Dr. Doupe himself. Dr. Doupe's evident sincerity and the hope expressed by Dr. Bell that even at this last minute some way might be found to provide the funds that would keep his friend and colleague in Winnipeg, persuaded Dr. Thorlakson that perhaps he ought to intervene. He said:

As I understand the problem, you need a three-year commitment of$10,000 annually to permit you to establish your home in Winnipeg and take an appointment as director of a new department of medical research at the University of Manitoba. You now face the necessity of accepting an offer from the University of Toronto because this money has not been made available. Perhaps there are other ways of resolving the problem.

I can tell you that we now have $7,500 in the Manitoba Institute for the Advancement of Medical Education and Research which I believe could properly be used to help in this situation. Within two or three weeks, I am sure it can be arranged that we will have in hand or in assured pledges twice this amount – that is, $15,000. If we could persuade the University to fund $15,000 over a three-year period to match our contribution, the $30,000 needed to fund your new department would be provided.

Tomorrow morning I will discuss this proposition with the Chairman of the Board of Governors of the University, Judge Berman. I believe he may find means to accept this plan and, if so, with funding assured, Dean Mathers will be able to seriously approach his arrangements for your appointment. In the meantime, I suggest that you postpone your plans to go to Toronto until the Dean has a chance to talk with you.

To Dr. Doupe, who had been struggling for a year to find the key to doors that it seemed impossible to unlock, Dr. Thorlakson's counsel came as a revelation. There was a pause. "And now," continued their host, "let us turn to other things. I know what Dr. Bell's tastes are, but Dr. Doupe, do you take soda or water with your Scotch?"

Dr. Doupe was duly appointed Director of the Department of Medical Research at the University of Manitoba, a position which he held until he was appointed Professor and Head of the Department of Physiology in 1948. Both in his profession and in his personal qualities he was a distinguished member of the Faculty of Medicine, recognized nationally for his role in medical research. He was appointed a member of the Medical Research Council of Canada and a consultant and panel chairman to the Defence Research Board. In 1960 he was awarded the Alumni Jubilee Citation for "distinguished achievement" and in 1966 the senior medical students chose him as first recipient of the Professor of the Year award.

Dr. Doupe died prematurely at the age of fifty-six on August 27, 1966. The sense of loss and the fondness and respect with which he was remembered are epitomized in the following tribute to Professor Doupe which appeared as a letter to the editor of the *Winnipeg Free Press* on October 8, 1966.

TRIBUTE TO PROFESSOR DOUPE

Sir: My wife and I were deeply saddened to learn of the passing of Professor Joseph Doupe, Winnipeg. The University of Manitoba Medical College and medicine at large will miss a great and gifted man.

Joe, as he was affectionately referred to by scores of students, was a superb physiologist and brilliant teacher. His lectures were extemporaneous, lucid and ruthlessly logical. His aim was to transform the slothful, illogical, confused mind of the neophyte into the alert, resourceful, reasoning mind of the graduate. He urged us to think, to inquire and to reason.

Joe was an iconoclast. He challenged many of our beliefs. Our basic premises shattered and fell. Then he rebuilt us, encouraging us to use our minds, to get our brains out of low gear and into high. In many instances he succeeded; those who failed Joe failed medicine.

The class of '66, of which my wife and I are members, honored Dr. Doupe by awarding him the first Professor of the Year trophy. This award will be given annually to the teacher who has most influenced the medical student in his four years of medicine. Joe was unanimously elected.

There are many incidents one can recall in which Joe played a central part. His oral examinations were the bane of our existence in the freshman year. His lavish parties will be remembered by all who attended. The critical question and central criticism of any work of research were put by Joe with unerring incisiveness. Half asleep, Joe was more alert than most of us wide awake.

It would not be an exaggeration to say that much of the progress at the University of Manitoba Medical College in the last 20 years was due to Joe's initiative, perseverance, encouragement and direction. As director of medical research he brought world-famous investigators to head other departments. He personally solicited much of the money with which to carry on the first-class research for which Manitoba is famous. Consequently, many of his students are widely known in their own right. The names of Cherniak, Israels, Zipursky and Cumming come quickly to mind. There are many others.

Joe's wit, generosity, genius and irreverence for blind faith has inspired and will continue to inspire those of us who were fortunate enough to know him. We join his students, colleagues and friends in extending sympathy to his family.

Drs. Keith and Phyllis Meloff,
Minneapolis

CHAPTER 24

Of Students and Teachers

During World War II most medical schools in North America were faced with many more applications for enrolment than they could accept. Manitoba was no exception. By 1943, the Student Selection Committee of the Faculty was flooded with nearly 400 requests for admission, a large number of which were from the United States. Under the circumstances most of the latter were almost automatically refused; but this still left 290 or more applicants from Manitoba and elsewhere in Canada clamouring for entry, when only sixty or seventy first-year students could be accommodated.

Inevitably, some criticism arose among the unsuccessful candidates about the methods of selection. Complaints reached both the Board of Governors of the University and the provincial government. The nature of their complaints was such that the Board felt it necessary in 1944 to establish an ad hoc committee from among its members to try to formulate guidelines for use of the Selection Committee of the Faculty. Emotions had been aroused and contentious letters appeared in the press. Claims were made that preference was given to applicants from doctors' families; and there were suggestions that racial discrimination entered into the selection process.

Like all his colleagues, Dr. Thorlakson was concerned about these sensitive issues. He was perhaps even closer to the problem than some, since Mrs. Thorlakson was a member of the Board of Governors of the University, and he had two sons in medical school.

In the spring of 1944 Dr. Thorlakson prepared a brief for presentation to the Ad Hoc Committee and the dean (which he later circulated to all members of the University Board), that injected a note of logic and realism into a situation that threatened to become unduly factious:

THE SELECTION OF MEDICAL STUDENTS
The responsibility of the Medical Faculty of the University of Manitoba is two-fold: the careful selection of medical students; and the thorough training of these students to the end that they will render a useful and creditable service to the community. At the moment we are concerned with only the first responsibility.

Certain broad principles must be laid down before arriving at a solution of this problem, which possesses many inherent difficulties.

1. The first point upon which there must be agreement is the necessity of limiting the number of students admitted to medical school. In every medical school certain controls operate to determine the number of students that can be provided with adequate facilities for training in the art and science of medicine.

There are many factors involved, such as teaching staff, financial support, laboratory and research facilities. However, the most important controlling factor is the volume of clinical material available for the practical demonstration of disease processes and their treatment. The value of a doctor to any community depends on his training and practical clinical experience in the diagnosis and treatment of disease, and his knowledge of public health. In Winnipeg there is a definite limit to the number of medical students who can receive clinical instruction in hospital in their two final years.

2. The second point upon which there must be agreement is that the basis for the limitation should be made common knowledge. The young student who is qualifying himself for admission to the medical school should have access to this information. It is obvious that this process of selection should continue even into the medical course itself.

3. It should not be difficult in a democratic community to reach agreement on the next point worthy of emphasis. Small financial means should not debar from admission an otherwise excellent candidate. This implies government subsidy for some individual students.

4. In the process of selection the relative importance of scholastic standing requires the most thorough study. This study should be based

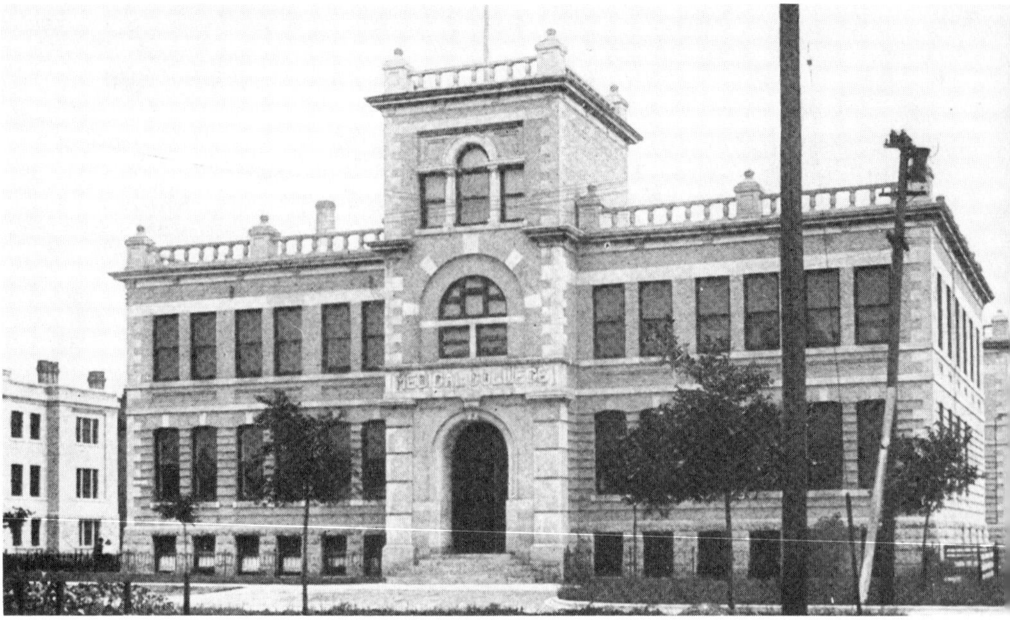

An early picture of Manitoba Medical College, Bannatyne entrance

on fairly complete knowledge and consideration of all the attributes which influence the moral character and professional ability of the candidate for medicine. In medicine the qualities of honesty, reliability and logical thinking, based on modern knowledge of disease and its treatment, are paramount to a greater degree than in almost any other group because the problem of life and even death itself is a matter of constant daily responsibility.

Before proceeding with the problem of laying down principles and rules that are to guide a committee on selection, there must be a definite stand taken on the following point: scholarship, by itself, is not sufficient guarantee of professional integrity and a high quality of unselfish service to the community. The records of graduates from our Faculty of Medicine prove this conclusively. Brilliance is an asset, but it is not the only factor in determining the fitness of the applicant to enter the profession of medicine.

5. In any field of public service, the predominance of any racial group in excess of its relation to the general population is not conducive to harmony, a sense of confidence, or generally improved social relationships within the community. Any group that insists that it is entitled to a disproportionate representation on the student body of any faculty in which restriction is absolutely necessary, lays itself open to a charge of a super-race complex. In the past, the committee that has accepted the onerous and thankless responsibility of selecting medical students has not been guilty of racial prejudice. On the contrary, it has adopted a practical attitude toward a problem upon which there can never be unanimous agreement as long as the principle of limitation is accepted as necessary and desirable. In the selection of medical students, the argument that a candidate should be considered a Canadian and his racial origin disregarded completely, has much to commend it. This attitude should be recognized and encouraged by the governing body of the University, but it represents a hope rather than a present achievement. In the final analysis, its recognition depends upon the ability and desire of the group concerned to blend itself without reservation into the fabric of Canadian life and custom. The committee in the past has adopted a rational, practical attitude toward this difficult problem. While its decisions in individual cases may be criticized, they have unquestionably been motivated by the desire to provide the West with a group of graduates that could best meet the special needs of this complex community.

6. It is fair and reasonable that students from Manitoba should receive preference. However, we should not go to the extreme of excluding desirable students from other sections of Canada, the British

Commonwealth or the United States, provided there are excellent reasons for their acceptance into the student body. By placing barriers against students from outside Manitoba, we would be giving the signal for the erection of barriers against our graduates entering the practice of medicine in other sections of the Dominion. In the long run, it is not an advantage to narrow one's horizon too much by viewing this problem from the purely geographical standpoint.

Examination of records and personal interview with the candidate enables the committee to determine if the student possesses the qualities of scholarship, character and personality, and citizenship which give promise of a high standard of attainment. Scholarship must take into consideration the candidate's ability to think and reason logically, as well as to memorize facts. The committee for selection has a serious responsibility. It should expect to receive the fullest measure of support from the Medical Faculty and the Board of Governors of the University of Manitoba. It is entitled to the confidence of the public which, in the final analysis, receives the benefits from the care and judgement exercised in the selection of medical students.

Apart from the local concerns about the method of selecting students, faculties of medicine in many universities were at this time engaged in a re-examination of the structure and effectiveness of medical education. The last great surge in the improvement of method and content in medical teaching had occurred in the years following the famous report of Abraham Flexner[1] issued in 1910, after a far-ranging survey of medical schools in North America. The body of medical knowledge had changed and expanded immensely during the ensuing three decades, resulting in greater demands on both teachers and students. It had become customary for the basic sciences to be taught by full-time teachers and researchers; but the clinical instruction continued to be directed and provided mainly by doctors in practice in the community, who devoted part of their time to academic affairs. The impending return of doctors who had been in the armed forces, many of whom could be expected to have an interest in postgraduate training, had to be planned for; and the pressure for admission to medical schools could be expected to increase in the postwar period.

In the spring of 1945, Dean Mathers circulated to faculty members a copy of the report of the Committee on Medical Schools, published by the Ministry of Health for Scotland. It recommended a number of principles that might be established to guide the organization method and curriculum of modern medical education.

Selected members of the Faculty were asked to prepare a commentary on specific sections of the Scottish report and make a presentation to Faculty Council, adding their own suggestions for improvement of programs or methods in Manitoba.

Faculty Council (which in effect consists of all members of the Faculty of Medicine) met on April 30, 1945, to hear and discuss the papers. Along with others selected by the dean, Dr. Thorlakson presented his exposition of the section of the Scottish report that had been assigned to him, setting the tone of his remarks by leading off with a quotation from it: "The organization of teaching is likely to be assisted if, (a) *informal meetings of all teachers* are held periodically for the discussion of the content of teaching and the correlation of teaching between departments; and, (b) *the views of the students* regarding existing deficiencies and desirable improvements are obtained regularly."

Dr. Thorlakson pointed out that the report gave much weight to an improved integration and coordination of the pre-clinical and the clinical phases of a student's training, and a closer dovetailing of the teaching provided by the various departments and teachers. He pursued the subject with suggestions for application of the principles in Manitoba:[2]

SUGGESTIONS

The following thoughts and suggestions are submitted to this meeting realizing that there are likely serious imperfections and impracticabilities in the recommendations and that modifications of one's viewpoint will be necessary in the light of the opinion of other contributors to this discussion.

MEDICAL DEPARTMENT AS COORDINATOR

As our main purpose and function is to educate and train general practitioners, the *medical department* should act as the central coordinating unit of the whole five-year course. In this department would be men well trained in functional anatomy, applied physiology and applied biochemistry, preferably recruited from specialists who had, in their junior years on the staff, served as instructors or done research work in these departments. In the hospital also, the medical department should be situated in the very centre of the teaching unit with adequate space for group conferences and consultations with other departments. There should be also many small examining rooms where histories can be taken *privately* by medical students or junior interns and checked by residents and the honorary attending staff. This diagnostic and consulting unit, attached to the indoor medical department, would also act as a clearing-house for general medical examinations and consultations from other departments.

Medicine and surgery should not be separated into two distinct departments as was the case twenty-five years ago. I do insist that a surgical operation is to be considered as only one step in the management and rehabilitation of the patient. An operation is neither the beginning nor the end of treatment, except in a small proportion of cases. If this attitude is sound with regard to general surgery, I suggest that it applies with equal force to other departments. The special diagnostic and therapeutic departments of surgery; urology; dermatology; eye, ear, nose and throat; etc., should not continue to function apart from the closest collaboration with a strong and well-organized medical department.

It is many years now since I advocated the appointment of a consultant in medicine to be attached to the surgical service and likewise a surgeon to be attached to the medical service, not for the purpose of occasional consultations but that, during any particular assignment period, they would have access to all the patients on that service.

On the surgical service, for instance, there would be regular ward rounds at which the medical consultant would attend. The students and interns attached to that service would have both the medical and surgical aspects of the case presented and discussed. The opportunities for instruction would be multiplied and each case fully utilized for demonstrating the patient as a problem in disordered function and disease, and not merely as a surgical case. There are many interesting acute and chronic medical problems on every large surgical service and I know, from recent ward rounds, that the medical department harbours many patients with minor and major surgical lesions associated with, or even unrelated to, the particular medical ailment which confines them to hospital.

It is recommended, therefore, that – as a matter of principle – we agree that the medical department assume the function of the main co-ordinating agency and influence of the medical school, and that this department be organized on that basis.

As the Department of Medicine should act as the hub of our system both in the college and in the hospital, so should the Department of Pathology hold a key position in matters of laboratory medicine as well as in combined medical, surgical and pathological conferences; examples of which are the clinical-pathological conferences on Saturday mornings and the tumor clinics on Wednesday mornings.[3] These two activities, in which the Department of Pathology has taken a leading part for many years, are two of the outstanding educational features of the week. Provided that the Department of Pathology is located in a central position, such as is provided in the proposed plan for the Winnipeg General Hospital, it can carry on its ordinary function as a laboratory more efficiently and with less waste of valuable time – time and effort that could go into developing more points of contact with some other clinical department. The relationships between the clinical departments and the Department of Pathology have, in the past, been most happy and have resulted in many fruitful and instructive discussions. The physical arrangement of our new hospital set-up should be such as to strengthen this particular link between departments . . . .

Three months after presenting this paper, Dr. Thorlakson was invited to address the incoming group of interns, some seventy in number, who on July 1 began their final year of basic training through practical experience on the wards of the Winnipeg General Hospital. His discourse reflected the philosophy and the principles which guided his own professional life:

TO THE INCOMING GROUP OF INTERNS,
WINNIPEG GENERAL HOSPITAL:
In considering the request that I speak to you today on behalf of the honorary attending staff of this hospital, I felt that the occasion would be of sufficient importance both to you and to the hospital that I should give some serious thought to the manner and substance of my remarks.

First, I want to take this opportunity of joining the Superintendent [Dr. H. Coppinger] in welcoming you to this hospital as interns. An innovation for this year will be regular joint meetings between the Intern Committee of the staff and representatives from the interns themselves. The purpose of these meetings will be to discuss your problems, assist in meeting the needs for your training and to do everything possible to help in organizing a better intern service for the hospital and a better hospital service for you as interns.

You are now members of the various medical, surgical and obstetrical teams of this institution. As Dr. Coppinger has so aptly put it on previous occasions, "You are working with us, not for us."

Success in the practice of medicine depends on many things. The value and importance of good teamwork cannot be over-emphasized. All of us rely on someone else for assistance in the form of consultations and ready access to expert laboratory and x-ray services. The members of the staff look to and rely upon the interns for their interest and intelligent cooperation. And both of us, staff and interns, depend greatly on the very capable and excellent nursing services of the hospital to assist us at all times.

You, as members of this hospital team, must play the game and give your best in the form of careful work and sustained interest in the many problems that present themselves to you. Half-hearted support and a lukewarm attitude may delay the work of the hospital and may postpone the recovery of a patient. Indifference and lack of diligence on your part *will* – not *may* – but *will* affect adversely your professional career and the esteem of your associates for many years to come. Remember that, as you go through life, you always carry your past record with you. If it is good, your load is lightened. If it is bad, it can prove heavy, cumbersome luggage.

Remember, too, that you have now – not next year when you graduate, but *now* – entered upon the serious business of the practice of medicine. You are serving your apprenticeship. You are laying the foundation for your whole future career. The knowledge and experience that you gain, the techniques that you master, will be part of your permanent armamentarium.

You have graduated from textbook medicine and surgery in which disease entities are presented and discussed as single problems. You have now entered upon the full-time job of bed-side diagnosis and medical care. You are about to translate the knowledge that you have acquired into practical experience. Remember that in the vast majority of the cases that you will encounter, you will not be dealing with a single disease entity. Primarily you are dealing with sick and maladjusted people with different social, economic and educational backgrounds. They may be cooperative or most difficult in their behaviour. An unpleasant mood of your patient must not be allowed to reflect itself in the loss of your mental poise and equilibrium. You must learn to be patient, tolerant and understanding.

Remember too, that medicine has, by force of circumstances, learned during the war years that emotional disturbances, motivation and anxiety all play important parts both in the causation and cure of disease. Psychosomatic medicine, with its moral concept of cause and effect, is here to stay, and the wise physician sees that he does not disregard its importance and its position in the field of diagnosis and therapy.

You must be genuinely interested in people and their reactions to their environment and not only in the organic lesions that may, at the moment, be the prominent feature of their illness. Thirty percent of your patients will be suffering from functional disturbances unrelated to any organic disease. They have unstable nervous systems. People, you know, are not as a rule very much concerned in the selection of their ancestors. Fully half of the remainder of your patients will have an organic disease aggravated by fear, frustration and fatigue. Heal the peptic ulcer, set the fracture, remove the malignancy but also soothe the frayed nerves. Reassure the patient. Give him confidence when this is justified but never leave him without hope. Be firm but never ruthless in your patient-physician relationships.

Your success, satisfaction and joy in the practice of medicine will depend upon your scientific knowledge and clinical experience but equally, in my opinion, upon your sympathetic understanding of the common frailties of human nature – and don't ever disregard this or consider it too lightly.

Avail yourself of the great wealth of clinical material in this institution. Study the records, check the laboratory and x-ray reports. Adopt a critical but not a cynical attitude. Make it your business to know why certain things are done. Ask questions of the attending physician and surgeon. He is apt to take for granted that you know more than you do except when he puts you to the test of your final examinations.

Examine the records of some of the men that have passed through this institution as interns. You will find them at Johns Hopkins University, at McGill, at the Mayo Clinic, in England, and elsewhere, making outstanding contributions to present-day medical progress. Without exception, these men made a noteworthy mark for themselves right here in this hospital. Amongst you are men made of the same stuff with sufficient will and determination and ability to achieve. Raise your sights – give this hospital the best that you have; take pride in your work. Remember the Indian proverb: "If you bring much, you will get much."

The management and staff of this hospital are anxious that your intern year will mark the beginning of a career that will bring happiness and satisfaction to you and relief from suffering and mental tranquility to many patients. This worthy objective deserves the best you have to offer – and no more, nor much less, should be expected of any of us.

Throughout this period, Dr. Thorlakson's well-recognized ability in planning and organization, and his dedication to high standards of clinical teaching, were called upon in the Department of Surgery to recommend ways of improving both the level of patient care and the quality of medical education. In the spring of 1946 he was asked by Dr. Oliver Waugh, then the Professor of Surgery and the Head of the Department of Surgery at the Winnipeg General Hospital, to prepare a special report indicating how the intern service in the Department of Surgery might be restructured.

Clinical teaching was provided for the interns mainly by doctors in private practice who were prepared to devote some of their time to academic affairs. The extent to which the undertaking to teach was honoured, varied with the demands on the time of the practitioner. Since the University payment to clinical teachers for the most part consisted of a very modest annual honorarium, the education of interns depended largely on the willingness of large numbers of doctors to voluntarily contribute their services from a sense of obligation to their profession and their alma mater, and for the intellectual rewards of University appointment. The physician-teacher was responsible for the care of his private patients and the "staff" patients on his service; the interns gave some assistance in the care of the private patients, and in the main provided the care of the "staff" patients under the guidance of their mentors.

Dr. Thorlakson examined the subject in all its aspects over a period of three months and, on May 21, 1946, presented his findings, including not only proposals for restructuring the intern service, but also setting out the philosophy and principles that should prevail in the conduct of this essential phase of medical education:

INTERN SERVICE (WITH SPECIAL REFERENCE TO THE SURGICAL DEPARTMENT)

The re-organization of the Intern Service, with special reference to the Surgical Department, has been under discussion now for three months. Meetings between the Intern Committee of the staff and representatives of the interns have been held. One meeting with the entire intern group was arranged. In addition, there have been meetings of the general surgery staff and also the honorary attending surgical staff dealing with this matter. The following is a consideration of some of the problems and is presented as a basis for discussion only.

The problem is one which involves more than the Winnipeg General Hospital. Its consideration involves the Faculty of Medicine, which is interested not only in the training of undergraduates but also in those seeking advanced training. Thus, the scope of any discussion must, of necessity, be broadened to include matters which are actually the responsibility of the dean and the medical faculty.

The Medical College should be more closely associated with the teaching hospitals in a program of postgraduate/clinical instruction. Under its active direction, the senior intern will be more interested in pursuing additional training leading to advanced work and the higher degrees in the profession. If the Department of Surgery undertakes the additional functions which are necessary, an increase in the supervision of the clinical instruction of our students, both undergraduates and graduates, becomes necessary. There might be created clinical professors of surgery who have clear-cut responsibilities and authority in the matters under their control and who would share direction of the department with the Professor of Surgery.

In the organization of the department, immediate consideration should be given to the recognition of outstanding service and interest in clinical teaching. This should be done by raising the status of many of the teachers to a position consistent with the volume of work they assume in teaching and the responsibility they share in the work in the public wards of the hospital. Consideration should also be given to those members of our staff who have served in the armed forces and also those who have taken extensive postgraduate training.

Prior to World War I of 1914–18, the intern staff of the Winnipeg General Hospital was composed of graduate physicians. The emergency at that time created a shortage of interns and in 1916–17, five men who were returned from overseas to complete their medical course were placed as junior interns in the hospital. In the following year, 1917–18, the majority of interns were undergraduates but by 1918–19 more interns were again graduates. It was in 1922 that the Medical College created an intern year out of the final college year.

Since the intern year is a college year, the Faculty of Medicine should establish a minimum of standards for the training of interns and continue the supervision of their students. The standards should be applied equally to interns spending one or more extra years in the hospital. This additional period represents an extension of the medical course and as such it is the responsibility of the Medical Faculty to maintain a proper level of requirements in this postgraduate work.

The following remarks are drawn up to indicate the position of the intern in his relationship to the patient, hospital and medical staff. The responsibility of the hospital and the attending physician to the intern is also included.

1. Responsibility of the intern to the patient: The care and welfare of the patient are the first concern of the intern and this involves an interest that cannot be measured by a working day of so many hours. The proper doctor-patient relationship, regarding continuity of interest and responsibility, should be established at this period in a doctor's training.

The patient must be met as soon as possible after his admission to determine the nature of his complaints and undertake his physical examination in order to obtain a tentative diagnosis. Routine laboratory tests ordinarily carried out by the intern should be completed at this time. Where the diagnosis is obscure in an apparently seriously ill patient, the assistance of the resident or senior on the service should be sought and the attending physician notified. Following the visit of the staff man, accompanied by the intern, the further care of the patient, as directed by the physician, is undertaken. This involves obtaining further information by physical and laboratory examinations which should be carried out in a reasonably proper time.

In a seriously ill patient, it should be arranged that the work be carried on by an alternate on the service familiar with the case. It is not reasonable to assume that this work can be carried out with maximum efficiency or benefit to the patient if it is delegated to the intern on routine call. Proper time for recreation is important and necessary, but prolonged absence from the ward without undertaking enquiry about seriously ill patients and other problems which have developed during the interval should be condemned.

The intern should seek to meet all private patients admitted to the service of his supervising surgeon in order to check their needs and direct, where indicated, any therapy or examination requested. A portion of the duties of an intern on a surgical service is to check preoperative orders. It should be part of his duty as well as his education to study in advance of an operation the surgical procedures and be familiar with the anatomy of the part involved. This preparation will provide increased interest in the operation and so eliminate the boredom which stems from a lack of knowledge and interest in the particular problem in hand.

2. Responsibility of the medical staff: In the hospital the actual care of the sick and the maintenance of scientific standards is the responsibility of the medical staff. In addition, this responsibility includes the education of the intern staff as a part of the policy of the hospital in which both groups serve. Within the teaching program, there are several important phases of intern instruction. Chief among these is well-conducted teaching at the bedside. This means systematic instruction by the attending physician with ample discussion of the history, the clinical and laboratory findings, the diagnosis and the treatment of the patient. To conduct such teaching properly is the duty of the attending physician who is in charge of the patients assigned to the intern.

Ample time should be provided to the intern for study and proper care to all patients. An excessively large service per intern is not conducive to good work, while excessive work, haste and fatigue may produce bad working habits and endanger the patient. Experience in the out-patient department, where circumstances are comparable to office practice, is an important part of the intern's training. It is desirable that this be under the supervision of a staff doctor.

Opportunities to attend and share in the usual clinical presentations and other organized medical functions, aside from work assigned on the wards, should be encouraged by the staff. These include such meetings as the Tumor Clinic, regular staff clinical luncheon presentations, intern lectures by staff doctors and journal clubs; as well as chances of observing fracture work, operations for interesting emergencies, autopsies of interesting cases and the like.

3. Responsibility of the hospital to the intern: The most important function of the hospital is to provide facilities where the patient may be given scientific medical care. Such an institution, if it offers internships, must have a well-organized program for the training of interns. This will improve the quality of the care available for the patient and thus enhance the primary function of the hospital. The purpose of the internship is to supplement the undergraduate academic instruction by a well-rounded experience of supervised clinical experience in diagnosis and therapy.

In accepting the training of interns, the hospital undertakes a serious responsibility, for this is a most important phase of medical education. A definition of his duties and privileges should be provided the intern by the hospital. The hospital should provide the intern with proper living quarters, food and an opportunity for healthful recreation. Provision for physical examination with roentgenological examination and immunization measures as indicated is part of the hospital's responsibility to the intern.

There should be a medical library readily accessible in the hospital available for intern use as well as for the use of the medical staff. It should contain reference books and a number of commonly used journals under the care of a librarian. [Twenty years later this was established in space adjacent to the medical cloakroom. On the door leading to the cloakroom and to the Intern's Reading Room and Library is the inscription, "This room was refurbished as a Reading Room and Library by Mr. and Mrs. F. Danchuk in memory of their son Dr. Edward Danchuk"].

4. Teaching on the surgical service: In considering appointments of junior interns to surgical services, as they are now constituted, it is recommended that they be placed on those services under supervision of a staff member. It is also recommended that junior interns spend four months on the surgical service, which includes general surgery, urology and orthopaedics. As general surgery is an important service which all interns should have, it is advised that in addition to the resident, two juniors should serve simultaneously on public surgery. Thus, a total of eight junior interns will be required to cover private, semiprivate and public surgery, orthopaedics and urology. It is recom-

mended further that arrangements be made so that each intern should devote two consecutive months on one surgical service.

The arrangement of the present vertical service within the hospital should now be modified to include Outdoor and Casualty. A continuous service throughout the year should obtain. The present intermittent service is not conducive to sustained effort in the field of clinical instruction. The staff man will take his intern group with him to the Outdoor and be responsible for Casualty and emergency admissions for that day.

It is recommended that the resident assume responsibility for emergency cases entering the hospital and associate himself with the senior intern on the particular service in the management of the case.

The resident, in effect, is the deputy of the chief of surgery and is directly responsible to him for the manner in which he supervises the public surgical services in the hospital. He is expected to assist in the training of the intern staff and to be available to them for advice and guidance. He will keep a record of the operations which the senior interns are permitted to perform and be responsible for proper allocation of cases. On these matters, he should consult with the staff surgeon in charge of the case. At the completion of his term of residency, he will be expected to come up for his degree in Master of Surgery (Manitoba). In addition to the emergency work, for which he will be in the main responsible, he may be permitted to admit patients on one-day-a-week under the Professor of Surgery. These cases will be his special problems in elective surgery and Saturday is suggested as his special day in the surgical Outdoor service.

CHAPTER 25

Professor of Surgery

In the summer of 1945, clouds began to gather that presaged an academic storm of a kind that occasionally besets universities. Perhaps faculties of medicine are particularly vulnerable from time to time to bouts of internal strife; for unlike most other major divisions of the university, at that time even senior academics such as the deans of medicine or the professors of medicine or surgery had part-time University appointments, and they continued their private medical practices. Inevitably, there were those who perceived this as a competitive relationship between those with University privileges and those with lesser, or no, academic rank. Occasionally there were episodes of tension that found the dean and his senior department heads engulfed in controversy, or caught in a crossfire of opinion, counter opinion, facts and rumours. The issues were sometimes clouded by clashes between the traditionalists and the pragmatists; and some well-intentioned individuals who found themselves drawn into the turmoil became the victims of confused and bewildering events. One such episode occurred in the Faculty of Medicine in 1945.

To understand the stresses described in this chapter, the reader who is unfamiliar with the system may be helped by a brief introduction to the nature and implications of a University appointment to the senior academic post in surgery.

The Professor of Surgery is the Chairman and Head of this important department in the Faculty. He is responsible to the Dean for all the academic activities with which it is concerned.

This includes the teaching of undergraduate and postgraduate students, programs of continuing education in surgery, and the encouragement of research in surgical subjects.

He presides at all meetings of members of the department, which in 1946 consisted of about forty practising surgeons. He selects and recommends surgeons for academic appointment, including the heads of the surgical sub-specialties (although the views of the section members are taken into account); he represents the department on the powerful Executive Committee of the Faculty; and he represents the department and the University at national and international conferences, often being asked to participate in their organization and direction.

Beyond the basic undergraduate level, training in surgery must of necessity largely take place in a hospital setting. Consequently it had become the custom for the Winnipeg General Hospital (the primary teaching hospital) to appoint the Professor of Surgery as Head of the Department of Surgery in the Hospital. Since teaching in surgery was also done at St. Boniface Hospital and Deer Lodge Hospital, a joint appointment between these hospitals and the University enabled the head of the surgical service at each of these institutions to act as the deputy of the Professor of Surgery with regard to academic matters in their respective hospitals.

The Professor of Surgery, therefore, had a high measure of responsibility, prestige and power, not only in academic affairs but also in the day-to-day operations of the teaching hospitals.

In addition to all this, his appointment with the University provided that he would still carry on his private practice.

Dr. Oliver S. Waugh, a highly respected neurosurgeon, had been appointed Professor of Surgery in 1939. Six years later he found his health was deteriorating; as a consequence, his capacity to fulfill his responsibilities was being strained. There were periods when he could not come to the hospital at all. At this time the number of surgical specialists was increasing rapidly. This brought pressure for increased hospital accommodation and an urgent need for active leadership in the Department of Surgery. Competition was keen for the highly utilized surgical resources in the Winnipeg General Hospital.

At the same time it was recognized that improvements were needed in the organization of the teaching services. In the absence of firm direction, it was difficult to effect recommended reforms.

In the early summer of 1945, Dean Mathers had a lengthy discussion with Professor Waugh about the problems in the Department of Surgery and considered the steps necessary to alleviate them. It was agreed that Dr. Waugh's health would not permit him to continue as Professor and Head; however, it was agreed that he would carry on temporarily and at the earliest appropriate time the Dean would initiate measures to find a successor.

The University's Department of Surgery consisted of all the qualified surgeons at both Winnipeg General Hospital and St. Boniface Hospital, a number of whom also had appointments on the staff at Deer Lodge (Veterans) Hospital. Probably close to a dozen members of the Department had the reputation, competence and experience to be considered for the position of department head. In the face of this, Dean Mathers decided not to take any hurried action.

The most influential surgeons on the Winnipeg General Hospital staff were Dr. Thorlakson and Dr. M.R. MacCharles, who were both very active in their practices, and were well-known and highly respected. Two other senior surgeons, Dr. G.S. Fahrni and Dr. C.W. Burns, were potential leaders. Indeed, these four men had been carrying a large part of the responsibility for organizing the teaching and the clinical work of the Department during Dr. Waugh's illness. They all held, of course, appointments in the Faculty of Medicine.

Nothing had been done by the end of September to provide the surgical service with the leadership it needed. Therefore, on the evening of October 1, 1945, these four senior members of the Department met to discuss the surgical service of the Hospital, particularly as it related to teaching. Illness prevented Professor Waugh from attending.

To these men it was evident that the lack of an active department head to provide firm leadership on a day-to-day basis was aggravating the normal strains and stresses of the hospital conditions for practising surgeons. At the same time, the educational arrangements for interns and residents were not as well-managed as either students or staff might desire.

The problems thus engendered were thoroughly discussed at

this meeting. It was essential that the teaching clinics in surgery should be scheduled for the month of October so that they could be posted for the guidance and information of the students. This task was completed at the meeting. On a similarly pressing matter, involving policy, they agreed that arrangements should be made that would allow surgeons returning from the military services to resume their General-Hospital and Faculty-of-Medicine appointments without delay. The meeting closed with a consensus that Dean Mathers ought to take early action on the appointment of a professor of surgery.

The University had an arrangement with the Department of Veterans Affairs under which some teaching of residents and interns was done at Deer Lodge Hospital. But things were not going very well in the organizational affairs of the Department of Surgery at that hospital either. The Hospital was without a surgical department head; and surgeons who would carry out a teaching role and who therefore required a joint appointment by the Hospital and the University, had not been named for the current year. A sense of unease and uncertainty seemed to shadow relations between the Faculty and officials of Veterans Affairs.

Since the educational placement of interns and residents had to be settled, Dean Mathers determined to go to Ottawa and discuss the difficulties with Dr. W.P. Warner, Director General of Treatment Services in the Department of Veterans Affairs. This he did on October 31, 1945. In the course of the meeting, he presented to Dr. Warner a list of nominations of surgeons in the Faculty who would like to do some of their practice at Deer Lodge and who would require appointment by the Minister to the Hospital staff, thus completing the joint appointment process. One of them would be the department head.

This initiative on the part of the Dean and the Faculty touched a tender spot. With respect to the Department of Surgery at Deer Lodge Hospital, Dr. Warner clearly expressed his view that the selection and appointment of the Chief of Surgery was the responsibility of the Minister and would be done by him on the recommendation of his senior medical staff. Further, Dr. Warner continued, no appointment of the Chief of Surgery at Deer Lodge had yet been made, but it would be attended to forthwith. Lt. Col. C.E. Corrigan had been selected for the position. When Dr. Corrigan's appointment had been officially announced, further appointments would be made to the surgical staff on his recommendation. Dr. Corrigan was Chief of Surgery at St. Boniface General Hospital.[1]

In closing the interview with Dr. Mathers, Dr. Warner expressed regret that there had been some internal problems in the Department that had caused delay in appointments; there were also some other difficulties with the Faculty of Medicine in Manitoba, but he hoped that they would be resolved. The Faculty nominations were not discussed in detail.

The procedure which had evolved for appointment of senior medical faculty and teaching hospital department heads was in fact unclear to some of those directly involved, and not quite acceptable to some of those who did have an insight into the system. It appeared that the Faculty executive made the selection and expected the University Board to confirm it. In turn, the Hospital Board was expected to make a corresponding appointment in administrative rank, and to grant rights of hospital practice.

Some felt that the rights and responsibilities in administrative affairs of the governing bodies of both institutions were being pre-empted by the medical staff. Training in administration (which would be rare indeed in a candidate for a faculty department head appointment) or demonstrated ability in management are qualifications unlikely to carry weight in the selection of an academic head. On the other hand, the actions and decisions of a senior medical department head in the University, but particularly in a teaching hospital, can have a marked influence on the financial and operational health of the institution. To some Board members of both the University and the teaching hospitals who were aware of the implications, strictly academic criteria for such appointments seemed to be inadequate.

The Faculty, however, were generally sensitive to the chartered rights of members of the University and the medical profession to self-government in academic and professional affairs, rights assumed by some as equally applicable to the management of the public institutions in which they function.

In 1943, University President Sidney Smith addressed the subject in a memorandum to Dean Mathers:

I have been wondering whether we could not devise better machinery for choosing Heads of Departments in your Faculty, and Heads of Service in the Hospital, where these posts are held jointly. It is undesirable that a small cabal of members of the staffs of the two Institutions should get together and make a selection, about which the Board of Governors of the University can do nothing except rubber stamp it. Would it be possible to have one or two laymen, including myself, from the Staff Committee of the Board of Governors, and yourself and one or two members of the Board of Trustees [of the Hospital] sit in with a joint Committee of the doctors on the Staff Committee of the Hospital and from the Faculty of Medicine?

This trial balloon launched by the President rapidly lost its buoyancy when it reached the Dean's office and apparently there was no formal response.

A further symptom of uneasiness over the procedure for Faculty appointments arose at a meeting of the Board of Governors in June 1944. Dr. A.W. Trueman had by this time succeeded Dr. Smith as President of the University.

It was reported as information at the meeting that the most recent five-year term of Dean Mathers was about to expire. (He had been appointed Dean of the Faculty of Medicine in 1931, and his tenure had been renewed regularly since that time.) A medical faculty member who sat on the Board of Governors immediately expressed the view that Dean Mathers should be reappointed, and made a motion to this effect. But University Faculty appointments are subject to consideration and recommendation to the Board by the President, and it appeared to Dr. Trueman and some Board members that this was an attempt by the Faculty of Medicine to avoid the customary review procedure, by-pass the President, and gain quick approval of the status quo. Objections to the motion were voiced, and it was withdrawn.

Dr. Mathers, who had been out of the city at the time of the Board meeting, was somewhat embarrassed by the controversy, and sent a conciliatory note to President Trueman on his return. He suggested that some of those present "may have confused the terms recommend, nominate and appoint"; that "the right [of the Faculty] to nominate or recommend was not being questioned"; but that, in his view, "appointment is quite a different thing and can rest with the Board only."

At the meeting of the Executive Committee of the Medical Faculty Council[2] in March 1946, it was finally determined that it was necessary to appoint a successor to Dr. Waugh as Professor of Surgery and on motion of Dr. Thorlakson, which was seconded by Dr. MacCharles, an Appointment Committee was established. With an unexpected irony, "to avoid subsequent charges of personal bias" it was agreed that the Committee would consist of the heads of all departments in the Faculty. This resulted in a large committee – eleven appointed members, and the Dean, ex officio. All the Committee members were attached to the Winnipeg General Hospital in some capacity, and seven were the heads of hospital departments.

The Appointment Committee elected the Professor of Ophthalmology and Director of the department at Winnipeg General Hospital, Dr. W.E. Campbell, as its chairman. The Committee decided that the chairman would send a letter to all members of the Faculty Department of Surgery (who were also members of the Hospital Department of Surgery at Winnipeg General, or St. Boniface General Hospital; and sometimes in addition at Deer Lodge). This letter announced the pending retirement of Dr. Waugh, and incorporated a brief questionnaire. The first question was, "Do you wish to be considered as a candidate for this post?" Replies were to be addressed to Dr. Campbell, and the committee would make a recommendation in due course to the Faculty Executive.

Response to the questionnaire showed a high degree of interest in the appointment. The Committee met, and from the aspirants they selected a group to whom formal invitations to apply were sent: Dr. Paul H.T. Thorlakson, Dr. M.R. MacCharles, Dr. C.W. Burns, Dr. Gordon S. Fahrni, Dr. C.E. Corrigan, Dr. Harry D. Morse, Dr. A.C. Abbott, and Dr. John Hillsman. All responded with applications.

At five meetings, all marked by divided opinion and vigorous debate, the Appointment Committee struggled with the problem of selecting one applicant who would be recommended to the Faculty Executive (and in turn recommended to the President of the University) as Professor of Surgery. A unanimous agreement was never reached. At the final meeting it was decided to take a ballot for first, second and third positions. The result: Dr. Corrigan had the majority of first-place votes; Dr.

Thorlakson and Dr. MacCharles respectively were runners up.

Here was a dilemma indeed! There was a generally high respect for Dr. Corrigan as a surgeon and as a teacher, so his selection as Professor would probably find acceptance among a majority of the Faculty members, but what about the well-established precedent that the Professor was always appointed as Director of the Department of Surgery at Winnipeg General Hospital? (Or conversely, as some would argue, the Director of the Hospital Department was always appointed Professor of Surgery.)

Dr. Corrigan was privately sounded out to see if he would move his primary base of practice from St. Boniface Hospital to Winnipeg General Hospital. But he had been Chief of Surgery at St. Boniface Hospital since 1939; he liked it there and he declined to consider a change. Nor did he consider this a necessary prerequisite for the senior faculty appointment in surgery.

The Appointment Committee could not arrive at a unanimous decision, since conflicting opinions were strongly held and vigorously defended. To complete their task, they decided to report to the the Executive Committee of the Faculty Council the results of their ballot, in which Dr. Corrigan stood first and Dr. Thorlakson second.

The latter part of June, when many members of the faculty were away, was not the most desirable time to deal with a matter of such importance. The Dean, however, decided to place the matter on the agenda of a meeting of the Executive of the Faculty held on June 25, 1946. With only half of the ten members present and voting, the Executive favoured Dr. Corrigan by a majority of one. Although the appointment would normally be expected to be made effective the first day of July, the beginning of the academic year, there must have been some doubt about this decision since the recommendation was not immediately forwarded by the Dean to President Trueman for his approval and submission to the Board of Governors of the University. Its substance, however, quickly became known to members of the faculty, and in particular to the members of the Department of Surgery.

The action of the Executive Committee resulted in a deeply divided faculty. One group held that if more members of the Executive had been present at the meeting, the recommendation of

Dr. Thorlakson would have been assured. There were mutterings that some votes may have been influenced by long-held prejudice rather than the merits of the immediate issue. The Dean himself, who was described by a distinguished colleague as a scholarly, soft-spoken, self-effacing man, must have looked with some misgivings at the prospect of the relative tranquility of his academic affairs being ruffled by the appointment of a man who had demonstrated an unusual ability to organize and innovate; who had carried out lesser academic assignments with a disturbing competence and creativity; who had exceptional influence in high places; and whose professional abilities were evidenced by his fully-booked surgical slates.

One must recall that at this time Dr. Thorlakson was founder and Director of the Winnipeg Clinic, which then had some thirty doctors as members, all of whom had staff appointments at the Winnipeg General Hospital; he had organized the Manitoba Foundation for the Advancement of Medical Education and Research, of which he was one of the two vice-presidents, the other being W.A. Murphy, Chairman of the Board of the Winnipeg General Hospital; he was Chairman of the Board of the Manitoba Medical Centre, which he had organized and brought to incorporation; he was a member of the Board of the Manitoba Cancer Relief and Research Institute, appointed to that post by the University of Manitoba; he had close relationships with leading members of the business community and with government. He was associated with the chairman of the Board of Governors of the University in the Manitoba Institute for the Advancement of Medical Education and Research, where Mr. Justice Bergman was a member of the Board of Directors. He held a number of other national and international appointments.

Some argued that Dr. Thorlakson would not have time to fulfill the responsibilities of the Professor of Surgery, and of the Chief of Surgery in the Winnipeg General Hospital. Nevertheless, past experience indicated that if he accepted an obligation, he carried it out with a resolution and resourcefulness that led to success. He had already submitted papers on changes which he believed would improve the Department.

If Dr. Corrigan had agreed to move his practice to the Winnipeg General Hospital and accept the post of Chief of Surgery there, his appointment as Professor and Head of the University

Department of Surgery would probably have been accepted without further question. But since he decided against this, there was a significant body of opinion in the Winnipeg General Hospital Department of Surgery that a surgeon at that hospital, where most of the teaching was done, could best fill the dual role.

On July 3, 1946, Dr. Thorlakson informed Dean Mathers of the views held by members of the Winnipeg General Hospital surgical staff, views which had been supported, in informal discussions, by the Chairman of the Board. He advised the Dean that before the Faculty Executive had reached a decision, Winnipeg General Hospital authorities ought to have been consulted. After all, the person selected would also require a General Hospital appointment. He suggested that this was the first occasion on which such consultation had not occurred.

Dean Mathers apparently chose not to contest these points. Rather, he took the deceptively narrow stand that on a purely University appointment he could not agree that such consultation was obligatory. In any case, he pointed out, four out of the five members of the executive who voted on the appointment issue were members of the medical staff of the Winnipeg General Hospital, and if they had thought the Hospital was being slighted, they surely would have mentioned it.

Nevertheless, the Dean agreed to call a special meeting of the Faculty Executive for July 5, 1946. During this meeting it was revealed that the Ad Hoc Appointment Committee established by the executive in April to deal with this matter had agreed, in their deliberations, that a teacher, in order to become a professor, need not be attached to one particular hospital; nor if appointed need he change his affiliation. The Faculty Executive decided that it would be desirable to have a joint conference on the issues with the Staff and Appointments Committee of the Winnipeg General Hospital. This was arranged for Thursday, July 11, 1946.

However, before the joint meeting was held, a meeting of the Staff and Appointments Committee of the Winnipeg General Hospital was hastily arranged for July 9, 1946. Chairman of the Committee was Dr. J.D. Adamson, the Professor of Medicine and Head of the General Hospital Department of Medicine. In addition to the Committee members, Dean Mathers, as an ex officio member, and Dr. Harry Coppinger, the Superintendent of the General Hospital, attended.

It is of interest that Dr. Adamson was Head of the St. Boniface Hospital Department of Medicine when he was appointed Professor of Medicine. He did not hesitate to resign from St. Boniface Hospital and move to the Winnipeg General Hospital in order to accept the appointment of Head of the Department of Medicine there.

Dr. Adamson opened the meeting by reading a letter addressed by Board Chairman Mr. Murphy to Dr. Coppinger, instructing him to have the committee proceed forthwith to select and recommend a qualified person to become the Head of the Department of Surgery in the General Hospital. In commenting on his instructions, Dr. Coppinger noted that the General Hospital Board – or some members of it – had the impression that a group in the faculty had held secret meetings and, ignoring the hospital, reached a decision about a position that had in the past been a dual appointment by the University Board and the General Hospital Board.

Dean Mathers intervened to affirm that the recommendation to appoint Dr. Corrigan as Professor of Surgery was strictly a University matter; and the General Hospital could appoint anyone they wished as head of their Department of Surgery. It was disclosed at the meeting, however, that the surgeons at the hospital did not accept this view, and indeed opposed the faculty action. For the moment, matters remained in this state of disagreement.

The conference between the Faculty Council Executive and the Staff and Appointments Committee of the General Hospital was duly held on July 11. The differences in points of view seemed to be as fixed as ever. A resolution said to have been accepted by the entire surgical staff of the hospital was presented to the meeting by Dr. Waugh, expressing the view that "it is highly desirable" that the Head of the Surgical Department at Winnipeg General Hospital be the Professor of Surgery. At this point, the members of the Staff and Appointments Committee asked permission to leave the meeting temporarily to consider their position. Having done this, they returned to express their support for the resolution of the Surgical Staff.

Dean Mathers then asked if a professor of surgery who was

not on the Winnipeg General Hospital staff were appointed by the University, would he have access to the teaching wards and services at the Hospital for academic purposes. Nobody present was prepared to answer this question, and it was suggested that the Dean put his enquiry by letter to the Hospital Superintendent. On this note, the meeting ended.

Promptly the next morning Dr. Mathers sent his letter of enquiry to Dr. Coppinger. "If the final recommendation of the Faculty Executive is for Dr. Corrigan," he wrote, "will he have entrée to Winnipeg General Hospital for purposes of planning, supervision and participation in clinical teaching?"

Despite Dr. Coppinger's urging to the Medical Executive Committee to formulate a reply, Dr. Mathers never did get an answer to his question. The only response was a letter dated July 16, 1946, from Dr. K.R. Trueman, then Secretary of the honorary attending staff, which said that "members of the Hospital Department of Surgery agreed to give full support to whoever is appointed Chief of Surgery at the Hospital"; that "he should be chosen from among the present staff members; and that it is highly desirable that this person should also be the Professor of Surgery."

In due course, the recommendation of the Faculty Executive for Dr. Corrigan, unchanged in any way by the controversy, was officially forwarded by the Dean to President Trueman for submission to the Board of Governors. At Dr. Trueman's request, Dean Mathers included a paper summarizing the events and circumstances leading up to the Faculty Executive recommendation.

The University Board was faced with an extremely difficult problem. They decided to follow the time-honoured procedure of appointing a committee to consider what should be done, and to meet with representatives of the Board of the Winnipeg General Hospital, since there was a concensus that dissension and dispute at the board level on such an important matter could not be allowed to develop. The Ad Hoc Committee consisted of Chairman of the Board of Governors Mr. Justice Bergman; President Trueman; and Mrs. H.M. Speechly, an active member of the Board with broad interests in community affairs, whose husband was a physician.

The Ad Hoc Committee with all three members present reported to the Board of Governors at a meeting held in the Broadway Building Boardroom on August 20, 1946, with ten members of the Board in attendance. Mr. Justice Bergman asked Mr. W.J. Parker to take the chair for this item of business; and Mr. Parker having acceded, Judge Bergman reported the Committee's findings.

With respect to the appointment of the Professor of Surgery in the Faculty of Medicine in the University, the Committee had met, as directed, with a committee of the Board of Trustees of the Winnipeg General Hospital on August 19, at which time there was a "full and friendly discussion of the entire question."

The Committee found that there had never been any agreement between the University and the Hospital to the effect that the University was obliged to appoint as its professor of surgery the person who had been appointed by the Hospital Board as head of its department; or that the Winnipeg General Hospital was obliged to appoint as its chief of surgery the person appointed by the University as its professor of surgery. Nevertheless, it had been a source of satisfaction to both the Hospital and the University that in the past it had been the custom that the same individual held both posts. It was the view of both the Hospital and University committees that this arrangement should continue. While this was so, it was noted that each body had full freedom of action with regard to the appointment it had to make, and the guiding principle for each body must be to appoint the best available man for the post.

Judge Bergman reported that after the Faculty Council Executive vote of June 25 became known, representatives of the Board of Trustees of the Winnipeg General Hospital had approached him, as Chairman of the University Board, asking that they be given an opportunity to make representation to the Board of Governors before the appointment of the Professor of Surgery was made. This led to the establishment of the Ad Hoc Committee.

He reviewed the action of the Medical Faculty Executive, and reported that at a meeting of the Executive held on August 19, Dr. Ian MacLaren Thompson, one of its members, had explained that if he had been present at the meeting of June 25 he would have voted for Dr. Thorlakson, resulting in a tie. In view of this it was moved that the Executive put forward the names of both Dr. Thorlakson and Dr. Corrigan (which would presumably require the University Board of Governors to decide the appoint-

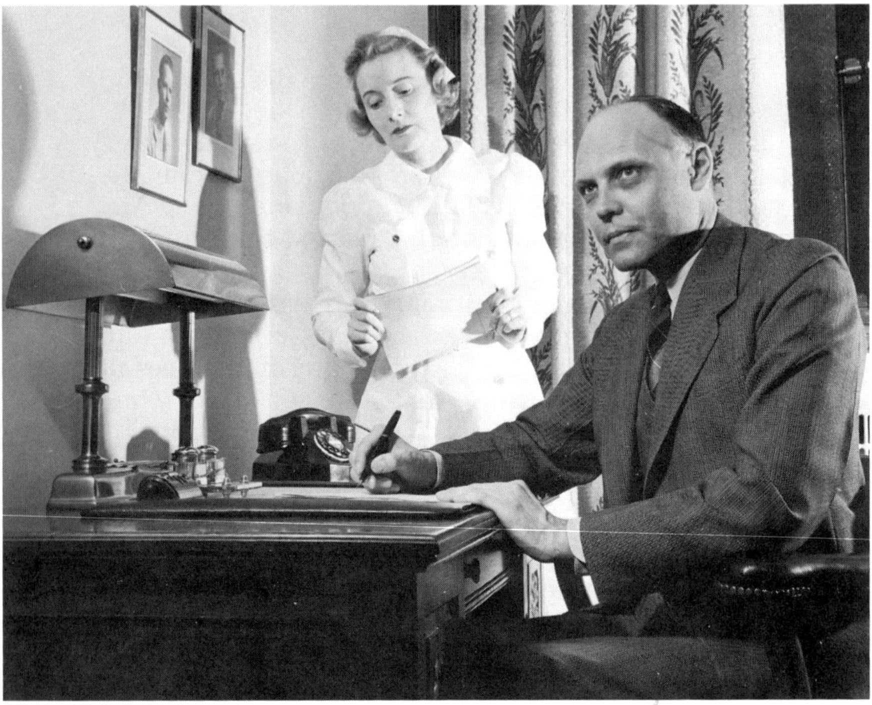

Professor of Surgery, 1946–47

ment). But this resulted in a vote of three for and three against, and the motion was defeated by the casting vote of the Chairman, Dean Mathers.

President Trueman then asked permission of the chair to read an extract from a letter which had been delivered to him during the meeting, dated August 20, from Dean Mathers, stating that in his casting vote he was not voting for or against either candidate, but against the procedure of submitting two names for consideration by the President and the Board.

The report of the Ad Hoc Committee concluded with the statement that in their opinion Dr. Thorlakson, whose abilities were well-known, was best qualified for the appointment as Professor of Surgery, and the Committee therefore unanimously recommended to the Board of Governors that this action be taken. After discussion, a motion to this effect was moved, seconded, voted upon and carried.

On August 24, 1946, Dr. Thorlakson received the following official notice from the University of Manitoba:

Dear Dr. Thorlakson:

I am directed by The Board of Governors of the University of Manitoba to notify you that you have been appointed to the position of Professor of Surgery in the Faculty of Medicine of The University of Manitoba; that your appointment dates from September 1st, 1946; and that your remuneration will be at the rate of $3,000 a year, payable in twelve equal monthly instalments.

Your appointment is subject to the provisions of The University Act and to all by-laws and regulations from time to time passed by The Board of Governors of the University of Manitoba. Subject thereto, the above terms are exclusive, and they cannot be varied except by The Board of Governors of the University of Manitoba, evidenced by a written communication to you signed by the Secretary of the Board. This notification supersedes all previous negotiations and communications, whether oral or written.

Your attention is drawn particularly to the provisions of The Tenure By-Law, which is printed on the reverse side hereof, and to the provisions of The Annuity By-law, a copy of which is enclosed herewith.

Dated the 23rd day of August, 1946.

F.W. Crawford
Secretary, Board of Governors

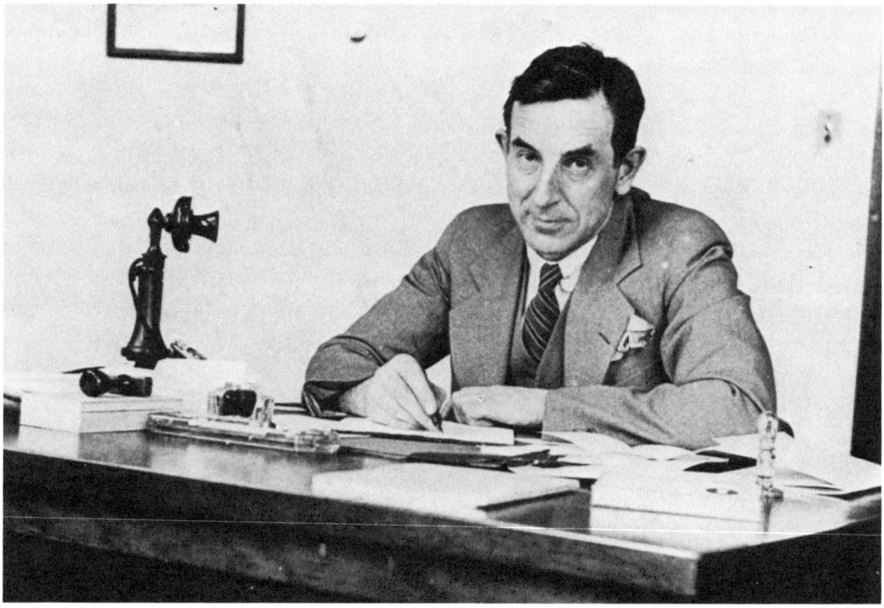

Dr. William Boyd, Professor of Pathology, University of Manitoba, 1915 to 1937

P.S. In view of the fact that you are appointed on a part-time basis, the last paragraph of the above communication does not apply F.W.C.

At its next meeting, the Board of Trustees of the Winnipeg General Hospital appointed Dr. Thorlakson Head of the Department of Surgery. It was hoped that the wounds inflicted by the controversy would heal and that a new era would be brought into being in the organization of both service and education in the Department of Surgery.

The feelings of many were expressed in the following letter from Dr. William Boyd, famed pathologist, formerly on the staff of Winnipeg General Hospital, and then the Professor and Head of the Department of Pathology and Bacteriology at the University of Toronto. Later, he was the first head of the Department of Pathology in the newly formed Faculty of Medicine in British Columbia.

Dear Thor:

Mike Hollenberg has just told me the great news. Heartiest congratulations and best wishes. For years I have wanted to see you get the Chair of Surgery, and now it has come to pass.

It is the best thing that could have happened to my old school, whose good I have so much at heart. I know that you will do great things for the Department, for you have made a success of everything you have turned your hand to.

Enid joins me in sending you our best wishes.

Ever yours,

Bill

CHAPTER 26

Conflict

Unhappily, Dean Mathers did not accept the decision of the Board of Governors of the University with respect to the Professor of Surgery. The Dean, as described by his successor, may have been "soft-spoken and self-effacing", but he also could exert great "determination and force" in gaining ends which he set out to achieve.[1] With the support of part of the faculty, Dean Mathers undertook a campaign of studied resistance to the appointment of Dr. Thorlakson as Professor of Surgery. The campaign was augmented by critical observations on the actions of the Board of Governors. The efforts of the Professor to carry out his responsibilities had a reception from the Dean ranging from indifference to disdain.

The dissidents took the stand that the University Board of Governors had been influenced in an unwarranted way by members of the Board of Trustees of the Winnipeg General Hospital; and that they had acted quite improperly by failing to follow the official recommendation of the Faculty Executive and the Dean. Any weakness in the methods or procedures under which that recommendation was reached were, from the standpoint of the objectors, irrelevant.

In retrospect, it appears that the Dean had procrastinated too long in dealing with the problems of the Department of Surgery. Earlier action, with firm leadership from the Dean's Office in the procedures to be followed in selecting the Professor, candid discussions with those directly concerned, and open communication with the President (and through him, with the Board) might have avoided some of the problems and made it possible to reach an amicable settlement.

President Trueman seems to have been equally equivocal in dealing with the situation. His position was difficult. He may have been willing to lend the weight of his office to an effort to bring the conflicting opinions to a concensus; but it might have been considered as an unwarranted interference in Faculty affairs if he had acted on his own initiative.

Dr. Trueman was a member of the Ad Hoc Committee of the Board of Governors that recommended the selection of Dr. Thorlakson as Professor of Surgery. He sent him a letter of congratulation after his appointment.

A few weeks later, when Dr. Thorlakson realized that Dr. Mathers was going to make his position on the Faculty as difficult as possible, he went to President Trueman to discuss the possibility of resigning. Dr. Trueman urged him not to resign, but to proceed with preparation of a plan to reorganize the Department of Surgery. It appears, however, that the President took no steps to persuade the Dean to cooperate in the decision of the Board; if he did, his efforts were unsuccessful.

By the end of September, the situation had reached a point at which Dr. Thorlakson was impelled to set out his position in a letter to Dean Mathers:

Dear Sir:

On Thursday, September 19, 1946, you called an emergency meeting of the members of the Faculty Council in order that you might present to them a carefully prepared statement, justifying your opposition to a decision made by the Board of Governors of the University.

Having delivered two statements, one official, and another unofficial, you immediately asked me if I had anything to say, thereby deliberately placing me on the defensive before my colleagues on the Faculty Council. Under such circumstances I declined your invitation to speak, but later in the evening made a brief statement concerning the events leading up to my acceptance of the appointment of Professor of Surgery.

Now after a careful review of the evening's proceedings, I regret that I am forced to the conclusion that your very masterly presentation was a direct, if veiled, attack upon me personally. More serious, however, are those sections in your report which can only be construed as an attack on the Board of Trustees of the Winnipeg General Hospital and upon the Executive of its Medical Staff. In your presentation you also attacked the Surgical Staff of the Winnipeg General Hospital and particularly the senior members – Dr. G.S. Fahrni, Dr. C.W. Burns, Dr. M.R. MacCharles and myself, when you said that we four had had a meeting and agreed that we would support that one of us who was selected for the Professorship of Surgery. The meeting referred to was called by Dr. O.S. Waugh to assist the Staff and Appointments Committee and the Board of Trustees of the Hospital to select a Chief for the Department of Surgery within the Hospital itself.

As the events of the evening developed, it was my impression as well as that of others, that you seemed most anxious to have the whole issue re-opened, for the purpose of bringing the condemnation of the faculty on the Board of Governors of our University.

Your attack on the actions of the Board of Trustees of the Winnipeg General Hospital is a matter of some serious significance. My information is that Mr. W.A. Murphy and his committee submitted certain facts to the Board of Governors, dealing with the very substantial contribution that this Hospital has made to the cause of Medical Education in this province over a period of sixty years. The General Hospital provides sixty percent of all the clinical teaching to the medical students of our university. The Board of Trustees commented on the excellent relationship that had existed between the University of Manitoba, the Medical Faculty and the Winnipeg General Hospital for years. The Board of Trustees could not understand why the Faculty should contemplate such a change in its relationship without discussing it with them – or at least advising them of such a change. Surely this would be a matter of ordinary courtesy. You have admitted at a committee meeting that the failure to discuss this with the Hospital was a "serious oversight."

The Board of Trustees of the Hospital did not take action or appoint its Chief of Surgery in the Hospital until the Board of Governors of the University had appointed the Professor of Surgery, even though this meant a serious delay in the re-organization which was necessary and urgent to meet the demands of the Medical College for clinical instruction for the term that was about to open.

By suggesting in your report that a group outside the University, namely, the Board of Trustees of the Winnipeg General Hospital, had brought undue pressure on the Board of Governors of the University, could only be calculated to cause a serious rift within the Faculty and to create friction and misunderstanding between the hospitals associated with the University.

If one sets out to be critical of others, one should be prepared to accept criticism. While listening to the presentation of your report, one got the impression that you felt yourself to be entirely without blame for the situation that exists. It may well be that you, Mr. Dean, are directly and personally responsible for the misunderstanding that now exists between the Board of Governors, the Board of Trustees of the General Hospital, and the Medical Faculty.

It is felt by many that steps should have been taken much sooner to deal with the appointment of a professor of surgery. Dr. O.S. Waugh proffered his resignation *two* years ago. You were, undoubtedly, aware that Dr. Waugh felt reluctant to make any permanent changes within the Department until a new director had been appointed. You repeatedly stated and complained that the Department of Surgery was not functioning efficiently under the circumstances, but yet you took no action to correct the situation until late this spring.

Furthermore, you withheld from the Professor of Surgery information submitted to you by students directly damaging to the reputation of the members, as teachers, of the Department of Surgery. This, you must admit, is not conducive to mutual confidence between yourself and members of the Surgical Department.

It was, I believe, unfair to emphasize the fact that the President of the University had dissociated himself from the procedure adopted by the Board of Governors, when you failed to add that President Trueman did associate himself with the final recommendation that was presented to the entire Board for consideration and action.

It is worthy of note that Dr. W.E. Campbell, Chairman of the special committee on selection set up to investigate the situation with regard to the appointment of a professor of surgery, did not transmit a recommendation to the Medical Faculty Executive and rather forcefully dissociated himself from the results of their deliberations.

When you called the first meeting of the Faculty Executive, Dr. I.M. Thompson had left the city on his holidays. When your personal recommendation was finally transmitted to the Board of Governors, it was late in the summer, when special meetings, not regular meetings, of the Board were held. It is a matter of opinion that such an important recommendation should have been in the hands of the Board of Governors earlier in the year, to give the Department of Surgery an opportunity to re-organize. The members of the surgical staff who had served in His Majesty's Forces required to be re-instated and to be given the proper recognition and status within the Department in view of their long absence.

When I received official notice of my appointment from the Board of Governors, you, I believe, had left the city. Dr. J.D. Adamson was already on his holidays, as was Dr. F.G. McGuinness. Dr. D. Nicholson, another member of the Executive, was about to leave for the East Coast. The President of the University was also away. From these dates until a few days prior to the opening of the College there was no possible chance for me to take the matter up with the Medical Council Executive. President Trueman wrote me a letter of congratulation from Toronto, and he was the first to return to the city, one week before the Fall session opened. I contacted Dr. Trueman as soon as I heard he was home. I explained to him that I had taken no steps towards preparing for the new term and felt that I could not take on the responsibilities of the Department until you, Mr. Dean, had acknowledged my appointment as Professor of Surgery and given me the necessary information regarding the Department. I assured him that as far as the Department of Surgery was concerned I had no doubt that a strong department could be set up, in view of the fact that never before in the history of our medical school have we had such a large group of keen, well-trained and experienced young surgeons prepared to work in the Department of Surgery. I did, however, point out to the President that unless I could be assured of your cooperation, there would be no use tackling the job, and for that reason suggested a meeting at which the three of us could discuss the situation together. A few days prior to the opening of the fall session, I received a letter from the President, stating that he had discussed the matter with you and that you had thought that such a meeting was premature. He conveyed to me your request that I call on you at your office, which I did the same day. As you were busy with other appointments, we agreed to meet the next day at noon. You were good enough to instruct your secretary, Miss Thompson, to give me the schedules of clinics and list of lecturers. I specifically asked you if you wished me to see what I could do to rearrange the course of lectures and to do what I could, on short notice, to re-organize the department. You assured me that you had never interfered directly with these matters, but had always left them entirely to the judgment of the Professor of Surgery.

I set to work on Friday, Saturday and Sunday, to familiarize myself with the information you had given me, in order that, as far as it was in my power, the returning students would not suffer from all the delays. Monday, the session opened at the College. It was on the third day, Wednesday, that I received the general notice of a special meeting of the Faculty to be held the following evening.

I made a point of calling on you the day of the meeting, and realized that you had *planned* to let me walk into a meeting which you had arranged, so that my standing in the Faculty would be jeopardized.

Being considerably disturbed about the situation and unsure what course I should follow in the interests of the school and the students, I decided to defer action until I had time to examine the proceedings of the evening, with as much calmness as I was capable of.

The next day, Friday, I received notice of an emergency executive meeting, schedule for Saturday afternoon, and decided to prepare a formal statement, which I presented to you on Saturday, and which I repeat here.

"I have been charged by the Board of Governors of the University of Manitoba with the responsibility for the supervision of the Department of Surgery in our Faculty of Medicine.

"I propose to apply myself to that task to the best of my ability and am prepared to devote the necessary time to develop a strong and well coordinated department of surgery. Furthermore, I am prepared to carry on until such time as my successor is appointed. Whenever that happens, and whoever that may be, I shall turn over to him all the information and plans available and support him whole-heartedly in the work of the Department."

I had hoped that you would perceive in this statement my sincere concern for the welfare of the Department of Surgery. Furthermore, I had hoped that the statement would indicate to the Executive my willingness to abide by whatever decision we finally reached between the Medical Faculty and the Board of Governors of the University.

I give my word of honour to the Faculty Council and to the Board of Governors of the University that whatever be the final disposition of this matter I shall abide by the declaration made to you in this communication. It is my firm conviction that the institution is more important than any individual, and that on that basis only can we re-organize a strong medical faculty. We must be prepared to readjust our attitude and our plans toward the many problems that face the medical profession as a whole, and this faculty in particular. It is to be hoped that by the closest cooperation between the Faculty of Medicine, the University of Manitoba, the Department of Health and organized medicine we may build a strong, progressive school of medicine and department of medical research, ready to serve the needs of the community in general and the requirements of the medical profession of this province and of western Canada in the fields of undergraduate and postgraduate instruction.

Yours truly,

P.H.T. Thorlakson, M.D.

In spite of the dissension, Dr. Thorlakson proceeded, with the full support and assistance of his colleagues, to prepare a plan for reorganization of the Department of Surgery, as requested by President Trueman and Dean Mathers. All the members were canvassed for suggestions that would improve the standard of teaching, and each sub-specialty in surgery was asked to prepare specific recommendations for its own section.

As the meetings and discussions were held, enthusiasm among the members of the Department grew. The feeling spread that a new era had begun that would bring unexcelled standards of surgical teaching to the University of Manitoba, the benefit of which would be felt throughout the Province.

In its final form, this Report for the Department of Surgery ran to 100 pages, and only a few points can be touched on here. It included a listing of every member of the Department, with University rank, and in some cases recommendation for promotion. It detailed the clinics and beds allocated for student instruction, and the actual teaching hours in each of the four hospitals in which surgery was being taught.[2] The head of each of the specialty sections – then only two (orthopedics and urology) reported on instructional plans in his unit, and outlined improved arrangements for undergraduate students and the resources needed for postgraduate study. Proposals were submitted by the appropriate specialists for the establishment of sections of neurology (including neurosurgery) and thoracic surgery. In all cases the development of postgraduate training (at that time very limited in Manitoba) was given consideration.

Dr. Thorlakson proposed a new course for undergraduate students, called the Fundamentals of Surgical Technique. He wrote:

> The purpose of such a course is to explain and emphasize the fundamentals of surgical technique rather than to teach any definite surgical procedures. This is, of course, done to some extent during the mammalian experiments in the Department of Physiology. But a course such as the one proposed [would] change the relationship between a student and a dog from that of an experimenter and a preparation to that of a doctor towards a patient. Instead of the living tissue [which he handles] being sacrificed at the end of the experiment, [he will be dealing] with tissue that is to live at the end of the operation; and not only to live, but to be observed and cared for. It is to be hoped that the importance of detail, such as gentleness, accurate haemostasis, asepsis, and [other elements of skillful care] will be self-evident to the student during the convalescence of the dog. Any complications that occur will be reported and discussed in the team, or even in the class. The instruction will centre around perfecting technique. . . .

Another important recommendation prepared by Dr. Thorlakson was a reorganization of the surgical staff at the Winnipeg General Hospital to permit private, semi-private and public patients to be made available for teaching purposes. This was a major change in concept, since before that only public patients (with minor exceptions) could be used for the instruction of students. This put a severe limitation on the training resources of the Faculty of Medicine. The proposed organization was known as a "vertical service," and had been approved in principle at a meeting of the surgical staff of the Winnipeg General Hospital on October 6, 1946.

Also included in the Report was an excerpt from a paper written by Dr. Thorlakson eighteen months earlier and published in the September 1944 issue of the Manitoba Medical Review. Entitled "Trends in Medical Practice," it gives an insight into his views of principles that should guide the development of both medical education and service.

EDUCATION AND RESEARCH

. . . To date the efforts of the medical schools to provide adequate postgraduate instruction for the doctors of Canada are extremely limited in scope and continuity of effort. This is not due to any lack of interest on the part of the teaching staff or a willingness on their part to sacrifice time and leisure to assist in such postgraduate activities. Lack of clinical facilities and lack of funds are in part responsible.

At least twenty-five percent of time and effort of our teachers should in the future be devoted to the continuation studies. Arrangement could probably be made to send our final-year students out into rural communities to be apprenticed for a time to practising physicians. The students would benefit by practical experience under this arrangement. The practising physician would not only come in contact with young, inquiring minds, which is in itself stimulating to all teachers, but would have the necessary relief to give him an opportunity to visit medical centres for courses of study. I would suggest that men of outstanding ability and sound judgment practising in rural Manitoba, who show special interest in students sent to them under such an arrangement, might be given the position of honorary lecturer on our faculty. What a great opportunity there is in broadening the sphere of influence and improving the standard of practice by such an arrangement.

The teachers should have available clinical cases in sufficient numbers to provide variety, and these need not necessarily be indigent or charity cases as in the past. With improved economic conditions and with increased numbers arranging the prepaid hospitalization at nine dollars a year for one and twelve dollars or slightly more for the family, we cannot expect to maintain our clinical teaching services on the number of charity patients that will present themselves to the hospital. The profession at large, as well as the authorities, should realize the vital necessity of maintaining teaching services on a high level of efficiency and excellence....

The whole problem of clinical teaching eventually may revolve around a plan to provide modern and expert laboratory, x-ray and consultation services to the man in practice, including the specialist. There is implied in this arrangement a distinction which is hard to maintain between the consultant as such and the specialist. I visualize the consultants in medicine and surgery in the future as men who have distinguished themselves in their special fields and who are willing to forego the advantages of the private practice and assume the combined responsibility of professorship, take charge of the active treatment on the teaching wards and accept appointments on official boards and tribunals which will supervise the implementation of policies which have been adopted by the profession and the Government with regard to health services to the public. They will hold positions of responsibility and trust in the community equal to that of a Supreme Court judge.

In view of the importance of proper nutrition to the normal development of the child and the maintenace of health in the adult, the Government of Canada should be urged to continue the nutritional laboratories that have been set up and, if necessary, to increase their number after the war. From such centres will come a better understanding of the nutritional requirements of the people of Canada....

Special Training

...It is our duty to develop plans by which increasing numbers of Canadian citizens will have access to improved facilities for medical care. This will mean some radical changes both in our method of training medical personnel and in our relationship with the public. This statement should not be interpreted as advocating complete abandonment of all the excellent and desirable practices that have been evolved in the past. It does, however, suggest an adjustment which may seem difficult for some of us, but the change is absolutely inevitable.

It is my conviction that the public does not demand cheap, but rather expert, medical service. Nor does the public wish to force upon the medical profession a system which will curtail its privileges or rights as individuals even though it expects doctors to practice within certain prescribed limits, depending upon their special qualifications and training....

GROUP PRACTICE

In discussing trends in medical practice, one should include some observations on the development of group practice. Cooperative medical practice will become more general. Medical men who have serviced with the armed forces and who have worked in teams and in military hospitals will wish to continue to enjoy the advantages of easy and freer consultations in private practice. . . .

IN FUTURE

. . . It is my belief that the medical faculty of each university in this country will have to re-organize its program so as to broaden its field of influence by more regular contact with every graduate in medicine. There must be better utilization of the clinical and laboratory facilities now available. Consideration must be given to the privileges that are granted by a license to practise. This might well be reconsidered every five years and special recognition given to the men who have rendered distinctive service to the community or who have qualified themselves as specialists by intensive postgraduate study and research.[3]

The Report on the Department of Surgery was sent to Dean Mathers on December 7, 1946. A budget estimate was requested to accompany the departmental proposal. In the course of a lengthy covering letter, Dr. Thorlakson pointed out that the cost would depend on the extent to which the reorganization plan was approved. In the absence of any direction on this point, he thought the very minimum for the Department of Surgery should be $12,000 a year, "and this could justifiably be increased to $25,000 or $35,000 as the recommendation of the Rockefeller Foundation is implemented."

Responsible people who have seen this report in later years have pointed out that implementation of its recommendations would have resulted in a substantial advance in the quality of education in surgery, and in the service of the University to the profession and the community.[4] However, it was not to be. There was no acknowledgement from the Dean or the President, and there is some doubt as to whether or not the material ever officially had the consideration of the Faculty Executive. There were indications that the Executive would not consider any proposals from the Department of Surgery as long as the state of conflict continued. Indeed, there were rumours that consultation referrals to the Winnipeg Clinic might suffer unless the difficulties were resolved.

In the face of these circumstances, Dr. Thorlakson concluded that he had no alternative but to resign. On January 10, he wrote:

Dear President Trueman:

I hereby proffer my resignation from the Faculty of Medicine of the University of Manitoba.

I wish to express through you, Mr. President, to the members of the Board of Governors, my appreciation for their confidence in appointing me to the professorship of surgery. I wish also to record my deep appreciation for the splendid support and cooperation given to me by the members of the Department of Surgery.

I have presented to you, Mr. President, and to Dean Mathers, a complete copy of all statements, letters and recommendations bearing upon the re-organization of the Department of Surgery. Included in this report are statements dealing with the relationship of the Department of Surgery to other Departments within the Faculty. Recommendations regarding postgraduate training and medical research are set forth. The plans for a medical teaching centre and our responsibilities as a Faculty of Medicine to rural medical practice are included. It is my belief that if these recommendations are carried forward, a strong, active teaching department can be developed.

I believe that the members of the Board might wish to know something about the progress that has been made to date in the Department of Surgery. I have, therefore, prepared and forwarded to Mr. F.W. Crawford, Secretary of the Board, copies of my report for them.

It is not my wish or intention to embarrass the Board of Governors in the middle of the teaching term. I shall carry on until my successor is appointed. I wish to assure you, Mr. President, and the members of the Board of Governors of my continued loyalty and support to the University.

Yours very truly,

P.H.T. Thorlakson, M.D.

The response came from the President on February 14, 1947.

Dear Dr. Thorlakson:

At the February meeting of the Board of Governors of the University, held yesterday afternoon, your letter of resignation was considered. The Staff Committee made the following recommendation which was accepted, namely, that your resignation should be tabled for the present in view of the fact that the Report of the Rockefeller Investigating Commission is now being considered and that there thus exists the possibility of some considerable changes in the organization of the Faculty of Medicine, and that when policies have been determined arising out of this consideration, your resignation will of course be then considered, and that in the meantime the Board should ask you if you will be so kind as to continue as the Professor Surgery to the end of the academic year.

I trust that this treatment of the matter will meet with your approval. I wish to reiterate what I wrote to you before, when your resignation first came to hand, namely, that I appreciate very much your statement that you do not wish to embarrass the Board by withdrawing in the middle of the term and that you are prepared to carry on until your successor has been appointed. There are many questions, as you know, which must be answered in relation to the organization and administration of the Faculty of Medicine. It is impossible for me at the present time to give you any hint of what decisions the Board may ultimately reach. You will be interested to know, however, that a strong committee of the Board has been appointed to consider the Rockefeller Report in detail and to act, if the Government so desires, as part of a joint committee between the Board and the Government which the Rockefeller Commission recommended should be created. It is also my own view that the Board committee should avail itself on all possible occasions of the professional advice which can be supplied only by the members of the Faculty of Medicine. I know it is your hope, as it is mine, that we may be able to add new strength to the Faculty of Medicine and to work out policies which will increase the effectiveness of teaching and research, and which will improve the relations between the Faculty itself and the Board. I appreciate too, your statement that whatever happens your interest in the Faculty and the University will be undiminished. I feel quite sure that, no matter what your own personal position in relation to the Faculty may turn out eventually to be, you will always be able to render a most important service to the University by your interest and support.

Yours sincerely,

A.W. Trueman
President

Dr. Thorlakson acceded to the request of the Board of Governors and carried on as Professor of Surgery until June 30, 1947, the end of the academic year. His resignation was accepted, effective on that date, at which time he was succeeded by Dr. C.W. Burns, one of his colleagues in the Department of Surgery at the Winnipeg General Hospital. At the request of Dr. Burns, he rejoined the Faculty in the fall of 1947 and was appointed Associate Professor of Surgery.

Mr. Justice Bergman resigned from his position as Chairman of the Board of Governors early in 1947 and was succeeded by Mr. W.J. Parker. Dr. Trueman resigned from his post in 1948 to become President of the University of New Brunswick. Dr. Mathers retired as Dean of Medicine in 1949.

In 1957 Dr. Thorlakson's contribution to the Faculty was recognized by appointment as Professor Emeritus of Surgery.

PART SIX

Medicine and Health Care

CHAPTER 27

The Treatment of Cancer

Sherman Black in 1982 was an active, keen-minded, golf-playing eighty-year-old, who was offering vigorous resistance to the best efforts of his wife and friends to convince him that it was time to give up driving his car to his winter home in Florida, and to persuade him that at his age he should travel by air, and let the pilot do the driving.

In 1943 Sherm and Lil (the names used by friends) began an episode in their life in which strength and faith were sorely tested. Sherman recently recalled it in these words:

After almost two years of tests following two hemorrhages of the bowel and two biopsies of the colon, it was determined that I had a malignant growth. My doctor, Dr. Stewart McInnes, referred me to Dr. Thorlakson, and I can well remember my first meeting with this man.

It was late May in 1945. We sat in his office and discussed my condition in frank, down-to-earth terms. He answered my questions honestly and clearly. He explained that he would operate twice, and perhaps three times; the first to establish a colostomy and explore; the second to take out the growth; and the third to re-join the bowel and restore normal function if that were possible.

I asked him what the chances were for a complete cure, and he said about seventy percent – providing the growth had not spread from the bowel to other organs. This inspired me to say, "By golly, that's good – better than two to one odds!" In those days, most people thought cancer meant the end of the line.

Dr. Thorlakson insisted that I go to the Winnipeg General Hospital, where he had specially trained staff to assist in the operation. I accepted his advice with confidence.

The first operation was on June 4, and it wasn't until July 8 that the colostomy was functioning well enough for the doctor to go after the growth. My private nurse attended this operation as an observer, in spite of the fact that she had been on duty all night. Weeks later she told me what she had seen. She said that there were quite a few doctors looking on, or assisting: Dr. Trueman, Dr. Isaac, Dr. McInnes, Dr. Stewart, and others.

The nurse watched them finally take a grey mass about the size of my fist from the opening, and heard Dr. Thorlakson say "I think we're going to be lucky." To which Dr. Trueman responded, "Lucky, Hell – superb surgery!"

At the third operation early in October the colostomy was closed, and I gave out a great shout of joy at my first normal bowel movement.

After every operation Dr. Thorlakson turned me over to other doctors in the Winnipeg Clinic for regular attention; but every day he, with his entourage, would travel the ward, as most of the occupants were patients of his.

He stopped at my bed very seldom, but the most memorable time was an occasion on which a piece of rubber tubing had slipped through the colostomy opening into my bowel. Each day my colostomy had to be drained and cleaned. My private nurse attended to this, and one day as I rolled over on my side during the draining I heard a "swish" and the tube disappeared through the hole. The nurse was upset. The intern said it would eventually pass through me. But my wife, when she heard of the accident that evening, made some phone calls. As a result Dr. Trueman came to see me that night.

The next morning, Dr. Thorlakson swooped into the room accompanied by his residents, the Head Nurse and a medical cart. They pulled up beside me. He said, "Something worrying you?"; slipped on his rubber gloves; and without any warning threw back the bed clothes, removed my dressing, pushed his finger into the bowel opening, swirled it around inside, and after a few seconds came up with the missing rubber tube. I was too stunned by this rapid action to react to the pain. "You'll be all right now," he said, and strode from the room followed by his retinue.

More than thirty-five years later, after he had been told by friends of mine that I was still around, he phoned and asked me to make an appointment with his nurse to see him, and we recalled together those operations. He had the particulars in his hand, which he had summarized from his records.

I have often thanked my lucky stars that Dr. McInnes referred me to this great doctor!

During the 1920s there was a growing concern in the medical community, not only in Manitoba but elsewhere in Canada, that, if any progress was to be made in the attack on cancer, special measures had to be taken among both the profession and the public. With notable exceptions, surgery was not very successful. Referrals to competent specialists were often too late to achieve the best results. Radio-therapy was being gradually introduced, but the indications for its effective use were just beginning to be established. Radium was in short supply, expensive, and carried some hazards for both patient and therapist. X-ray therapy was available only in the larger centres. Chemotherapy was essentially unknown. Both professional education and public understanding in the field were relatively limited, and among the population at large questionable information was frequently disseminated.

In 1928 a small group of professional and lay people in Manitoba began to advocate the funding of an organization which would be concerned with cancer from all points of view – medical, social, economic and humanitarian. Education, prevention and research would be emphasized. The organization would act as a coordinating, informational and fund-raising agency.

The idea found favour with Dr. E.W. Montgomery, then the Minister of Health for the Province, and in 1930 legislation was passed chartering the Manitoba Cancer Relief and Research Institute. Dr. P.A. McDonald, a staff member at the University of Manitoba, was recruited as the first executive officer of the Institute and its physicist. He gave distinguished service and innovative leadership to the Institute for more than twenty years.

The University of Manitoba was empowered to appoint a member to the Board of Trustees of the Institute, and in 1941 they named Dr. Thorlakson to the position for a three-year term. This was renewed triennially until the Institute was succeeded by the Cancer Treatment and Research Foundation on March 30, 1957. At that time the Manitoba Medical Association was invited to nominate a member for appointment by the Government to the Advisory Board of the new Foundation, and they nominated Dr. Thorlakson. He was duly appointed by Order-in-Council dated November 27, 1957. He was also a member of the Cancer Committee of the American College of Surgeons for a number of years in this period.

Thus both in Dr. Thorlakson's surgical practice and in the formulation of policy, cancer was an old antagonist, with which he had been in combat for many years. Much was still unknown about the causes and the intrinsic properties of cancer. But within his own experience he had seen an ever increasing proportion of patients saved by the deeper insight and improving resources available to the surgeon.

At the national level, the Canadian Cancer Society was founded in 1947, with the active support of the Honourable Paul Martin, then Minister of National Health and Welfare. Its role was to coordinate the work of the provincial affiliates, concern itself with national policies, and provide expertise and direction in fundraising and public education. The Society was particularly charged to use every means to encourage early diagnosis, which would improve the rate of successful treatment. On the medical side, the National Cancer Institute was established to screen all cancer research projects in Canada and allocate funding for those they approved, primarily from money raised by the Cancer Society and its agencies in the provinces, and from federal grants.

This activity at the national level induced the provinces to reexamine their programs. In Manitoba, the benefits of early diagnosis were considered to be particularly lacking in the rural parts of the Province. This became a matter of concern to the Government and to the Union of Manitoba Municipalities. They raised the problem with the Manitoba Cancer Relief and Research Institute. In response, early in 1949 the Institute proposed that special cancer clinics be organized at the Winnipeg General Hospital and the St. Boniface General Hospital, to be staffed by appropriate specialists. Any resident from rural Manitoba suspected of having cancer would be able to come directly, or be referred by his or her doctor, for free diagnostic service. The Government was prepared to fund these clinics through the Institute to the extent of $80,000 annually.

Although some doctors had been involved as individuals in formulating the plan, apparently there had been no formal advance discussions with either the medical staff organizations in the hospitals, nor with the Manitoba Medical Association. Announcement of the plan brought a negative response from both the Medical Association and the staff organization at Winnipeg General Hospital, in defence of the status quo, and on the ground that "free" clinics supported by tax funds were a first step towards "socialized medicine." This label, though interpreted in different ways, tended to arouse strong emotions, both pro and con.

On May 17, 1949, Dr. Thorlakson was elected a member of the Board of Directors of the National Cancer Institute of Canada, and was immediately appointed a vice-president of that body. He served as President of the National Cancer Institute in 1951–1952. To his normal concerns as a practising surgeon, and as a member of the Board of the Manitoba Cancer Institute, of the Manitoba Medical Association, and the medical staff of the Winnipeg General Hospital, a national influence was added.

As early as April 15, 1949, shortly after the Institute's clinic plan for free diagnosis had been announced, Dr. Thorlakson had expressed his views:

> The prevalence and ravages of cancer have reached such proportions that the laity have become thoroughly aroused. This has resulted in a general public demand for action, and large sums of money are now available from various governmental sources. Humanitarian consideration alone dictates a policy which extends equal privileges to all the citizens of this province. . . .
>
> The plan that has been submitted discriminates against residents of the City of Winnipeg. This, to me, is grossly unfair and defeats the primary purpose and objects of the Institute. This Institute must not recognize any intra-provincial barriers if it hopes to accomplish the greatest good to the greatest number of cancer victims.
>
> It is proposed to organize a cancer diagnostic service in the two large teaching hospitals. I have no disagreement with this recommendation except that I do not think it goes far enough. It is, however, a beginning. Details of the plan should be formulated, setting up a panel of qualified specialists in the City and Province who would have the opportunity of using the facilities of these hospitals on every occasion for the diagnosis, and later the treatment, of cancer patients.
>
> To summarize, it is my contention that the Institute should sponsor a plan which includes all cancer patients in Manitoba and all qualified physicians and surgeons. The "detection centre" should be the physician's office. The selection of the patient for further diagnostic study should stem from the general practitioner who should have the privilege of sending his patient to a selected, qualified specialist from a list approved by the Institute.
>
> One further point of tremendous importance in this connection, which must be thoroughly understood by all concerned, is that the

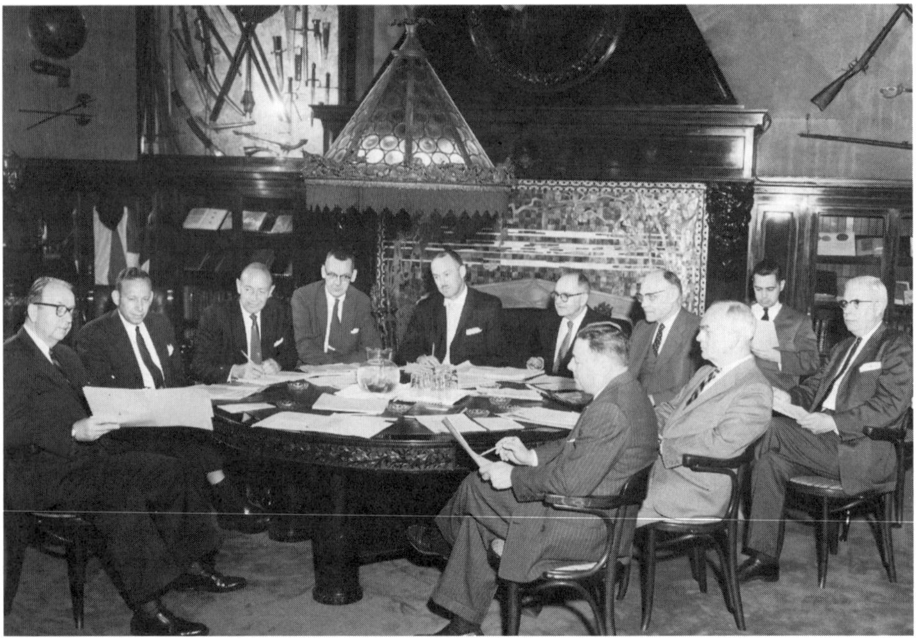

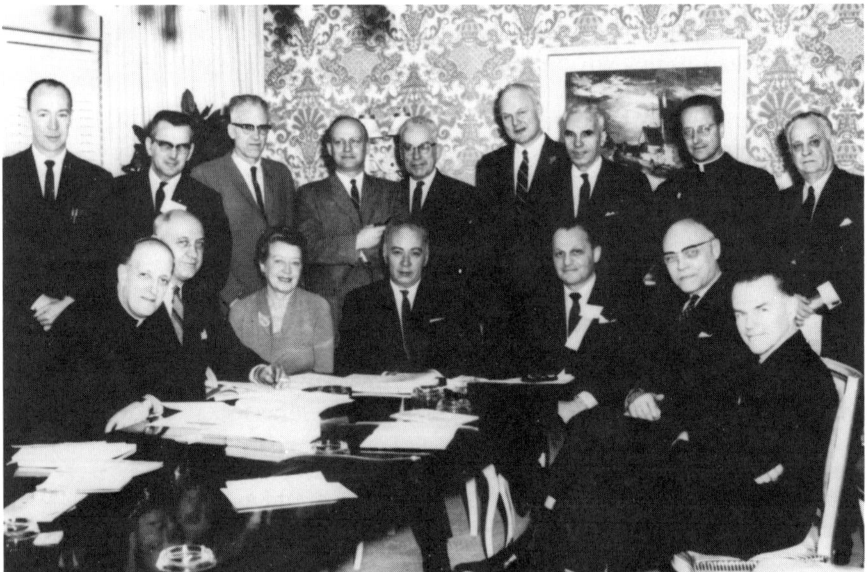

Meeting of the executive members of the Committee on Cancer of the American College of Surgeons held in the Rare Book Room at the College Headquarters in Chicago on June 6, 1958. From left (clockwise): Drs. Murray M. Copeland; Charles Eckert; Howard E. Snyder; Ian MacDonald; R. Lee Clark; James B. Mason; Paul H.T. Thorlakson; Eugene E. Miller; Harold R. Hennessy; Ernest M Daland; and Danely P. Slaughter. (Photo: Oscar and Associates, Chicago.)

In 1952 the directors of the National Cancer Institute met in Quebec City to hono the centenary of Laval University. With the directors is Monsignor Ferdinard Vandry, Rector of Laval University.

term "free" is a misnomer. Nothing is "free" which in the final analysis is paid for by the taxpayers. In this case it is merely another form of prepaid health insurance.

Both the Manitoba Medical Association and the Winnipeg General Hospital Medical Staff appointed committees to deal with the plan for special diagnostic facilities. On July 4, 1949, Dr. Thorlakson offered his suggestions to the Chairman of the Hospital Committee, Dr. Frank Mathewson:[1]

The following communication is in the nature of a suggestion to your sub-committee of the Executive of the General Hospital staff dealing with the proposed diagnostic cancer clinics.... This suggestion is drawn up in the belief that it would be prudent . . . to make some sort of arrangement with the Cancer Institute which will at least meet with their objectives....

It appears necessary that some sort of diagnostic service be offered. Rather than set up a completely new organization, it is recommended that we expand somewhat the present tumour clinics. Our tumour clinic, instead of functioning as a conference, will have to be altered to function as a diagnostic clinic to classify the cases that present themselves.

Similar arrangement could be made with the clinic at St. Boniface General Hospital, and perhaps elsewhere, especially in the Brandon General Hospital.... [Dr. Thorlakson's recommendations were:]

1. That some central organization be created to which these cases can be referred. This is an essential requirement of the Institute.

2. The patients are to be examined by a group of interested and qualified people.

3. It should interfere only slightly with present medical practice.

4. It uses existing arrangements. It does not create a new organization or set up a select small group that might be considered as experts, above their colleagues in dealing with this disease.

5. It can be fitted into any general plan that may be evolved in the future by the Manitoba Medical Service for dealing with these cases. All medical services [are] to be paid for by the Cancer Institute on a basis acceptable to the medical profession, the Cancer Institute, and the Manitoba Medical Association.

6. Funds available will be spent to assist *the patient who has cancer*.

The special committee of the Manitoba Medical Association, however, did not favour the plan. "A Cancer Diagnostic Clinic," they said, "is an anomaly, as the diagnosis of cancer cannot be divorced from the diagnosis of every other disease. Moreover, cancer diagnosis cannot be separated from treatment. In fact, the diagnosis of cancer is usually either made or confirmed at operation."

Prominently involved in the ensuing debate was Dr. Thorlakson. Powerful forces pressed in upon him, engendered by the opinions of his medical colleagues at the National Institute; the concerns of the local medical organizations; the possible effect of change on his own surgical practice and that of his associates; the expressed feelings of influential friends who were opposed to "socialized medicine"; his own humanitarian instincts; and sympathy with the objectives of the Manitoba Institute, if not their precise proposal. He struggled to devise an acceptable compromise.

His views were expressed at a joint meeting of the Executive Committee of the Manitoba Medical Association and members of the Board of the Cancer Relief and Research Institute. He first recalled the statement by the Honourable Paul Martin that, while it is up to each province to find its own solution to the cancer control problem, "the objective is always that of free treatment."

Dr. Thorlakson pointed out that this objective had not been accepted by the doctors. Therefore, he said:

> It would seem to be a mistake to organize cancer diagnostic and treatment clinics in the [teaching] hospitals under the supervision and control of the Cancer Relief and Research Institute. This does not preclude the organization of cancer services within a hospital under the complete control of its medical staff and administrative officers, and financed by funds from Government.
>
> These services should be directed toward providing free services to indigent patients; a complete registry and follow-up system for all patients, both public and private, to be coordinated by the Institute; in the larger hospitals, radiotherapy services under the supervision of the Institute; and the organization of professional study groups within the departments concerned.

He noted the importance of the family physician in early recognition of cancer, and the carrying out of its investigation and treatment in some cases. "But in our present state of knowledge," he said, "cancer is first and foremost a challenge to the surgical profession." He said that the Institute should concentrate its efforts on those activities to which it has contributed so substantially in the past: lay education, operation of a central registry, coordination of a central pathology service and operation of the radiotherapy service.

The Government, however, continued to get complaints about diagnostic services in rural Manitoba. The Manitoba Medical Association continued to oppose the Cancer Relief and Research Institute plan for free diagnostic clinics, and the debate between proponents of the varying points of view was vigorously pursued.

The Government and the Union of Municipalities were pressing for some action. Probably at the suggestion of the Minister of Health and Public Welfare (The Honourable Ivan Schultz), Mr. I.B. Griffiths was appointed Chairman of a special committee of the Board of the Cancer Relief and Research Institute to consider what could, or should, be done.[2] Dr. Thorlakson was asked to make a submission to this committee. He therefore drafted a comprehensive proposal which was forwarded to Mr. Griffiths and the medical members of the Institute Board on February 25, 1950. It ably presented views which were widely held at this time:

> The problems of providing improved cancer diagnostic services for patients from rural Manitoba has now been considered and discussed for almost a year. Several plans have been submitted, each containing some excellent recommendations. However, no one plan has been submitted which can be accepted in its entirety.
>
> In our attempts to bring about centralized control of these services within the Institute, we have committed the error of treating the prospective patient with cancer as a mere pawn in the scheme of things. It is not enough for an individual to learn that he may have cancer. He thereupon loses his right as a free citizen. He is told where he must go for further investigation. If he exercises his freedom of choice of doctor and consultant directly, without reporting to an examining board appointed and paid for by the Institute, he forfeits the financial assistance provided, and for which he has already been taxed!

The second error that would be committed by adopting the plan first presented is to ignore completely the fact that excellent facilities are already available to the patient at a reasonable cost. Any new plan should, in the first place, utilize existing services, and supplement them only where need arises.

In the third place, the plan that has been presented by the Institute does not comply with the policies laid down in its annual reports. The following quotations (1948) represent a fair statement of the situation, and incorporate principles of procedure that the Institute should adopt and the medical profession could endorse:

"A very large number of cancer deaths can be prevented by increasing the availability and efficiency of *general education, diagnostic and treatment services*. This, then, is a major responsibility of a Cancer Institute. Since the *end result* of the fulfilment of this responsibility *is the improvement of all medical practice,* it follows that the work of a Cancer Institute, if properly conceived and executed, *should constitute one of the main structural supports of all medical service.*"

"This concept of a Cancer Institute is quite different from the popular idea of a special institution caring only for a special disease. Since cancer is closely integrated with many other conditions, both in diagnostic and treatment procedures, technical and economic efficiency require that its handling be in institutions *which diagnose and treat not only cancer, but also all the allied conditions*. Only in this way can the diagnostic and treatment procedures necessary for the handling of cancer, be utilized to give the maximum benefit to the maximum number of people, which, after all, is the ultimate objective of social service."

Again in the discussions on this problem much has been made about the fact that similar charity cancer diagnostic clinics are available in many places in Canada and the United States, and that they have been recommended and endorsed by the American College of Surgeons. It should be added that only in the areas of large populations are they really successful, and as a rule they come directly under the control and management of the hospital authorities and their medical staff. A third organization, while it may support the work financially, does not become involved in the actual practice of medicine, as is envisaged in the Institute's plan. By the plan, the Institute intends to take over space in the hospital, pay the medical staffs, and set up a place to practice medicine. This the Institute should not undertake.

I have carefully studied all the recommendations that have been presented. It is my opinion that a satisfactory solution can be reached if each party concerned will now re-examine its position in the light of all the discussion that has taken place. The proposals which I will enumerate are not new or original. No new set of circumstances is created which complicates a difficult situation. The best interests of the patient are safeguarded. The cooperation of all the doctors of Manitoba is assured. The taxpayer is protected, in that his money will be spent for the patient with cancer. The aims of the Manitoba Cancer Relief and Research Institute are fulfilled, and the Union of Rural Municipalities would have achieved their main objective, namely, of making available to the citizens of rural Manitoba the modern scientific facilities for the early diagnosis of cancer, backed by the experience of the entire medical profession of Manitoba.

I submit that the following considerations are basic in any plan that we may devise to improve cancer diagnostic services for patients from rural Manitoba:

1. At all times, the welfare of the patient suffering from cancer should be our first and foremost consideration.

2. In view of the difficulties inherent in the problem, it should be agreed at the outset that any plan that is adopted be regarded as a social experiment. By this agreement, all parties would undertake to carry out the provisions of the plan for a three-year period. At the end of this time, the plan would be automatically discontinued should the Union of Rural Municipalities, the Manitoba Medical Association, or the Manitoba Cancer Relief and Research Institute decide to withdraw their support. It must be a full partnership arrangement.

3. The importance of early recognition of any disease must be borne in mind and emphasized. The creation of facilities for the early diagnosis of cancer, whilst it will remain our chief concern, should be regarded as part of this larger concept. A presumptive diagnosis of cancer should not be made, even in the presence of suggestive symptoms, until the result of investigations is known. In other words, the patient who seeks medical advice should not be considered primarily as a cancer suspect until certain preliminary essential steps leading toward a diagnosis are taken by the physician or surgeon whom he first consults. The ordering of these investigations depends so much on the doctor who first sees the patient that the plan must envisage the fullest cooperation of all doctors practicing in Manitoba.

4. By encouraging patients to seek earlier medical advice, and by eliminating as far as it is practical the fear of costs, we shall thereby employ more fully the excellent public educational program and statistical surveys that have been conducted by the Manitoba Cancer Insti-

tute and its staff. To find ways and means of providing improved diagnostic facilities appears to be the next logical step.

5. If all the foregoing is conceded, then how should we proceed to bring about further improvements in cancer morbidity and mortality?

6. The continued education of the public regarding the early signs and symptoms of cancer is important. In Manitoba the Manitoba Cancer Institute has given leadership in this field. The Canadian Cancer Society and the medical profession by their public meetings and radio talks will continue to advise the public regarding the early signs and symptoms of cancer.

The education of the medical profession about the newer methods of diagnosis and treatment of cancer will bring earlier relief to the patient. All doctors in Canada are being constantly given information about cancer by means of lectures, demonstrations, tumour clinics in hospital, scientific articles in medical journals, by monographs sent out by the National Cancer Institutes of Canada and the United States and by our medical schools. These active educational programs both for the laymen and the profession should in themselves bring about better results. Our particular plan for Manitoba should recognize and utilize these powerful forces that have been and are being used to create a better understanding about the problem of cancer.

7. The following suggestions are, in my opinion, fundamental to the success of any plan, and embody already established and accepted principles in the practice of medicine in Canada:

A. The patient should have free choice of doctor and consultant. (Let me observe that this is still a free country. Patients should not be herded into designated channels for their medical services on the threat that otherwise they will not receive the benefits of so called free medical services.)

B. Unless the patient is indigent, the individual should make a direct financial payment for the services rendered. (Surely we have not reached the stage in Canada where the state taxes the individual, assumes full financial responsibility and then tells the individual that the services are entirely free).

C. The Manitoba Cancer Institute should undertake to pay from public funds:

1) The total costs of diagnosis for cancer in patients from rural Manitoba who are indigent. (This provides for the patient who cannot

provide for himself, and will assist the teaching hospitals to carry out their special function of training medical personnel.)

2) Fifteen dollars ($15) to the doctor who carries out the initial examination, properly recorded and submitted to the files of the Cancer Institute, for all patients from rural Manitoba proven to have cancer. This serves two purposes: The patient and family doctor are directly in touch with the work of the Institute early in the course of the disease; it also pays the doctor who does the initial work, and makes him a member of the team. (In estimating this fee, we recognize the fact that the doctor will on occasion send in clinical reports on patients suspected of having cancer who later are found not to have cancer. This patient will pay the original fee of examination. No single doctor in rural Manitoba will see many cases of cancer during the year. The fifteen dollars for the positive cases is a small fee for the extra work necessary to fulfill his part in our total plan.)

3) Five dollars ($5) for each follow-up examination requested by the Institute.

4) As many patients will be referred to a consultant for special investigation before the diagnosis of cancer or even the suspicion of cancer can justifiably be made, the Manitoba Cancer Institute should undertake to pay fifteen dollars ($15) for the initial examination if cancer is present, properly recorded and submitted to the Institute, and also pay for that *portion* of the special x-ray investigation necessary to demonstrate the presence of cancer (for example, in cancer of the kidneys, intravenous or retrograde urography); and thirty-five dollars ($35) for any special procedures (including endoscopies and biopsies leading to the proven diagnosis of cancer).

5) Furthermore, the Manitoba Cancer Institute should undertake to pay the hospital diagnostic costs excluding the charges for the ward or bed for all patients from rural Manitoba proven to have cancer. This provision is made to discourage ambulant patients from *demanding* hospitalization for convenience and for board and room privileges. Surely $5 a day should be the minimum that the independent and free citizen should pay for these specialized services. At least let him pay for his room and board and not be forced into already overcrowded hospitals to get the *full benefit of so-called free service*. Let us help the patient to help himself. We should not go so far with our misdirected benevolence that we cure people of their disease and keep them alive so that our government can tax them to death!

6) The Manitoba Cancer Relief and Research Institute should under-

take to establish a diagnostic centre or centres in Manitoba to which patients or their clinical records may be referred by any doctor in Manitoba for opinion or advice and organized to provide the following facilities and services:

a) Registration of all cancer patients in rural Manitoba.

b) A systematic follow-up for all patients with cancer from rural Manitoba.

c) Pathological service for all patients from rural Manitoba suspected of having cancer.

d) An information bureau to keep physicians and patients informed about the services provided by the plan.

e) A special diagnostic centre or centres to which patients or their clinical records may be submitted for opinion and advice, including such special investigation as is agreed upon by the Special Committee acting for the Institute and the profession, and paid for by a system which incorporates the basic principles previously enumerated in this letter and others that will, no doubt, be submitted by the members of the Special Committee.

f) A list of consultants who are prepared to undertake the diagnosis and treatment of difficult and serious cases of cancer involving special fields.

In conclusion, let me suggest that all parties contributing, in one way or another, to the success of these negotiations consider the project as a social experiment, based on the work that has already been done by the Manitoba Cancer Institute, by the hospitals of Manitoba, and by the medical profession. Members of the medical profession have, in the past, been ready to devote much time and thought, often to the point of sacrifice of income and leisure, to develop plans for improved medical care for their patients, including the many patients in and outside our public hospitals for which no monetary reward was in sight. This attitude still prevails, and will continue unless the people of this country are forced to take the stand that financial security, based on the taxing powers of the state, is the important consideration, and not the individual's ability to plan, to work and save and to adapt himself to the particular needs of any situation.

The members of the Medical Committee of the Manitoba Cancer Institute should accept the responsibility for the mistakes and failures that have so far attended our efforts to bring about a satisfactory solution of the problem. This is not intended to be a criticism against any individual or group of individuals. It is merely a recognition of the fact that disappointment, many arguments, and even frustration were to be expected because of the very nature of the problem. It has involved a large number of busy people with differing points of view, and they could tackle it only in spare moments and at long intervals. The plans of the Institute, in our enthusiasm, proceeded to their present stage of development without the approval of the medical profession and without the approval of the Medical Committee of the Institute. This should not be allowed to happen again. In whatever plan is finally adopted, let us be sure that it is entered into in the form of a partnership about which not only the Manitoba Cancer Institute and the Government, but also the medical profession are fully informed and in reasonably full agreement. Therein, and therein only, lie the best prospects for the patient who now or in the future may be suffering from cancer.

ADDENDA:

In the course of discussions on the subject during the past year, I have been told that there are doctors who are not qualified to diagnose or treat cancer – that certain doctors are carrying out procedures on cancer patients which they are not trained to do, and so forth. In this connection, I would state most emphatically that any scheme which automatically or by design excludes certain registered practitioners is, in the long run, not a good plan. We are not the licensing bodies for Manitoba. Let us not become involved in that problem at the moment. If individuals who are so definite in their opinions about such matters would be frank enough to register their objections and complaints to the proper authorities such as the Manitoba College of Physicians and Surgeons, the Faculty of Medicine of the University of Manitoba, or their elected representatives of the Manitoba Legislature, or with the Manitoba Medical Association, then their criticisms and advice could be examined in the open and, if necessary, corrected. At this juncture when we are trying our best to work out a plan to assist the cancer victim, we should avoid confusing the issue by introducing into the scheme measures to regulate the practice of medicine. I deal with this matter in some detail because, frankly, I have been alarmed by statements made to me by doctors and laymen on this subject. I suspect that the views of the laymen have been largely influenced by some doctors who adopt a hypercritical attitude toward their professional associates. From this attitude comes the suggestion that consultants should be drawn only from the staffs of the university teaching hospitals. I submit again that this is a very short-sighted policy, and is neither wise nor workable.

The highly respected representatives of the Union of Manitoba Municipalities on the Board of the Cancer Institute, Percy Beachell from Rosser and Oswald Mackay from Alexander, must have been astonished and dismayed at the trouble that stemmed from their simple hope that the diagnosis and treatment of cancer among rural residents could be improved.

Essentially no change took place in the diagnostic and treatment services for cancer until the Institute was succeeded by the Cancer Treatment and Research Foundation in 1957, by act of the provincial legislature. The objects of the Foundation were "to conduct a program of diagnosis of, treatment of, and research in, cancer," including specifically "the establishment and operation, or the assistance in the establishment and operation, of clinics in hospitals or institutions for examination and diagnosis or treatment or both of persons in the province afflicted, or suspected of being afflicted, with cancer, or with any other disease or condition for the examination of which the clinics may thereafter become equipped. . . . "

* * *

Benito, Manitoba
October 28, 1982.

Dr. P.H.T. Thorlakson
Winnipeg Clinic Research Foundation
Winnipeg, Manitoba

Dear Friends:

Enclosed is a cheque for one thousand dollars ($1,000) in memory of my dear husband, Clifford Harvey.

Dr. Paul Thorlakson operated on Cliff 28 years ago for cancer. Cliff passed away in September [1982]. Dr. Thorlakson's sons have both examined him in previous years. I am very grateful to all the Thorlaksons.

Cliff was so dear to me and I miss him very much.

Thanking you sincerely,

His wife,

Dagmar E. Harvey

CHAPTER 28

A Provincial Health Plan

In 1940, the results of the medical examination of young men volunteering for service in the armed forces made it evident that there was a good deal to be desired in the health status of the people of Manitoba. It was apparent that the problem needed to be attacked on two fronts. The public health service needed to be reorganized and upgraded to direct more resources to the prevention of illness, to the control of environmental conditions that were detrimental to health, and to the encouragement of positive measures to improve physical fitness. At the same time, steps needed to be taken to provide better medical and hospital services throughout the Province. An informed independent opinion was clearly needed to formulate a comprehensive plan to meet these health service needs, and to provide the planning expertise and the objectivity that were essential to an effective development.

Dr. F.W. Jackson (Deputy Minister of Health), who had practised in rural Manitoba before joining the Provincial Service, had received international recognition in the field of public health, and was a member of the Sub-Committee on State and Provincial Health Studies of the American Public Health Association. It was natural, therefore, for the government to turn to that body to conduct a study in Manitoba. Late in 1940, with some financial support from the Commonwealth Fund,[1] the Province made a contract with the Association to prepare a report and recommendations to be used as a basis for a long-term program of health service development encompassing the whole province. The project was immediately initiated under the personal direction of Dr. Carl E. Buck, Doctor of Public Health, field director of the Association, and an experienced health program planner. Dr. Buck and his staff made a comprehensive survey of provincial health resources and facilities in Manitoba in 1941.[2]

The report and recommendations were issued in the fall of 1941. They dealt with the public health side of the program, and essentially recommended the establishment of the province-wide public health service through a system of full-time local health units. The report also recommended a separate study of hospital needs in the Province. This undertaking was in due course assigned to the Welfare Supervision Board, a body established by Manitoba statute to carry out investigations at the request of the government. The Board had the assistance of Graham L. David, Hospital Consultant of the W.K. Kellogg Foundation, and Dr. E.W. Williamson, Associate Director of Hospital Activities of the American College of Surgeons. After a study lasting almost two years, the report of the Welfare Supervision Board recommended a plan of hospital development in rural Manitoba. Essentially it called for the formation of hospital districts throughout the province that usually would encompass a number of municipalities, to provide a hospital service graded in size and scope according to community need. This might vary from a ten-bed "medical-nursing unit" to a regional secondary level referral hospital. They also recommended development of the Manitoba Medical Centre as a major training resource for the health professions, and a provincial referral resource for complex illness.

It became apparent in the course of these intensive studies of the health care system that the close relationship between social and economic well-being and the health of the individual made it desirable to examine the social welfare program. Consequently, the American Public Welfare Association was asked to make a study of Manitoba's social services. Mr. Howard L. Russell, Director of the Association, made his final report to the Government with respect to this project, on September 20, 1944. His most interesting recommendation advised that as a pilot study there should be set up in one district a combined administration of health and social services, to test the effect of integrated direction of these related programs. If this project were successful, the principle could be applied in other health units.

It is a tribute to the dedication, insight and vision of Dr. F.W. Jackson, the Deputy Minister, and to the leadership of the Honourable Ivan Schultz, the Minister of Health and Public Welfare from 1944 to 1952, that action was taken in an orderly and informed manner to implement most of the recommendations resulting from the excellent studies that had been done. Indeed the developmental scheme that was put forward by the Government in the fall of 1944, and enshrined in legislation early in 1945, was probably the most carefully prepared and the most comprehensive health plan devised in any Canadian province. It was directed mainly at the health needs of rural Manitoba, where most of the shortcomings were to be found. The program provided for a significant increase in preventive services and the promotion of health through establishment of the local health units; for special arrangements to increase the number of physicians in rural centres; for an improved hospital service; and for the location of laboratory and x-ray facilities in rural hospitals that would serve the diagnostic needs of physicians practising in the surrounding region. Dr. Jackson wrote:[3]

> Before the Government's health proposals were made public, the Honourable Ivan Schultz . . . discussed them with the Manitoba Division of the Canadian Medical Association. As soon as the legislation was drafted it was made available to the legislative committee [of MMA] and discussed both with them and the executive of the Association. Any changes which did not conflict with government policy were made; even the most minor alterations in the draft legislation were cleared with the Association's legal advisor before the bill was finally presented.

During this period, Mr. Schultz and Dr. Jackson not only met with Medical Association officers; they also visited the district meetings of the Manitoba Medical Association, to ensure that local practitioners understood the plan that the Government was proposing, and to give them an opportunity to voice their opinions and suggestions directly to the Minister.

Probably typical was the meeting on Thursday, January 25, 1945, called especially by the Winnipeg Medical Society after selected members had studied the draft legislation, at which Mr.

Shultz and Dr. Jackson presented the plan to Winnipeg doctors.

Following the introductions by the Chairman, Dr. P.H. McNulty, and a brief statement by the Minister, Dr. Jackson described in detail the proposals regarding public health and the preventive medical services. The discussion was opened by Dr. C.H.A. Walton, who read a prepared statement in which he drew attention to the necessity of safeguarding the interest of the medical personnel involved and the impact of the program on private medical practice. He suggested that there should be some provision for research in the field of prevention.

The Minister followed with a description of the proposals to improve diagnostic facilities in the rural parts of the Province, resulting in a lively discussion led by Dr. Digby Wheeler, a leader in the specialty of radiology.

Dr. Jackson then detailed the plans to encourage doctors to practise in the country, and outlined the assistance that would be offered in arranging for municipal councils to contract with physicians on either a fee-for-service, capitation or salary basis. Dr. A. Hollenburg read a prepared paper on this topic.

The Honourable Ivan Schultz completed the specific consideration of the provincial plan with a discussion of the section on hospital accommodation, followed by a prepared commentary by Dr. Bruce Chown.

There was a strong feeling among the doctors that the Government's intentions could only succeed if the facilities for medical education were substantially improved. This, of course, was a basic purpose of the Manitoba Medical Centre, and Dr. Thorlakson had been asked to express the profession's views on this essential subject. Until now, there had been no public recognition by government of the obligation to support this fundamental need. Dr. Thorlakson made it clear in his address that this requirement could not be overlooked. He spoke as follows:

I wish to take this opportunity to congratulate the Minister of Health, the Honourable Ivan Schultz, and his Deputy, Dr. F.W. Jackson, on taking the initiative in submitting a definite plan for improved medical care in this province. No individual or group of individuals can hope to produce a plan that will, from the beginning, be acceptable to everyone. I am confident that the outline, "Basic Health Proposals of the Province of Manitoba," has been submitted for two reasons; first, to make a contribution to this rather complicated problem; and second, to stimulate constructive and helpful criticism.

Dr. F.W. Jackson, because of his wide contacts in the Province both with the profession and the public, has had a better opportunity than any other individual to study this problem in its entirety. He has studied and worked hard on this subject for many years. While there is bound, by the very nature of things, to be some disagreement, the profession should study the proposals seriously and sympathetically. While changes will undoubtedly be made as the result of free and open discussion, the address given by the Honourable Minister over the radio two weeks ago will constitute a landmark in Manitoba's medical progress. It is the duty of organized medicine to support the Government in any measure that will give the people of this province more equitably distributed medical services, provided it improves the standard of medical care while the status of the physician is maintained.

It cannot be urged too strongly that the success of any system depends primarily on the training and experience of the doctor and the opportunity he has to keep informed of the advances of medical science. No new system of medical practice will succeed unless greater emphasis is placed on medical education and medical research. These are the two main pillars which assure proficiency and progress in medical care. The most important single factor is the qualification and training of the doctor. A criticism of the Government's "Basic Health Proposals" is that no provision is made, in the outline at least, to provide increased and improved teaching facilities. The Government is aware of the fact that the salaries paid to our preclinical instructors are quite inadequate and that our teaching staff is overworked and underpaid. It is well known that many medical men who could be excellent teachers and instructors have entered practice only because of the lack of facilities and the poor incomes which they would receive if they followed this very high and important calling. Yet it is proposed to supply this new system, which will require additional medical personnel, without first giving serious thought to the urgent needs of that institution which educates and trains that personnel.

It has been estimated that 45 to 50 new doctors must graduate and remain each year to supply the needs of Manitoba under this new plan. If this estimate is correct, are we going to increase medical student enrollment by fifty to seventy-five percent? In our public wards, the clinical facilities for teaching are even now insufficient to meet the needs of our present enrollment of students. After the War, greater emphasis is to be placed on better undergraduate and more postgraduate instruction. Committees have been at work organizing courses of instruction but as yet neither the Government through its Department of Health, nor the University of Manitoba through its Faculty of Medicine, nor organized medicine, has presented any plans for the development of adequate teaching facilities. This, ladies and gentlemen, forms the groundwork for our whole system of improved medical service. We are building an elaborate superstructure before we have strengthened the foundation. This appears to be an opportune time to urge Government and organized medicine to accept their share of the responsibility of arranging for adequate clinical facilities and to act upon a resolution that was passed unanimously at the last meeting of the Manitoba Division of the Canadian Medical Association.[4]

In addition to training doctors, there is the additional responsibility of the Government, through the University, of providing adequate teaching facilities for the training of the non-professional staff necessary to carry out effectively any scheme for improved medical services. If the standard of medical care is to be raised, there must be well-trained laboratory and x-ray technicians, social workers, nurses, dietitians and medical stenographers in sufficient numbers to adequately staff the proposed health units and hospitals. No steps should be taken to introduce a new system of medical service unless this trained personnel is made available from the outset. In his preface to the health broadcast, Mr. Garson, Premier of Manitoba, strongly indicated the early need to assemble the elements of medical personnel and the equipment required in order to get this health scheme under way.

The next point I would like to draw to your attention is that no funds have been set aside to support fundamental or clinical research. The debt that the medical profession and the public owe to the research worker can never be properly computed. Any plan of improved medical services must include a provision for adequate support of our research worker. This will require the fullest understanding between the Department of Health and the medical profession. The value does not rest alone with the positive results of research but also with the great stimulus that is derived by the doctor from the association with men and women trained to carry out scientific research. Surely, in this new day of medical progress, the people of Manitoba are not going to be satisfied to enjoy the advantages of new medical discoveries without making some contribution to their development.

As the late Sir Frederick Banting said in 1938, "Canada cannot continue to export a large proportion of its trained minds who are graduates of our universities." From now on, Manitoba cannot allow this annual exodus of men and women seeking an opportunity to carry out systematic research. It must be made possible for them to find this opportunity at home. In the University of Manitoba, adequate remuneration and facilities for the research worker are long overdue.

The meeting was considered to have been a great success by all who were present. It demonstrated the importance of open and frank communication between Government and the medical profession with regard to matters which could become highly controversial. As the minutes recorded, "The Hon. Mr. Shultz and Dr. Jackson presented their plans and took part in the discussion in their usual masterly and lucid manner. The standard of discussion was of a very high order, both as to adverse criticism and constructive suggestions. . . . The organization of this meeting, the presentation of the case and the discussion by our own medical representatives reflected a great deal of credit on our public men and on our own medical speakers."

Legislation to bring all these measures into effect was introduced in the provincial legislature in March 1945, and passed in the estimates of the Department of Health and Public Welfare. It had a far-reaching effect on the health and well-being of the people in all parts of the Province.

CHAPTER 29

Manitoba Medical Service Incorporated

A satisfactory method of applying insurance principles to alleviate the financial burden of illness for all Canadians had been sought for more than half a century before our present national health care plan was inaugurated.

As early as 1928 the federal government asked interested agencies to thoroughly investigate the possibilities. In 1930 the Canadian Medical Association created the Standing Committee on Economics. One of its functions was to formulate a health insurance plan that would be acceptable to the medical profession. In 1934 this committee issued a comprehensive report setting out the principles under which such a plan might operate.

During World War II, health insurance became a major issue of public policy. In principle it was endorsed by all political parties. In 1943, in what Dr. Thorlakson described as a "precedent-shattering statement," the CMA announced that "the Canadian Medical Association approves the adoption of the principles of health insurance . . . [and] favours a plan . . . which will secure the development and provision of the highest standards of health services, preventive and curative, if such a plan be fair both to the insured and to all those rendering the services." The CMA included a timely warning. "It is obvious," it noted, "that any plan of health insurance which is not supplemented by a program to ensure better nutrition, better housing, and the reduction of worry and anxiety, particularly for those of low or uncertain income, will fail in its objectives."

Dr. Thorlakson noted these landmark statements by the Canadian Medical Association in his "History of Prepaid Hospital and Medical Care in Manitoba" – a paper which he was invited to present at the annual meeting of the American Association of Medical Clinics in New Orleans in October, 1960.

During the hard times of the 1930s, illness was often the final blow that turned financial difficulty into catastrophe. Medical and hospital charges, modest as they were, simply could not be paid in many instances. It was clear that regular payments of small sums were needed to build insurance funds to pay the costs of illness. Some unions in Winnipeg (in particular the Firefighters Union) pioneered by adding a premium for medical services into their monthly union dues.

In 1938, a public, non-profit agency known as the Manitoba Hospital Service Association was incorporated to provide a prepayment vehicle for hospital care. It later became associated with Blue Cross. Meanwhile, in advance of the CMA endorsement of a health insurance plan, a committee of the Manitoba Medical Association was formulating a prepayment plan for medical care, subsequently known as the Manitoba Medical Service (MMS). This doctor-sponsored plan was incorporated by an act of the Manitoba legislature on March 31, 1942. The MMA Committee continued its study of the structure and operating requirements of the plan, and with Dr. E.S. Moorhead as its Executive Director it opened for business on October 1, 1944.[1]

Although sympathetic to the purpose of this enterprise, Dr. Thorlakson had some forebodings about its viability in its initial form. His practice, when contemplating a major project in affairs for which he was responsible, was first to seek the advice of experienced and successful experts in similar fields; as his plans progressed he continued to seek advice from knowledgeable people. But he had noted in the case of the MMS, which was entering a sector of the insurance business that was known to have special hazards, the medical committee had apparently failed to consult professionals in the field of casualty insurance. The Committee had worked hard, however, and had designed its own program.

When Dr. Thorlakson read the details of the plan as announced at the beginning of October 1942, it was evident that his concerns were well-founded. His views were clearly expressed in a paper, published in the *Manitoba Medical Review* for November 1944:

The Manitoba Medical Service (A Criticism and a Recommendation)

In the establishment of a charitable institution it has always been taken for granted that the services of the medical profession were obtainable at little or no cost. Doctors have been ready to assume responsibilities in connection with the medical aspects of these charities. As a rule, the medical services have been rendered without remuneration or there has been a token payment to cover incidental expenses. The aggregate value of such services to the community must, over a period of years, represent a very substantial contribution.

The Manitoba Medical Service is apparently based on the understanding that doctors are willing to extend their charitable services to include not only the indigents but all employed people in the community. The increased cost of medical care, which has nothing to do with an increase in medical or surgical fees – (for these are being lowered below the level of twenty years ago while everything else is going up, including taxes) is to be borne by the medical profession. The committee will decide how much your bill is to be discounted. Furthermore, as this scheme continues to grow and serve a larger number of citizens, the Committee will take over the responsibility of supervising and controlling medical practice by scrutinizing all doctors' accounts. By reviewing the case after all tests have been completed and the results known, they will have power to disallow certain charges because, in their opinion, some of the examinations might have been avoided. No other group in the community would think of thrusting themselves between the doctor and his patients to this extent and expect to get away with it.

The Association has gone into operation before many of the difficulties have been satisfactorily ironed out. At this very moment while the public are buying the contracts, the Committee is still grappling with a large number of unsolved problems. The official announcement from the Committee at the recent meeting of the Manitoba Medical Association was that "a lot of these difficulties had been by-passed. . . ."

One reason given for the haste in launching the plan immediately was the fear that the Dominion government scheme of health insurance would make the position of the doctors untenable. Early this year it was known that there was no reason for this fear, or for this haste.

The members of the profession have been told that they would be fortunate to receive, during the first two years, sixty percent of the accepted (minimum) schedule of fees. It is admitted by some that only forty percent of the medical bills may be paid. . . .

During the recent annual convention of the Manitoba Medical Association, the General Secretary, Dr. T.C. Routley, said that in answer to lay groups who demanded the right to control any scheme of health insurance for the people of Canada, he would like to state emphatically that the medical profession would not tolerate any outside interference with the medical aspects of the plan; that they, and they alone, were qualified by training and experience to undertake this phase of the work. During that very hour we heard that a group of doctors, unaided by any expert with experience or special knowledge of insurance principles, were embarking upon a plan to organize a sickness insurance society. This independent step was taken in complete disregard to the fact that we have in Canada a very large and important group of men who have made a lifelong study of insurance problems.

How would the medical profession react to an announcement by the insurance companies of Canada to the effect that they would no longer require doctors to supervise the medical aspects of their insurance problems?

Many of the members of the Committee are medical specialists; and they all subscribe to the opinion that in a difficult medical or surgical situation, a man specially trained to deal with that problem is required. Sound principles that govern human conduct and attitudes under one set of circumstances should, with equal force, apply to others. In one of the most important steps taken by our profession in this province, no expert has been consulted and we are to be advised and governed by a group who possess little or no experience in sickness insurance. . . .

If the members of the medical profession are convinced that this is a sound venture, then they should be prepared to subscribe a sufficient sum to launch the scheme in a businesslike manner. There are, no doubt, one hundred medical men in Winnipeg who have, before this, made investments of $1,000 each in a speculative venture; and they would be prepared to do so again if they could be assured that the plan was a cooperative enterprise in which the public, the larger corporations, the municipal authorities, were prepared to assume some financial responsibilities for its success. But no, the doctors insist on assuming the whole burden themselves, and continue in a direct way to provide medical relief to a large section of the community at fifty percent of a reduced schedule of fees. If there is such a great demand on the part of the public for an insurance plan of this kind, then substantial support should be forthcoming to aid the medical profession to embark upon such an experiment. . . .

The financial aspect of the problem is by no means the most serious infringement upon the direct relationship between the doctor and his patient. . . . The Association proposes to limit the amount of investigation that may be carried out on a given case. Permission must be obtained before certain procedures can be carried out . . . ; [but] when a group abrogates this power to themselves without proper authority approval, . . . the profession should resent such intrusion into the accepted doctor-patient relationship. . . .

There are many commendable features in this scheme. The members of the Committee have been given an arduous task. The Committee was originally authorized to canvass the local situation and to recommend and bring before the Manitoba Medical Association a plan that would enable people in the low income groups to budget for unexpected and altogether unpredictable illness. The members of the Committee deserve credit for the amount of work they have done. . . . The scheme has been launched by a group of doctors who feel that they have given it their best thought and consideration. The correct thing to do now is to support it, on the understanding that further study based on experience will make it possible to strengthen and consolidate the work of the Committee by the introduction of sounder insurance methods. . . .

On a blustery winter evening in early 1954, Dr. Thorlakson was just finishing his customarily late dinner at home when the telephone rang. It was Dr. P.H. (Pat) McNulty, a past-president of the Manitoba Medical Association who was the current Chairman of the Manitoba Medical Service. He enquired whether it would be convenient for him to come over to get Dr. Thorlakson's advice about a number of rather urgent matters.

Assured that he would be welcome to come immediately, he drove at once across the city. It turned out that he wanted to discuss the Manitoba Medical Service. The troubles – mainly financial – that had hovered over the MMS from the beginning had reached a critical point. Policy changes were needed, and the Board wished to invite Dr. Thorlakson, whose concerns were well known, to stand for election as Chairman of the Board of Trustees. With some hesitancy, but with a strong feeling that he had a duty to the profession and to the public to lend his support in these times of difficulty, he acceded to the request of Dr. McNulty and his colleagues. In March 1954, Dr. Thorlakson was elected as the Chairman of the Board of the Manitoba Medical Services, Inc.

During the ensuing weeks he spent long hours in discussion with Dr. J.C. MacMaster, who had become Executive Director of MMS in 1948. He studied reports and documents on the MMS operations; and he explored the MMS problems as seen by medical colleagues, non-medical members of the Board, and others. On April 20, 1954, he addressed a meeting of the Board – his first as their chairman. This statement was published in full in the MMS newsletter and distributed to all members:

Gentlemen:

It is now a month since you elected me to be the Chairman of the Board of Trustees. During that month I have given much thought to the general duties and responsibilities of a chairman. I have, as chairman, also given much consideration to my personal duties and responsibilities to the medical profession and general public; and also to our collective responsibilities as a board of trustees toward the public on the one hand, and to the Manitoba Medical Association, the members of which have nominated most of us to this board.

For the coming year, you look to me for leadership. Accordingly, I would ask your indulgence while I express some ideas that I have developed and which should, in all fairness, be mentioned at this time. I realize only too well the many problems that have beset my predecessors in this office and on this board, and I am also aware of the great things they have accomplished against great odds, much criticism, and opposition. I pay my respects to the public representatives now on the Board, and to the pioneers who ventured into the hitherto unknown field of medical economics, and to the members of the medical profession at large. We have reached our present position because of their signal and generous contributions. Therefore I address myself to this task in all humility, and with a fervent prayer in my heart.

The primary responsibility of the members of the medical profession is to attend the sick; to instruct the future practitioners of medicine; to associate themselves actively with public health agencies; and to offer counsel, advice and instruction to patients on all matters relating to the prevention of disease; to continue the education of the physician by experience and practice, by reading and by attendance at local and national medical meetings; and finally, to identify themselves with all responsible agencies concerned with the problem of providing sickness insurance, in order that the burden of illness will not threaten the future financial security of the individual or family. If the doctor does all these things conscientiously and within the limits of his competence his future position in society is assured, irrespective of reasonable change that may occur in the social structure.

On all matters dealing with public policy and finance as it relates to the practice of medicine, the profession should place itself in the strongest possible position to advise but not to control; otherwise we will in the long run alienate public confidence and support. By education, training and experience the average doctor is ill-equipped to engage in business or commercial enterprise. Any financial success may be attributed more to hard work, long hours and professional training than to special business ability. If this is so, this medically dominated board would appear to be on dangerous ground in assuming too easily that good fortune will crown with success our future efforts, however well-intentioned they are, in the field of prepaid medical care. Prepaid medical and hospital care is one of the most important political and financial problems of the day. It may be argued with some justification that medically sponsored plans saved our people from state medicine. Now we must take care that we operate them in such a manner as not to invite socialized medicine. Our plans must be sound and solvent, yet sufficiently flexible to meet the medical needs of the community in a manner that meets the requirements of the patient and at the same time gives due consideration to the circumstances under which the services are rendered. . . .

With each advance of civilization, the individual becomes more and more affected by or dependent upon the collective action of society. The success and happiness of the whole group govern to an increasing degree the success and happiness of the individual. To this extent we become "our brother's keeper"; not in the strict, narrow sense of charity toward the weak and poor, but in the broader sense of the maintenance and preservation of our way of life. Herein lies our philosophy regarding the provision of prepaid medical care and hospital services.

Our society is dedicated to the principles of individual freedom and of free enterprise, restricted only by the bounds of decency and the protection of the public weal. In this society, no insurable group should be able to demand complete and all-inclusive service without some immediate personal and financial responsibility simply by presenting a card. Human nature being what it is and medical services being what they are, there is opportunity for over-utilization and over-servicing (not necessarily deliberate or dishonest) by both contracting parties. A small but fair restriction should be placed on demand for, and the provision of, such services. No community in the world is sufficiently wealthy to offer unrestricted hospital and medical services to all the people all the time, under any scheme that has yet been devised. There is no mathematical measurement that can be applied to the quantity or quality of the services required or rendered. In no other field of human endeavour is personal integrity of greater necessity and value. But, no matter how important personal integrity is, one cannot afford to take this attribute for granted.

The correction of excesses and the strengthening of our plan lie in the steady improvement of our methods of doing business, and placing such restrictions as are necessary to protect the equity in the contract of the insured. We should return to our first objective, that is, to provide a plan of prepaid medical care for all those in the low income group and to protect them against the financial calamity of catastrophic illness. Is our present plan accomplishing this objective? Decidedly not! Our all-inclusive Plan B is the greatest single bargain on the market today. Our well-to-do citizens recognize this and are joining in large numbers. These are the very people who have been educated by us to the value of periodical health examinations, the necessity of early diagnosis, and the value of tests. These people can easily be accommodated by the MMS but surely not on the basis that we have carefully chosen for the average artisan or the struggler in the lower income group. Other policies are being sold to the public which deny certain classified services to the individual unless he enters hospital; and he feels abused if a hospital bed is refused him so that he can get more than the value of his contract. He wants bed and board thrown in with the need for investigation. These are not isolated cases. Blue Cross keeps one medical man busy checking the hospital records for these abuses, yet he only discovers the most flagrant instances.

The next proposition that I would submit is that the medical profession in the long run cannot by itself afford to underwrite the health of the community or even part of it. For this reason, I disagree with the official attitude that medically sponsored and controlled plans are the answer to socialized governmental medicine. All our political parties are committed officially to national health insurance. The difference is only one of timing. . . .

Finally, while we should seek and ask for a wide measure of cooperation with government and industry in solving the difficult problem of providing adequate and efficient medical services to the people of our communities, we should expect the cooperation of the medical profession and the public in keeping the costs within reasonable bounds. This can only be done by adopting the principle of co-insurance, whereby the individual is obliged to pay a modest sum toward the initial cost of hospitalization, or medical or surgical care, in addition to his paid premium. This places responsibility on the individual alone, and where this rightly belongs in every country where freedom of choice and freedom of action are cherished and proclaimed as a right. It is the only way of controlling over-utilization and preventing steady and marked increase of premium rates. By way of precedent, notice the co-insurance charge levied by the provincial government for x-ray and laboratory services at the time of rendering the services; and this device is acceptable to people who have already paid their premiums through tax deduction. That such a device is even urged by some of our own subscribers is a matter to be noted. To illustrate, on the ninth of April [1954] a delegation from labour and management of a major business in the City had a meeting with Dr. MacMaster, our Executive Director, in this boardroom, to discuss present and future policy of

MMS, especially with respect to premiums. In this discussion it was emphasized by labour that grave danger existed through over-utilization and over-servicing; and this group tendered a remedy: co-insurance.

On the topic of cooperation with the Government, it is relevant to ask what our policy should be in the event of exploratory conversations or enquiries on behalf of the Government. Can we go on alone? I do not believe we can. Nor does the Canadian Medical Association. . . . There is an understandable fear that government participation means political control. Quite apart from the adverse effect that would have on professional competency and initiative, there is good reason to believe that the public would suffer from the standpoint of efficiency, cost and quality of service. In a discussion about such an important issue, one must avoid, as far as possible, sentiment and broad generalization. There are examples in which government participation has not meant political interference or government control. The Sanatorium Board of Manitoba receives both government and private support. There is no government interference. The service which the patient with tuberculosis receives is of a high order of excellence. Again, the National Cancer Institute of Canada is the trustee for funds which support the work of Canadian cancer research scientists engaged in the investigation of the cause and cure of cancer. The National Government provides almost fifty percent of these funds. . . . As a member of the executive of the National Cancer Institute for four years and the President for one year I can, from first-hand knowledge, say that there has been no government restriction or interference with its policies at any time. . . .

I would like to digress for a moment to mention deficits. It is a matter of record that a disparity always exists between MMS income and the medical claims filed against it. To bridge this gap in the early days of MMS, an ingenious pro-rating principle was adopted to carry the plan through emergency situations or crises. But after ten years of experience, pro-rating is still applied to claims and we are virtually announcing every month that a state of emergency exists, and would even appear to have existed for 120 months! In short, the temporary has become the permanent. Once a year, with one sweep of the pen this board can cancel out all debts to doctors. While it is true that this power is assigned to the Board by the terms of the agreement with the doctor, it is nevertheless a situation that causes uneasiness to some of us. It is probably without parallel in business or commerce anywhere on this continent. Do we realize that more than $3.25 million have been struck off since 1944? . . .

In accepting the chairmanship of the Board of Trustees one month ago, I warned you that you have committed a grievous error in judgement, because while I have always been a strong and persistent advocate of prepaid medical insurance, I have in the past differed sharply with many of the policies adopted by the Board. However, I shall endeavour to direct the affairs of this organization to the best of my ability and within the prescribed limits of a chairman, leaving the active direction and management to our very capable executive director and his excellent staff. It shall be my guiding principle to endeavour to interpret the wishes of the majority of the members of this association rather than inflict my personal convictions on you.

However, the Executive and the Board of Trustees have a twofold duty which they must discharge with fairness and with justice. One concerns the medical profession alone, and the second, and possibly the paramount, duty must always be to safeguard the health and welfare of that large group of citizens who place their confidence in us.

The next major statement on MMS affairs by Dr. Thorlakson was his report at the annual meeting of the Manitoba Medical Association on October 13, 1954. In his address he first noted that the MMS was in its tenth year of service. At the beginning of his report, he paid tribute to the members of the first board and its first executive director, Dr. E.S. Moorhead. Then he said:

However, every progressive and successful organization must critically assess the decisions of the past in the light of subsequent experience; [and] to improve our effectiveness and efficiency we must make necessary changes in policy and procedure. . . . The MMS was organized for the purpose of collecting, at stated intervals over the year, a sufficient premium from prospective patients to compensate prospective physicians and surgeons for their professional services. By this token, active membership is restricted to members of our profession engaged in active private practice. It is in no way another general medical association to which all registered physicians and surgeons can belong or take part in its active management. As the medical members of the Board are all elected by the MMA it behooves the parent body to select representatives who are in active practice and who can speak for this section of the profession. Notwithstanding what I have just said, special circumstances demand special consideration. There are members of our profession who are not engaged in active competitive practice and yet whose judgement and contribution we value highly. We should be able to include them in our committees by special arrangement. The re-classification of physicians here suggested brings us to another topic – group life insurance for doctors.

While MMS must always have for its principal purpose the arrangement and payment of medical services on behalf of subscribers, there are subsidiary objects in its constitution and these can properly be used. It is proposed, for example, to use MMS as an instrument through which group benefits can be secured for physicians – all physicians if possible. Group welfare includes such elements as retirement pensions, group life coverage, disability insurance and so on. A physicians' retirement pension program has been under study by our medical economists, and when income tax legislation is favourable, we shall probably be in a good position to implement this program. There is, however, one phase of the social security program which has been established as from October 1, 1954 – group life insurance.

Doctors in the class of full and active members are eligible for this coverage. On behalf of associate or non-contributing members, we are requesting group coverage and hope to use MMS as the instrument through which these physicians will also acquire group life protection.

Under group life coverage there is now an enrollment of seventy-five percent of eligible physicians under sixty-five years – a response that must gratify those responsible for the pioneering and negotiating of this contract. They well deserve our thanks.

Now that the MMS has come of age and has on its board members who have devoted much time and thought over the years to its special problems and also have an experienced and well-trained staff, the time has arrived to reconsider the working relationships between the MMA and the MMS.

At the present time all matters of policy are referred to the parent organization before action can be taken by the Board of Trustees of the MMS. In effect, this means that a body, largely selected by the membership of the MMA, can spend weeks and months in arriving at a decision on policy and procedure and then must refer it to the Executive of the MMA for approval or disapproval. If the members of the Executive of the MMA are to give the matter full consideration, then it must have time, possibly to refer it to one of its sub-committees, before it can come to a decision. If the original decision is upheld, then two large bodies of busy medical practitioners have spent much time arriving at the same conclusion. Or again, should the parent body reject the recommendation of the Board of Trustees of the MMS, it then, in effect, represents a vote of lack of confidence in the members elected by your association. What is more important, it retards the introduction of necessary changes. This deliberate slowing up of the machinery can cause serious discouragement and a sense of frustration to a group of men working hard to promote the welfare and success of the MMS. There is little reason to expect that one body of doctors sitting around a conference table is likely to arrive at a wiser decision than the first group of doctors sitting around the same table in the MMS boardroom. To me, this arrangement wastes the time of two groups of busy doctors who are already giving a great deal to the affairs of organized medicine. The interests of the MMA are adequately safeguarded by the fact that the Board of the MMS are nominated by the Executive Committee of the MMA and elected by our membership and that these representatives are being constantly changed.

The report went on to discuss a number of MMS operating problems related to the authority and powers of the Board; the decisions about fees; what appeared to be abuses of the comprehensive coverage in Plan B; and the need for experience rating for high user groups. It closed with a tribute to the members of the Board, the Executive Committee, and to Dr. MacMaster and the staff.

Dr. Thorlakson presented his last report to the medical members of the MMS during his term as chairman, on March 20, 1956. His two-year tenure of office had been marked by strenuous efforts to identify the management and financial problems that had been evident during the first decade of MMS operations. Having identified the causes of difficulty, they were discussed thoroughly and openly with the appropriate people, and specific steps were taken to introduce policies that would correct, or at least improve, the health of the operation. Experience rating based on actuarial analysis was introduced; public and professional relations were improved; and due to Dr. Thorlakson's strong stand in the matter, the pro-rating of medical accounts, initially proposed to be seventy-five percent in 1955, was actually increased to eighty-five percent. Net operating revenue had improved; and the chairman refused to accept the principle that doctors' accounts should be arbitrarily reduced to provide funds for a "reserve."

Dr. Thorlakson's report on his second year as chairman is a strong record of change and achievement that laid the foundation for the successful years that followed. This report to the thirteenth annual meeting of the MMS (quoted in part) was presented on March 20, 1956:

The prepayment of medical care is a permanent feature of our medical-economic existence. The means by which the benefits of modern scientific medicine are to become available to an ever increasing number of our citizens under a contributory prepaid system are receiving intensive examination by the public and the profession. Basic principles of policy and procedure have been established and are available for application by any health insurance agency. The MMS must now implement them for the benefit of the patient and the community.

Fiscal Policy

The MMS has pioneered in the field of comprehensive care on a fee-for-service basis with free choice of doctor to the patient. In our program, the patient has available to him any physician and surgeon practising in Manitoba. He has access to the general practitioner or specialist of his choice. A high standard of public service has been achieved. In spite of this record, the MMS has been subjected to criticism both from within and outside the profession. This is a good and encouraging sign. It denotes increasing interest in the affairs of the organization. Both the public and the medical profession are vitally concerned with the practical application of voluntary prepaid medical insurance. Freedom to disagree and to criticize is essential during the evolutionary stage when repeated adjustments are necessary. The immediate question that confronts the MMS is, To what extent can its policies and methods be improved to meet the reasonable expectations of the profession and of the public in the field of prepaid medical care?

Let us first examine the position of the medical members of MMS. No reasonable person will deny that the doctors serving MMS have a just grievance. They know that financial solvency is being maintained by automatically writing off, each year, large debts to the participating physicians and surgeons for services they have rendered on a substandard schedule of fees. We have persisted in this method of financing during a period of unexcelled prosperity. Who could not balance his accounts if he was permitted to write off all his just debts at the end of each year, only to begin all over again to acquire new debts? This is surely unrealistic, unfair and unnecessary. We have been circumventing the ordinary laws of bankruptcy. Pro-rating of physicians' accounts should be used in emergencies, when the profession would wish to share with the entire community the financial effects of a disaster or epidemic but surely not as a continuing way of carrying on the affairs of a successful organization during these years of plenty. *It is a damaging precedent which can only boomerang to the discredit and disadvantage of the profession.* It is a public acknowledgement that the fee schedule can be manipulated at will and the profession will officially and without protest accept this arrangement. It, unfortunately, implies that the doctors themselves consider their remuneration more than adequate. How can we seriously object if other organizations or a government agency ask for the same privilege? Our apologists say that this is our private concern and what we do in the conduct of our business affairs does not concern others. The truth is that our methods are being closely scrutinized and are being used as a basis for commercial organizations in setting up their schedule of fees. The greatest disservice that any member of the profession can render to his medical colleagues is to suggest that the doctors should accept and be satisfied with the present financial arrangements.

The MMS must be prepared to take losses when they are necessary but not, as in the past, accept them as a normal method of conducting its affairs. The public does not expect this of us; nor do they understand this type of fiscal policy. Nor should we expect the average citizen to give us any credit for our failure to pay a just fee for services rendered to the participating physicians. There is a vast distinction between charity to the poor and altruism towards those not needing or wanting it. In our MMS planning we must employ a flexible combination of realism and humanism.

The MMS has come of age. It is entitled to, and must have, experienced advice and direction. The methods employed in conducting the affairs of the organization have been examined by two separate groups of experts in the field of prepaid medical plans. They have submitted practical recommendations. Today, the Board of Trustees of the MMS can assure the public and the profession that we now have a group of energetic, capable administrators who are prepared to implement corrective measures which will place the MMS on a sound economic basis. . . .

So far, I have dealt only with one side of our relationship with the medical profession; that is, with the medical members of MMS. With the growing importance of MMS, it is paramount that we establish proper lines of communication between the MMS and other medical organizations, especially the executive of the MMA. We must also agree on responsibility for establishing medical policies to be used as a guide by the MMS Board of Trustees.

These matters are under consideration by a joint committee consisting of the officers of the MMA and the Executive of the MMS, and definite progress can be reported. There is agreement that all matters concerning the affairs of another medical organization must, in the future, be transmitted only through official channels and not through someone who happens to be on the two boards or executives.

Regarding the method by which medical policy should be established, it is fair to state that the majority of the sixteen medical members of the Board of Trustees were under the impression that, having been elected to the MMS Board by the entire medical electorate, they were directly responsible to the entire profession.

The MMS Board of Trustees, legally a completely autonomous body equally responsible to subscribers and medical members, must at all times know that in the discharge of its dual obligations it has the support of an informed profession. When, as individual members of the medical profession, we criticize the MMS, we must admit, in all fairness, that the MMS has been and will be exactly what we make it. The MMS has never had adequate directives from the profession regarding medical policy. No machinery or regular procedures have been set up in the past to ascertain the opinions of the medical electorate. . . .

A recent meeting of Blue Shield Prepaid Medical Plans of America, in Chicago, was devoted largely to "professional relationships." Nine Manitoba doctors attended. We learned that many medical societies have a "professional policy committee," the composition varying, of course, from state to state. Our delegates were of the opinion that this idea was worth exploring for our Manitoba plan.

Some Highlights of 1955

The Board of Trustees can look back with some satisfaction on the year 1955. Substantial progress has been made in several areas of our responsibility. The year 1955 has been, in some respects, a transitional phase in the story of MMS and is probably the turning point in its history. The members of the Executive, the Board and the Administration have worked hard. Many important meetings and private interviews have been held during the year.

The activities crowded into the year cannot easily be measured. An enumeration of the projects cannot tell anything of the coordinated planning behind them. The highlights of the year are as follows:

1. Research reports were analyzed by actuarial and underwriting consultants.

2. The sales staff was strengthened.

3. An Actuarial Division was established, headed by a full-time actuary.

4. The subscriber contract was revised and ratified by the Board in October 1955.

5. A new non-group comprehensive plan was presented and approved.

6. Experience rating of groups was adopted.

7. The principle of controlled extra billing (supplementary fees) for subscribers in the higher income brackets was approved by the Board of Trustees.

8. The principle of co-insurance was approved by the Board of Trustees but the specific method recommended to implement this fundamental principle in sickness insurance failed to receive general acceptance by the profession.

9. Subscriber utilization statements were authorized for monthly distribution and this has already had some interesting results. Patients have actually offered to pay to the MMS and to the doctors the twenty-five percent pro-rated deduction.

10. The absence of an employer contribution was deplored and steps were initiated to correct this serious defect.

11. Ratio of medical to non-medical members of Board was reconsidered.

12. Increased labour representation on the Board has been discussed and generally approved.

13. Municipality interest in MMS coverage is increasing.

14. Joint MMA-MMS discussion took place on policy by senior officers of both organizations.

15. Meetings were held in the boardroom with representatives of the press and of labour.

16. Direct contact with senior management officials in the city has been made. The services available to employees by MMS have been stressed. As a result, employee enrollment in these firms has increased, resulting in a wider distribution of risk.

17. A public relations committee has been established.

18. Trans-Canada Medical Plans: national uniform in-hospital program approved; national plan for coverage of dependents of armed services personnel approved.

19. Blue Shield Commission of USA: affiliation continued and meetings attended.

20. Department of National Health and Welfare: cooperation was offered conditionally.

21. At the request of the Manitoba government, a brief on membership and financial data for the period 1944–55 was submitted.

22. There has been an encouraging increase in enrollment. Today, twenty-six percent of the residents of Manitoba are enrolled with MMS, and fifty-three percent of the population of Greater Winnipeg is being served by MMS.

23. Unpaid balance to doctors for services rendered to December 31, 1955, $1,315,938. This creates a total of $5,800,000 deficit to doctors since MMS was established.

This has been an important and difficult year for the MMS. Substantial improvement will become evident as the new arrangements become operative. There is always a lag period between planning and performance. It has been a hard year for our staff. Many extra burdens have been placed upon its members. They have accepted them without complaint and have discharged their duties with unfailing courtesy and efficiency. To Dr. MacMaster and his staff may I offer the appreciation of the Board of Trustees. The Manitoba Medical Service was terminated on the introduction of the government's Medical Service Insurance Plan on July 1, 1968.

* * *

'TIS NEVER TOO LATE. . . .

With its roots in the Manitoba Medical Service Inc., the United Health Services Corporation Limited was formed in 1958 to provide its clients with such benefits as the extra cost of private hospital rooms, special nurses, and similar expenses not covered by the provincial health insurance plan. In the intervening years the services have been broadened, and the Corporation is commonly known today as Manitoba Blue Cross. Dr. Thorlakson was a member of the Board of this organization when it was established and Chairman between 1959 and 1961.

On May 14, 1986, the Corporation held a testimonial dinner at the Westin Hotel in Winnipeg to honour its former board chairmen, three of whom are still living and were present at the dinner: Dr. W.D. Bowman, Dr. Norman I. Corne and Dr. Thorlakson. Each guest was presented with a handsome bronze plaque, embossed with his photograph and an inscription. Dr. Thorlakson's reads as follows:

Presented To
Dr. Paul H.T. Thorlakson
In Recognition
And Appreciation For
His Dedication
And Valuable
Contribution As Chairman
Of The Board
Of Directors Of
The United Health Insurance
Corporation Limited
1959–1961

May 14, 1986. K.V. Bittner, President

CHAPTER 30

Wide Horizons

It is not uncommon in the social history of man to observe that the introduction of a new idea or a practice varying from the norm is first looked upon as a radical and perhaps threatening deviation from tradition, subject to sanctions by the peer group. But with the passage of time, action that in the beginning was controversial is first tolerated, then applauded, and finally is held to be an exemplary mark of social progress. Thus it was with group practice in medicine.

In the years following World War I, when clinic groups were organized in which doctors shared their professional activities and their resources, the organized profession looked askance at this departure from traditional solo practice. Three decades later, in 1955, the Canadian Medical Association reported that a survey of group practice in Canada revealed that there were 127 group practices in Canada in 1949. This had increased to 187 in 1955. The number of groups of three or more doctors had increased three-fold in the United States in the same period. Unions and other "consumer" organizations, and indeed the highest levels of government, began to see advantages in the delivery of medical services through organized groups. In 1962, United States President John F. Kennedy made the following statement in the course of a message to Congress:

> Experience in many communities has proven the value of group medical and dental practice, where general practitioners and medical specialists voluntarily join to pool their professional skills, to use common

facilities and personnel, and to offer comprehensive health services to their patients. Group practice offers great promise of improving the quality of medical care, of achieving significant economies and conveniences to physician and patient alike, and of facilitating a wider and better distribution of the available supply of scarce personnel.[1]

On June 20, 1961, the Government of Canada created the Royal Commission on Health Services, with Mr. Justice Emmett M. Hall of Saskatchewan as its Chairman. Judge Hall quickly became interested in the potential of group practice as an efficient way of delivering medical services under the plan that the commission would recommend. He took two immediate actions to explore the possibilities. He appointed Professor J.A. Boan of the University of Saskatchewan at Regina to make a special study of the nature and significance of group practice and its place in the future development of health services. And he invited Dr. Thorlakson, as its most experienced and active proponent in Canada, to submit a brief to the Commission. The brief was called, "The Provision of Medical Services Through Group Practice."

Dr. Thorlakson presented his brief at a meeting of the Commission held in Montreal on April 16, 1962. He began by expressing some of the essential principles he believed should underly a national medical services plan. He then went on to describe in concise and explicit terms the place of group practice in service to the community; in improving the standards of medical care; and in broadening medical education.

The records indicate that the Brief and the informal remarks that accompanied it sparked an animated question and discussion period, and aroused a lively interest among the commissioners. A few selections from the Brief provide examples of its content:

A comprehensive medical care plan should be based on the following principles:

1. Availability to every citizen.

2. Government financial assistance on a flexible scale according to need.

3. Retention of a measure of personal financial responsibility.

4. Freedom of choice by both patient and physician.

5. Acceptance and participation in administration but not complete control by the medical profession.

6. Freedom from government monopoly and domination but subject to government audit.

7. Separation of x-ray and laboratory insurance premiums from other hospital and medical insurance costs.

8. Utilization of the resources and experience of the Canadian insurance industry. . . .

We should look carefully at some of the provisions of the Australian plan in which the patient pays his doctor directly. The Australian Insurance Plan pays ninety percent of the patient's medical and hospital bills. . . .

Government aid should aim to avoid hardship and relieve unnecessary suffering; it should not go beyond this and discourage thrift, self-reliance, independence and free choice. . . .

I challenge anyone who says that there will be no difference for the patient or the doctor if and when a completely government-sponsored and government-controlled scheme of collecting premiums, supplemented from the general tax fund, is instituted and the bills for medical and surgical services are sent to a government agency. . . .

The standard and excellence of medical care . . . is directly proportionate to the standard of medical education and research carried on in the province or the country. . . . One doctor in a community can be a health educator and can continue to educate himself; two or more doctors, working together, can carry out these functions much better. Medical education in its fullest sense does not end within the Faculty of Medicine in the University or in the University teaching hospital. Every hospital, large or small, should be a teaching centre; every privately organized medical group or clinic should be a teaching and investigative group. University affiliation and recognition are desirable but should not be a primary requirement. . . . This is one of the many reasons why group practice should be extended; it should provide some of the advantages that accrue to medical staffs of university hospitals, namely, continuing group education and group criticism. . . .

Undoubtedly we need, and will need, more doctors; but what we will need more and more in the future is better teamwork and less wastage of trained personnel. . . . The sharp separation of specialists and general practitioners should be discouraged. The doctor of the future, in any category, should have specially trained technicians who will carry out some of the routine procedures which the doctor now performs. These assistants, including secretaries, will be able to concentrate on many details to which the doctor can now give only passing attention. The doctor will diagnose, direct, supervise and follow the results of treatment. . . .

There followed a complete description of the nature of group medical practice, together with short accounts of the work of two Manitoba examples outside Winnipeg: the group at Flin Flon, described by Dr. Percy Johnson, its senior member; and the Hamiota Medical Group, portrayed by Dr. J.E. Hudson.

The preface to Professor Boan's Report on Group Practice for the Royal Commission is an indication of the interest in Dr. Thorlakson's contribution: "Special mention must be made of Dr. P.H.T. Thorlakson of the Winnipeg Clinic. He not only provided the Commission with his views on group practice in a brief and in conversations both formal and informal; but, through his tireless devotion to the cause of better medicine through group practice, [he also] made it possible to meet and talk to other physicians interested in group practice both in Canada and in the United States." The reference to "other doctors interested in group practice" relates to a journey by Chief Justice Hall to an event in Portland, Oregon.

At the beginning of October 1962, the American Association of Medical Clinics (of which Dr. Thorlakson was a member) held its two-day annual meeting in Portland. They were interested in expanding the Canadian membership in the organization, and they had invited Dr. Thorlakson to encourage the attendance of as many Canadian doctors as possible who were involved in group practice. This he did, and about twenty doctors from Canada arrived for the Portland meeting. Among them was Dr. Arthur D. Kelly, General Secretary of the Canadian Medical Association.

Shortly before the meeting, Dr. Thorlakson learned that Chief Justice Hall was in Vancouver. Aware of his keen interest in considering alternate ways of delivering medical services, and recalling the animated discussions they had shared on the subject of group practice, Dr. Thorlakson telephoned the Royal

Commission Chairman to invite him to Portland to hear first-hand the dissertations and discussions drawn from the experience in group medicine of both Canadians and Americans.

Chief Justice Hall accepted this invitation, and he and Mrs. Hall motored from Vancouver to listen to the conference speakers and converse with the delegates. The presence of the distinguished chairman of the Royal Commission added a special and unexpected dimension to the meetings and provided him with a unique opportunity for face-to-face discussion with the leading practitioners of group medicine in North America.

During the conference, Dr. Thorlakson presided at a meeting of the Canadians present to consider the invitation of the American Association for increased Canadian membership. The discussion indicated that, although the offer of membership in the American Association of Medical Clinics was appreciated, there was a general feeling that circumstances were different in Canada, and that a Canadian organization was required to meet Canadian needs. Consequently a committee was named, with Dr. A.C. Abbott, senior member of the Abbott Clinic in Winnipeg, as Chairman and Dr. T.A. Lebbetter of the Winnipeg Clinic as Secretary, to explore the possibilities and purposes of a Canadian group practice organization; to consider its relations to other medical bodies; and to draft a constitution. If the response was favourable they were to proceed to create a formal association of Canadian group clinics.

The response from prospective members was strongly affirmative, and the Canadian Association of Medical Clinics was formally created at a meeting in Ottawa some months later. Dr. Abbott was elected as the first President, and Dr. Lebbetter as the first Secretary, of the new organization.

Throughout his life Dr. Thorlakson had shown an active interest in community affairs, but as he gradually relinquished his surgical practice he found time to increase his participation in non-medical activities. He continued, of course, his involvement with the Winnipeg Clinic and the Winnipeg Clinic Research Institute, and with medical affairs generally. But the five-year period beginning in 1962 (when Dr. Thorlakson was sixty-seven) saw him engaged to a greater extent in fields less directly related to medical practice.

For example, he devoted more time to his interest in educational concerns (see chapter 32). He was appointed to a number of official or semi-official bodies, including the Manitoba Hospital Commission; the Civic Development Association; the Informal Committee for Manitoba on Bilingualism and Biculturalism; and the National Executive Council of the Pan-American Games Society. He became a member of the Board of Trustees of United Way. He was elected to the Board of Directors of the Great-West Life Assurance Company. He addressed both non-medical and medical organizations ranging from the Rotary Club of Winnipeg to the Twelfth Middle East Medical Assembly at the American University in Beirut, Lebanon. He received the Community Service Award from the City of Winnipeg and the Golden Boy's Good Citizenship Award from the Manitoba Travel and Convention Association.

As Canada's centenary approached, Dr. Thorlakson looked forward to 1967 with the growing sense of exhilaration experienced by Canadians everywhere. This festival year would be a time when national pride and patriotism could be expressed without inhibition.

Dr. Thorlakson's advice was sought by many who had responsibilities for centennial projects and programs. For his own part, he accepted the appointment of Chairman of the Canadian (Icelandic) Centennial Committee. In addition to the local Icelandic celebrations, he represented the Canadian Icelandic community on a number of formal centennial occasions. Among these was the presentation of a commemorative bronze plaque to the people of Canada from the Canadians of Icelandic origin. This plaque carried a suitable message in the Icelandic language in a central panel, and was flanked on either side by the same sentiments, expressed respectively in English and in French. To even the most casual observer one thing stood out: it took only about two-thirds of the space to convey the message in Icelandic as it did in either English or French.

The presentation ceremony took place in Ottawa, and the gift was accepted by the Prime Minister, the Right Honourable Lester B. Pearson. In responding to Dr. Thorlakson's presentation address, after a gracious acknowledgement of the gift, and of the great contribution to Canadian life made by the Icelandic settlers and their descendants, the Prime Minister noted, with

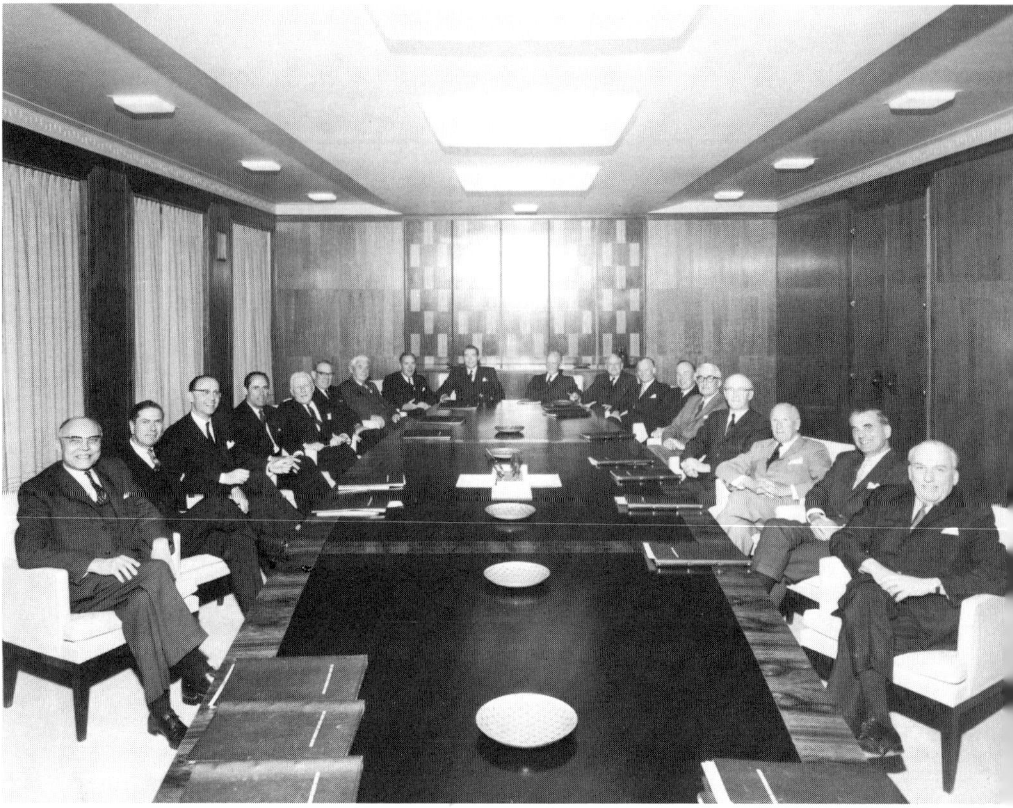

*Great-West Life Assurance Company Board of Directors meeting on June 10, 196
The directors are clockwise from the left: P.H.T. Thorlakson, M.D.; Donald M. Elliman, New York; G.T. Richardson, E.H. Moncrieff, H.S. Foley, Vancouver; Rhys M. Sales, Oakville, Ontario; H.W. Manning; J.E. Morrison (Executive Vice-President); D.E. Kilgour (President); Joseph Harris (Chairman of the Board); J.A. MacAulay, Q.C., (Vice-President); P.S. Bower; A.S. Leach; P.A. Chester; George McLean; H.E. Sellers; W.P. Walker, Toronto and W.C. Riley.
Executive Officers: D.E. Kilgour, President; J.E. Morrison, Executive Vice-President; P.S. Bower, Vice-President and Treasurer; George Aitken, Vice-President and Comptroller; E.A. Palk, Vice-President and Director of Agencies; R.O.A. Hunter, Vice-President and Secretary; A.E. Loadman, Vice-President and Actuary; W.L. Benson, Director of Group Sales and Administration; F.A.L. Mathewson, M.D., Medical Director; R.C. Barnsley, Director of Research.*

wry humour, that "their contribution would be enhanced by millions of dollars if they could just convince the Government to keep all the national records in Icelandic!"[2]

As a measure of Dr. Thorlakson's breadth of interest, examples of his other centennial-year activities is revealing. On the subject, "One Hundred Years of Medicine in Manitoba," he was the guest speaker at a meeting of the Dietetic Association of Manitoba, and of the Home Economics Association. He participated in the inaugural meeting of the Manitoba Chapter of the Vanier Institute of the Family, and introduced the guest speaker, his friend, Dr. Wilder Penfield. At a meeting of the Canadian Association of Medical Clinics in Toronto, he was chairman of a panel which discussed "Group Practice in University Affiliated Hospitals." On invitation from the Canadian Medical Association, Dr. Thorlakson wrote a thoughtful preface to its published report entitled, "Group Practice in Canada," prepared after four years of study by a committee headed by Dr. E. Kirk Lyon. He was the dinner speaker at a Symposium on Cancer Chemotherapy in Montreal, his topic being, "A Century of Medical Progress." He delivered an address at a dinner given by the Icelandic community in Manitoba on the occasion of the Centennial visit of His Excellency, Asgeir Asgeirsson, President of the Republic of Iceland. To close the year, he visited Mexico, where he had been invited to address the Ninth Western Medical Meeting held at the University of Guadalajara.

Following the meeting in Guadalajara, Dr. and Mrs. Thorlakson flew the hundred kilometres to Puerto Vallarta, a resort town on the Pacific Coast. There they settled in comfortably for a period of rest and relaxation before going on to Mexico City, where they would spend Christmas.

Sunset at Puerto Vallarta is a splendid sight. As the sun touches the horizon, apparently enlarged and arrayed in brilliant orange, yellow and red, it suddenly appears to speed its departure and with an astonishing haste seems to plunge beneath the waves of the Pacific. Since there is virtually no twilight at this latitude, in just a few minutes the transformation from day to night is complete.

One evening, Dr. Thorlakson strolled alone to the beach to watch this impressive phenomenon. As the spectacle ended and darkness closed in, he stretched out in his beach chair and con-

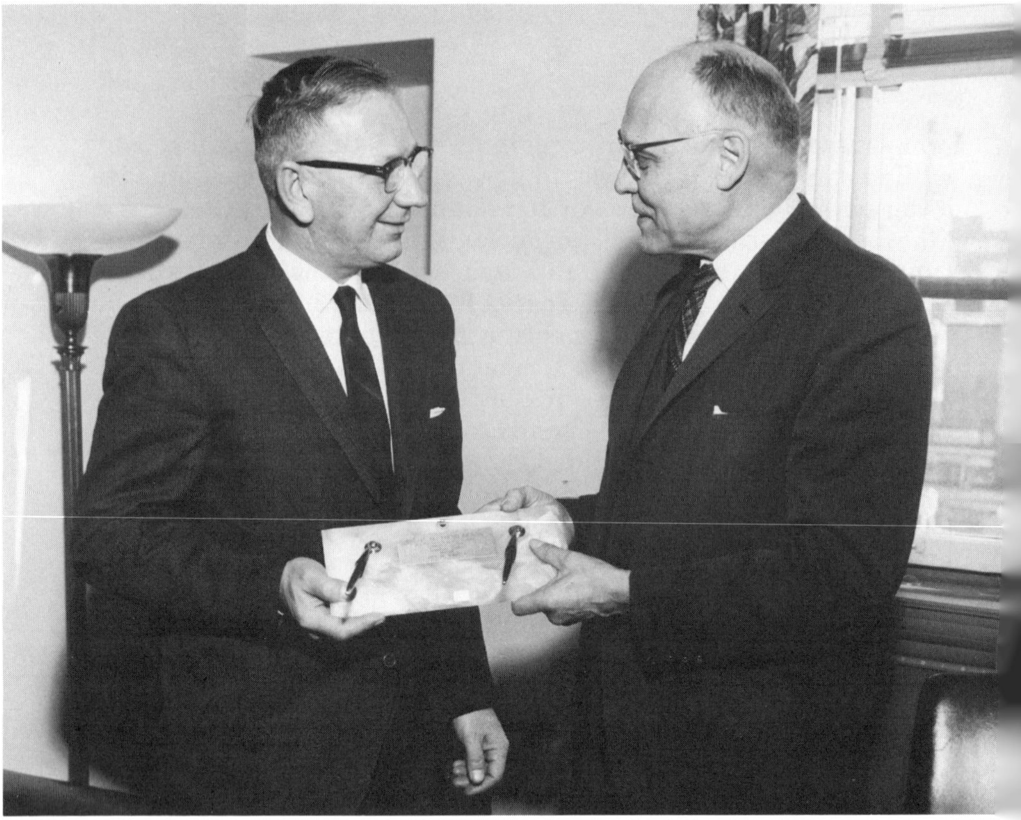

Winnipeg's Mayor Juba makes a presentation to Dr. Thorlakson in appreciation his outstanding community service (December 24, 1962).

templated the events of the past year, a year that would end while he and Gladys were still in Mexico. He thought about the letter he had received earlier that day from the Chairman of the Manitoba Centennial Commission, Maitland Steinkopf, Q.C., extending an invitation to tour the Centennial Concert Hall complex, which was not yet quite complete.

He considered his own commitments for the coming year. He would have to make arrangements for the meeting of the Board of Directors of the Canadian Association of Medical Clinics, which would meet in Winnipeg the next spring at the International Inn, partly to do the final planning for the annual meeting to be held in Vancouver in June. This reminded him that the long-term schedule of the Association called for the 1970 annual meeting to be held in Winnipeg, at which time he would be president.

It was at this point, on the Pacific sands of faraway Mexico, that the Great Idea was born. Why not turn the 1970 meeting into an international conference, with doctors in group practice from all parts of the world congregating to share subjects of mutual concern. It was an exciting prospect. If it could be done successfully, it would be one of the most significant events of the Manitoba centennial year! Group practice was growing in Europe, Japan, South America, Australia, the United States, Canada . . .

He walked briskly back to the hotel to talk to Gladys.

On his return to Winnipeg in the latter part of January, 1968, Dr. Thorlakson lost no time in telephoning his good friend, the Chairman of the Manitoba Centennial Commission. Mr. Steinkopf renewed his invitation to give Dr. Thorlakson a personally guided tour of the Centennial Concert Hall. An appointment was made to meet a few days later.

As they walked through this splendid building, in which skilled workmen were installing the final furnishings and fittings, Mr. Steinkopf pointed out the special features of its design. He spoke of the careful thought that had been given to the important matters of acoustics and aesthetics. They admired the statue of Queen Elizabeth II, from the studio of Leo Mol, standing in the corner of a storeroom awaiting its placement on a pedestal in the courtyard.

As Chairman of the Centennial Commission, Mr. Steinkopf

had experienced the difficulties frequently faced in reaching an acceptable decision on a project involving three levels of government and wide public interest. He spoke not with complaint, but with gentle humour, about his experience.

Following the tour, they had lunch together, and it was then that Dr. Thorlakson outlined to Mr. Steinkopf his idea of organizing a world conference on group medicine to be held in Winnipeg in 1970. As they talked, their enthusiasm for the project grew. Mr. Steinkopf pointed out that even before the planning could formally begin, it was essential to make a reservation for the facilities of the Concert Hall, and have accommodation blocked out with the hotels for the hundreds of rooms that would be needed. He offered to send a man over the next day who was experienced in the organization of large meetings. This man would arrange these first steps, and he could continue to be available to Dr. Thorlakson for advice and assistance on the organization necessary to arrange a world-class congress.

The advisor duly arrived. It turned out to be Mr. Morley Decker, an executive assistant in Mr. Steinkopf's office. In business-like fashion, he explored the available dates in 1970 at the Concert Hall, reviewed them with Dr. Thorlakson, and forthwith all its facilities were booked for April 26 to 30, 1970.

Next came discussions with the hotel representatives, and arrangements were made to allocate 1,000 rooms for delegates and their families.

With these essentials taken care of, the challenge of turning an idea into a reality could begin in earnest. During this flurry of activity Dr. Thorlakson met with the Manitoba doctors in group practice and described his Manitoba centennial project as he conceived it. Their response was to offer enthusiastic support and assistance.

The Board of Directors of the Canadian Association of Medical Clinics, with representation from across Canada, met at the International Inn in Winnipeg in February, 1968. Again, Dr. Thorlakson put to them his idea of a great international meeting to take the place of the regular annual meeting of the Association in Winnipeg in 1970. And again, the response was unanimously favourable, "provided he would take the responsibility for its organization."

They suggested that he ought to explore the proposal with the

Canadian Medical Association, the Department of National Health and Welfare, and the American Association of Medical Clinics. This required a trip to Ottawa, Toronto and Chicago (where the executive of the American Association of Medical Clinics was meeting). In each place he received encouragement for the project.

Two months later, in April, the Canadian Association of Medical Clinics held its annual meeting in Vancouver. Once more, Dr. Thorlakson presented the idea and reported the initial steps that had been taken toward its realization. Not only did the Association (along with its associated body, the Medical Group Management Association of Canada) agree to officially sponsor the international meeting, but they also advanced $25 per member as a loan to fund some of the promotional expenses. (This loan, which amounted to $11,437, was repaid in full from Congress revenues.)

During the Toronto visit, the advice and assistance of Dr. Arthur F.W. Peart, who had become General Secretary of the Canadian Medical Association in 1966, was especially helpful. Dr. Peart felt sure that the Canadian Medical Association would endorse the Congress, and he would see that it was placed on the agenda of the next Executive meeting.[3]

About this time, Mr. L.R. (Bud) Sherman accepted an appointment as public relations adviser for the Congress. Mr. Sherman, who was experienced in the fields of journalism and broadcasting, had been elected to the House of Commons as the Member for Winnipeg South in 1965.[4] Out of his experience he was able to offer Dr. Thorlakson very helpful support in relationships with the press and broadcast media, and with government agencies, during the early stages of organization.

Mr. Sherman was appointed to the position of Executive Director of the Congress on February 1, 1969. The pressure of organization was building up and full-time assistance in planning and coordination was urgently needed. Dr. Thorlakson recalls a discussion with his new executive director after one particularly difficult day. "Whatever you do," said Mr. Sherman, "as the Congress draws closer and the problems multiply, don't panic!" To which Dr. Thorlakson replied, "Bud, I've had forty years of dealing with crises in the operating room, and there is one thing you can be sure of: I won't panic!"

When Mr. Sherman decided to stand for election to the Manitoba Legislature some months later, he found that the demands on his time did not permit him to continue his work with the Congress organization. He was succeeded as executive director by Mrs. Dora Sorell, an experienced and highly recommended convention manager from Montreal. Her skilled direction and detailed written operational plans contributed much to the smooth coordination of events. Mr. D.R. MacFarlane, a Winnipeg consultant in communications, became the public relations coordinator.

With the advice of Mr. Decker, eleven active committees involving the substantial commitment of eighty-five busy people were formed. Each had its own chairman; but as general chairman, Dr. Thorlakson was an ex-officio member of all of them. They took responsibility for ensuring the success of all aspects of the congress.[5]

The Canadian Association of Medical Clinics, and the Medical Group Management Association of Canada, were the official sponsors of the Congress. It was endorsed by: the Canadian Medical Association; the Association of Canadian Medical Colleges; Association des Medicins de Langue Française du Canada; the College of Family Physicians of Canada; the Royal College of Physicians and Surgeons of Canada; the Canadian Hospital Association; and the University of Manitoba.

Thirteen international vice-presidents of the Congress were appointed, each of whom was a distinguished member of the medical profession in his own country.[6]

It was decided to send a promotional letter and an invitation to participate to doctors of renown and to medical societies of various kinds throughout the world. The messages were to be conveyed in both English and French.

The basic draft was done in English, and in order to ensure that the French version would be of international standard, Dr. Thorlakson consulted the Department of External Affairs in Ottawa. They referred the material to a translation centre at Laval University in Quebec.

Up to this time, the conference had been named The First International Congress on Group Practice. Word quickly came back from Laval that doctors didn't "practice" in France, nor, in the sense intended, elsewhere in Europe; and consequently there was no acceptable, one-word, translation of "practice" and it would be wise to re-consider using the term.

The hazards inherent in planning international events were revealed during the preparation of overseas publicity. Obviously, a change was necessary, and the official designation, First International Conference on Group Medicine was agreed upon.

In the summer of 1968, the first Information Bulletin was prepared, and 50,000 copies were distributed around the world. The External Affairs Department in Ottawa gave its full cooperation. Canadian Embassies, Trade Commissions and other government offices in about eighty countries received the Information Bulletin and an official letter requesting their assistance in publicizing the Congress to the departments of Health, Medical Associations, Medical Faculties and Medical Journals in their respective regions. Within six weeks, enquiries from countries as widely separated as Peru and Finland, Rhodesia and Thailand, Denmark and Australia began to come in. In all, there were enquiries from forty countries.

In October 1968, Dr. and Mrs. Thorlakson went to Japan to attend the Sixteenth Biennial Congress of the International College of Surgeons, which was held in Tokyo and Kyoto. During the Congress, Dr. Thorlakson was made an honorary fellow of the College.

The meeting provided an opportunity to discuss with Dr. Taro Takemi, the President of the ninety-thousand-member Japanese Medical Association, the possibility of a delegation coming to the Congress in Winnipeg. Dr. Takemi was subsequently appointed one of the vice-presidents of the First International Congress on Group Medicine.

After the Tokyo meetings, Dr. and Mrs. Thorlakson went with other Canadians to Hong Kong and Thailand. At each place meetings were arranged with members of the health departments and local physicians to promote the Congress.

During the next eighteen months, Dr. Thorlakson travelled the world to arouse interest in attending the Congress and interview prospective speakers. In June 1969 he visited Toronto, Montreal, Chicago and Rochester (Minnesota). In September he attended the annual meeting of the Association of American Medical Clinics in New York. In November he attended the meeting of the Association of Schools of Allied Health Professions in Washington. There he also spoke with officials of the Department of Health, Education and Welfare.

January 1970 found him in Vancouver and Victoria, where he met with Dr. Hugh L. Keenleyside, who kindly agreed to open the Congress sessions with an address called "Socio-Economic Changes Affecting World Health Care."

In February, in part by courtesy of Air Canada for flight accommodation, he was off to London, Paris, Bonn, Oslo, Montreal and Ottawa, meeting with key medical people and professional associations in a final drive to settle Congress details and promote attendance. He was back in time for the last, strenuous, six weeks of preparation.

In addition to the distinguished speakers and delegates, this congress was exceptional in another way. At the invitation of Dr. Thorlakson, the president and general chairman, His Excellency, The Right Honourable Roland Michener, C.C., C.D., Governor-General of Canada, graciously agreed to act as the Honorary President. On being apprised of this, the Senate and the Board of Governors of the University of Manitoba invited His Excellency to accept the degree of Doctor of Laws, Honouris Causa, to be conferred at a special convocation of the University at the Centennial Concert Hall on Sunday, April 26, immediately prior to the official opening ceremonies of the Congress, scheduled for 8 p.m. The Governor-General was pleased to consent to these arrangements.

It was evident, as some 2,000 delegates and guests gathered in the Concert Hall on Sunday evening, that this was no stiffly formal and austere occasion of the kind that not infrequently marks the opening exercises of conferences and conventions. A sense of joy and pleasurable anticipation was present everywhere. The smiles and the animated conversation in the foyer indicated the sense of exhilaration created by the event, and a general satisfaction that this international occasion, for which so many had worked so hard, was at last actually under way.

No one was disappointed. The formal entrance of the Governor-General, wearing the scarlet robe and hat of a candidate for the doctorate about to be conferred by the University; the Chancellor and the President clad in their robes of office; and the ancient ritual of the convocation; all provided an impressive reminder of the place of the University in the professional and social structure of every nation.

The convocation ceremony was followed by the welcoming remarks of the chairman, Dr. Thorlakson, and by brief greetings from The Honourable James Richardson on behalf of the Government of Canada; from The Honourable Edward Schreyer, Premier of Manitoba, on behalf of the Government and people of the Province; and from Alderman Robert Taft, on behalf of the City of Winnipeg. A message was read from Dr. J. Monier, Paris, France, President of the World Medical Association, extending good wishes for the success of the conference, and expressing regret at his unavoidable absence.

The chairman then invited the Governor-General to address the meeting. In a thoughtful and witty speech, His Excellency provided an appropriate introduction to the conference sessions which would begin the following morning, and formally set the Congress on its way. These duties were carried out with a felicity of style and manner that delighted the audience and set a tone that prevailed throughout the events of the coming days.

The theme of this First International Congress on Group Medicine was New Horizons in Health Care. The program dwelt on the social and economic philosophy of health care; the place of group medicine in delivery of medical services; and the nature and extent of its present development in many countries of the world. A session was devoted to university-based group medicine. Another dealt with the economics of health care delivery in group practice. Research and education in relation to group medicine, and the role of allied health professions, were examined.

The proceedings were published at the conclusion of the Congress in a 350-page book entitled *New Horizons in Health Care*. The papers still make inspiring and informative reading.

The total registration at the Congress was 950. The delegates came from twenty-one nations; and fifteen of the allied health professions were represented.

The organization of an international event of this kind is a monumental undertaking. Dr. Thorlakson was full of praise in public and in private, for the dedication and devotion with which literally hundreds of people at home and abroad contributed time and talent to making the Congress a success. In par-

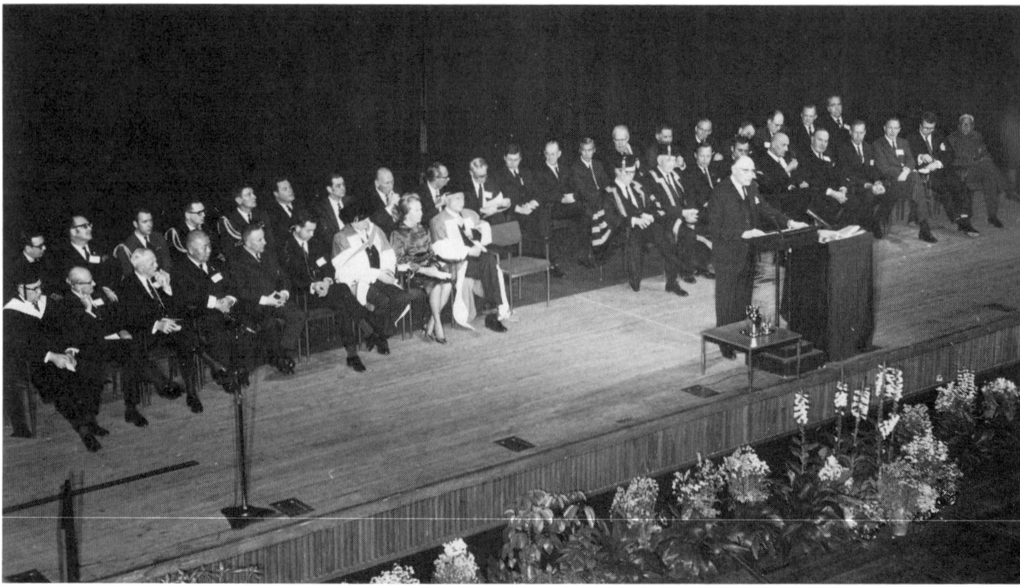

First International Congress on Group Medicine. Mr. L.J. Hughes, Registrar, University of Manitoba; Mr. B.R. Wolfe, representing the Metropolitan Corporation of Greater Winnipeg; Captain Emond, Personal Aide-de-Camp to His Excellency, The Governor-General; Major David Girling, Aide-de-Camp to His Excellency, The Governor-General; Colonel D.M. Gray, Aide-de-Camp to His Excellency, The Governor-General; Mr. Esmond Butler, Private Secretary to His Excellency, The Governor-General; Dr. L.L. Lovshin, President, American Association of Medical Clinics; The Honourable Maitland B. Steinkopf, Chairman of the Manitoba Centennial Corporation and Chancellor of Brandon University; The Very Reverend W.C. Lockhart, President of the University of Winnipeg; Dr. Stanley S.B. Gilder, Editor of the World Medical Journal and representing the World Medical Association; Dr. C.H. Vipond, President-Elect, Canadian Association of Medical Clinics; Mr. D.S. Grant, President, Medical Group Management Association of Canada; Dr. T.W. Fyles, Dean, Faculty of Medicine, University of Manitoba; Dr. Walter C. MacKenzie, representing the Association of Canadian Medical Colleges; Dr. J. Léger, representing the Association des Médecins de Langue Française du Canada; Mr. L.R. Adshead, President, Canadian Hospital Association; Dr. R.M. Matthews, President, The Canadian Medical Association; Dr. J.T. MacDougall, representing the Royal College of Physicians and Surgeons of Canada; Dr. C.H. Murphy, representing the College of Family Physicians of Canada; Dr. O.A. Schmidt, President, Manitoba Medical Association; Professor A.S.R. Tweedie, University of Manitoba; Dr. M.O. Kent-Hughes, Vice-President from Australia; Dr. Alton Ochsner, Vice-President from the United States of America; Dr. Taro Takemi, Vice-President from Japan; Dr. Gustave Gingras, Vice-President from Canada; Dr. Jacques Beaupère, Vice-President from France; His Honour, The Lieutenant-Governor of Manitoba (The Honourable Richard S. Bowles, Q.C.); Her Excellency, Mrs. Michener; His Excellency, The Governor-General of Canada (The Right Honourable Roland Michener, C.C., C.D.); Dr. Paul H.T. Thorlakson, President of the Congress, at the podium; Dr. Peter D. Curry, Chancellor of the University of Manitoba; Dr. H.H. Saunderson, President of the University of Manitoba; The Honourable James Richardson, representing the Government of Canada; The Honourable Edward Schreyer, Premier of Manitoba; Alderman Robert Taft, Acting Mayor of Winnipeg; Dr. J.C. Cameron, Vice-President from the United Kingdom; Dr. Juljan D. Czapski, Vice-President from Brazil; Dr. C.F. Borchgrevink, Vice-President from Norway; Dr. K.H. Metzner, Vice-President from the Federal Republic of Germany; Dr. P.R. Trivedi, Vice-President from India.

ticular he recognized the work of all the Committee Chairmen; and he particularly acknowledged Dr. R.E. Beamish,[7] Chairman of the Program and Facilities Committee; Dr. C. Hollenberg, Chairman of the Public Relations Committee; and Mrs. J.M. Gillies, Chairman of the Ladies' Committee. The excellence of their work was the foundation on which the success of the Congress was built. But Dr. Thorlakson did not forget the assistance of such friends as Dr. M.M. Pierce, prominent in the musical life of Winnipeg, who volunteered to arrange for music and other entertainment for the Congress banquet and other social events. Nor did he fail to pay full tribute to the work of the staff serving the Canadian Committee on Arrangements, and the General Chairman's office.

The work of winding up the Congress affairs and publishing the record of its proceedings took some eight or nine months. A complimentary copy of *New Horizons in Health Care* was sent to each of the 950 registrants, all committee members, exhibitors, members of the news media and contributors to the promotional funds. As a result of reports from observers at the Congress, a few days after its conclusion Dr. Thorlakson received a phone call from officials of the Department of Health, Education and Welfare in Washington, who advised that they were sending a cheque for $10,000 to purchase copies of the proceedings; a tangible, thrilling tribute indeed! Complimentary copies were sent to deans of medical faculties and medical libraries throughout Canada and the United States, and in many other countries as well.

Dr. Thorlakson was fond of saying, "What I like doing doesn't tire me." Nevertheless, it must have been with some feelings of relief, mingled with an immense sense of satisfaction, that nine months after the Congress he rose to address the final meeting of the Canadian Committee on Arrangements – a dinner meeting held at the Winnipeg Inn on February 4, 1971. At this meeting, he said:

The purpose of this dinner meeting is to thank you, and – through you – the many other individuals who helped to plan the First International Congress on Group Medicine and to pilot it through some tough and rocky channels to ultimate success. Another reason for this gathering is to present each one of you with a specially bound and numbered copy of the proceedings, of which there are only twenty-six. Next I will submit an audited statement of the income and expenditures. Finally, I want you to help me put the First Congress to bed!

This reminds me of a story which appeared recently in the United Church paper, *The Observer*. A minister asked a little boy if he said his prayers before going to bed. "No," replied the boy, "my mother says them." "What does she say?" asked the minister. "She says," responded the boy, "'Thank God he's in bed!'" And them's my sentiments!

It was Ralph Waldo Emerson who said, "A great institution is the lengthened shadow of one man." Certainly the bringing about of the First Congress on Group Medicine, and its impact in many parts of the world, rests on the man who directed its course from beginning to end.

One suspects that Dr. Thorlakson may have had mixed feelings about a headline in the Winnipeg Tribune above an excellent account of the purpose and nature of the Congress, by Manfred Jager. The headline reads, "Dr. Thorlakson, the Grand Old Man of Medicine." Years, as valid measures of age, he never really accepted. Nevertheless, the fulfilment of the idea of an international conference, born three years before on the Pacific Coast of Mexico, is an even greater achievement when one recalls that the Congress occurred just a few months prior to Dr. Thorlakson's seventy-fifth birthday.

And indeed the idea became an institution. Even before the first Congress was over, invitations were being given to attend the second one, which was planned for Rio de Janeiro three years later. Subsequently, congresses on group medicine have been held triennially, in Paris, Berlin, Tokyo and Dallas, Texas. Meetings are already scheduled for Vienna in 1988 and Helsinki in 1991. Dr. Thorlakson has had an interest in them all. He delivered the opening address at the Second Congress in Brazil; and, in a related field, delivered the address officially opening the Scientific Section of the Fifth World Conference on General Practice in Melbourne, Australia on October 1, 1972. In spite of his eighty-nine years, he attended the Sixth Congress on Group Medicine in Dallas, Texas, in April, 1985, where he was appointed Honorary Chairman of the meeting. He was present at every session of the Congress, including the banquet and dance, and provided a historic and inspiring link with Group Medicine during the years of its development.

There is a diverting sidelight on the Australian engagement, illustrating the problems of protocol that plague the organizers of international events. The Chairman of the Organizing Committee of the Melbourne Conference was Dr. M.O. Kent-Hughes, who had been a vice-president of the First World Congress on Group Medicine in Winnipeg. On behalf of the Fifth World Conference on General Practice, he had invited Dr. Thorlakson to be a special guest of the Conference president, and to deliver a paper on the effective use of skilled professional and technical persons, working as a health team under the direction of, or in association with, the physician. This presentation was scheduled for the second day of the Conference. All these arrangements were completed in May. In mid-August, Dr. Thorlakson received the following urgent message from Dr. Kent-Hughes:

Dear Dr. Thorlakson,

Please excuse the lateness of this invitation, but we have just heard that His Excellency the Governor of Victoria will not be able to open the Exhibition Meetings on Sunday, October 1. Our Governor-General, His Excellency Sir Paul Hasluck, will be opening the Conference ceremony on Tuesday, October 3, and I understand it is considered inappropriate for both the Governor-General of Australia and the Governor of Victoria to attend the Conference, although the invitations were extended for separate occasions.

My committee would be most grateful if you would honour them by officially opening Our World of Tomorrow Exhibition to be held at the Masonic Centre of Victoria, 300 Albert Street, East Melbourne, on Sunday, October 1, at 2:30 p.m.

The opening address on that day will be delivered by Mr. Leonard W. Weickhardt, Chancellor of the University of Melbourne. The title of his address is Society in the Year 2000, and he expects to speak for about thirty minutes. We have allowed a time of approximately ten minutes for the official opening remarks, making the session about forty-five minutes. . . .

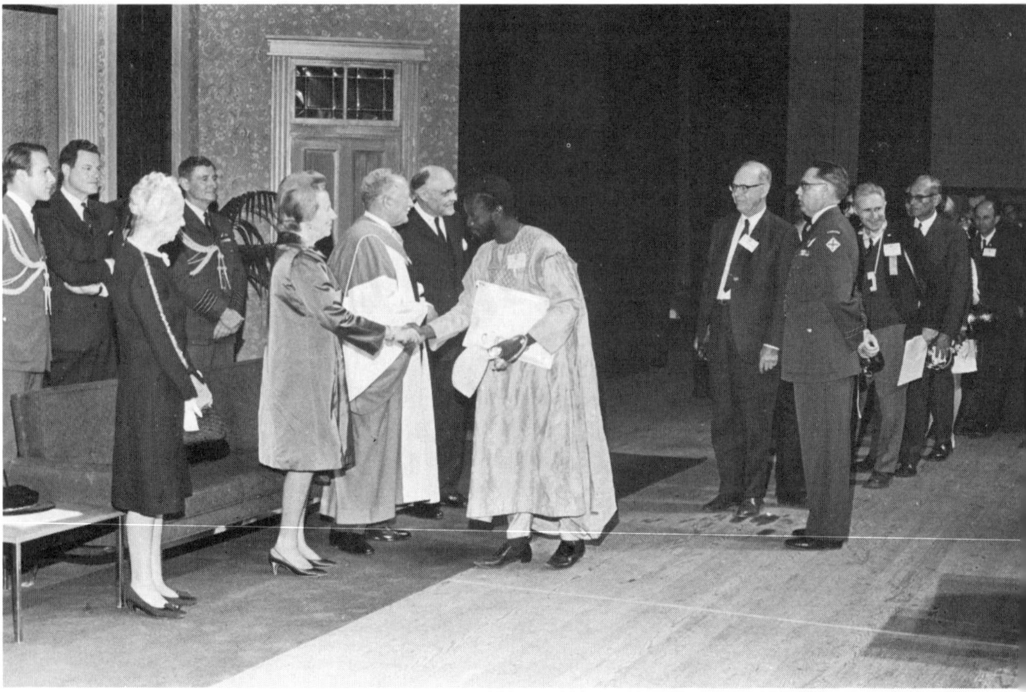

His Excellency The Right Honourable Roland Michener, C.C., C.D., and Her Excellency Mrs. Michener, accompanied by Dr. and Mrs. Thorlakson, greet the delegates to the First International Conference on Group Medicine. Here Mrs. Michener is welcoming Dr. Simon Be'Daya-Ngaro, Director of Public Health, Bangui, Republic of Central Africa.

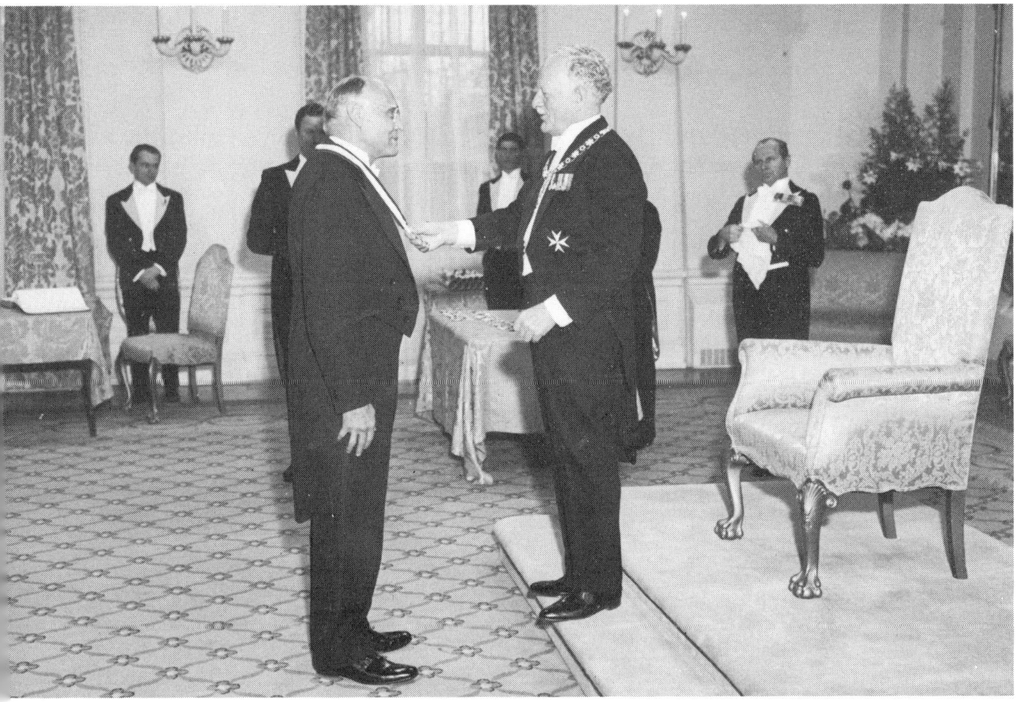

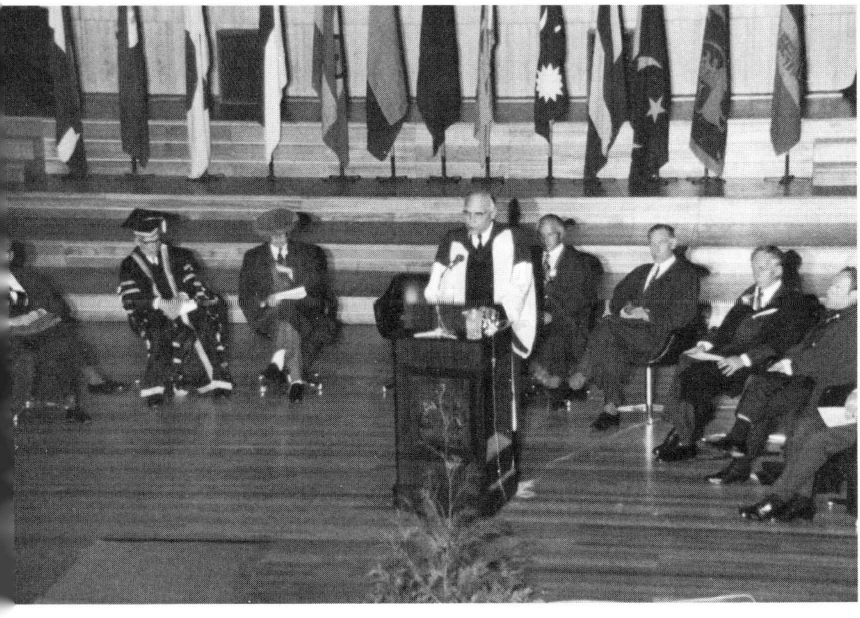

ı March 31, 1971, Dr. Thorlakson was installed as a Companion of the Order of ɪnada by His Excellency, Governor-General Roland Michener, C.C., C.D., at an ɪestiture at Rideau Hall in Ottawa.

·. Thorlakson opening the scientific sessions of the International Congress of mily Practitioners in Melbourne, Australia, October 1, 1972

I would be most grateful if you could let me know as soon as possible if you would accept the Organizing Committee's invitation to officially open the Exhibition.

Most sincerely,

Monty Kent-Hughes

In such circumstances only one answer was possible. Dr. Thorlakson promptly air-mailed his acceptance, and set about re-arranging his schedule.

PART SEVEN

For Culture and Community

CHAPTER 31

The Icelandic Community

RECOGNIZING THE CANADIAN MOSAIC

A few years ago, in a letter from his sister Margrethe (Mrs. Haraldur Sigmar, of Kelso, Washington), Dr. Thor was reminded of incidents from their childhood in Selkirk. She wrote:

> Do you remember that Mother would have us sit around the big dining room table Saturday mornings, each with his tablet and pencil, and write Norwegian, each according to his age, and she would teach us to read Norwegian and memorize favourite verses and songs? I think you had a copy of your tablet in your *skrin* [an Icelandic word signifying a chest for treasured possessions]. Because of those lessons I always wrote my letters in Norwegian after I left home, and she could write to us in her mother tongue.
>
> And then we had to learn the catechism in Icelandic; and we were confirmed by Dad in Icelandic. So learning the three languages was no problem and has come to good use, and we have learned from our parents to know Norway and Iceland with their culture and traditions.

The Thorlakson family home at Selkirk abounded with the chatter and laughter of children during those years. They enjoyed that privilege accorded especially to members of large families, the gift of sharing each one's joys and sorrows, successes and disasters, whether small or large, which weave the fabric of life for all of us. Each of the children played a musical instrument, and family orchestral and choral entertainment was enjoyed by those who played and those who listened. Visitors were warmly welcomed, and conversation might be in any one of three languages. Both parents encouraged this for they knew, from the breadth of their own knowledge and experience, that facility in more than one language may not only be an advantage in communicating with one's neighbours, but that it is also the key to entering a whole new world, rich with intellectual treasure, that otherwise is largely inaccessible.

It was to be expected, then, that Dr. Thorlakson would subscribe to the general principle of multiculturalism; that he would respect linguistic ability; and that he would favour the social philosophy of a Canadian mosaic rather than the American policy of total assimilation of newcomers – the "melting-pot" policy. He had a concern and an instinctive sympathy for the frustrations of Canadians who were French-speaking when they met with indifference or opposition in their efforts to protect the French language and culture.

In medicine, the "two solitudes," about which Hugh MacLennan wrote so vividly nearly half a century ago, revealed itself in the organization, by doctors of French heritage, of the Association des Médecins de Langue Française du Canada. Membership in this body largely replaced a relationship with the Canadian Medical Association which professed to speak nationally for all Canadian doctors.

In 1940, in a period when differences between the French and other Canadians were aggravated by World War II, Dr. Thorlakson thought the medical profession ought to make some unifying effort in its own field. On June 11, 1940, he wrote to the General Secretary of the Canadian Medical Association, Dr. T.C. Routley. His letter reads in part:

> To be a truly national organization, the Canadian Medical Association must appeal to all racial groups in Canada. For reasons which seem fairly obvious, the present organization fails to include the second largest of these racial groups: the French-speaking Canadians. Any national organization must take into account the fact that Canada is officially a bilingual country. Therefore at the meetings of such an organization the two languages should have equal status.
>
> The language difficulty is probably the main reason why French-speaking Canadians do not find the general meetings of our society helpful to them. It also explains why, in Quebec Province, a French-

speaking medical society, and not the Canadian Medical Association, is the one to which the majority of our French-speaking colleagues feel they can best give their allegiance.

Dr. Thorlakson went on to recommend the organization of a French language division of the Canadian Medical Association, with a bilingual secretary, to serve French-speaking doctors from all parts of Canada. He proposed that whenever the CMA met in the cities in which there are considerable numbers of doctors whose first language is French (he cited as examples Montreal, Winnipeg and Edmonton) joint meetings of the two divisions should be held. This progressive suggestion was not followed.

Twenty-two years later, in a paper entitled "We Must Build Bridges," Dr. G.W. Halpenny of Montreal again took up the cause of bilingualism in the CMA. "This two-fold medical heritage is a rare and valuable legacy," he wrote. "Unfortunately, its wealth cannot presently be used for the benefit of our nation, as the barrier of language has quite effectively placed it beyond our reach. . . . However it is very gratifying to find, at long last, a general awakening of interest in bilingualism. . . . It would be a great medical triumph if Canada on her 100th birthday possessed a single national medical organization. . . . "

It has now become common practice to have simultaneous translation of papers and discussion at professional meetings with a national or international audience. This, of course, is not a substitute for the individual's ability to express his thoughts in both French and English. Nevertheless, it does make attendance at these professional meetings useful and informative to an extent not otherwise possible.

Although he was prepared to do what he could to support English-French bilingualism, Dr. Thorlakson was firmly of the opinion that to confine the discussion to these two language groups was to take far too narrow a view. Well versed as he was in English, Norwegian and Icelandic, his life enriched with the heritage from all three cultures, he was an early public advocate of multiculturalism.

On September 4, 1963, the Central Region of the Canadian Council of Christians and Jews sponsored a seminar in Winnipeg on French-English relations in Canada. The keynote speakers were the Reverend Father Ludger Guy, Dean of St. Boniface College, and Dr. Thorlakson.

Father Guy opened the proceedings with a cogent argument for community and provincial understanding of the need of the Franco-Manitobans to preserve and develop their use of the French language, and to encourage knowledge and appreciation of their French cultural heritage. He cited the University of Manitoba as an example of sensible and fair support of biculturalism. "The University of Manitoba," he said, "is officially English but within it there is a French minority – St. Boniface College – and we are given the status we would like to have everywhere. . . . "

The next speaker was Dr. Thorlakson. He had in mind a broader concept than just French-English relations. This was revealed in the title of his address: "Canada, a Multicultural Nation."

> It seems to me that the basic problems in this general area stem from the conviction, held by some, that future cultural developments in Canada must be firmly based on a dual English and French national heritage, and that our ten provincial education systems should, without delay, accept and implement this concept. He noted that during nearly 100 years of Confederation, there had been a failure on the part of politicians, educators and members of the clergy to come to terms with this issue. Too often discussions of the subject had been marked by rancour and prejudice rather than insight and understanding.
>
> How different, refreshing and encouraging is the viewpoint expressed by the Honourable Guy Favreau, Minister of Immigration and Citizenship, speaking in Winnipeg on August 15, 1963, to a group of new Canadians from thirteen different countries, after they had taken the oath of allegiance. The Honourable Mr. Favreau said: "Group immigration has been the germ of life in this country. . . . Canada is justly proud of its pluralist culture. Many individuals and nationalities have enhanced Canadian traditions. I have no doubt that the many ethnic groups represented here today will, in time, also add appreciably to the cultures and traditions of our country.

Dr. Thorlakson expressed the view that the teaching of a second language in our schools should begin when the children are very young, a principle which has become widely accepted after two decades of public debate on the subject. Although he conceded that in most communities the two languages offered would be English and French, he advocated that no restriction be imposed on the choice of a second language in which instruction would be offered. "Let [the student] have the widest choice," he argued. "If he chooses to learn Chinese, Spanish, Hebrew or Russian as a second language he should be encouraged to do so." Dr. Thorlakson questioned the rationale of requiring children of Ukrainian ancestry, living in a Manitoba community predominantly populated by immigrants from the Ukraine, to learn French as a second language rather than that of their forefathers.

Dr. Thorlakson's multicultural perspective was well supported among ethnic societies and in the ethnic press. Across the country the doctrine of "the Canadian mosaic" gained prominence. Canadians discovered a newly awakened pride in the traditions they or their forefathers brought with them from abroad, and which had an influential part in moulding the character of Canadian society.

On July 19, 1963, on the recommendation of Prime Minister Pearson, the Government appointed the Royal Commission on Bilingualism and Biculturalism. During the commission hearings across Canada, it became evident that although English and French might be acceptable as the languages that made Canada officially bilingual, the concerns of other language groups and the rights of other ethnic segments of Canadian society were important issues. When the Commission report was issued in 1968, Book Four of the study was devoted entirely to a discussion of multiculturalism, with specific recommendations that the Government ought to formulate a set of policies which embodied principles applicable to this wider field.

A document entitled "Response to Book IV of the Report of the Royal Commission on Bilingualism and Biculturalism," was tabled in the House of Commons by Prime Minister Trudeau on October 8, 1971, and this appears as an appendix to Hansard for that date. It was a clear acceptance of the multicultural position. The first paragraph states the case:

> [The government] believes the time is overdue for the people of Canada to become aware of the rich tradition of the many cultures we have in Canada. Canada's citizens come from almost every country in the

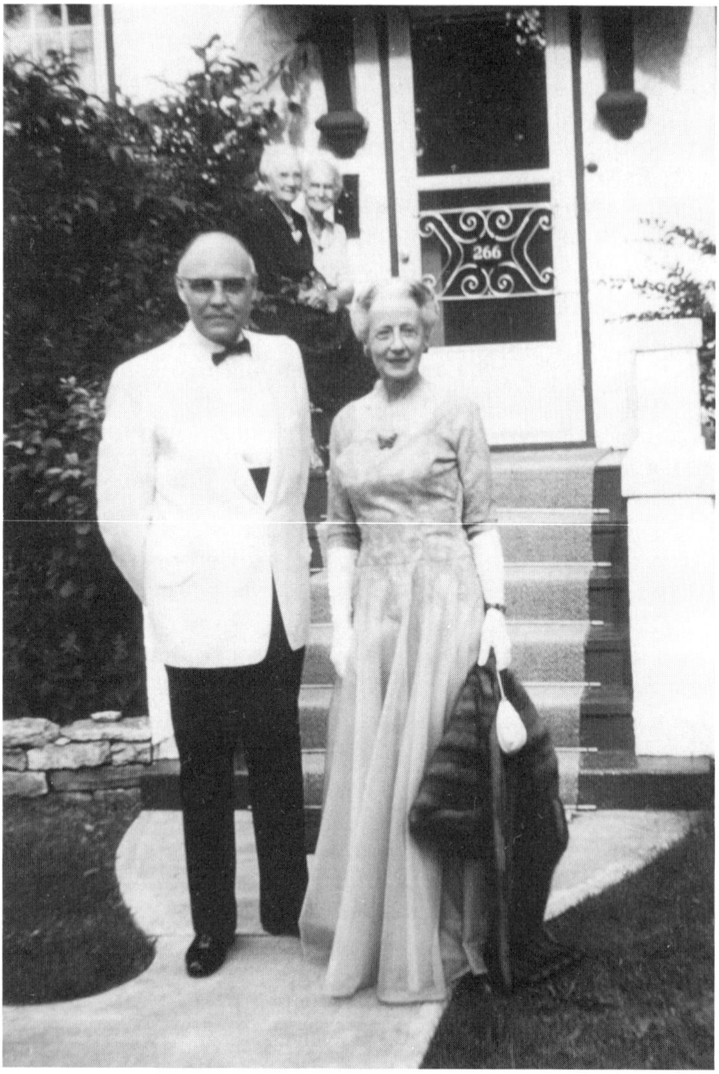

Dr. and Mrs. Thorlakson leaving to attend a reception at Government House for Princess Elizabeth and Prince Philip, prior to attending a command performance of the Winnipeg Ballet (1951). The group became the "Royal" Winnipeg Ballet two years later.

world, and bring with them every major world religion and language. This cultural diversity endows all Canadians with a great variety of human experience. The government regards this as a heritage to treasure and believes that Canada would be the poorer if we adopted assimilation programs forcing our citizens to forsake and forget the cultures they have brought to us.

Dr. Thorlakson was appointed a member of the federally organized Canadian Consultative Council on Multiculturalism in 1973. In 1975 he was asked to organize meetings of the eleven-member Manitoba group on the Council, to review and make a report on the activities and cultural accomplishments of societies in Winnipeg having English, Italian, Métis, Jewish, Mennonite, and other backgrounds.

He continued to give special thought to the responsibilities of Canadians of Icelandic origin under the new national policies. The following excerpt from an important statement on the subject in an address given at Arborg, Manitoba, on January 25, 1974, is representative of the message Dr. Thorlakson conveyed:

In considering the true meaning of multiculturalism, which is a purely Canadian concept, we must ask ourselves how we, as Canadians, can participate in and contribute to this new official approach to a problem with which we have struggled for over 100 years.

It is important for us of Icelandic or partly Icelandic descent to remember that from the very first days of their arrival 100 years ago the Icelandic people were committed to the preservation of their ancient and honoured heritage.

Furthermore, by common consent, it was agreed that this objective would be steadfastly pursued and accomplished within a Canadian context. This, they declared, was the basis of good citizenship. But when we are speaking about Icelandic culture, we must bear in mind that we are not dealing with a completely indigenous national product. Icelanders have always been great travellers. The European influence has always been important. The love of books has been characteristic of the Icelandic people from earliest days. Icelanders are great readers of foreign books and many can read them in the original languages. But Icelandic culture is not limited to language and great literature, prose or poetry. Sculpture, painting, fine jewellery, the creation of beautiful national costumes, and the cooking of food are also important. Also included is folklore that deals with sea monsters, outlaws and the "huldufolk" or "hidden people," who are said to live exactly like all Icelanders; they attend church and raise sheep but are invisible except under very strange circumstances. Haraldur Olafsson said, in a recent roundtable discussion in Iceland, that "culture" also refers to how we (in Iceland) went about surviving in this country. . . . "

The Icelandic language is the classic language of northern Europe. For 1,000 years, this small island nation, Iceland, has preserved Old Norse, which is now the Icelandic language and which was spoken in half of the British Isles, and over large areas of northern Europe, a thousand years ago. Much of this Old Norse language has been incorporated into the modern languages of these countries. The Icelandic language has a close kinship with Anglo-Saxon, which forms the basis for the most forceful and effective speech in modern English. Early explorations and discoveries of North America are recorded in the Icelandic Sagas. Icelandic is a required subject in advanced studies in the English language at several universities in Great Britain and in the United States of America. . . . The Chair of Icelandic Language and Literature at the University of Manitoba is helping to preserve and nourish the rich heritage and culture which dates back in a continuing, unbroken form to an early period of western European civilization. . . .

This, then, is part of the Icelandic heritage. This is the cultural treasure chest which those of Icelandic origin, both young and old, can explore for their own edification and enjoyment. . . . [1]

THE CHAIR OF ICELANDIC LANGUAGE AND LITERATURE AT THE UNIVERSITY OF MANITOBA

"One of the most interesting and stimulating stories in the history of this University is that of the establishment of the Chair of Icelandic Language and Literature, endowed by the generosity and self-sacrifice of the people of Icelandic descent." Thus began an account of this achievement by Dr. Hugh Saunderson, published in 1961 by the University of Manitoba Press.

He referred to the long-standing concern of the Icelandic people in Manitoba to retain their ancient language and rich literary heritage as a living part of their development as Canadians. This had been a motivating force in their community from the time the first settlement was established, in 1875. As early as 1884, Mr. Freeman B. Anderson, who two years later became the editor of the second Icelandic newspaper to be published in Winnipeg, was advocating the establishment of a school for the preservation of Icelandic culture in North America. From 1901 until 1926, Icelandic was taught at Wesley College – now the University of Winnipeg. With studies at the high-school level, the Jon Bjarnason Academy was established in Winnipeg in 1913, with the Reverend Runolfur Marteinsson as principal,[2] continuing until 1940.

Dr. Saunderson recalled that after the establishment of the Icelandic National League in 1919, a league policy was proposed to support professorships in Icelandic at centres of learning in the provinces and states in which a substantial number of Icelanders lived. In 1926 the League approved a resolution that $100,000 be raised, with the interest on this fund designated to support the teaching of Icelandic. However, no action was taken at that time.

In 1932, Dr. B.B. Jonsson, in an address to the Icelandic National League, advocated the establishment of a centre for Icelandic Language and Culture at the University of Manitoba. Shortly after, a distinguished scholar from Iceland, Dr. Sigurdur Nordal, spoke to a group of younger Winnipeg Icelanders at the home of W.J. Lindal – later Judge Lindal – advocating the study of Icelandic in association with the study of Old English.

It was not long before Mr. Asmunder P. Johannson, a Winnipeg contractor, arranged a number of meetings at his home to explore plans for a chair of Icelandic at the University. Among those attending were Mr. Justice Bergman, Reverend Rognvaldur Petursson, Einer P. Jonsson and Dr. Thorlakson. Interest in the project continued, but no definite action was taken.

In 1942, the Board of Governors of the University set up a committee consisting of the President, Dr. Sidney E. Smith;, Mr. Justice Bergman, Mrs. H.M. Speechly, Mrs. P.H.T. Thorlakson and Mr. W.J. Parker, to study the project and report to the Board.

The first money actually received by the University toward the establishment of a chair, Dr. Saunderson reports, was a gift of $5,000 in 1945 from Dr. Thorlakson in memory of his father, the Reverend N.S. Thorlakson. Later that year Mr. A.P. Johannson, who had initiated the meetings in 1934, confirmed his gift of $50,000 if others would contribute at least an equal amount. Shortly thereafter a third gift, $3,000, was received in the form of a bequest from Mr. Magnus Hinrickson, of Churchbridge, Saskatchewan, the father of Mrs. Lindal.

Early in 1944, Mr. Justice Bergman (who by this time had become Chairman of the University Board of Governors) and Mr. A.P. Johannson asked Dr. Thorlakson to accept the chairmanship of a fundraising committee to provide for the establishment of the Chair of Icelandic Language and Literature. Determined that this effort should not be marred by factionalism, Dr. Thor-

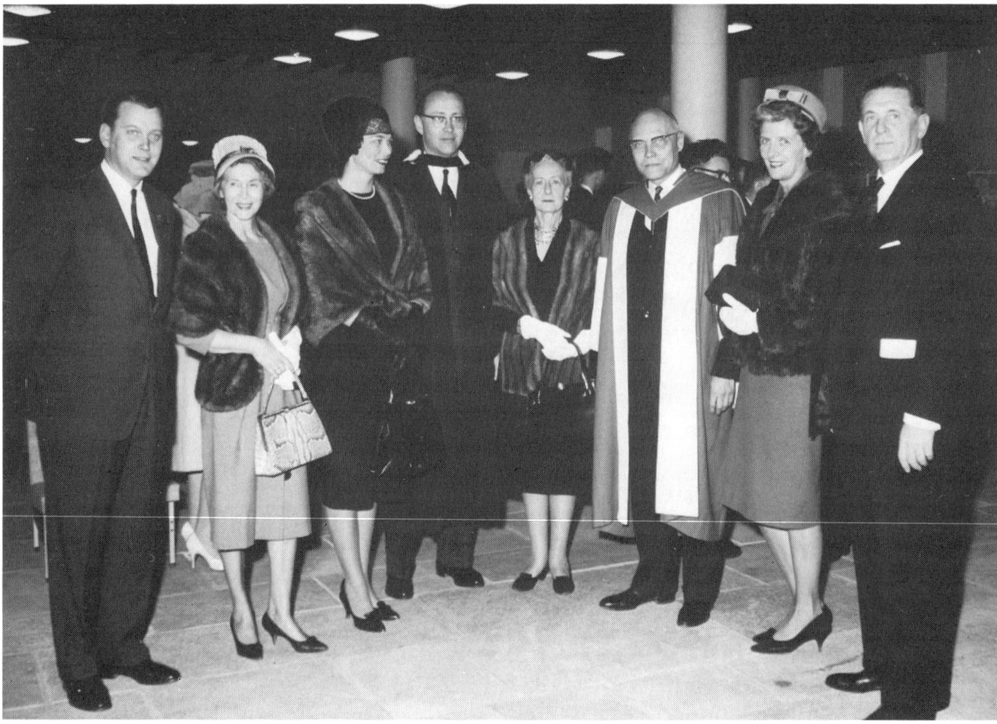

At the convocation of the University of Iceland, Reykjavik, on October 7, 1961 (its fiftieth anniversary) Dr. Thorlakson was awarded the honourary degree of Docto of Medicine. Above are some of the distinguished guests, left to right: Dr. George Johnson, Manitoba Minister of Health; Mrs. M. Hallgrimsson, wife of the Canadian Consul to Iceland, sister of the Honourable Thor Thors, Icelandic Ambassador to the United States and of The Honourable Olafur Thors, Prime Minister of Iceland; Mrs. George T. Richardson (nee Tannis Thorlakson); Mr. George T. Richardson, Chairman of the Board of Governors, University of Manitoba; Mrs. Paul H.T. Thorlakson; Dr. Thorlakson; Mrs. George Johnson; M Hallgrimur F. Hallgrimsson, Canadian Consul to Iceland.

lakson agreed to assume this responsibility only on condition that every Icelandic organization in North America, as well as the two Icelandic weekly newspapers, committed themselves to support the campaign in every way possible, and ensure total community participation.

Regular meetings of the organizing committee[3] were held on Sunday afternoons, in the beginning at Dr. Thorlakson's home at 114 Grenfell Boulevard, but later at 45 Home Street, where the very able committee secretary, Miss Margret Petursson, resided.

A welcome guest at the first meeting held by the Committee was the late Skuli Johnson (1880–1955), Rhodes Scholar, from 1915 to 1926 Professor of Classics at Wesley College and from 1927 until the time of his death professor of classics at the University of Manitoba. In consequence of a suggestion he made at that meeting, the objective of $100,000, originally agreed upon by the Icelandic National League, was raised to $150,000, and eventually to $200,000.

The Committee agreed from the beginning that the minimum contribution to the fund should be $1,000. Each individual or group contributing that amount or more would be recorded as a founder in a published list. Eventually, four categories of founders came to be recognized: (1) individual founders; (2) organization founders; (3) recognition founders (When a group of people collectively contributed $1,000 or more in the name of someone, living or dead, whom they sought to honour, they established a recognition founder.); (4) group founders (many people interested in supporting this project were not able to become individual founders, but by joining with others in a district or community they became group founders.)

Hence donations were solicited on as broad a basis as possible, from farmers and fishermen, doctors and judges, lawyers, merchants, artisans and teachers. It was stipulated that if the Chair were not established by June 17, 1952, all money collected would be returned with interest to the donors.

The campaign was formally launched in the spring of 1948. By early 1949, it had made enough progress that the Committee was sure it would be a success. Something over $100,000 had been collected and deposited with the University, and the enthusiastic support made it evident that the goal of $200,000 could be reached.

One or two examples may convey a sense of the dedication to the success of this enterprise that permeated all parts of the Icelandic community. During the early stages of the campaign, two Foundation Committee members, along with Einar P. Jonsson, editor of *Lögberg,* spent a weekend making calls in an Interlake community on behalf of the campaign. Toward the end of the afternoon, as they were relaxing over coffee and cake in a farm kitchen before setting out for Winnipeg, they received a telephone message asking them to stop at another farm before leaving the area. The caller was a retired farmer who lived with his wife in a modest cottage they had built for themselves after turning over their farm to their son. After placing more coffee and cake before the visitors, the farmer and his wife presented them with a cheque, already made out, in the amount of $1,000. Known to be people of strictly limited means, they would not have been pressed for a donation.

From this weekend of activity, the Foundation funds were augmented by six cheques, each of $1,000, and two for $500 each, a total of $7,000.

Further afield, Mrs. John David Eaton of Toronto made a substantial gift in memory of her father, Frederick Stephenson; and a generous contribution was made by the Government of Iceland.

By early spring of 1951 there was on deposit with the University of Manitoba the sum of $155,000. Of the remaining $45,000 to be obtained, $20,000 had already been pledged. With accumulated interest the final amount was $219,132.72.

On Friday evening, March 30, 1951, a concert for the Icelandic community was held at the Playhouse Theatre in Winnipeg. At the close of the musical portion of the evening Dr. Thorlakson spoke briefly, after which the late Dr. A.H.S. Gillson, then President of the University of Manitoba, announced the establishment of the Chair of Icelandic Language and Literature for the session 1951–1952. This chair is unique in two respects: it was the first endowed chair to be established at a university in Western Canada and, so far as is known, the only one in the country ever to have been made possible through the contributions of an entire ethnic community.

Dr. Gillson invited Dr. Alexander Johannesson, Rector of the University of Iceland, to visit Manitoba to provide advice on the establishment of the department. On his recommendation, Professor Finnbogi Gudmundsson, a scholar from the University of Iceland, was appointed first incumbent of the Chair. He took up his position in November, 1951. The Centre for Icelandic language and culture became a reality, and the hopes and aspirations of leaders in the Icelandic community for almost two decades were finally realized.

Professor Gudmundsson served for five years, and then decided to return to his homeland, where he holds the position of Head Librarian in the National Library of Iceland. He was succeeded as Professor and Head of the Department of Icelandic Language and Literature at the University of Manitoba by Professor Haraldur Bessason, Cand. Mag., University of Iceland.

At a testimonial dinner in honour of Dr. and Mrs. Thorlakson held by the Icelandic National League at the Royal Alexandra Hotel in Winnipeg on April 30, 1953, Mr. Arni G. Eggertson, Q.C., paid tribute to Dr. Thorlakson's outstanding contributions in the fields of medicine and public life. With regard to his efforts on behalf of the Chair of Icelandic Language and Literature, Mr. Eggertson commented:

In this campaign for the establishment of a chair in Icelandic Language and Literature there were difficulties to overcome besides those of raising money. During the years there were many contentious issues which arose requiring the services of a diplomat and a combined Admiral-General. There was not one occasion when Dr. Thorlakson did not eventually steer his committee into the placid waters [of unanimity]. He also took the leading part in personally canvassing for contributions to this fund which involved long weekend journeys to various parts of this province, to neighbouring provinces and states, and to the Pacific Coast. All of these trips were performed without a cent of expense to the endowment.

On these journeys it was a delight to see and hear Thor perform. He never took no for an answer and by some subtle power of concentration on [the potential donor] he seemed to lead him to a positive response; and it was only after he had partaken of his subject's hospitality and extended his thanks for the $1,000 cheque and coffee that his host realized that he had actually parted with $1,000 for culture.

I often wondered why Thor always insisted on the wife being present at these interviews and extractions. He undoubtedly knew of the plight of the husband if she had not been consulted. You will now understand what I mean when I say Dr. Thorlakson is an industrious person. I venture to say that with such versatility and powers of persuasion Thor would have been successful in any endeavour to which he directed his energies.[4]

The banquet room at the Royal Alexandra Hotel was filled, not only by members of the Icelandic community, but with other friends, all of whom wished to pay tribute to Dr. and Mrs. Thorlakson for their contribution to the life of their city and province. Among the many speakers, Dr. A.H.S. Gillson, on behalf of the University, expressed gratitude for Dr. Thorlakson's efforts in establishing the Chair, which enriched the University culture "with the treasures that come from Iceland." He had warm words of praise for Mrs. Thorlakson and her devotion to the University as a member of the Board of Governors.[5]

The high point in the evening came with the investiture of Dr. Thorlakson as a commander of the Icelandic Order of the Falcon. The ceremony was performed by the Icelandic Consul, G.L. Johannsson, on behalf of the President of Iceland.

Thirty-five years later, in 1985, another committee was formed to raise funds for the continuing support of the Department of Icelandic Language and Literature at the University of Manitoba. This led to a renewed appreciation of the success of the initial campaign chaired by Dr. Thorlakson. "Never before," said the editor of *Lögberg-Heimskringla* in the issue of November 15, 1985, "had the Icelandic community in North America been as united in its effort to accomplish one major goal. This was mostly due to the ability of Dr. Thorlakson to motivate people and organize them."

On November 3, 1985, some thirty Manitobans of Icelandic origin met to express appreciation to Dr. Thorlakson for his leadership in founding the Chair of Icelandic Language and Literature. They invited him to accept the position of Honorary Chairman of the second campaign for funds on its behalf. He was pleased to be able to accept this invitation and provide a living link with the creators of this testimonial to the cultural heritage of the Icelandic people.

THE BETEL HOME

When the Ladies Aid Society of the First Lutheran Church of Winnipeg was formed in 1896, one of its concerns was the welfare of elderly Icelanders in the City. The ladies soon realized that their efforts would be more fruitful if they could bring these needy people together under one roof. Having reached this sensible decision, they pursued their vision persistently and diligently until it was eventually realized. Money, of course, was very scarce. But, as a remarkable evidence of faith in their cause, four years later, in 1900, they set aside $50 from their limited funds "towards the erection of a Home for elderly Icelanders in Canada."

By 1914 they had enlisted the active interest and participation of a number of men prominent in the Icelandic community, seven of whom joined with eight of the ladies to form a committee to advance the project. The fund for the "old people's home" had been increased to $3,000, and after gaining assurance that the Icelandic Evangelical Lutheran Synod would continue the promotion of their plan, they deposited this amount with the Synod treasurer.

The Synod promptly named a board of directors to whom responsibility for the project was assigned. At the first Board meeting Dr. B.J. Brandson, an eminent Winnipeg surgeon, was elected Chairman. A warm-hearted, kindly man, he served in this capacity for thirty years.

The Board began its work by renting a house early in 1915 at 854 William Avenue, Winnipeg, which could accommodate up to ten people. It was soon found, however, that these quarters were inadequate; and after a few months an unoccupied boarding house in Gimli was purchased, in which twenty-six elderly persons could be cared for. But the needs continued to grow, and in 1917, with the help of a bequest from an elderly Winnipeg recluse named Jon Helgason, the Board was able to buy the Lakeview Hotel, a three-storey stone structure ideally situated overlooking Lake Winnipeg at the end of First Avenue in downtown Gimli. The move to the Lakeview Hotel site by what we now know as the Betel Home, was completed on December 12, 1917.

From the beginning, the atmosphere at the Betel Home has been that of an extended family rather than an institution. Even today the supervisor of the Home is distinguished by the Icelandic title *husmodir* – mother of the family, an expression with connotations of warmth and affection.

Throughout the 1920s, with a modest charge to residents able to pay, and donations to the Pioneer Memorial Fund, which helped in the maintenance of the Home, gratifying progress was made. But with the economic depression of the 1930s there came a marked increase in the number of applicants seeking admission, many of whom were virtually devoid of financial resources. Reluctance to turn away anyone in genuine need resulted in serious overcrowding, and strained the endowment income of the Home to the limit. Donations dwindled to a mere trickle. No funds were available for major repairs, or for the replacement of worn-out equipment.

The Depression years were followed by the shortages and restrictions of World War II. In 1944, the difficulties besetting the Home were compounded by the death of the longtime Chairman of the Board, Dr. Brandson. His widow, Mrs. Adalbjorg Brandson, who shared her husband's concern for Betel, succeeded him on the Board, and served faithfully and fruitfully until her health deteriorated.

By the spring of 1953, three people with a special interest in the welfare of the residents became convinced that conditions in the Home had deteriorated to the point where redevelopment was absolutely essential. This "triumvirate" consisted of Dr. George Johnson, who, despite the heavy demands of a large family practice in Gimli and the surrounding district, always made himself available to respond to the medical needs of the Betel residents; the Reverend Harald Sigmar, Pastor of the Lutheran Church in Gimli, Chaplain of the Home – and a nephew of Dr. Thorlakson; and Mrs. Augusta Tallman, then the *husmodir* who had known Dr. Thorlakson since they were children together in Selkirk.

These three people considered what might be done. Major planning, building and fundraising would certainly be necessary. For a project of such magnitude it seemed that the first step should be to strengthen the Board of Directors (now having only four members), by the appointment of an able, experienced, knowledgeable individual from among the Icelandic people, who had a high profile in the community, and who could organize and head a re-development program. In the mind of each, after a moment's thought, one person stood out as meeting the criteria. The chaplain was the first to speak. "What about Uncle Thor?" he asked. There was instant agreement from his two colleagues. They were aware of his many commitments. "But," said Dr.

Johnson, "if the need is put to him, I think he will do it."

The proposal was put to the directors, who welcomed it. They agreed that Mrs. Tallman's brother, Skuli M. Bachman, the treasurer, would speak to Dr. Thorlakson on their behalf, inviting him to become a Board member, and head the re-development program. Mr. Bachman promptly made an appointment to meet Dr. Thorlakson. He gave a graphic account of the difficulties being experienced at Betel, and the urgency of action to improve and expand the facilities.

Dr. Thorlakson agreed to think over the invitation to join the Board. He sought the views of Dr. Johnson about conditions in the Home, and its requirements for more and better space. All that Mr. Bachman had described to him was confirmed. Considering all the circumstances, it must have seemed to Dr. Thorlakson that here was a case in which, clearly, "new occasions teach new duties." Despite his many obligations, he decided to accept membership on the Board of Directors and carry out the tasks that they might ask him to do.

No sooner had this news been conveyed to the Board, than he received a letter from the capable and far-seeing *husmodir,* Mrs. Tallman, expressing a faith and confidence which a man of feeling could not betray. The letter was written on June 10, 1953:

Dear Thorbjorn:

I cannot resist the urge to write a note to say how grateful and happy I am to hear that you are joining the Betel Board of Directors.

At this time the Home is particularly in need of just such counsel – wise, kind, and of high authority, which your presence on the Board will bring to it. I have learned to love this Home, and I realize how greatly its work is needed.

It should now be assured of a very fine future. With kindest regards and wishes, I am

Very sincerely,

"Jennie"

At his first Board meeting, Dr. Thorlakson was thoroughly briefed on the building deficiencies. He was taken on a tour of the Home, met many of the residents and saw at first hand the

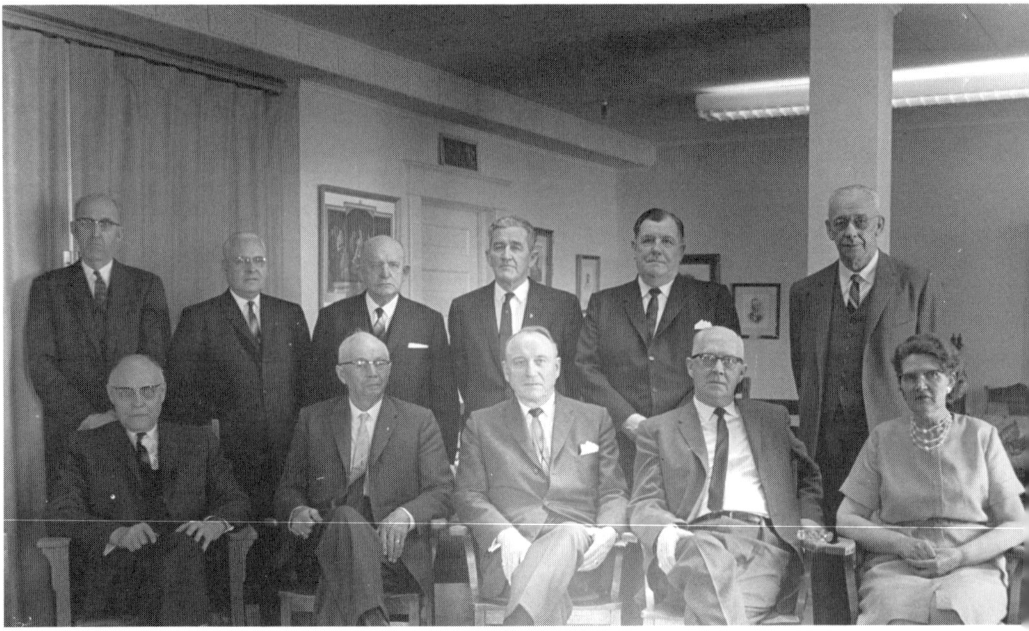

Betel Foundation Board, about 1960. Standing, left to right: John Guttormson, Lundar; Lincoln Johnson; Arni Eggertson; Mayor Barney Egilson, Gimli; Bill Johanneson; Skuli Backman. Seated, left to right: Dr. Thorlakson; S.V. Sigurdson, Riverton; Grettir Eggertson, Board President; Victor Jonasson, Secretary; Sigga Hjartarson, Matron of Betel Home, Gimli.

urgent need for renovation. It was also apparent that the Home should be enlarged to meet the requests for admission by many persons in need of care. With the general nature of what ought to be done in mind, he asked his old friend, F.R. Lount, the builder of the Winnipeg Clinic, to visit the Home and provide an estimate of the cost of the necessary renovations and additions. The first priority would be to eliminate the existing fire hazards.

Ultimately the renovations of the old building and a fifty-bed new extension provided accommodation for about 100 residents, including twenty-four infirmary beds.

In 1955 the Synod approved a fundraising campaign and Dr. Thorlakson was named Campaign Chairman. Estimates indicated that about $250,000 was required. To launch the campaign, Dr. Thorlakson published in the December 1955 issue of *The Parish Messenger* (a Synod publication) an account of the needs for expansion and renovation, and the nature of the work that was planned, appealing not only for the support of church members but of the whole Icelandic community.

In the meantime, on the basis of Mr. Lount's estimates, Dr. Thorlakson approached the Central Mortgage and Housing Corporation for a mortgage loan to finance the construction. They were agreeable, but stipulated that the mortgage must be countersigned by the provincial government. Dr. Thorlakson lost no time in meeting with Premier Douglas L. Campbell and the Honourable R.W. Bend, Minister of Health and Public Welfare.

With commendable foresight Premier Campbell expressed his reluctance to set a precedent that would commit the Province to the guarantee of mortgage loans to religious institutions. It would be far more satisfactory, the Premier pointed out, and more practical for the Province, to make an outright grant toward the cost of the construction.

At that time there was no legislation permitting grants to help build homes for the aged and infirm; but Premier Campbell and Mr. Bend promised that they would introduce the enabling legislation at the next session of the Legislature.

The result of the conversation was the enactment, in 1956, of the Elderly Persons' Housing Act. It provided authority for grants-in-aid for construction of all approved institutions of this nature in Manitoba, and was of inestimable benefit in improving care for elderly Manitoba citizens.

Betel Home received a grant from the Government of $42,500. Balance of the construction cost was covered by contributions, so that no interest charges had to be paid, and operating costs were accordingly lower.

On Sunday, November 18, 1956, Premier Campbell laid the cornerstone of the new building in the presence of 300 guests. Building proceeded rapidly, and on Sunday, June 2, 1957, the Reverend V.J. Eylands, D.D., President of the Icelandic Evangelical Lutheran Synod of America, dedicated the new wing.

In 1957 Dr. Thorlakson was elected Chairman of the Board of the Betel Home and served on it until 1959. The last paragraph in his chairman's report to the Icelandic Lutheran Synod on June 3, 1958, bears testimony to his interest in the personal well-being of the residents:

> At a recent meeting of the Board we set up a special Committee on Religious and Recreational Services under the chairmanship of the Reverend J. Fullmer, Chaplain of the Home. Now that we have adequately attended to the physical needs of the residents, we must apply ourselves to their personal problems. The manner in which we approach this responsibility will largely determine the success we achieve in creating a happy family of old folks. They should be assisted and encouraged to pursue their interests and hobbies. Above all, they need love, companionship and understanding combined with the necessities of food, shelter and recreational diversion. May Betel always be known as "The Home of the Happy Sunset."[6]

THE CANADA ICELAND FOUNDATION

The Canada Iceland Foundation became a legal entity in 1958 under the patronage of His Excellency Asgeir Asgeirson, then President of Iceland, and The Right Honourable Vincent Massey, Governor General of Canada from 1952 to 1959. The late Judge Walter J. Lindal conceived this organization, and was its founding president. Dr. Thorlakson was the first vice-president.

Its primary purpose was to foster and strengthen cultural bonds and mutual understanding between Canada and Iceland. To this end, it proposed, for example, to promote an appreciation of the related Canadian and Icelandic heritage in the fields of representative government and the rule of law; to give scholarships to students studying Icelandic at Canadian universities; to encourage the recognition of Icelandic as a credit course in postgraduate and honours courses in English; to arrange cultural exchanges between Canada and Iceland; and to support other events that would contribute to shared experiences between the people of Iceland and Canada.

Each of the charter members of the Foundation had pledged an annual contribution of at least fifty dollars, but in view of the extent of the plans these contributions seemed to provide only a modest beginning.

Canada Council Grants in the fields of the arts, humanities and social sciences had been initiated in 1957. With the support of some members of the Foundation, Judge Lindal proposed that a petition be forwarded to the Canada Council asking for funds to help finance the Foundation's program.

Dr. Thorlakson took issue with the supporters of the plan to petition the Canada Council for funds. "If I were a member of the Canada Council considering such an application," he said, "I would immediately raise two points: first, what are the specific aims and objectives of the Foundation; and second, what other sources of financial support are available to this new foundation?" His principle concern, he continued, was not with the present, no matter how satisfying it might be that there was spontaneous and enthusiastic endorsement of the plan:

> Herein lies the real danger. What assurance have we that this initial enthusiasm will last? Will the people who are young now, but will be sitting in the councils of the Foundation twenty years from now, understand and support the propositions which we now accept without hesitation?
>
> I am convinced that our first and most urgent need is not to appeal for funds from the Canada Council. We should, nevertheless, register with them . . . a statement of purpose and a tentative prospectus. Having done this, we should set about seeing what actual support in terms of donations from our own group is available. . . .

Some two and a half years later, in an address to the Icelandic Canadian Club on February 21, 1961, Dr. Thorlakson referred again to the Foundation:

> The most recent ambitious venture into the field of cultural interests has been the formation of the Canada Iceland Foundation. This orga-

nization has had a modest but significant beginning. Eventually it could become a great rallying point for all those organizations and individuals who aim to foster an interest in the great cultural heritage which belongs to the people of Iceland and which will, for an unpredictable period, continue to make its contribution to Canadian life....

In the years ahead the Canada Iceland Foundation should develop into a well-endowed organization able and ready for effective and constructive action....

To provide guidance and support in Iceland for the Canada Iceland Foundation, the Board of Directors was able to establish an advisory committee composed of men of influence and public stature: Armann Snaevarr, Rector of the University of Iceland; Bjarni Benediktsson, Minister of Justice; Gudmundur Vilhjalmason, Manager of the Iceland Steamship Company; Vilhjalmur Thor, Manager of the National Bank of Iceland; Gylfi Gislason, Minister of Education; Hallgrimur F. Hallgrimsson, Honourary Canadian Consul to Iceland; Sigurdur Nordal, Professor at the University of Iceland, and former Ambassador to Denmark; and the Most Reverend Sigurbjorn Einarsson, Bishop of Iceland.

On June 20, 1963, Judge Lindal was in Iceland, where he met with the Advisory Committee. He spoke, no doubt eloquently, about the work the Canada Iceland Foundation hoped to do to maintain and strengthen the bonds between the people of the two countries. The Advisory Committee members gained the impression that the Foundation proposed to make fluency in the Icelandic language a prerequisite to receiving any benefits under its programs. Such a condition, the Committee felt, would unduly obstruct the achievement of its objectives.

Separated by 3,000 air miles from the Foundation members whom they were appointed to "advise," which precluded a meeting in person, the Advisory Committee members felt that they ought to make a written statement of the views they had expressed to Judge Lindal, so that they would be available to the officers and members of the organization.

A few weeks after Judge Lindal's visit, Professor Nordal was delegated to draft a letter to him, which was signed by every member of the Advisory Committee. An excerpt from the letter illustrates the tenor of its message:

Dear Fellow Countryman:

In this letter we want to put on record a few of the matters we discussed on June 20 when we had the pleasure of meeting with you. We look on this letter primarily as a brief salutation from the Advisory Committee to your colleagues in Canada – the Canada Iceland Foundation – with whom we have not had an opportunity to discuss matters in person.

There is no reason to speak at length here of all the endeavours of Icelanders in North America to preserve their identity and maintain ties with their ancestral land. We prefer to proceed directly to the question: What is the attitude of the people of Iceland toward the younger generations of Icelandic descent on the other side of the ocean, who know little or nothing of the Icelandic language but are nevertheless conscious of their origins and for that reason desire to cultivate ties with Iceland and the Icelandic people?

If these kinsmen of ours believe that, insofar as the people here at home are concerned, contacts are dependent upon language alone, this is a complete misunderstanding. Two things should be clear to every reasonable individual: Icelandic cannot continue to be the mother tongue of the younger generations as it was for the older. On the other hand, there will come to be fewer and fewer of them who speak Icelandic, or even understand it. Secondly, the descendants of the Icelandic settlers are first and foremost Canadians (or Americans) and have a duty to be good citizens of their adopted countries. We Icelanders readily admit making the same demand on the children and decendants of foreigners who become Icelandic citizens. Nevertheless there are excellent opportunities for cooperation between these younger generations and Icelanders here at home and, under the circumstances, the role of the Canada Iceland Foundation can exert a profound influence on the future. . . .

The letter goes on to extol the importance of the establishment of the Chair of Icelandic Language and Literature at the University of Manitoba, and to make a number of specific suggestions for improved communication in the fields of scholarship and education, and through visits to the homeland and other individual contacts. It applauded the formation of the Icelandic Canadian Club in 1942 and other activities of the Icelandic-Canadian community. The letter illustrated the wisdom of providing means for opinions from Iceland to help shape the Foundation's policies.

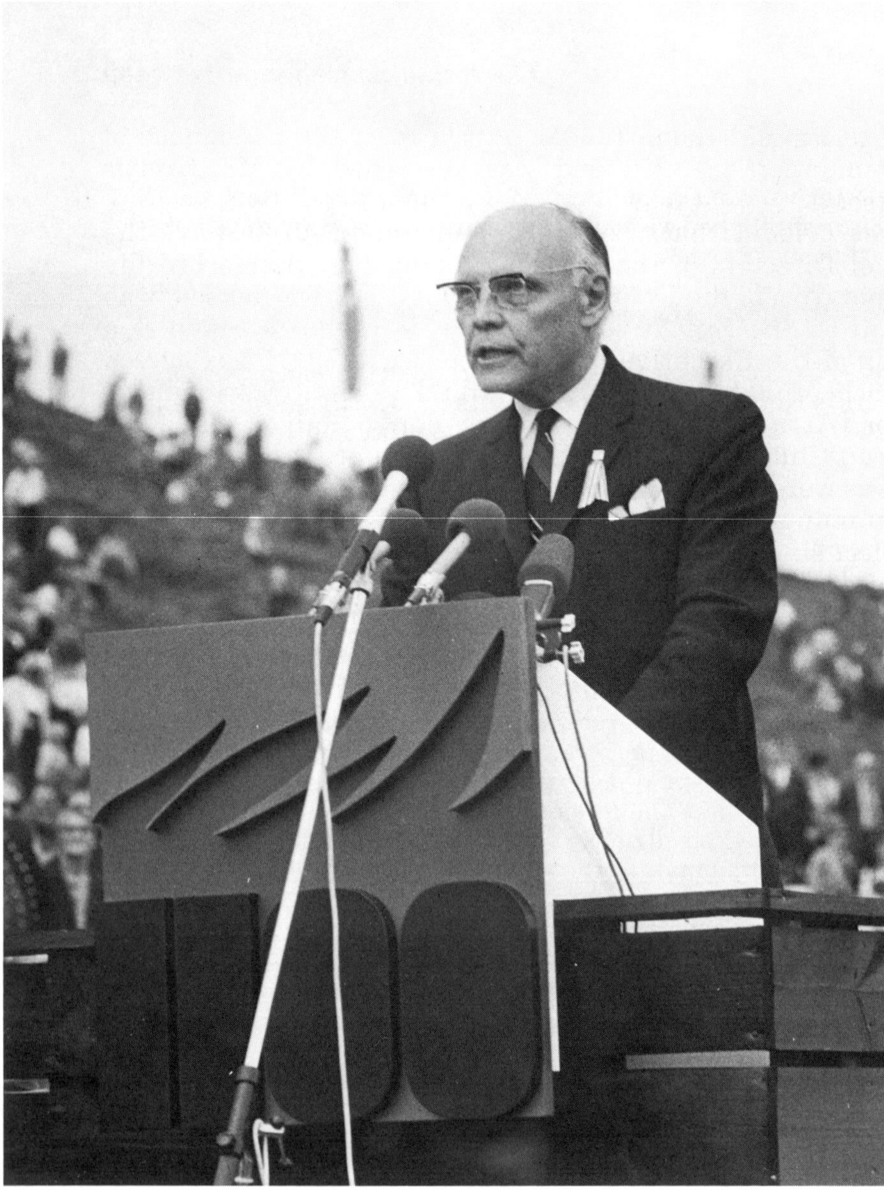

Dr. Thorlakson extending greetings on behalf of the Government and people of Canada at ceremonies on July 28 and 29, 1974, celebrating the eleven-hundredth anniversary of the settlement of Iceland. He was speaking on the site of the Lögberg (the Law Stone) at Thingvellir where the Parliament of Iceland – the Althing – met for about the first three centuries of its existence, that is, from about the year 930 to 1260. Dr. Thorlakson found it a moving experience to participate in this historic event, rooted in the ancient tradition of Icelandic parliamentary government.

Due to illness, Judge Lindal retired from the presidency of the Foundation in 1972 and was succeeded by Mr. Grettir Eggertson.

It was evident that it would be advantageous to have the Board of Directors of the Canada Iceland Foundation broadly representative of the Icelandic community. Dr. Thorlakson, who was still on the Executive Committee, initiated this step at a meeting of the Executive on December 21, 1972. It was agreed that each of eight organizations would be invited to name a director. At a joint meeting in the parish hall of the First Lutheran Church on Victor Street in Winnipeg, all these organizations were represented and the plan was endorsed, with the understanding that the basic Board of eight directors would then elect six additional directors to constitute a Board of fourteen persons. Dr. Kris Kristjanson was elected President.

Dr. Thorlakson was one of the elected members, and was named to the Executive Committee. He has continued to take an active part in the affairs of the Canada Iceland Foundation, latterly as the Honorary President.

CHAPTER 32

The Manitoba Council on Education

In the mid-1950s there arose a feeling in nearly all parts of Canada that it was time to make a complete overhaul of Canada's educational structure: its form, its content, its plant and equipment, its standards, and its priority among the essential requirements of the nation in a changing world.

Originating with a group of interested people in Toronto, and supported by the Canadian Teachers' Federation, the conviction arose "that a wider public understanding of Canada's educational needs and problems would be a major step in their solution." Ultimately their work culminated in the First Canadian Congress on Education, held in Ottawa from February 16 to 20, 1958, at which 850 delegates from nineteen national organizations having objectives related to education met in plenary and workshop sessions to discuss such varied subjects as financing, education; higher education; education for leisure; organization and curricula; role of the home in education; special needs in education; teachers – quantity and quality; buildings and equipment. Chairman of the Conference was the famous Montreal neuro-surgeon, Dr. Wilder G. Penfield.

The Conference was considered to be so beneficial that the delegates decided that similar conferences on education should be organized in each of the provinces; that the Second National Conference should be held two years later; and that some of the conclusions of the workshops approved at the plenary sessions should be presented to Prime Minister Diefenbaker and his government as recommendations. All these commissions were in due course carried out. There is no doubt in the minds of professionals in education that this conference and its successor held two years later in Montreal had an immense influence in moving public perceptions of the needs in education out of the Victorian era and into the twentieth century.

Little had been done in Manitoba to prepare for the demands on educational resources consequent on the postwar "baby boom." A royal commission chaired by R.O. MacFarlane (formerly Manitoba's Deputy Minister of Education) had reported in 1958, making broad recommendations for change in the educational system in the Province. Probably the most controversial sections were those that recommended reducing the school administrative units in Manitoba from nearly 2,000 to about sixty; and those that clearly stated the need for improved buildings and equipment, staffed by teachers with higher qualifications – all of which implied the allocation of more money in the provincial budget.

Similarly, the needs for adequate funding of the universities had not been accepted by government and the public. Full-time university enrolment in Manitoba increased from 4,900 in 1957–58 to 13,426 in 1967–68. This was a time when universities everywhere were faced with demands for new courses to keep pace not only with growth in the student population but with the generation of new knowledge. These were matters of concern to all levels of society, and it was not sufficient to leave governments and the professional educators to struggle with the problems by themselves.

Among the individuals approached in connection with the formation of a Manitoba affiliate with the Canadian Conference on Education was Dr. Thorlakson. At a preliminary meeting of the representatives of a number of interested organizations held on April 8, 1959, Dr. Thorlakson expressed the opinion that lay people would be much more interested in supporting the proposed Manitoba Council if the three older organizations (i.e., the Manitoba Education Week Association, the Manitoba Educational Association and the Manitoba Teachers Society) expressed, preferably in writing, their desire for lay support; and they should indicate clearly not only that a Manitoba Council on Education would be a help, but also the specific ways in which it could be useful.

In a letter on June 26, 1959, to Dr. W.C. Lorimer, Superintendent of Schools for the City of Winnipeg (and subsequently Deputy Minister of Education), Dr. Thorlakson stressed that "it is important at the outset to have specific and immediate objectives. Lay cooperation and support must be predicated on strong leadership and direction and advice from professional educators." He also emphasized what he felt should be the coordinating role of the proposed Manitoba Council: that it should not attempt to usurp the work of other organizations in the field of education, but should act as a consultative body to coordinate, guide and influence the activities of all when such help was desirable.

With a membership of more than twenty-five provincial organizations as well as individuals representing virtually all elements within the Province, the Manitoba Council on Education, affiliated with the Canadian Conference on Education, came into being on December 10, 1959. Dr. P.H.T. Thorlakson was elected President of the provincial organization, and Mrs. James A. Richardson was named Honorary President. The other officers were: Mr. Justice (later Chief Justice) G.E. Tritschler, Vice-President; Dr. Hugh H. Saunderson, President of the University of Manitoba, Vice-President; Mr. R.O.A. Hunter, Secretary of the Great-West Life Assurance Company, Secretary, and Brigadier General N. Elliot Rodger, Treasurer.

The first project undertaken by the Manitoba Council on Education was organization of a provincial conference to discuss the question, "What must we teach our children in our schools?" At the request of the Executive, Dr. Thorlakson appointed a conference organizing committee of eight, four lay members and four professionals, headed by Mr. Justice Tritschler.[1] He then invited Dr. Wilder G. Penfield, of Montreal, to be the keynote speaker.

Dr. Thorlakson left the city for a few weeks. On his return he found that the response to invitations to participate in the conference, scheduled for Saturday, February 27, 1960, at the University of Manitoba, had been so enthusiastic that after accepting 1,010 applications, the Committee had to turn down another 120 due to lack of space.

More than 1,000 people were gathered in the conference facility at the University of Manitoba at 9:30 a.m. on Saturday, February 27, 1960 when Dr. Thorlakson, President of the Manitoba Council on Education, opened its first conference. Following the brief opening formalities, Dr. Thorlakson introduced the famed keynote speaker, Dr. Wilder Penfield,[2] whose talk was entitled, "Education Seen in Long Perspective."

In the words of one very interested observer, Dr. Hugh M. Ross,[3] Dr. Penfield's address "set the tone for many of the subsequent discussions. The refreshing personality of this eminent neuro-surgeon soon had the entire audience enthralled."

The report of the meeting prepared by Dr. Ross and published in the Manitoba Medical Review for June-July, 1960, records some of Dr. Penfield's thoughts:

> He stressed that the resources of the mind [are] infinitely more important than the natural wealth with which a generous Creator has so liberally endowed our country. . . . Money is not all that is necessary to provide better education in Canada. We must examine the defects in our educational system [and here Dr. Penfield referred to the recommendations by the Royal Commission in its 284-page Report on Education in Manitoba].
>
> Dr. Penfield emphasized that the school is only one element in the larger process of education. The development of the child requires contributions from the home, society and his church. . . .

Dr. Penfield discussed the importance of ability to communicate in more than one language, and remarked on the relative ease with which children of four or five years can acquire a second language if they have the opportunity for total exposure to it on a regular basis. "The acquisition of grammar and vocabulary can come later," he said.

Chairman of the afternoon panel discussion was Mr. Justice A.M. Monnin. Panel members were Miss Helen Marsh, Editor of the Dauphin Herald; Dr. R.O. MacFarlane of Ottawa; Dr. D.W. Penner, pathologist and Chairman of the St. Vital School Board; and Miss Sybil Shack, Principal of Lord Roberts School, Winnipeg.

The theme, "What Must We Teach Our Children in Our Schools?" provided ample opportunity for expression of a wide variety of opinion. It produced a lively, informative, stimulating and thought-provoking session. There was general agreement that the Conference was a great success.

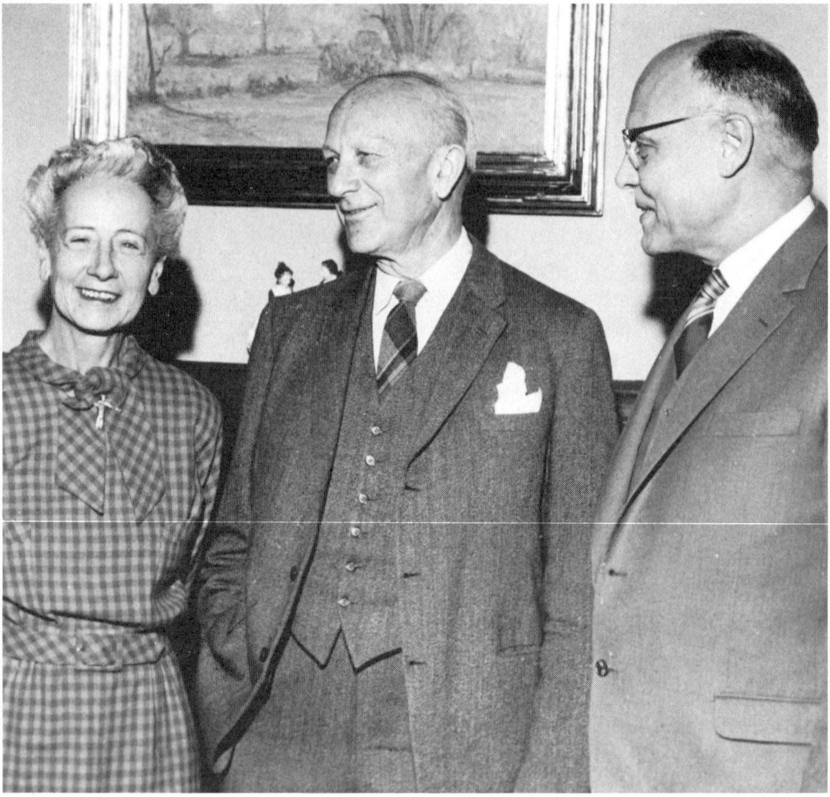

As President of the Manitoba Council on Education, Dr. Thorlakson invited Dr. Wilder Penfield to be the keynote speaker at a conference organized by the Council held in Winnipeg in February 1960. Dr. Penfield is shown here as the honoured guest at a reception held at the home of Dr. and Mrs. Thorlakson.

Under Dr. Thorlakson's guidance as President, the Second Manitoba Conference on Education was held in Brandon on Saturday, March 11, 1961, modelled on the first; it was equally as successful.

For this occasion, Dr. Thorlakson invited as the keynote speaker Dr. Malcolm G. Taylor, a well-known and highly respected scholar, a prolific writer in the health field, the Research Consultant to the Royal Commission on Health Services, and in 1961 President of the University of Calgary. His subject was "The Horizons of Education." Again, this address set broad parameters for consideration of educational programs, and was an inspiration to the twenty workshop groups of some thirty-five people each, who examined specific questions relating to the Conference theme, "Continuing Education."

Dr. Thorlakson undertook two other important responsibilities as President of the Manitoba Council on Education. At the Second National Conference on Education, held in Montreal in February, 1962, he was Chairman of the forum called "The Citizen in Education" – one of seven forums of 200 to 300 delegates each, which were in turn broken into workgroups of about twenty-five persons for discussion of specific topics pertaining to the general forum theme.

To publicize educational needs, he addressed the Rotary Club of Winnipeg on April 26, 1962. He reported on the work of the Manitoba Council on Education, the national conferences, and in particular the last national conference held in Montreal two months before, attended by 2,000 people. He noted that the forum chairmen and their rapporteurs worked long hours preparing statements for the final plenary session. "These summaries probably should not have been presented as recommendations," he said, "but rather as a compilation of views and opinions. It is, I believe, on this score that the Canadian Teachers' Federation have voted to withdraw their support of the Canadian Conference as presently constituted. The teachers, as professional people, are unwilling to be committed by recommendations or resolutions based on expressions of opinion unsupported by careful study or experience. This point of view, I think, is understandable."

The National Conference organization was disbanded in June 1961 by vote of its Standing National Committee, turning over its mission to other established professional groups.

On June 17, 1964, a public announcement was made that the Manitoba Council on Education would follow the precedent set at national level, and terminate its affairs. It turned over all its remaining funds to the Manitoba Education Week Association.

On the whole, it appears that these national and provincial projects, which brought several thousand Canadians together to focus their attentions on the strengths and weaknesses in our educational systems, were successful. They gave education at every level a new importance in the minds of all thoughtful Canadians. Certainly funding at every level of government was immeasurably improved, administration was modernized, and the quality and quantity of professional and physical resources reached new heights. It is worth noting that although there was substantial professional support, a major share of the responsibility for these achievements was carried by volunteers, selected from the ranks of busy, highly committed people. Dr. Thorlakson was a typical example.

In thinking about the enormous contribution made by voluntary participation of this kind, one is reminded that the giving of time and talent for the public good has some of the attributes of the quality of mercy, as described in Portia's words in "The Merchant of Venice":

The quality of mercy is not strain'd,
It droppeth as the gentle rain from heaven
Upon the place beneath: it is twice bless'd;
It blesseth him who gives and him who takes:
'Tis mightiest in the mightiest: . . . "

CHAPTER 33

University Chancellor

At a joint session of the Senate and the Board of Regents of the University of Winnipeg on February 7, 1969, Dr. Thorlakson was elected Chancellor of the University. Though young as a university (its charter was granted on July 1, 1967) it had roots reaching back almost a century in the educational life of what began as the Red River Settlement.[1] Dr. Thorlakson succeeded the first chancellor, Mr. R.H.G. Bonnycastle,[2] who, after little more than a year in office, died from a heart attack just minutes after landing his private plane near the junction of the Waterhen and Long Island Bays on Lake Winnipegosis. He was en route to a nearby hunting lodge with a long-time friend, G.W. Malaher.

The new chancellor was duly installed at a convocation of the University, with some 2,000 people gathered in the Civic Auditorium, on Sunday, May 25, 1969. He was presented to the Convocation by a senior member of the University Senate, Dr. Gordon Blake, Professor of Economics. The Very Reverend Wilfred C. Lockhart, President and Vice-Chancellor of the University of Winnipeg, and recently the Moderator of the United Church of Canada, administered the Oath of Office:

> I, Paul Hendrik Thorbjorn Thorlakson, accept the office of Chancellor of the University of Winnipeg and will seek, as its titular head, to the utmost of my ability, to uphold the principles and purposes of this University as set forth by its founders and affirmed by its statutes. I will at all times defend its rights, maintain its freedom and promote its unity and welfare, so help me God.

It was an obligation Dr. Thorlakson took seriously and which he honoured throughout his nine years in office.

At the conclusion of the installation ceremony, Dr. Thorlakson addressed the Convocation:

The Board of Regents and the Senate of the University of Winnipeg have conferred a great honour upon me. To them, I express my deep appreciation and pledge that such talents as I may possess will be used towards helping to build a progressive and influential centre of higher learning – one that will be strong and responsive to the needs and expectations of our students, of their parents, and of society.

On our university campus, we have Manitoba Hall and Wesley Hall. These historic names are constant reminders of the early pioneering days, when it took a great deal of vision and fortitude to found colleges in a settlement of a few thousand people; Manitoba College founded in 1871, and Wesley College founded in 1888, later became United College, which was destined to become a University in the heart of this growing metropolis.

As monuments to the faith and foresight of our predecessors, we also have Sparling Hall, Bryce Hall, Ashdown Hall, Riddell Hall, and Graham Hall. Less than an hour ago, the Minister of Youth and Education, the Honourable Donald W. Craik, laid the cornerstone of a new building which is being erected on the Campus, and which will be known as Lockhart Hall. This is a most deserving and fitting tribute to a man whom we wish to thank, and honour, for his qualities of heart and mind, and for his courageous and effective leadership of the affairs of this institution for fourteen years.

Under Dr. Lockhart's guidance United College was elevated to university status.

Because of the many progressive developments in education in Canada, it behooves every adult citizen – both young and old – to be well informed of the academic, administrative and financial problems and difficulties facing our educational institutions, and to care enough to do something for them. Our personal and collective involvement in education promises to become one of the most exciting and challenging Canadian adventures during the remaining years of this century. It is, therefore, with a sense of keen anticipation that I look forward to my association with the University of Winnipeg.

The purpose of this convocation is two-fold – to honour four distinguished Canadians and to confer degrees upon the students who have successfully completed their course of studies at the University of Winnipeg.

In the process of learning, you have gained a foundation of knowledge upon which you can continue to build for the rest of your lives.

You have acquired a sense of values and adopted attitudes which you will continue to develop. In your further pursuit of knowledge, you will – I hope – be constructively critical of some of the presently accepted ideas, and be helpful in finding workable solutions to some of the explosive and perplexing problems which confront us today.

To each graduate, I extend my good wishes and express the hope that life will present you with ever-widening and challenging opportunities.

At the Baccalaureate Service this morning we sang a hymn of guidance, "O God of Bethel." The third verse reads as follows:

Through each perplexing path of life
Our wandering footsteps guide;
Give us each day our daily bread,
And raiment fit provide.

May God grant that you and I will be true to ourselves, prepared for the responsibilities that lie ahead, and worthy of the academic gowns which we wear on this day.

The 1960s were years of unrest and protest against the status quo among university students everywhere, but particularly on some campuses in the United States. Occasionally, violet confrontations occurred. There were reports that radical student leaders were orchestrating protest activities among university and college students throughout North America, from a central headquarters in Chicago.

In Canada, there was a marked increase in activities of a political nature in student organizations, and "demands" for students representation on the governing bodies in the universities; but in this country confrontations were limited and there seems to have been only one instance of major damage to university property, when students at Sir George Williams University in Montreal occupied a computer centre.

At the University of Winnipeg, President Lockhart and the Board of Regents maintained a policy of open discussion with student representatives about any problems or proposals affecting them, and as early as 1966 it became the practice to name students to some of the important standing committees of the Board. Consequently, while the University of Winnipeg was not without its instances of strain, student leadership was generally responsible and opportunities for discussion with administrators were readily available.

It was within this framework that less than a week after his election as Chancellor, and almost four months before his formal installation, the officers of the University of Winnipeg Students' Association, through the President, asked for a meeting with Dr. Thorlakson, presumably to explore his attitudes with respect to student aspirations for a greater participation in University administration. Dr. Thorlakson was quick to respond, and the first of a number of meetings with student representatives took place in the boardroom of the University on February 19, 1969.

After reviewing some of his earlier discussions with the Students' Association and discussing the nature of their concerns, Dr. Lockhart introduced the Chancellor:

In introducing your Chancellor I am not going to give you an extended "who's who." You are, I am sure, much more anxious to hear something about his methods of approach to problems, his attitude of mind at the conference table.

First the background of heredity and environment: The man who has been selected for this high office is half Icelandic and half Norwegian. He spent his boyhood years in Selkirk, Manitoba – not far from a city, and close to the wonders of nature in rural Manitoba.

His father, a Lutheran minister, always spoke to him in Icelandic and taught him the virtues of the good life; his mother lavished affection and soft-pedalled administration in Norwegian; and on the streets he learned English "as she is spoke." This trilingualism is an undoubted asset.

Your Chancellor works hard, has worked hard all his life. He claims that a change is as good as a rest and has put this into practice the half century I have known him.

Whether by nature or constant practice, or both, he has mastered a much-needed attitude of mind. His type of thinking can be expressed in a well-known quotation from Latin – words of wisdom which were adopted as the motto of Wesley College: *Felix qui causas potuit cognoscere rerum*. [He is fortunate who is able to ascertain the reason for things.]

One of his teachers in Selkirk, now gone to her reward, was fond of telling how often it happened that this high school boy would come to her during recess and ask her to explain more clearly something in the lesson which seemed to him a little blurred. They discussed it from every angle and, as a result, she proudly admitted, the point became much clearer to both of them.

That type of inquiring mind is needed at all times; it is imperative in the world of today, and college halls are no exception.

Your Chancellor reads *The Uniter* [the student newspaper]. So do I. He at times may not agree but he does not wring his hands in despair. He sits down and asks himself: Why do they express those views or use that language?

He seeks an answer; and the answer may come from the very people whom he at first felt prone to severely criticize.

The Chancellor has often said, "I learn from those with whom I disagree, even from my opponents; they often bring out a point of view I may not have seen before." On the other hand, he is careful to add, "Sometimes I have to discount my closest friends; they may be anxious to say what they think I'll want to hear." Fawning is not to the taste of this man.

Your Chancellor has another asset. He, like former Prime Minister John G. Diefenbaker, does not allow himself the luxury of hate.

To ascertain the reason for things: That has been and will be the approach of your Chancellor to all conflicts of views and positions taken.

Members of the staff, in this as in other universities, will often find it difficult to understand the position taken by some of the students. That applies both ways. On such occasions a man with the approach of your Chancellor will do much to build the needed understanding. Then a sound, a correct decision should be reached.

Your University chose wisely. It is an honour to present to you the Chancellor of the University of Winnipeg, Dr. Paul H.T. Thorlakson.

Dr. Thorlakson began by expressing his pleasure at becoming associated with the University of Winnipeg and his confidence in its future role in higher education in Manitoba. He noted the qualities of friendship and goodwill that characterize the spirit of the University and its reputation for academic excellence. He then proceeded to express some of the principles he believed should prevail in discussion by – and with – the Students' Association about University government:

I believe the administrators of the University realize that rules and regulations to be followed by students must be presented to and discussed with representatives of the student body and receive their cooperation before being put into force.

I understand that the University of Winnipeg has a good working relationship with the students in terms of their involvement in University government, particularly at the committee level where they can be most effective.

The University of Winnipeg has encouraged freedom of expression

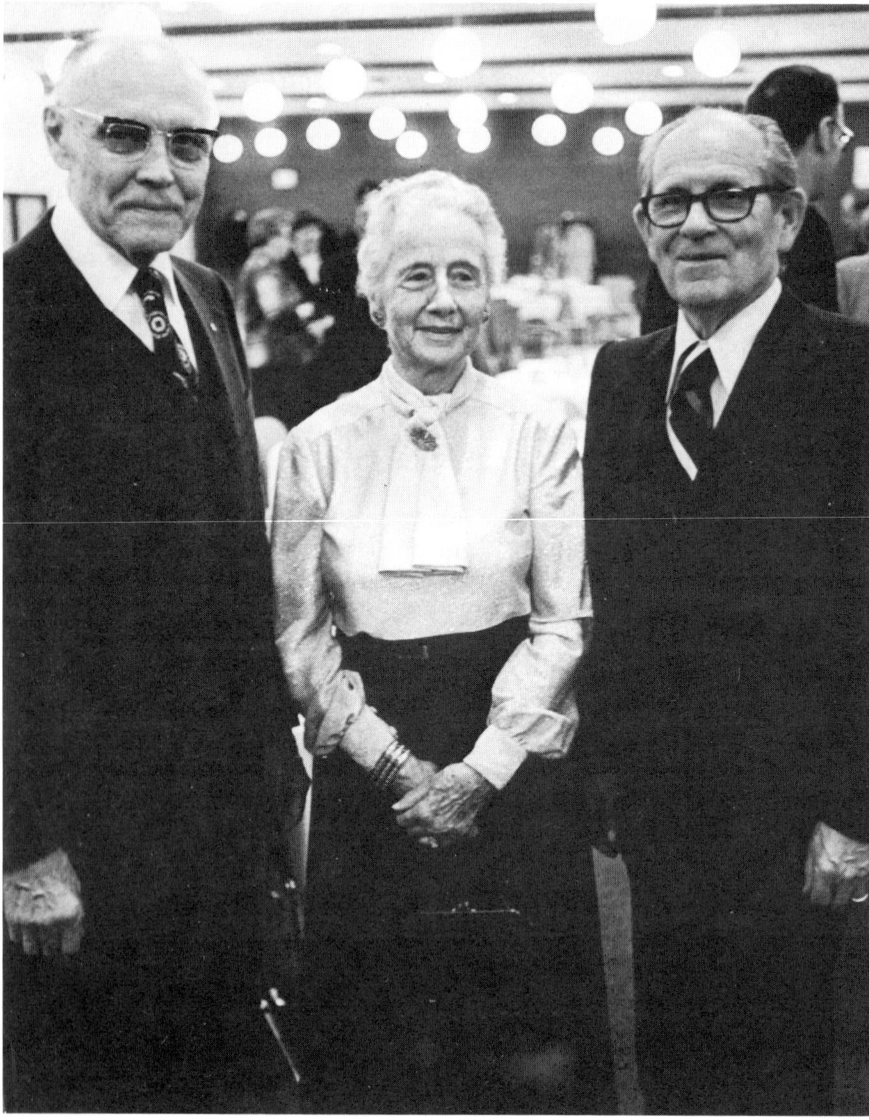

Chancellor and Mrs. Thorlakson with the Very Reverend Doctor Wilfred Lockhart, former Moderator of the United Church of Canada, Principal of United College, and the first President of the University of Winnipeg.

on the part of the individual student and members of the Faculty. A university, in my opinion, must not officially take on a political position in regard to national or international problems. The university is a place where there should be a constant dialogue between people of all points of view. The university must take a position which allows for all points of view on any issue to be presented and discussed.

My working philosophy has always been to encourage dissent and free discussion, and on many occasions in the past I have found myself on the side of the dissenters.

I understand the impatience of youth. Their ideas, energies and enthusiasms should be channelled – by them – into creative and constructive directions and, hopefully, within the existing structures of society.

I have no patience with arrogance, ruthlessness and destructive actions on the part of anyone. These lead to anarchy. We are only too painfully aware of the effect which anarchy and a disregard of the democratic process has had on the lives of millions of innocent people who have been victimized by power groups.

Mrs. Thorlakson and I are looking forward to our association with the University of Winnipeg. We are happy to be back where the students are, even when they dissent! But, let me add a note of caution – destructive behaviour and lack of consideration for others just serve to harden the public attitude against those who display these characteristics. In the reading of history, they must learn that a state of anarchy does not advance the cause of education, of freedom, of justice or of human progress.

The results that are obtained by representatives of the student body on working committees, with the administration, or even with Senate and the Board of Regents, will be determined in part by their attitude and capacity for understanding and appraising the many important problems that face the administrators.

Dissent has its place but, unless it is accompanied by constructive and cooperative action, it serves no useful purpose.

This pre-supposes that there is a spirit of understanding and cooperation on all sides and at all levels. The art of successful negotiation is usually acquired by application and experience, not by emotional outbursts.

Members of the older generation, who have the major responsibility of directing the affairs of a university, have all experienced the joys and frustrations of youth. While we look old, even very old, to the students, we can – and do – think young most of the time. It seems only yesterday that I was standing in your shoes and looking at the "old fogies" who were probably only ten, fifteen or twenty-five years older than I was. We try to live our lives again when we observe the joy, the exuberance, the vitality, the idealism and even the impatience of young people.

Authority still has a place in the lives of people everywhere, but it is not the absolute authority and the unquestioned obedience of a few decades ago. Now the old and the young must speak frankly to each other, they must work together in order to improve the lot of the student and, in the process, reduce the anxieties and burdens of the much over-worked President and those closely associated with him.

The moderates – who occupy a central position and form the majority of the members of our society, of our University administration, the faculty, and the student body – function as the balance wheel between lack of action and excessive action.

In all meetings of this kind, it was Dr. Thorlakson's style to listen attentively to what others had to say and then offer his own thoughtful, relevant, well-directed comments on the subject under discussion. It is a mark of respect too often neglected in situations in which controversial matters are being considered. Courtesy has a great influence in bringing about a meeting of minds with respect to even the most vexing questions.

When officers of the Students' Association were pondering subjects of special concern, with the concurrence of the University President the Chancellor was sometimes invited to meet with them informally – usually by way of Dr. Thorlakson inviting them to be his guests at lunch. Perhaps the most notable occasion of this kind occurred when he took them to lunch at the Manitoba Club to meet Chancellor Peter D. Curry of the University of Manitoba.

There is little doubt that this unusual rapport between the Chancellor and the spokesmen for the students contributed much to the spirit of reason and responsibility that was experienced at the University of Winnipeg throughout these eventful years.

Dr. Thorlakson understands the value of ritual in our lives, and as Chancellor he was firm in maintaining the colourful ceremonies of the University in the granting of degrees, at whatever level. Despite his own recognition by so many institutions of higher learning, he never lost his sense of the thrill experienced by students who were receiving their first degrees. It was in the spirit of sharing in a joyful occasion that he participated in the sometimes lengthy convocation ritual. During his term as Chancellor, despite many other obligations he was only absent from Convocation once, when he was addressing a medical meeting in Australia. Several thousand graduating students appeared before him in his nine-year tenure, and as they came forward to receive their degrees, each received a warm handshake from the Chancellor, usually accompanied by a personal word of congratulation.

With equal attention to detail, Dr. Thorlakson carefully prepared the remarks it was his duty to provide on all and sundry occasions, both formal and informal. Each address was tailored to the occasion, with an economy of words that marks the well-ordered mind.

A few samples are given in the following pages. The messages they contain, shaped especially for the students in his audience, reflect the character of the man who delivered them.

A month after the first meeting between the Chancellor and the representatives of the University of Winnipeg Student's Association, and well before his official installation as Chancellor, he was invited by the Association to be their guest at a dinner they were hosting for the graduating class of 1969.[3] Dr. Thorlakson was asked to address the Class:

It was a surprise and an unexpected honour for me to be elected to the chancellorship of the University of Winnipeg. This appointment is a sobering, albeit a stimulating and exciting, challenge.

My recent elevation to this high office reminds me of a remark made by that great Canadian physician, the late Sir William Osler, upon his appointment to the Faculty of Medicine at Johns Hopkins University in Baltimore in the year 1889. The University had increased its entrance requirements and had set new and higher standards of medical education and training. Sir William Osler said that he was pleased to be admitted to the University as a professor because he doubted that he could qualify for admission as a student!

Mrs. Thorlakson and I are looking forward to participating in the activities of the University of Winnipeg. We are happy to be back again where the students are. A great part of our lives has been spent in close association with university students and faculty. To be part of the University of Winnipeg family is an honour and a privilege which we value highly.

It is exactly fifty years ago, this year, since we graduated from the Universtiy of Manitoba. The graduation exercises were held in the Walker Theatre, now the Odeon Theatre. Mrs. Thorlakson received a

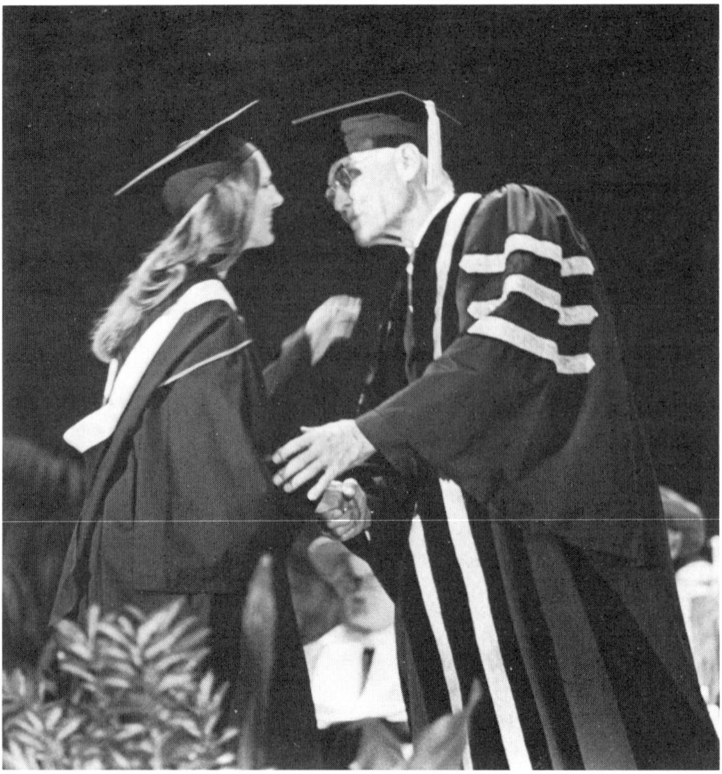

Chancellor Thorlakson reaches out to kiss his granddaughter Patricia when, as one of the graduating students, she came forward to receive her Bachelor of Arts degree.

Bachelor of Home Economics degree and I received a doctorate in medicine. To you, who are about to graduate, the year 1919 must seem a long time ago but, surprising as it may be, we share with you much of the enthusiasm, the idealism, the hopes and even some of the impatience of youth.

I know it is the desire of our President, Dr. Lockhart, the members of the Board of Regents and the Senate, the Faculty and the Graduates that the University of Winnipeg will continue to move forward and become an increasingly exciting centre of learning and research. Recent events in Canada, and in many parts of the world, have emphasized the urgent need for research in the field of human relations and in the analysis of factors which determine human behaviour. This has become the most important and pressing issue of our time.

The origins of the University of Winnipeg date back to the pioneer days in Manitoba and the Northwest Territories – a period of exploration, of expansion and the building of a new nation.

The pioneering spirit was also exemplified in the founding of colleges and universities. These institutions of higher learning have exerted a powerful, motivating force in the process of national expansion and development.

The definition of "pioneering" is "to discover and to explore in advance of others" or "to open new ways for others to follow."

The pioneering days, therefore, are not over, and surely the pioneering spirit is not dead. Every graduate of the University of Winnipeg is a potential pioneer. Strengthened by your interest and support, after you join the ranks of the alumni, your university will explore, expand and establish new frontiers of knowledge.

This is the quest which all of us who belong to the University of Winnipeg must pursue in a spirit of mutual understanding and trust. We must show respect and tolerance for the opinions of those who disagree with us and, above all, maintain a sense of balance and a reasonable sense of humour in our approach to the solution of difficult and vexatious problems.

These are the distinguishing hallmarks of educated men and women, the needed attributes of mature citizens and potential leaders.

On behalf of Mrs. Thorlakson and myself, I want to thank the University of Winnipeg Students' Association for inviting us to this delightful dinner.

To the members of the Graduating Class of '69, I wish to say that I am looking forward to sharing – with each one of you – the excitement and the satisfaction of your graduation day on Sunday, May 25.

In response to the continuing need for increased accommodation for the steadily rising enrolment, the Board of Regents approved plans for a fine new building facing on Ellice Avenue, ultimately named Lockhart Hall. Construction began in 1968. The formal opening ceremonies took place on Sunday, May 10, 1970, in the course of which the Chancellor addressed the distinguished guests and friends of the University gathered:

For centuries, it has been generally accepted that a university is one of our most enduring institutions but, in recent years, we have come to realize that it is a very fragile institution. Within the last ten years, in some places, we have seen fearful evidence of its vulnerability. Our long-cherished beliefs in the indestructibleness of these ancient strongholds of learning and freedom are suddenly being challenged both from within and from without.

In case some of you may think this is a modern phenomenon, let me remind you that the first chancellor of Oxford University was appointed in the thirteenth century. It is said that his main function was to control unruly students. Six of the first eight chancellors of that venerable and proud institution were beheaded. When I first heard of this method of solving their chancellors' tenure of office, shortly after my election to the chancellorship of the University of Winnipeg, I experienced certain misgivings. Possibly this has made me overly cautious about what I say in public as a chancellor.

Many years ago, recognition of the services of former principals was established on this campus by naming new buildings in their honour. Hence, we have Bryce Hall, Sparling Hall, Riddell Hall, and Graham Hall – and, for good measure, we have Manitoba Hall and Ashdown Hall. The Policy Committee of the University of Winnipeg wisely decided to follow this precedent. When Dr. Lockhart was told of the recommendation to name this new building Lockhart Hall, he resisted the proposal but was finally persuaded by his friends to allow his name to stand. When the Policy Committee subsequently submitted the name Lockhart Hall to The Board of Regents and to the Senate, it was enthusiastically and unanimously approved.

There are so many reasons why this new addition to our university is named Lockhart Hall. The list of Dr. Lockhart's achievements and his record of community service is long and impressive. I shall mention only a few of his interests and activities. In addition to his arduous duties as Principal of United College, he served as President of the Rotary Club of Winnipeg in 1965–66. He is a member of the Province of Manitoba Local Government Boundaries Commission. In 1967, Dr. Lockhart was elected Moderator of the United Church of Canada. This was a most important, responsible and time-consuming assignment. Under Dr. Lockhart's very able guidance, United College became the University of Winnipeg on July 1, 1967.

In this time of uncertainty – particularly for unversity presidents – a most reassuring incident occurred at the annual grads' farewell of this university. In my opinion, the crowning moment of the event came after the retiring president of the Students' Association, Mr. George Van Den Bosch, spoke about his experience during his term of office and his relationship with President Lockhart. George admitted that President Lockhart and he had, at times, some differences of opinion. However – at the conclusion of his address – he said that, if he could be granted a wish, it would be that future presidents of the University of Winnipeg would be men of equal integrity. On hearing these words, the students gave Dr. Lockhart a rousing ovation. In this university, the name Wilfred Lockhart will always stand for integrity and progress.

I know I speak for everyone here today when I say that the name chosen for this new building – Lockhart Hall – is a most appropriate and well-deserved honour. We trust it will convey to Dr. Lockhart the high regard and affection which everyone connected with the University of Winnipeg has for their president, and also the esteem of the citizens of this community.

Dr. Wilfred C. Lockhart, distinguished churchman and academic, was appointed Principal of United College in 1955, coming to Winnipeg from his position as Minister of Kingsway-Lambton United Church in Toronto. For a number of years he had been Padre of Hart House at the University of Toronto; had been the first secretary of the Canadian Committee of the World Council of Churches; and at the time of his appointment at United College he was the Chairman of the church's Board of Colleges and Secondary Schools. He was thoroughly familiar with the problems and the possibilities at United College, and he undertook the leadership of this historic institution as a challenge and an opportunity to return to daily contact with students and faculty.

Under Dr. Lockhart's leadership, United College increased its stature in every direction: in enrolment, in faculty, in administrative organization, in buildings and equipment, and in financial strength. It was, of course, an era in which there was a surging growth in post-secondary education throughout Canada. During the Lockhart years, United College shared fully in this movement, and on July 1, 1967, it achieved the full status of a university.

Dr. and Mrs. Lockhart made a great contribution to the life of the church, to academic affairs and to the province during their years in Manitoba, and there was general regret when in 1976 Dr. Lockhart found it necessary to retire from the strenuous demands that had been made upon him.

To seek a successor, a search committee under the leadership of Dr. Thorlakson was set up in June, 1970. In January 1971, it was announced that Dr. H.E. Duckworth had been chosen. Dr. Duckworth, a distinguished Canadian physicist, was then Vice-President (Academic) at the University of Manitoba, and the current President of the Royal Society of Canada. He had also served as Dean of Graduate Studies at McMaster University, and – a particularly happy circumstance for the whole University community – he was himself a graduate of Wesley College.

The new President arrived on campus at a time when excitement was building for the celebration of the centennial of the first of the founding colleges of the University of Winnipeg, Manitoba College. The festivities began on October 8, and were climaxed by the installation of the University's second President and Vice-Chancellor, Dr. Duckworth.

The events of Friday, October 8, 1971, which launched the celebrations, were described by Dr. Thorlakson at the unveiling and dedication of a centennial plaque at the site of the Rock of Remembrance on the University grounds facing Portage Avenue.

> This morning the Centennial Cavalcade, consisting of a University float and a fleet of automobiles provided by General Motors of Canada, took representatives of the University of Winnipeg to the City Hall where His Worship, Mayor Stephen Juba, made a presentation of proclamation to our President, Dr. H.E. Duckworth – a proclamation heralding the University of Winnipeg Centennial Week. The proclamation reads, in part: "Now therefore, I, Stephen Juba, Mayor of the City of Winnipeg, in the Province of Manitoba, do hereby proclaim October 10 to 17, 1971, as the University of Winnipeg Week, requesting all citizens to take due note of this, and govern themselves accordingly."
>
> The cavalcade then proceeded on its twenty-seven-mile route, first down Main Street to Nesbit Hall, the original Manitoba College building in Old Kildonan. A copy of the proclamation was nailed to the door, commemorating the founding of Manitoba College in 1871. The cavalcade next paid a visit to St. Boniface College in remembrance of that

institution's contribution to early Manitoba education.

Dr. Duckworth and our group then called at the office of Dr. Ernest Sirluck, President of the University of Manitoba, honouring the association of St. John's College, St. Boniface College and Manitoba College in the founding of the University of Manitoba in 1877, and to recognize that our students received their degrees from the University of Manitoba for ninety years prior to 1967. Mr. W.J. Condo, Senior Vice-President of the University of Manitoba, presented Dr. Duckworth with a scroll which expressed congratulations and best wishes for the next 100 years.

The procession continued to St. Paul's College and St. John's College on the University of Manitoba campus to honour the role that these institutions played in Manitoba's educational history. And, finally, we arrived back home fifteen minutes ago. . . .

The plaque being unveiled today commemorates the historical event which occurred in 1871. The massive rock on which the plaque will be placed is, I think, symbolic of the strength and fortitude of the pioneers of 100 years ago. In establishing Manitoba College, they formed an educational institution which has proved as enduring as this huge piece of Manitoba granite, sculptured as it is by the forces of nature. It is a most appropriate symbol to express our gratitude for the past and our hopes for the future.

We are indebted to Mr. Duncan Robertson of the Winnipeg Supply and Fuel Company for providing us with this magnificent piece of granite from their Gull Lake quarry. Many of you may be amazed to learn that the weight of this rock is twenty-five tons.

It was an inspired thought when the Reverend Dr. David Owen, professor emeritus of philosophy, suggested the placement of this Rock of Remembrance on the campus site.

On Saturday, September 25, 1971, the University of Winnipeg had the honour of hosting a luncheon, at which Her Royal Highness, The Princess Margaret and her husband, Lord Snowdon, were present, on the occasion of the formal opening of its neighbour, the new Winnipeg Art Gallery. The Chancellor welcomed the distinguished guests:

Your Royal Highness, Lord Snowdon, Mr. Premier, Mr. Minister, Mr. Aitken, ladies and gentlemen: This is a great day of celebration for Winnipeg, and for all of Manitoba. We have looked forward to this for a long time and many people have worked diligently and patiently to make it possible. The presence of Her Royal Highness, The Princess Margaret and her husband, The Earl of Snowdon, increases immeasurably the pleasure and significance of this occasion.

There are at least two universal methods of communication – music and art – in which there are no national boundaries and which, in their own way, represent a universal language. We need *more* such methods of communication because written and spoken words too often confuse and obstruct good relations between individuals, groups and nations.

In this connection, I believe it is appropriate for me to tell a story which I heard two weeks ago in London, on my way home from Russia, about the problem of communication. This concerns an Oxford don who travelled around the ancient University city on his bicycle. One day, he had a blowout. He repaired the tire, replaced it, and then took out his pump. A student came along and stopped to watch the professor working the pump. After a moment or two, he thought he should point out to the professor that the *front* tire was flat but he had the pump connected to the *rear* tire. To which the professor replied, "I've always been under the impression that they communicated."

Wherever one travels, either behind or on this side of the so-called iron-curtain, one hears essentially the same classical and modern music from the concert stage and in other places of entertainment. Hundreds of millions of people around the world listen to the same music over their radios.

Similarly, wherever one travels, one may see paintings displayed, and other works of art, which have, over the centuries, been produced by master artists and craftsmen of many nations. Today, we are, in fact, celebrating and paying tribute to the universality of fine art by the opening of the new Winnipeg Art Gallery.

On behalf of the Board of Regents, the Senate, the Faculty, and the Student Body of the University of Winnipeg, it is my privilege to welcome Her Royal Highness, The Princess Margaret, The Earl of Snowdon, and other distinguished guests to this luncheon.

In October, 1975, His Grace the Bishop of Iceland visited Winnipeg to take part in the Canada-Iceland Centennial Conference. During a conference event at the Manitoba Theatre Centre on October 5, a special convocation of the University of Winnipeg was convened for the purpose of conferring the degree of Doctor of Divinity, *honoris causa*, on this distinguished guest. On these occasions, the Chancellor, of course, officially awards the degrees, but the President and Vice-Chancellor is the presiding officer.

At an appropriate point in the program for the evening, The Chairman of the Conference, Dr. Kris Kristjanson, (President of the Canada-Iceland Foundation) announced the Convocation, and invited Dr. Duckworth to open the proceedings. Dr. Duckworth addressed the meeting:

The University of Winnipeg is grateful to the organizers of the Canada-Iceland Centennial Conference for giving us the opportunity during this evening's program to hold a special convocation, for the purpose of awarding the degree Doctor of Divinity (*honoris causa*). Because of the circumstances of the occasion the academic party is small in number, but we are greatly honoured that it includes the President of the University of Manitoba, Dr. Ernest Sirluck, the President Emeritus of Acadia University and sometime Professor of Wesley and United Colleges, Dr. Watson Kirkconnell, two distinguished churchmen of Icelandic descent, Dr. Valdimir Eylands and Dr. Philip Peturrson, and a distinguished alumnus of the University, Dr. Wilhelm Kristjanson. The rest of us are the regular officers, that is, the Chairman of the Board of Regents, Mr. William Norrie, the Dean of Theology, Dr. George Taylor and the Registrar, Mr. Richard Bellhouse, in addition to the Chancellor and myself.

With these acknowledgements and explanations, Mr. Chancellor, may I respectfully request you to take your place at the podium in order that Dean Taylor may present to you the candidate for the degree.

Following the awarding of the degree, on behalf of the Canada-Iceland Foundation, Mr. A.P. Johannson presented a plaque to the University of Winnipeg in honour of the occasion, which Dr. Duckworth acknowledged in the following terms:

As I said at the luncheon yesterday, the University of Winnipeg greatly values the long and significant association which it and its founding colleges have enjoyed with the Icelandic community. For example, the first Icelandic student to obtain a degree in Manitoba was a student of ours. This year, ninety years later, we re-elected for a third term to the University's highest office Chancellor P.H.T. Thorlakson. And in the intervening ninety years we have had a remarkable succession of Icelandic students and members of staff – much too numerous to attempt to name – who have contributed enormously to the development of our academic strength and reputation – and, I might add, are continuing to do so.

Because of this valued association I accept the plaque with special pleasure and I assure you that it will be accorded a suitable place of honour. Although the inscription on the plaque only carries the voyage of discovery to Labrador and Newfoundland, we're grateful that later

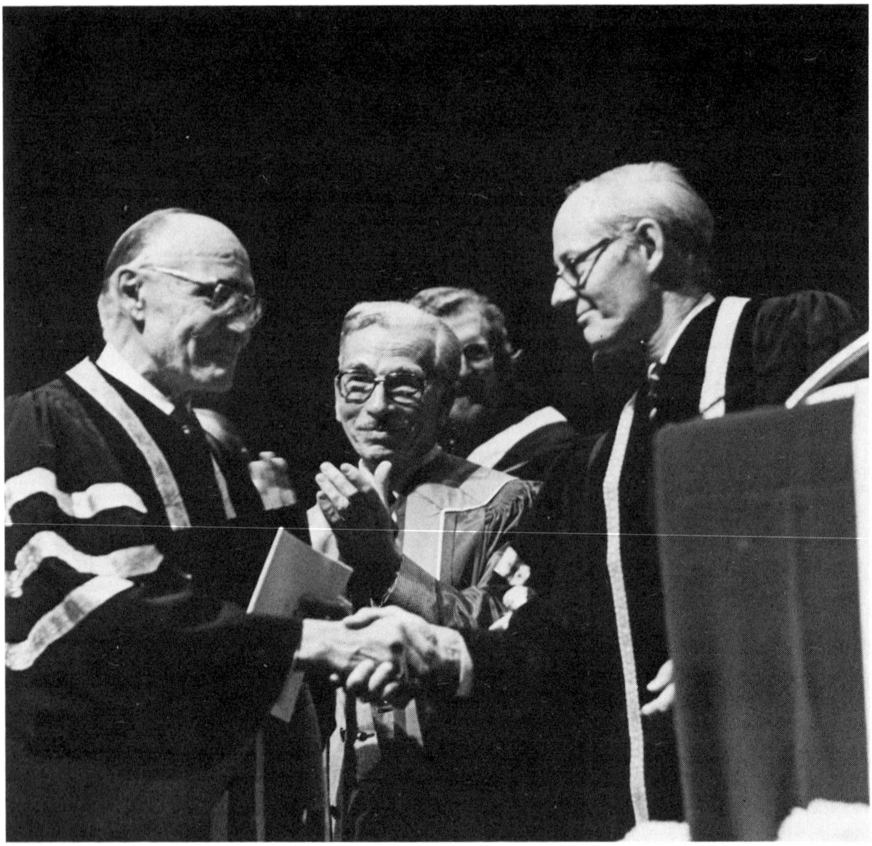

Words of appreciation and a warm handshake from University of Winnipeg President Harry Duckworth at the close of the last convocation in Dr. Thorlakson's nine-year term as Chancellor.

generations pushed further west to discover and to share with the rest of us – "this other Eden, demi-paradise. . . . "

After nine years in office, Dr. Thorlakson, at age eighty-four, felt that he could not accept another three-year term, and retired from the position of chancellor on February 7, 1978, "full of years and honours." The evening of December 9, 1977, was devoted to a festive occasion for tributes to him by the members of the University, and from his fellow chancellors – Mrs. Isabel Auld of the University of Manitoba, and Mr. Stanley Knowles of the University of Brandon. Dr. Duckworth presided. The accolades were many, expressing sentiments deeply felt and sincerely stated.

Although Mr. W. James Millar spoke on behalf of the University of Winnipeg Alumni Association, he had first met Dr. Thorlakson when he was President of the Students' Association. He spoke in part as follows:

Guests, Ladies and Gentlemen: You will hear tonight, I believe, much about the honours and achievements earned by our chancellor. These are the milestones in the life of a truly great Canadian. I wish however to spend a few moments on the qualities that are not very often recognized in certificate, award or degree. I refer to the great humanity, charm and concern that Paul Thorlakson displays for his fellow man.

My association with Dr. Thor goes back to my student days and has continued over many committee responsibilities and occasions in the ensuing years. Before meeting the Chancellor, I felt as a student politician of the late sixties that one was expected to have some preconceived notions about the administration of a university. Some of them were right, some of them weren't. My preconceived notion was that the position of chancellor was basically an honorary one. Not unlike the Canadian Senate it was a retirement award for having distinguished oneself during one's productive years. But our chancellor took his job very seriously and as his life's achievement would warrant, he gave it his all. It was not retirement but simply another phase of a supremely productive life.

The Chancellor was always a source of great inspiration to me. For example, on several occasions and in connection with certain committee responsibilities, we had lunch together. The Chancellor, unfailingly, felt there were sound medical reasons for feeding a starving student, and he insisted on paying. Fortunately, by this time I learned, as we all have, to defer to his judgement in all things. . . .

Dr. Lockhart often stated that the nickname Thor which was favoured by many of his friends was not a shortened form of Thorlakson but a shortened form of "thorough." I always considered this comment apt since there is no aspect of the university community which did not deserve and receive his close and conscientious attention. The Board, the Senate, the Students' Association, the Alumni Association, the Library, the building committees, the Entrance Scholarship Program, Athletics, Convocations and the list goes on. No project was too large or too small to attract his interest. . . .

I am sure I speak for all the alumni when I say it has been an honour and a privilege to work with you, sir, and although your direct connection with the University will soon be coming to an end, your friends will remember you. In testimony to the esteem in which the Alumni Association holds your service to the university, we have chosen to place, in the library, six volumes of *Tresor de la Langue Française*. In selecting an appropriate way to recognize your great contribution to our university it was important to settle on a prominent and popular vehicle to carry your name. We have done so. The *Tresor de la Langue Française* promises to be on daily and prominent display in our reference library a hundred years from now. This monumental dictionary of the French language of the nineteenth and twentieth centuries will comprise approximately fifteen volumes. When completed it will doubtless be accepted as the French equivalent of the prestigious Oxford English dictionary. . . .

Dr. Duckworth then invited Mrs. Thorlakson to unveil the portrait of the Chancellor, painted by Canadian artist Thomas R. McDonald. The portrait having been duly examined and admired, it was time for Dr. Thorlakson to respond:

Mrs. Thorlakson and I have enjoyed many very pleasant gatherings during our association with the University of Winnipeg. During the past nine years, we have met many wonderful people and we have made many new friends.

We would be less than human if we did not confess that we will miss this association but we can assure you that we will have only the happiest memories. Should we get lonesome and wish to make direct contact again, we have a surprise for President Duckworth – in case he thinks he has seen the last of us. We may just register next fall as mature students at the University of Winnipeg!

It has been my good fortune to be chancellor of the University of Winnipeg during an exciting period of its development. I would like to refer briefly to some of the achievements, all of which are a great credit to the Board of Regents, the Senate, the academic staff and the administrative officers of this institution:

1. Lockhart Hall was formally opened in May 1970.

2. The centenary of the founding of Manitoba College was celebrated in 1971 and the big – 25 ton – Rock of Remembrance in front of Wesley Hall is a constant reminder of our one hundredth birthday.

3. The University of Winnipeg established the Institute of Urban Studies focusing on housing, community planning and land use.

4. The University opened its Theatre Arts Program, thereby establishing itself as part of the city's theatre community.

5. The part-time courses scheduled at convenient locations were introduced and have effectively expanded the influence of the University. More and more people are turning to part-time studies to obtain a degree while continuing to work.

6. A course of studies, designated as University at Two, is scheduled from 2 to 3:30 p.m. on the campus for the convenience of married women.

7. In 1972, the University of Winnipeg established a *first* in Canada by providing tuition-free courses for senior citizens.

8. An important academic event was the commencement of the master's program in English, history, public administration and religion to be jointly offered with the University of Manitoba.

9. Of great significance was the introduction of cooperative programs with Red River Community College.

10. The Entrance Scholarship Program was successfully launched in 1973 and continues to expand.

11. Student representation on the Board of Regents, the Senate and many committees was arranged.

In addition to all these milestones, we entertained royalty at luncheon in Riddell Hall after the official opening of the Winnipeg Art Gallery.

Here, I would like to express my sincere admiration for President Duckworth and his associates. The University of Winnipeg is indeed fortunate to have its affairs guided by such an eminently qualified group of people.

The Alumni Association is very active in its support of the Univer-

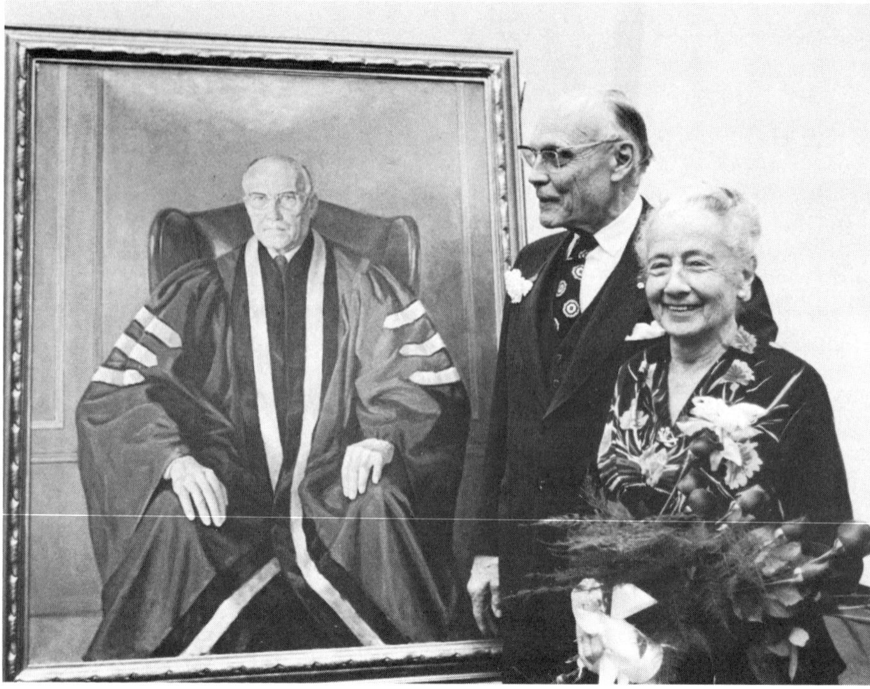

At a special reception in the evening of December 9, 1977, the University of Winnipeg paid tribute to Dr. Thorlakson's nine years of distinguished service as the University's second chancellor. A highlight of the occasion was the unveiling of a portrait of the Chancellor in his robes of office, painted by Canadian artist Thomas R. MacDonald. Along with that of the first chancellor, Mr. R.H.G. Bonnycastle, it now graces the wall of the approach to the President's offices on the third floor.

sity. As one of the honorary presidents, I have attended annual class reunions. Graduates have come from long distances to see their former classmates and to visit their alma mater. This demonstrates the continuing "family feeling" which permeates the University.

I wish to single out the students of our University for special mention. During my term as Chancellor, I have come in contact with student representatives on the Board of Regents and on various committees. I have been impressed by the manner in which they conducted themselves and presented their points of view. Granted, I may not have always agreed with their suggestions but this has not prevented me from respecting their opinions. I have noted how our young students matured and developed confidence as they advanced through their years of study, and I have seen the look of satisfaction on their faces as I shook their hands and wished them well at Convocation.

It is a pleasure to have with us on this occasion Mrs. Isabel Auld, Chancellor of the University of Manitoba, and Mr. Stanley Knowles, Chancellor of Brandon University. This is typical of the cooperation that exists between the three Universities.

Now, for the portrait – I am greatly relieved to see the likeness of myself but, of course, I am not the best judge of what I look like to other people.

When the artist, Dr. T.R. MacDonald of Hamilton, Ontario, made some of the early strokes with his brush on the canvas, he would peer at me from time to time around the edge of the canvas frame. I asked him what he expected of me and he replied: "I want you to look wise, benevolent and like a man of action." I responded by saying that this would be almost impossible because, at that moment, I was experiencing a severe attack of shingles! . . .

The association that Mrs. Thorlakson and I have had with the University of Winnipeg has been very gratifying and stimulating. It brought us back, after a lapse of some years, into a University circle. Gladys was a member of the Board of Governors of the University of Manitoba for twelve years during the period when the University was in the process of recovering from the disastrous effects of the Great Depression; and I, for a number of years, was a teacher in the Department of Surgery of the Faculty of Medicine.

Many nice things have been said about Mrs. Thorlakson and about me this evening, and we are both most appreciative of the hospitality and honour extended to us.

On behalf of Mrs. Thor and myself, I wish to offer our grateful thanks to everyone at the University of Winnipeg who has accorded us such unfailing kindness and friendliness during these past nine happy years.[4]

Knowing the man, it is unlikely that any of his friends believed that Dr. Thor's retirement from the post of Chancellor of the University signalled the end of his interest and participation in community affairs. There would be more to the Thorlakson story. Indeed this book records tributes and honours that came to him until he was well past his ninetieth birthday. But the future is hidden from us; and this seems to be a fitting point at which to end the record of the "achievements and adventures" – truly the Saga – of this distinguished Canadian whose roots extend far back into the history of both Iceland and Norway.

Dr. Thorlakson had the capacity to be successful in any career he might have elected to follow. He chose to be a surgeon, and he achieved an eminence in his profession that gained international recognition. He had a talent for leadership that enabled him to attract the interest and support of people from all walks of life to aid and advise him in his remarkably successful achievements outside the practice of medicine. In the care of his patients he was unstinting of his skill and his time; his manner was kindly, his direction firm; his response to their concerns and anxieties was calm, considerate and reassuring. He turned these exemplary qualities to the service of health care organizations, to cultural affairs and to education. His insight and his character influenced every project with which he was associated. Yet the firmness of his resolve in pressing toward the goals of his public undertakings was infused with an underlying humanity that found its most revealing expression in the lifelong love and tenderness that he shared with Gladys, and his quiet pride in the achievements of his children, and his grandchildren. The world is a better place because of his life and work.

PART EIGHT

Epilogue

CHAPTER 34

A Private Life in Vignettes

This book has been devoted almost entirely to an account of the professional and public life of Dr. Paul H.T. Thorlakson. This life was so rich and full, so influential in shaping the development of medicine and the health services, and so significant in the city and province which has been his lifetime home, that the story of his family has had to be generally untouched. Nevertheless, the deeply-felt bonds of affection and empathy with wife, children and grandchildren – and most recently, great-grandchildren – were integral and treasured parts of his being. They gave an added dimension to all that he did, and provided perspective and balance when the pressure of affairs was heavy. Despite his involvement in the stream of outside events, a gift for the management of time permitted him to be a central figure in the life of his talented, close-knit and fun-loving family.

Since their marriage on November 10, 1920 Gladys Maree Henry – Mrs. Thorlakson – wife, mother, confidante and constant companion, has shared all the ebb and flow of events in Thor's life. At the same time she has been able to maintain her own identity, develop her own personality, and pursue her own special interests. First came her family responsibilities. But she also participated actively in University and Alumni Association affairs, and in social and community events. Her ability to organize and to manage, well-recognized when as a young woman she so ably carried heavy responsibility for the success of the Chatauqua in Manitoba and Saskatchewan, was regularly called upon in support of family and community enterprises.

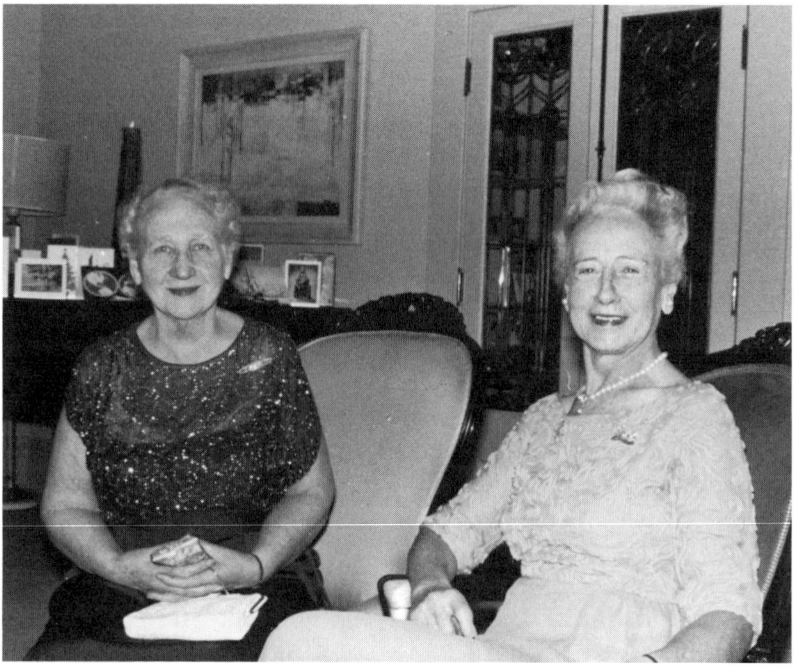

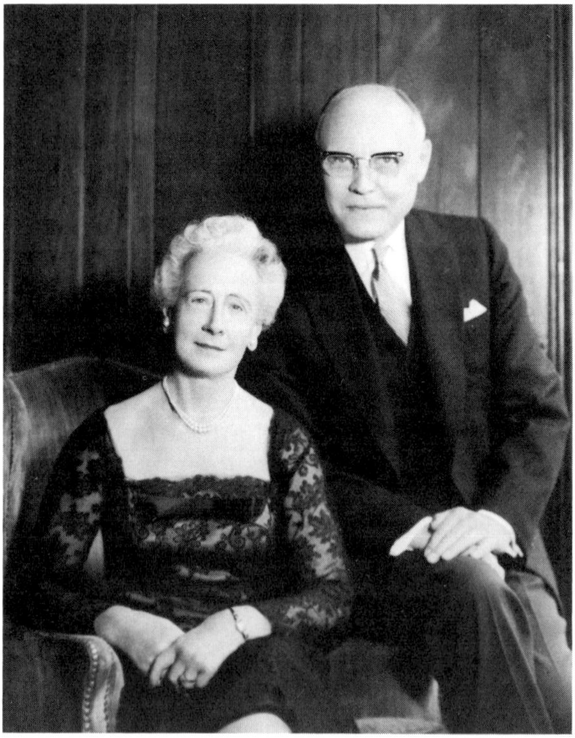

Mrs. Muriel Richardson and Mrs. Gladys Thorlakson were photographed during chat at a Christmas gathering of the families at Mrs. Richardson's home.

Thor and Gladys in their home at 114 Grenfell Boulevard (about 1965)

The Thorlaksons have three children: one daughter, Tannis, who is the wife of George T. Richardson; and twin sons, Ken and Bob, who became surgeons and who are members of the Winnipeg Clinic. The years have added eight grandchildren and four great-grandsons to the immediate family.

There has always been a warm-hearted, responsive and regular sharing of experience between Gladys and Thor and the members of the family circle, both young and old. This is illustrated continuously in the family memorabilia, from which six examples have been selected to provide some sense of the family ties that sustained and renewed the spirit, and gave special character to the public life, of the man presented in this volume.

JOURNEY TO CHURCHILL

On June 26, 1939, Dr. and Mrs. Thorlakson, Kenneth, Robert and Tannis, and Mrs. Thorlakson's sister Florence (known in the family as Frankie) began a trip from Winnipeg to Churchill and return by lake steamer, canoe and train. Kenneth, then in his teens, was appointed logkeeper for this journey, and the following is an excerpt from his record:

Hudson Bay! The fist of ocean thrust into the North American continent, grasping in its clutch tributes from a million square miles. Swing-door between the meadowed lowlands of the Old Land and the hostile north tundra of the New Land.

This was our goal. Our journey was to lead us down the muddy waters of the Red River and the shallow length of Lake Winnipeg by steamer; along wild, wooded shores, across treacherous lakes, and past thundering falls and swirling cataracts of the mighty Nelson by canoe; on steel bands over frozen muskeg by "iron horse" to the mouth of the serpentine Churchill and the broad expanse of Hudson's Bay. Three weeks of brilliant sunshine, flaming sunsets, magnificent scenery, exhilarating fresh air.

After weeks of extensive planning in which the adventurous, overly enthusiastic elements of the family vied with the sober, more logical factions, our big day, Monday, June 26, arrived amid ringing alarm clocks, splashing showers, clattering shoes, and the persistent ringing of the telephone. Orderly confusion broke into a wild stampede. This, in spite of long and careful preparation!

The taxi rolled up at eleven o'clock precisely. Fifteen minutes later the front door swung open and a motley-attired family surged into the sinking cab.

After making stops for last minute indispensables, we tried to make up in speed for precious seconds lost.

We arrived at the dock on the Red River below Drewery's Brewery in a cloud of dust and holding wind-blown hats against feverish brows, ankled into the boat, – the S.S. Keenora. Leisurely the boat left an hour later.

We were finishing dinner when the boat left its moorings at the Drewery Dock. Nan and Grampa Henry and Mary Dyck came as far as Selkirk with us. En route we caught glimpses of grain-sown fields through the green foliage on the banks. The "Keenora" moved past old St. Andrews church.

We looked with mild interest, accepting without appreciation the present peaceful environment, forgetting that not so long ago the Indian considered this Red River Valley his unchallenged hunting ground. This historical panorama passed before us as we were carried down the river to the modern mechanised locks. Perhaps this structure too at some further date will be pointed out to the tourist as an outmoded device of the period.

Arriving at Lockport, we disappeared from view down into the locks. The river is much narrower below this point. The numerous fishing boats and anglers gave credence of the presence of fish. (Mary had to give her 13 cows to Tannis in a game of country white cows they were playing because there was a cemetery at her side of the boat.)

Lower Fort Garry, whose walls have stood unchanged for a century, looked like a thick ribbon of rock among the works of nature. Many of Mother's friends, who were at a luncheon there, came out from the Fort to wave to us.

The "stone fort" was the hub from which Hudson's Bay men controlled vast Rupert's Land. Paved highways have replaced prairie trails, automobiles have taken the place of dog-teams, meticulously attired gentry of today have replaced the buck-skin clad trader of yesteryear.

Approaching Selkirk the ship signaled our arrival with a hoarse bleat of the horn and we sailed through the new draw-bridge. A large portion of the town's younger generation was draped along the dock or splashed about in the water. Being a blistering hot day, Tannis, Bob and I would gladly have joined them. More freight was taken on, including chickens, and a large boiler and a load of bricks destined for the new Indian School at Cross Lake, which is being built by the Dominion Government to replace the school that was burned down twenty years ago. There is a young newlywed couple on the boat by the name of Stevens on their way to serve the church at Cross Lake.

Nanny and Grampa and Mary got on the Winnipeg Electric bus for Winnipeg and we proceeded down the river. We had a long chat with the Captain, Mr. V.C. Hokanson.

As night fell we entered Lake Winnipeg. Two beacons, placed diagonally across the river, had guided the skipper to the mouth of the Red River. Even on the darkest night he is able to steer a course, in or out of the narrow channel by keeping the two lights, constructed at different levels, in line. Twinkling lights from summer cottages dotted the distant shores at Ponemah and Matlock.

After watching our entrance into Lake Winnipeg at about 9:40 p.m., we turned in.

TUESDAY, JUNE 27, 1939 (SECOND DAY)

We were awakened at 4 a.m. by the howling and yelping of huskies on the shores tethered to the trees. The reason for this commotion turned out to be the departure for the northern fishing stations of a large fishing fleet owned by Mr. Sigurdson. From Hecla we continued our journey to Gull Harbour, a summer resort six miles farther north on Big Island (Hecla Island). Here several vacationists disembark with their luggage and two crates of hens which are to supply their owners with new-laid eggs during the summer. One obliging hen has already laid an egg in the crate during the night and is cackling over her achievement in true barnyard fashion.

A dense fog shrouded the lake; consequently the boat moved along cautiously over the calm waters. The fog-horn sounded repeatedly during the morning, much to the annoyance of my sensitive brother Bob. Eventually we were brought to the dock at Jack Pine Bay. Several cords of Jack Pine and Spruce were heaved, log by log, in through the steamer's side for its furnace.

Turning a deaf ear to the protests of all, Frankie and Tannis enthusiastically donned abbreviated bathing suits. The fellow passengers crowded to the rails and one toe in the icy waters warned the swimmers of discomforts to come. In a face saving operation they plunged into the liquid ice. (June 27th) Not to be outdone the rest of the family, including Mom, went in for a swim at the next port of call which was Snake Island.

The next leg of our journey took us to Berens River on the east shore of Lake Winnipeg. We tied up at the new HBC's dock and were met by Mr. Leslie, the manager of the HBC post. After showing us his future house under construction, he directed us down the path toward Mrs. Kemp's "Log Cabin Inn." Mrs. Kemp's son Dick had been a fellow passenger on the S.S. Keenora. He was returning home from Montreal where he was attending school. Dick was very fond of his two dogs, Nig and Beaver, and when he saw them from the boat running along the shore towards the dock he cried because he was so happy to see them again.

Mrs. Kemp, a lively and ambitious lady, is developing a tourist camp at Berens River begun by her husband who died about four years ago. After a visit we started on our way back to the boat. It showed signs of leaving without us and we were forced to scramble over slippery rocks and past amused natives in a most undignified manner in order to catch it.

The Captain piloted the ship across the small bay to another landing where freight was unloaded belonging to Oscar, a fur trader headed for his post at Reindeer Lake. Now this Oscar is quite a fellow about these parts as vouchsafed by Mrs. Kemp. We, however, met him under unfavourable circumstances because he was inebriated all the time aboard ship. He is a successful trader. His cargo consisted of 200 sacks of flour and about 100 parcels of other merchandise for his trading post. When all these goods were delivered on the dock a terrific wind arose and threatened rain. Bob and I decided to assist the plucky Métis and Indians in the work of conveying the pile of goods to shelter in the log storehouse up the hill. Some rain fell on the flour but no serious damage was done.

WEDNESDAY, JUNE 28, 1939 (THIRD DAY)

As the entrance to this harbour is shallow and treacherous, we were unable to leave the dock until early dawn this morning. The ship's engineer, Mr. Anderson, whose home is in Arborg, was good enough to show me around the engine room. Our next port of call is the trading-post and Indian Reserve center at Grand Rapids, situated near the mouth of the Saskatchewan River. The river has its source in the Rockies and empties into the north-west corner of Lake Winnipeg.

About an hour before our departure, the stoker, fireman, engineer, waitresses, and cooks organized a square dance on the dock, and a member of the ship's crew gave his interpretation of the "Irish Washerwoman" with foot and fiddle. The natives joined in, and entered into the spirit of the dance with keenness and great enjoyment. This was the first time that a boat had called here since last October.

THURSDAY, JUNE 29, 1939 (FOURTH DAY)

At 6 a.m. we were rudely awakened by loud clanging of bells and sharp raps on doors. We were informed that we have arrived at Warren's Landing at the mouth of the Nelson River. This gave us an hour and a half to dress, have breakfast, collect and pack our belongings, and transfer them to the Chichame (pronounced Chi-kay-mee).

On the dot of 7:30 a.m. we took leave of the Captain (Hokanson), the mate (Sigurdson), the purser (Tom Pierce) and the engineer (Anderson).

The Chichame is a small tug driven by a Diesel engine which transports passengers and freight up and down the Nelson River between Warren's Landing and Rossville, a distance of twenty-five or thirty miles. Fortunately we had a warm sunshiny day.

The river between Warren's Landing and Norway House is very wide, comparatively shallow, and peppered with rocky islands. As we weaved past islets and hidden shallows a gentle easterly wind vacuumed away the wisps of cloud from the sky and left the sun in undisputed sovereignty. Entering a narrow channel we wound our way between flanking wooded shorelines. Passengers and freight were unloaded at the Mission, Play Green Inn and the historic HBC post of Norway House. Then we crossed Little Playgreen Lake to Rossville, site of the United Church Mission and center of the Indian Reserve.

We were greeted on the dock by Dr. Turpel and Nurse Thomas who led us over the rock-slabbed surface of land to the 14 bed hospital. It was spotlessly clean and so situated that from every window one obtained a beautiful view of land and water. There was an x-ray machine, used chiefly in the diagnosis of tuberculosis. The hospital was staffed by a doctor and three nurses. The rest of the help were local Indians and Métis.

On our way back to the HBC Fort of Norway House across Little Playgreen Lake, the stewardess from the S.S. Keenora, assisted by Dad, served lunch on the boat. Dad had the misfortune to have his clean gray flannels sprinkled with pickle juice!

The Fort, situated on Little Playgreen Lake, derived its name from the fact that it was constructed by a group of Norwegians who had been brought over by the HBC to build a road to the mouth of the Nelson River. Norway House was at one time an important divisional point and distributing center for goods that were transported from York Factory on the Bay into the interior. It was here that Sir George Simpson resided and conducted the affairs of the "Northern Council" of the Hudson's Bay Company. In the old Council House the chair used by Simpson still remains.

In the grounds inside the fort was a sun dial made by Sir John Franklin, the Arctic explorer. It was left at the Fort by his wife when she came through with a search party looking for him.

The original HBC post was built at Montreal Point near Warren's Landing by the group of Norwegians brought over by Lord Selkirk, but it burnt down. That year the Post was built about thirty miles further north at the present location of Norway House. Bachelor's Hall was the residence of the clerks, and is now used by the wireless telegrapher,

Mr. William Crannett, who brought down a message to the wharf this morning sent by Grampa Henry notifying us that Bob and I had passed our exams without one "supp." This was a great relief, and we started upon our northward journey with light hearts.

Round about 1840 the Wesleyan missionary, Rev. James Evans, was establishing missions in the North-west and it was while he was working in the Norway House Territory that he devised the system of syllabic characters which are still used for writing in the Cree language today.

FRIDAY, JUNE 30, 1939 (FIFTH DAY)

Playgreen Inn, our hostel for the next two days, is situated on Fort Channel of the Nelson River. It was built in 1921 by Mr. J.W. Low. It has accommodation for seventy-five guests. The morning was spent leisurely around the Inn. Just before lunch we hiked back to the rocky ridge situated about three-quarters of a mile behind the house.

This has been a restful day. During the afternoon we looked over our supplies and equipment and met Jim Begg, our head guide. This six-foot Cree had been recommended to us as the most competent guide in the North country. At the suggestion of Mr. Learmouth, the Hudson's Bay Factor, we added a third canoe and two Indians (now six) to our party. Two canoes meant four people in each, which with our bedding and other supplies was quite a large load. Jim Begg had sent word over the night before that he wished to "sample us down" in the canoes in order that he might decide how to distribute the load. It was during this "sampling down" process that we found we needed the extra canoe.

After the final details had been arranged Dr. Turpel took us by boat into Little Playgreen Lake, over to Forestry Island where Mr. and Mrs. Durant received us most hospitably.

Mr. Durant is in charge of the Forestry Service. Apart from a three year period around 1928 he has been in this part of the country since 1918. There is an eighty-five foot observation tower on the island. Frankie, Bob, Tannis and I climbed the tower and had a wonderful view of the surrounding country. On the way down at the seventy-five foot level, my coloured glasses decided to descend ahead of me and corkscrew down to the rocks below. They broke in a thousand pieces. Coloured glasses are very necessary here as the glare of the sun on the water is hard on one's eyes.

During our stay at Norway House we bought several articles of Indian handicraft – many coloured, beaded gauntlets, wristlets, mocassins, head-bands. We also bought a harness which Bob and I wore when we helped carry some of our baggage over the portages.

Saturday, July 1,1939 (sixth day)
Up bright and early this morning. Beautiful sunshiny weather. Our six Indians arrived shortly with the three canoes. We were soon packed and ready, so we set off immediately for the Fort. About halfway to the Fort we saw the demolished remains of the last York boat which carried freight from Oxford House to Norway House. This boat was beached ten to fifteen years ago. It is unfortunate that this relic of the past – the last boat to do duty of this kind, thereby closing a period in the transportation of this country – was not salvaged and kept on exhibit at the Fort by the HBC. Its ribs jut out from the surface of the water to mark its grave.

At the Fort we took on our tents and food supplies, took leave of Mr. Learmouth, and headed our canoes towards the north. We were paddled across "Little Playgreen Lake" down the Nelson River for about five miles. We landed at an old deserted dock about 11 o'clock. Some of our men had not eaten since 4 a.m. as they had a long distance to come to the Fort, so they were ready to have lunch. We ourselves seemed to be always hungry at this latitude. Our bill of fare consisted of pork and beans, bread and butter, jam, pickles and coffee. This does not conform with Mother's idea of a diet for growing children, but time and place changes everything, even our daily habits. Dr. Turpel informed us that he saw practically no patients with indigestion amongst the people up here, nor in twelve years had he seen a case of acute appendicitis. Probably partly cooked meats and fish, eaten out in the fresh air, is what nature intended for our stomachs.

While we were finishing our lunch the men prepared poles. To these poles they tied the canvas floors of our tents for sails, which they set in the hole of the crossbar on the bow of the boats. As we pushed away from the dock we unfurled our sails and with a fair south wind our little flotilla glided down the Nelson River.

About 4 o'clock we could hear the roar of the first falls, Sea Falls, situated about twenty miles below Norway House. This proved to be an easy portage. As the wind had died down we had to go back to our oars and paddles. By this time the weather had changed completely. The sky was overcast with black threatening clouds, and before we had gone a mile the first few drops began to fall. Jim Begg, our guide, decided to pitch camp immediately. The three canoes were beached on the sloping rocks and in just no time our tents were pitched, our bedding under cover and our campfire lit. We seemed to have been very fortunate in our crew, they are all very quick and alert, clean and tidy.

We used one of our tents for an eating house before spreading our bedding. Our supper consisted of canned fried sausage (Pat Burns variety), bread and butter, scrambled eggs, strawberry jam and canned peaches, a sumptuous repast eaten to the tune of the pitter-patter on our tent top. By 8 o'clock we were set for bed with our mosquito bars in place. Mother, Frankie and Tannis in one tent consisting of a low canvas roof, under which they suspend their mosquito bars. All four sides are open. This is not a bad idea for summer as they get the full benefit of all the breezes. And, so to bed.

This brought to a close the first day of our canoe journey. We tucked ourselves in warmly between our blankets and fell asleep to the tune of the distant waterfall, and to the closer hum of the mosquitoes.

Good-night.

SUNDAY, JULY 2, 1939 (SEVENTH DAY)

My gosh! What mosquitoes. Compared with these, our southern variety fade into insignificance. A few of them got under our nets during the night and had apparently gorged themselves at our expense. Someone had said that one mosquito holds up the curtain while the others file in. At any rate they are as companionable as a pack of wild cats, they truly eat you alive. Yesterday Dad asked Jim if he had a gun along. Jim said yes. Dad asked if he could bag some wild ducks along the way. Jim replied, "No, the gun isn't for ducks but to shoot mosquitoes!" However, in fact, we have not been troubled greatly with mosquitoes so far so we can't complain.

We were awakened by Jim at 6 o'clock and as soon as we were dressed, preparations were immediately begun for our first breakfast on the trail. We washed our face and teeth at the edge of the river, leaning over the edge of a convenient flat rock.

At 6:30 our men had finished their own breakfast, went over to the edge of the camping ground, seated themselves in a circle and conducted early Sunday service and prayer. I wonder who are the heathens on this trip? By 8 o'clock we were in our canoes and off.

Today has been a most thrilling day for us. We have made several short portages past waterfalls and rapids. This is surely a canoeist's paradise. We have already found it necessary to change our ideas of the Nelson River. In reality this first section of the river is made up of a series of lakes connected by numerable channels. The entire waterway is strewn with rocky, pine covered islands. We have had several showers of rain today, which forced us to nose our canoes into the reeds. The guides would then cover everything (and everybody) in the canoe with rubber tarpaulins and canvas. In this way everything in the canoe is kept dry and we proceeded on our way after each shower.

We discovered that when the Indians think it is time to eat they always asked us if we wanted to "boil a kettle," so that from now on we do not have breakfast, lunch and dinner as is the custom at home, we simply "boil a kettle" and eat, whenever the spirit moves us. We had our mid-day "boil kettle" at Sugar Falls.

About 4:30 the sky looked very black, and it seemed as though we might be in for a long rain so we decided to land and pitch one tent for cover. A roaring camp fire was immediately started, and after a brief conference with Jim Begg it was decided to "boil another kettle" here. Our supper consisted of fried corn beef (very good), hot canned spinach and butter and canned apricots. The odd corners of our stomachs, which seemed to be harder to fill each day, were packed with bread and honey.

After this the wind, which had been blowing from the west, veered around to the north, the clouds began to break, the rain stopped and the air became distinctly cooler. It was now decided that we push on and try to reach and cross "Pipestone Lake" before nightfall. Tannis, Bob and I had a good workout on our paddles and Dad spelled off one of the rowers on the oars.

We passed a group of Indians who were busy repairing their outboard motor. They were returning to Cross Lake with their children who had been attending the United Church Mission School at Rossville. This was on the Pipestone River about 6 p.m. (Pipestone River is apparently a small section of the Nelson River which enters Pipestone Lake). At 7:30 we paddled into Pipestone Lake and as it was quite calm we crossed it. At this point the lake was five miles across. We were told that travellers can be windbound here as long as two days because the lake can get very rough making it unsafe to cross in canoes. It was beautiful on the lake, the sky had cleared, and the sun was setting in the west.

Pipestone Lake receives its name from a soft slate coloured rock from which the Indians carve out with a knife the bowls of their pipes – the pipes of peace. The stems are made from the branches of the wild honeysuckle which has a hollow centre about ¼ to ⅓ of an inch in diameter.

At 9 p.m. we had picked out our camp site on an island near the mouth of the river which takes us out of this lake, and situated about five miles south of Cross Lake. Everything on the island was soaking wet from the rains, but it was surprising how quickly our men had hewn out a camp site and pitched our two tents. Every man had his own task and sets to it immediately he sets foot on shore. It is interesting to see how quickly they made a camp fire, even after a drenching rain. One man scurries up along the shore and brings back three or four dead trees from which he makes small shavings with his sharp axe. The inner part of the tree is of course dry. Another man goes up under some of the large pine trees, breaking off some small dry twigs which are sheltered from the rain. In this way a roaring fire is begun in just a few moments and after a chilly ride across the lake we gathered ourselves around its welcome warmth. By 10 o'clock we were all settled under mosquito bars for the night; and are we sleepy and tired after a long day! And thus ended our second day in the wilderness.

MONDAY, JULY 3, 1939 (EIGHTH DAY)
We left our island encampment about 8:30 a.m. after a good night's rest and a substantial breakfast. I marvel at Mother's and Frankie's appetite for breakfast at 7 o'clock in the morning, as they sit on hard granite rock for a chair. We reached Cross Lake at 9:45 a.m.

Our next point of call was at the Hudson's Bay Company post across the Bay where we were received and welcomed most hospitably by Mr. Jack Denton the Manager (and his niece Miss Una Carver). By this time the sun was beating down upon us unmercifully and were we glad to be taken in under cover at the Company home. Mother and Frankie were feeling a little ill from the sun, in fact Mr. Denton said that Frankie looked as though she had been on a binge but hadn't had much fun. She (Frankie) was put to bed and by six o'clock had made a complete recovery except that her nose was still very red – from the sun! We met again Mr. and Mrs. Stevens who were getting settled in the manse of the United Church of Canada. . . .

TUESDAY, JULY 4, 1939 (NINTH DAY)
We had a real breakfast this morning at Mr. Denton's and set out again on our journey refreshed and rested. We had taken leave of Mr. Denton at the docks and so you can imagine our pleasure at seeing him catch up to us in his canoe and outboard motor a few miles above Whitemud Falls. Mr. Denton towed our three canoes behind his for the rest of the trip to the Falls where we all stopped for a lunch. During the morning Edward told us that if we tied a pail to the bow of the canoe and threw it overboard that the pail would fill with water, sink into the strong under-current and pull the canoe downstream. He also told us the same idea was used in the early days by the men on the large York boats in that they tied large logs to a rope weighted down with rocks and allowed the current to carry the boat downstream while all the crew slept. . . .

WEDNESDAY, JULY 5, 1939 (TENTH DAY)
We were aroused about 6:30 by Jim Begg announcing through the tent flap that the day was going to be fine. We had breakfast, packed and were out by 8 o'clock. We hadn't travelled very far before we came to Hill Rapids which meant another portage. While the men were carrying our supplies and canoes over the ridge four of us walked around the point to the falls. The rock formation at this point was rather interesting. There were huge boulders, igneous rocks, mostly granite, with many intrusions. There was one particularly large slab on the surface

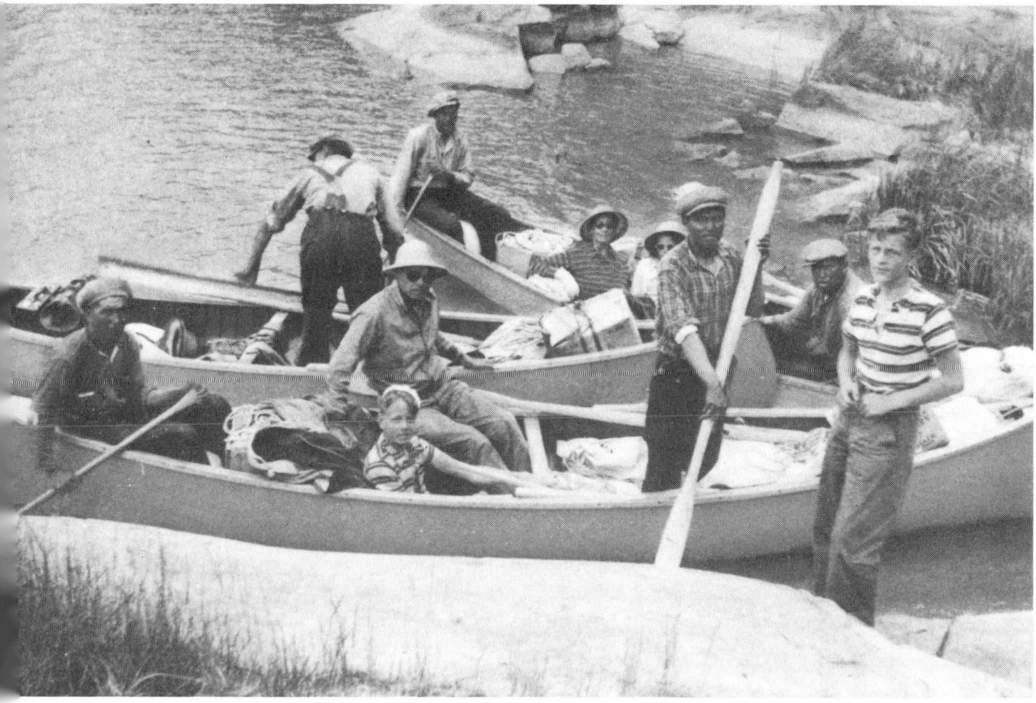

ing just run a stretch of rapids on the Nelson River, the canoes have been aded in readiness to proceed on the next leg of the Thorlakson family journey iscovery in the North.

of which there were large parallel grooves running in a north-south direction, which at first sight suggested glacial scour. Bob, however, thinks that the markings are of more recent origin and probably due to ice weathering. About a mile below the rapids our guide spotted an Indian who was probably fishing for sturgeon. Dad took one of the canoes up the river and returned shortly with a fifteen to twenty pound live sturgeon which had just been taken out of the nets. He paid a dollar for the fish. Sturgeons are caught that weigh as much as 150 pounds, so this was not a large one but it was just the right size for our party. We had a rather long overland portage by foot, but the guides took the canoes and supplies through the rapids. We paddled up a small stream for quite a distance before our portage. At one spot we saw the deep hoof marks of a moose. At another point there was evidence of recent activity by the beavers. There was evidence here of large scale transportation operation from the earlier days. Across the muskeg in the centre of the portage were old logs and at one end were some old dilapidated log buildings.

THURSDAY, JULY 8, 1939 (ELEVENTH DAY)

This had been a very exciting and eventful day on our cruise down the Sipiwesk Lake, which derives its Indian name from the fact that it is half river and half lake. We saw mink over on the bank scampering for cover. A little further down we saw a large moose in among the reeds at the water's edge. These animals are being forced out of the woods by the vicious bull flies which are pest number two at this time of the year. While we were having lunch a ground hog came out of its burrow near our campsite. At high noon the sun was fiercely beating down upon us so our guides built us a wigwam-shaped leafy arbor. This was made of young poplar trees; the upper half had branches laden with leaves. These branches were woven together to form a perfect shade overhead. This was supplemented further by a piece of canvas on the south exposure.

After lunch a favorable wind came up again so we set sail once more. Think of our consternation when we discovered by 4 o'clock that we were lost in Sipiwesk Lake. The channel that we were on was taking us to the eastward instead of to the northwest. In other words the sun was at our backs instead of in front of us. If you look at the map and examine Sipiwesk Lake you can easily understand how an inexperienced traveller could be lost for days wandering about the islands and inlets of this bizarre body of water. With the assistance of our aerial maps (which had been sent down to Dad by special messenger to the boat from the office of the Minister of Mines and Natural Resources, the Hon. Mr. John McDiarmid), our guides and Dad had us back up into the main current by 8 o'clock.

FRIDAY, JULY 17, 1939 (TWELFTH DAY)
At 7 o'clock this morning the whole family betook themselves down to the edge of the water and went in for a morning plunge. By 9 o'clock we were packed and ready to go and set the bows of our canoes into the Nelson River towards the north east. We soon came upon some fishermen who were busily engaged in pulling in their nets. Apparently the sturgeon fishing has not been very successful this year. We next landed at Cross Portage where we met Mr. Freeman, a partner in the firm of Johnson and Freeman, traders in this territory. Mr. Freeman arranged to have one of his men transport by horse and cart our heavy equipment and supplies across the portage.

From Sabomin Lake we went through a narrow winding creek, not more than eight feet wide, bounded by tall reeds, and in its still waters there was a luxuriant growth of water lilies. At the edge of this creek we came upon a variety of white lily which none of us had seen before. . . .

SATURDAY, JULY 8, 1939 (THIRTEENTH DAY)
It is now 9:30 in the morning and we are still in bed under our mosquito bars. It has been raining most of the night and there is a steady pour this morning. The lake is quite rough and it is quite possible that we may not be able to cross it in our canoes today. Under these circumstances it is better to remain in our beds under cover until hunger drives us forth. We three men are in one tent and the ladies in the other. We are wondering what breakfast we can take to them. Times have certainly changed since Grandfather was a boy! In those good old days the ladies would have been worrying about *our* breakfast.

The rain stopped and the sun came forth in a blaze of glory about 11:30 o'clock. After a brief conference it was decided to have a swim and "brunch" (a combination of breakfast and lunch) and then be on our way down Landing Lake. As we had about only twelve miles to travel, and as our train did not go through Thicket Portage until 12 midnight, we had plenty of time on our hands. . . .

We landed at the dock about 7 o'clock. Dad, Frankie and the six guides walked up to the Village of Thicket Portage. As it had rained heavily the road was slippery and muddy. Dad made arrangements with Mr. Peterson, the manager of the Johnson and Freeman store, to have a team sent down for the rest of the family and the baggage. Mr. and Mrs. Peterson had kindly invited us to stay in their house until the train time. Mrs. Peterson and a Mrs. Baldwinson served us a cup of good hot Icelandic coffee, sandwiches and cake. Dad also visited Mr. and Mrs. Miller whom he had met on the trail up from the lake. When he saw how tanned Dad was he said, "When I saw you in the W.G.H.

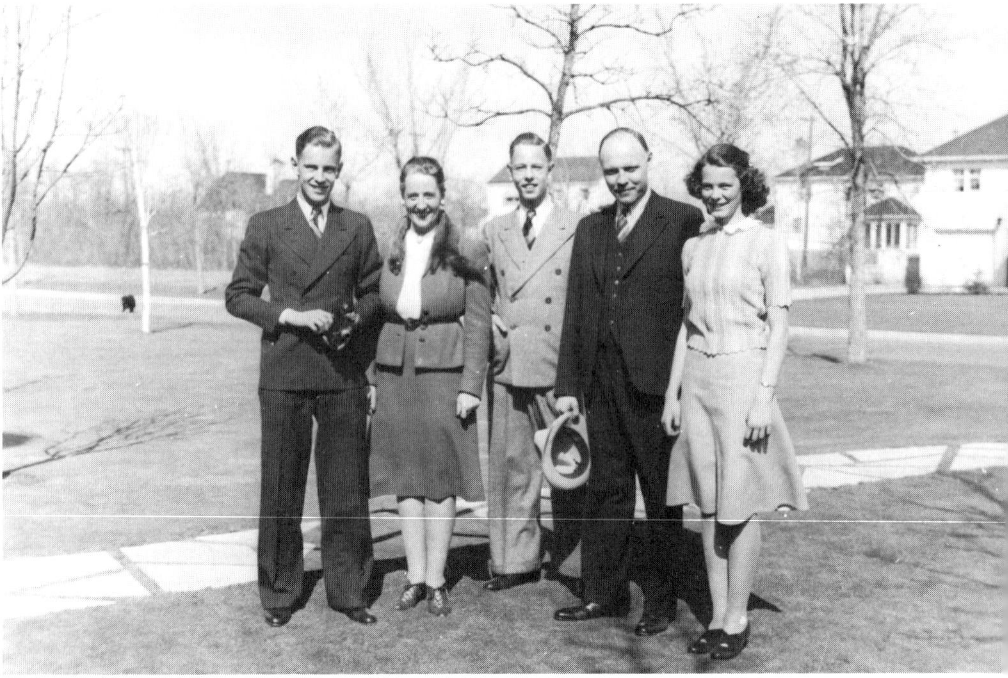

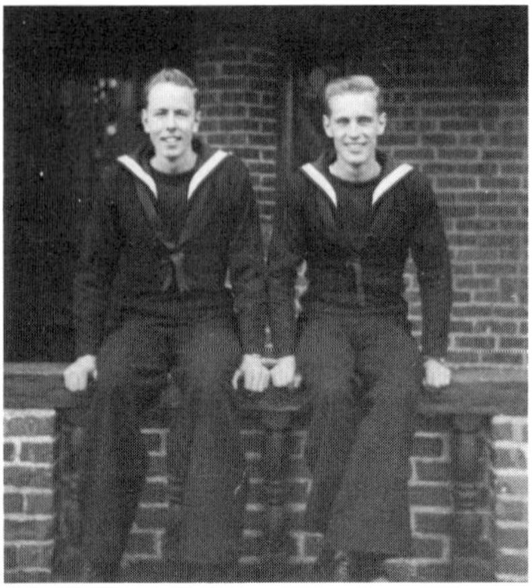

Home from church, left to right: Bob, Gladys, Ken, Thor, Tannis

After completing their first year in medical college, Ken and Bob joined the Roy[al] Canadian Navy in 1944.

you were a white man." Mr. Miller runs a general store and is the local postmaster.

Dr. Kjarton I. Johnson from The Pas arrived at Thicket Portage during the evening on his open gas car. A trunk on the front of his "car" contained his medical equipment and supplies. Dr. Johnson makes this trip twice a month to attend to the sick along the railway line. Dr. Trimble at The Pas is the Chief Medical Officer for the CN Railway in these regions.

Our guides stayed at the store until train time and then loaded our baggage onto the train. They seemed genuinely sorry to see us leave, we felt sorry also for they had been responsible for our care and comfort on what could otherwise have been a miserable experience. Bob and I stood on the steps as the train began to pull away. One of our guide friends ran alongside the train calling out repeatedly, "Bobby Boy, I will never forget you, I will never forget you." . . .

The adventurers continued from Thicket Portage to Churchill by train and, after holidaying for ten days at Flin Flon, went back to Winnipeg, which was reached at the end of July.

SIXTIETH WEDDING ANNIVERSARY

On November 9, 1980, the sixtieth wedding anniversary of Dr. and Mrs. Thorlakson was celebrated at a reception held at Briarmeade. Dr. Kenneth Thorlakson proposed a toast:

On behalf of the family, I wish to thank you all for coming out to Briarmeade this afternoon to share with our family this celebration of Mother's and Dad's sixtieth wedding anniversary.

Sixty years ago, the young Manitoba couple, "Dr. Thor" from Selkirk and Gladys Maree Henry from Killarney were married in Calgary, Alberta, at the home of the bride's parents, Robert and Elizabeth Henry. The groom's parents, the Reverend Niels and Erica Thorlaksson, had travelled from Selkirk to be present. The groom's father performed the holy rights of matrimony. This was the beginning of one of the happiest and most successful marriages, as everyone here today can attest.

There are many similarities between today's celebration and the one on that afternoon so many years ago. For instance we are gathered in a family home, one as noted for the warmth of its hospitality as was the home of the Henrys.

Today the weatherman has arranged a little snow, a gentle reminder of the blizzard which struck Calgary on that day in 1920; but he has also provided a little Manitoba sunshine to grace the occasion.

According to this morning's forecast, Winnipeg is the only city in Canada where the sun is shining today. Pierre Trudeau must have arranged this especially for us Westerners!

The Stampeders are in town today to represent the city of Calgary; a city which has exploded into prominence, but which on that day in 1920, because of the blizzard, could only generate enough gas pressure to barely heat its homes and hotels.

There are some differences in the two events. In 1920, western pioneer parents were there. In 1980, the great-grandchildren of these pioneers are here. Also, today's celebration is on November 9 (one day early). After all, as Karen's husband Frank Somers points out, Dr. Thor has to be down at the Clinic seeing patients tomorrow!

I know that Mother and Dad treasure the statement made by David Richardson when he spoke on behalf of the grandchildren on the occasion of their fiftieth wedding anniversary. What he said in part, I am sure he would agree, should be said again today, and I quote:

"We have been very fortunate that our grandparents live in the same city. Throughout the years they have played an active part in our lives and aided our development. They have attended school closings, sports events, and out-of-school activities. Even when it was not convenient they made us feel that it was the very thing they wanted to be doing at that time."

It is small wonder that these past sixty years have been happy and rewarding years. Those of us here today admire the thoughtfulness and devotion which Mother and Dad have had for each other.

There were other qualities which they shared with their family and their many friends. In our family home, as in our grandparents' homes on both sides of the family, there was active participation in community affairs as well as a keen interest in books and learning, in music, in travel and a great affection for animals.

There was a great awareness of one's cultural background. Three young grandchildren (David, Hartley, and Derek) were taken to their country of origin by their grandfather, who later, in 1974 addressed the government and people of Iceland on behalf of the government and people of Canada to commemorate the arrival of the first settlers in Iceland in 874.

The love of books and learning was evident outside the home by Mother's twelve years on the Board of Governors at the University of Manitoba and Dad's Chancellorship of the University of Winnipeg.

There was great affection for animals. How can Bob, Tannis or I forget that summer in 1930 when we arrived in the family Huppmobile at Ponemah Beach with a Boston terrier, two cats, two rabbits, a

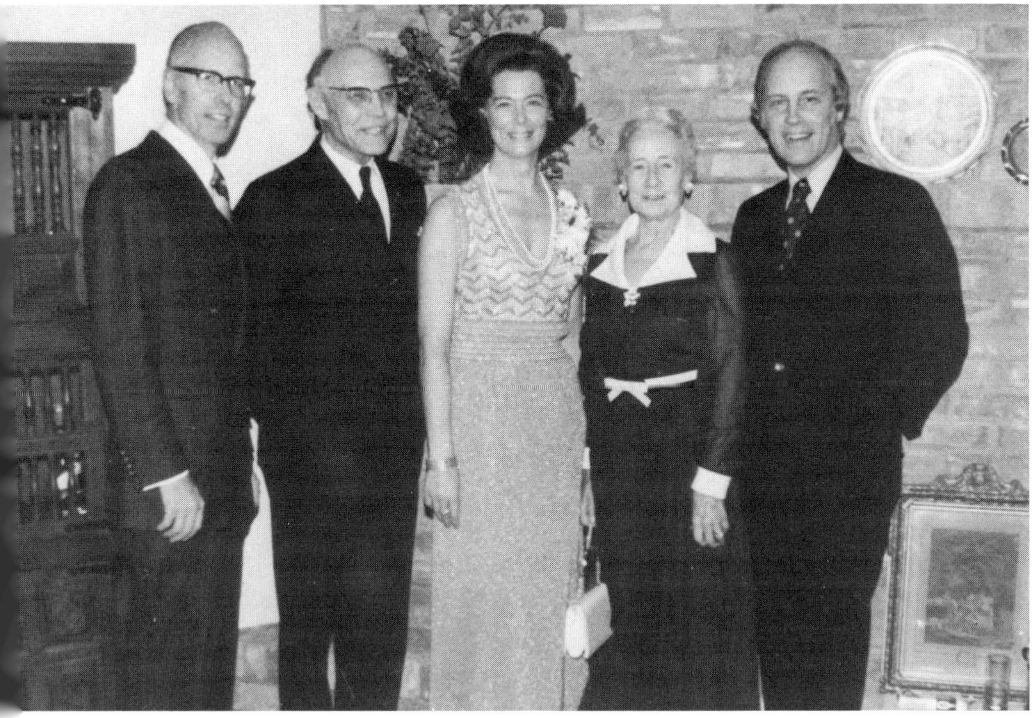

nnis on her twenty-fifth wedding anniversary, with her parents and
r brothers.

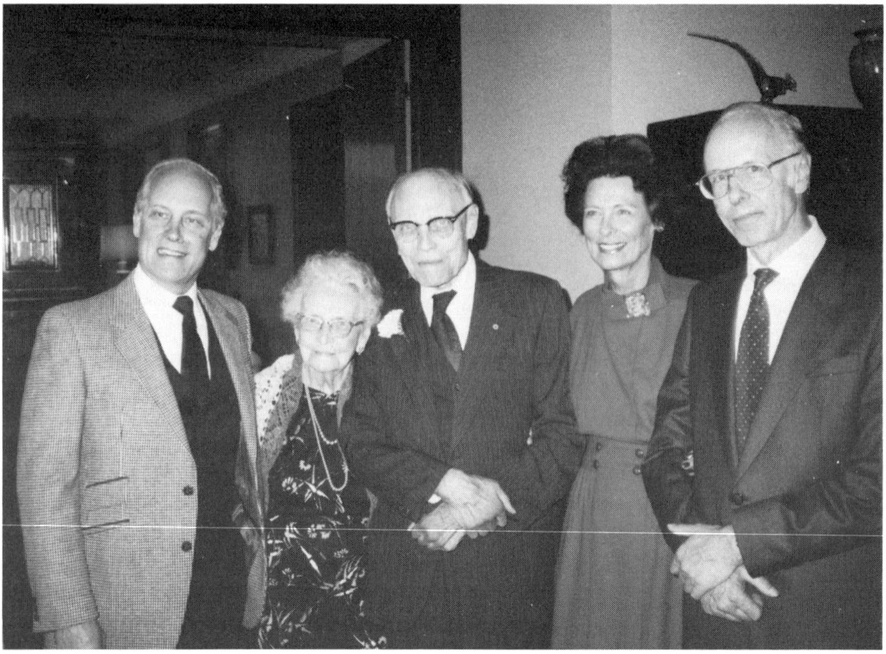

Dr. Thorlakson's ninetieth birthday was celebrated at Briarmeade, the home of Mr. and Mrs. George Richardson. Enjoying the party are Dr. Thorlakson and his sister Margrethe Sigmar of Seattle, with Robert, Tannis and Kenneth.

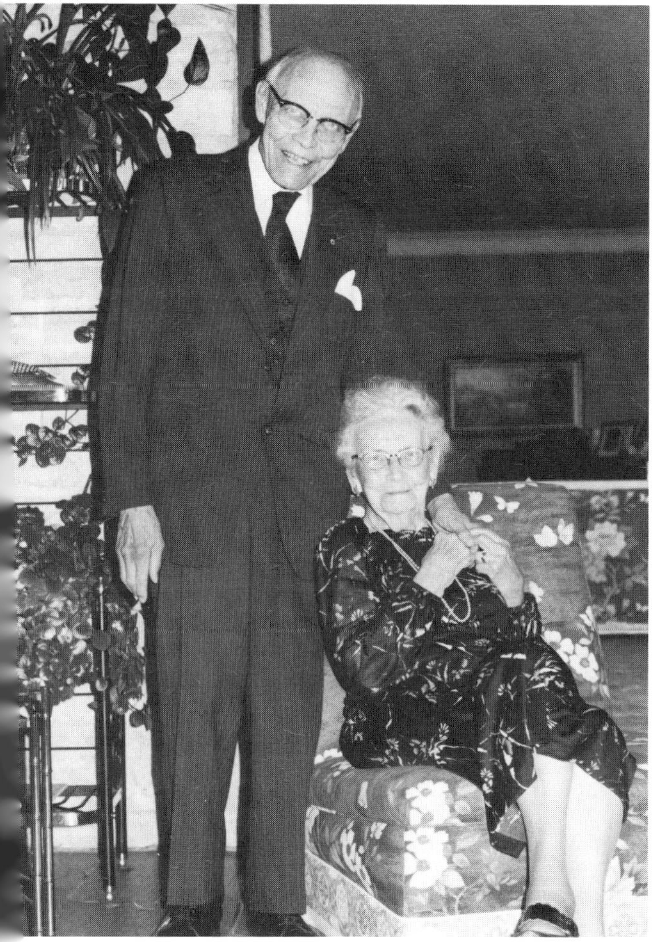

Thorlakson's sister Margrethe, age 94, came
n Seattle for his birthday celebration, to which
contributed a delightful speech.

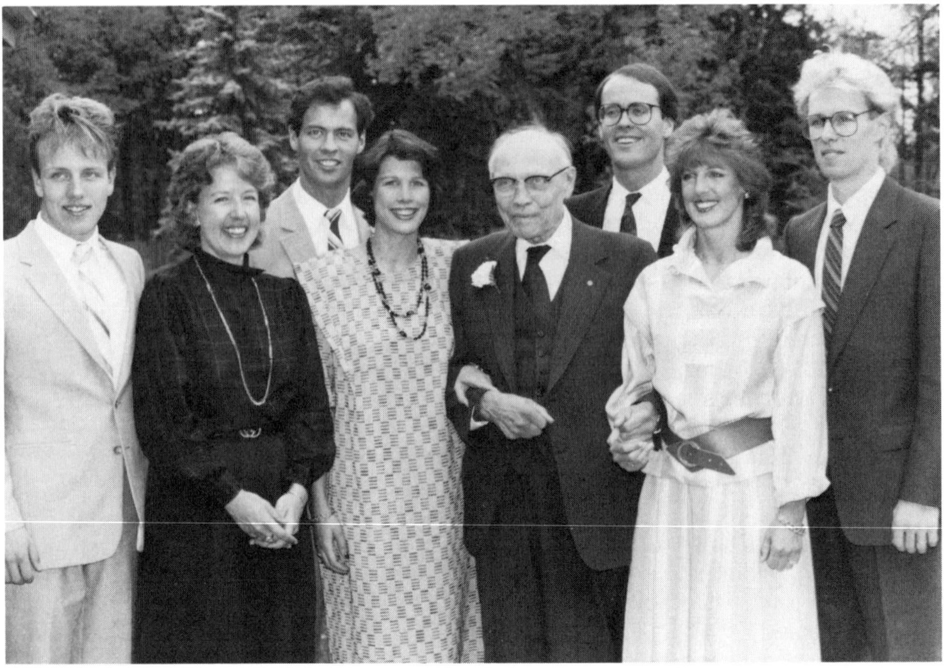

Dr. Thorlakson with his grandchildren on his ninetieth birthday. Left to right: Ian and Carla Thorlakson, David, Karen and Hartley Richardson, Patricia and Derek Thorlakson.

canary and a guinea pig! There was always a dog or two chasing alongside our bikes and horses on which we learned to ride and to compete. Today, some of the grandchildren are as at home in the saddle as Mother was, as a girl on her cutting-horse Bonnie.

There was always music in the home, as manifest by the sweet (and sometimes not so sweet!) sounds of the violin, the piano and of singing.

Mother and Dad shared a great interest in other countries of the world and travelled extensively. The Far East held a special attraction because Dad's brother, our Uncle Tavi, was a missionary in Kobe, Japan, and Mother's sister, our Aunt Florence, taught school in Canton and Shanghai.

This legacy has continued. Tannis and George travel extensively to all parts of the world. Bob and Fran as well as Lorna and I lived for five years in Britain. The grandchildren have lived for various periods in France, Switzerland, Australia, Italy, and now England.

But perhaps the greatest virtue of the couple we honor today was their respect and love of people – their close friends, colleagues and good neighbors.

Every one here this afternoon has a special place in the hearts and memories of Mother and Dad.

Mom and Dad, we, your family and your friends, are grateful to you for sharing some part of these wonderful sixty years with each one of us.

We congratulate you on your sixtieth wedding anniversary, and hope that you may be granted many more years with us in health and happiness.

Ladies and gentlemen, would you all join with me in a toast to Dr. and Mrs. Thorlakson . . . Gladys and Thor . . . Grandfather and Grandmother . . . Mother and Dad.

"SAID MY MUSE . . . 'LOOK IN THY HEART AND WRITE'"

Pamela Richardson, the daughter of Mr. and Mrs. George T. Richardson, and Dr. Thor's grand-daughter, gave early evidence of a fine mind and a happy and generous disposition. In school, she enjoyed learning, and valued her friendship with other children and her teachers.

But at the age of nine, she was diagnosed as a diabetic, and by her early teens her sight was gone. Nevertheless, Pamela was courageous and persistent, and scarcely faltered in her studies. She attended the Collegiate Division of the University of Winnipeg, passing her grades with flying colors. She was able to travel, with pleasure, to other parts of Canada. Nevertheless, with the passage of time the burden of her increasing ill health grew heavy, and Pamela died in 1980.

In 1968, while she was in grade eleven, Pamela submitted an entry in the High School Historical Research Essay Contest of the Red River Valley Historical Society. She was a first place winner, and her essay was published in the summer, 1968 edition of the Society's bulletin, the "Red River Valley Historian." The subject: "Dr. P.H.T. Thorlakson, Member of a Great Family Heritage."

In this well-researched and well-documented biographical essay, Pamela wrote of her grandfather's life and accomplishments, both personal and professional. Quoted below are some excerpts from her essay; stories of his early life, and observations on Dr. Thor's attributes and character as they presented themselves to the perceptive intellect and sensitive spirit of his sixteen-year-old grand-daughter:

. . . Many unconnected incidents in Paul's youth portray his character. One of the most shocking experiences was the time he first heard his older brother Octavius say "damn." Paul realized swearing was a great sin. He went out and sat on a woodpile in the backyard of the parsonage and conjured up a vivid picture in his imagination of his mother and father and their other five children sitting comfortably up in heaven peering down in the nether regions and witnessing the tortures of this poor degenerate soul who had fallen from grace and foresworn his prospects of eternal salvation. Octavius redeemed himself by becoming a missionary in the foreign field.

Paul's older sister and friends were making Christmas flowers one night around the living room table when the parsonage bell rang. Paul opened the front door. The visitor was the young and handsome president of the Lutheran League, Mr. B.S. Benson. After the young ladies' excitement had died down and work had resumed, Mr. Benson called Paul over to him. Mr. Benson gave Paul twenty five cents to get a bag of chocolates at the confectionary. Paul brought home a big paper bag filled with the best chocolates. The purchase of these chocolates made a great impression on Paul's young mind – to him it seemed incredible that any man would spend a whole quarter for chocolates on a bunch of girls! . . .

The day before a meeting of the Ladies Aid Society had been arranged, Paul's mother had injured her knee, but Mrs. Thorlaksson insisted on attending. She suggested that Paul drive her on his sled be-

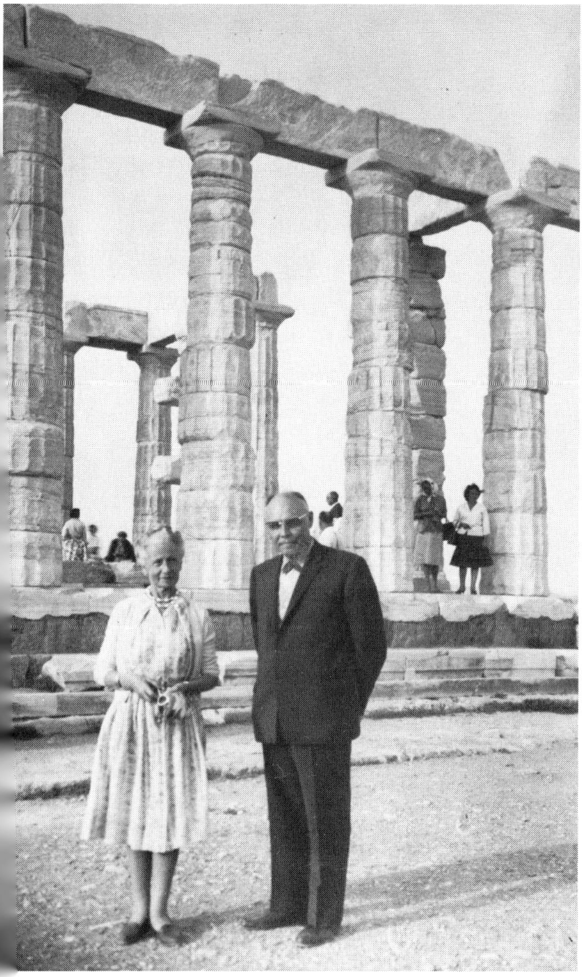

r. and Mrs. Thorlakson visited the Temple of oseidon at Sounion during a brief stay in reece en route to Beirut, Lebanon, where he d been invited to be a guest speaker at the welfth Middle East Medical Assembly at the merican University. His subject was Regional Enteritis."

cause at that time he was the proud possessor of a large and powerful husky dog by the name of Quick. Paul ran as hard as he could to keep up with the sled as they travelled across town. Suddenly the road took a sharp turn and Mrs. Thorlaksson was dumped into a deep snowbank. Her peals of laughter rang loud as she lay in the soft snow and absolved Paul from any responsibility for the accident.

Following the stories of her subject's youth, Pamela wrote in some detail about him under the headings "career and accomplishments"; "family"; "publications"; "travels"; and a "concluding summary". A sense of her youthful writing skill, and an author's struggle to retain objectivity in writing about someone she loves, shines through her narrative:

Paul has three brothers and two sisters. Octavius, the eldest son, is a Lutheran minister and was a missionary in Japan for twenty-five years. Margrethe was a school teacher prior to her marriage to the Rev. D.H. Sigmar who, at one time, was the president of the Icelandic Lutheran Synod. Frederick graduated in medicine from the University of Manitoba and subsequently specialized on opthalmology. Halfdan recently retired from the position of Comptroller of the Hudson's Bay Company in Vancouver. Erika, the youngest member of the family, married an attorney, Mr. Harold Eastvold of Seattle. . . .

Dr. Thorlakson has travelled to numerous places to reap new knowledge, give papers, and discover new people and lands. . . . [In Lebanon, he] and his wife walked over the excavated ruins of the ancient cities of Byblos and Baalbek. They spent five days visiting the Holy Places of the New Testament in and [beyond] the Old City of Jerusalem, in the Hashemite Kingdom of Jordan. Included in the tour were Bethlehem, Bethany, Jericho, the River Jordan, the Dead Sea, the Mount of Olives, the Garden of Gethsemane and the Way of the Cross.

They cruised for seven days on the Aegean Sea visiting several of the islands. Rhodes, the Isle of Roses, was the site of one of the seven wonders of the world, the Colossus of Rhodes, and a stronghold of the Knights Hospitalers of St. John of Jerusalem. By ship they then went through the Dardanelles, across the Sea of Marmora and up the Bosporus to Istanbul, Turkey. . . .

As I conclude my essay with a summary of this man, I feel a strong sense of pride, respect and love for him. To say that Dr. Thorlakson is loved by all who know him is far from being sentimental and inappropriate. The love and gratitude people feel for this man is genuine. In doing an essay on William Worrol Mayo, I dedicated the biography to Dr. Paul Thorlakson in this way: "This essay is respectfully dedicated to my dear, wonderful grandfather, Dr. Paul H.T. Thorlakson, whose genuine interest in history has always inspired mine and without whose help this essay could not have been possible."

Yes, it is true, this man about whom I have so glowingly written is my grandfather! I am prejudiced, but in no way have exaggerated; his traits are self-evident. He has always given me a broader outlook on history. . . . Without his many articles, I could not have reaped such a personal account of his life. He is articulate in speech and an interesting, descriptive writer.

Grandpa enjoys and takes all he can from life, but he always gives much in return. He is a dedicated doctor and in his seventies still finds much to interest him. I literally and truthfully say he can do almost anything – play a skillful game of cribbage or bridge, delve into his mind for a segment of interesting and informative knowledge and still on the average put in a full working day, until last year due to his extensive travelling, lectures and speeches. . . .

I have remained as a writer until the end, and kept the secret of my identity, as grand-daughter, until now because I wanted to write just true, unbiased facts and save my feelings and opinions to the end. It gives me a great deal of pleasure to tell you about my grandfather. I hope if you do not know him now, you will feel as if you do. At sixteen, I realize I am subjective, and have access to a wonderful, educated man. My grandfather does not know I am writing this essay, because if I told him, I would hope he would be proud, but I know his modesty would soften some of my statements and opinions. So as not to seem too sentimental, which sometimes bores a reader and makes truth seem hazy, I will stop by saying, "Grandpa, I love you, with a pride for your dedication and devotion. Thank you for making my heritage part of your quest."

FOURTH VISIT TO ICELAND

Of Dr. Thorlakson's five visits to Iceland, this was the only one on which Mrs. Thorlakson did not accompany him. It was her contention that this visit should be a project exclusively for her husband and those of his grandsons old enough to make the trip, David Richardson, eighteen at the time, Hartley Richardson, sixteen, and Derek Thorlakson, twelve years old. On June 10, 1971, Dr. Thorlakson wrote to Mrs. Thorlakson from the Hotel Holt in Reykjavik:

Dear Gladys:

We have been in Iceland for one week. Already we have travelled and seen more of the country than on any previous visit. No tour leader has

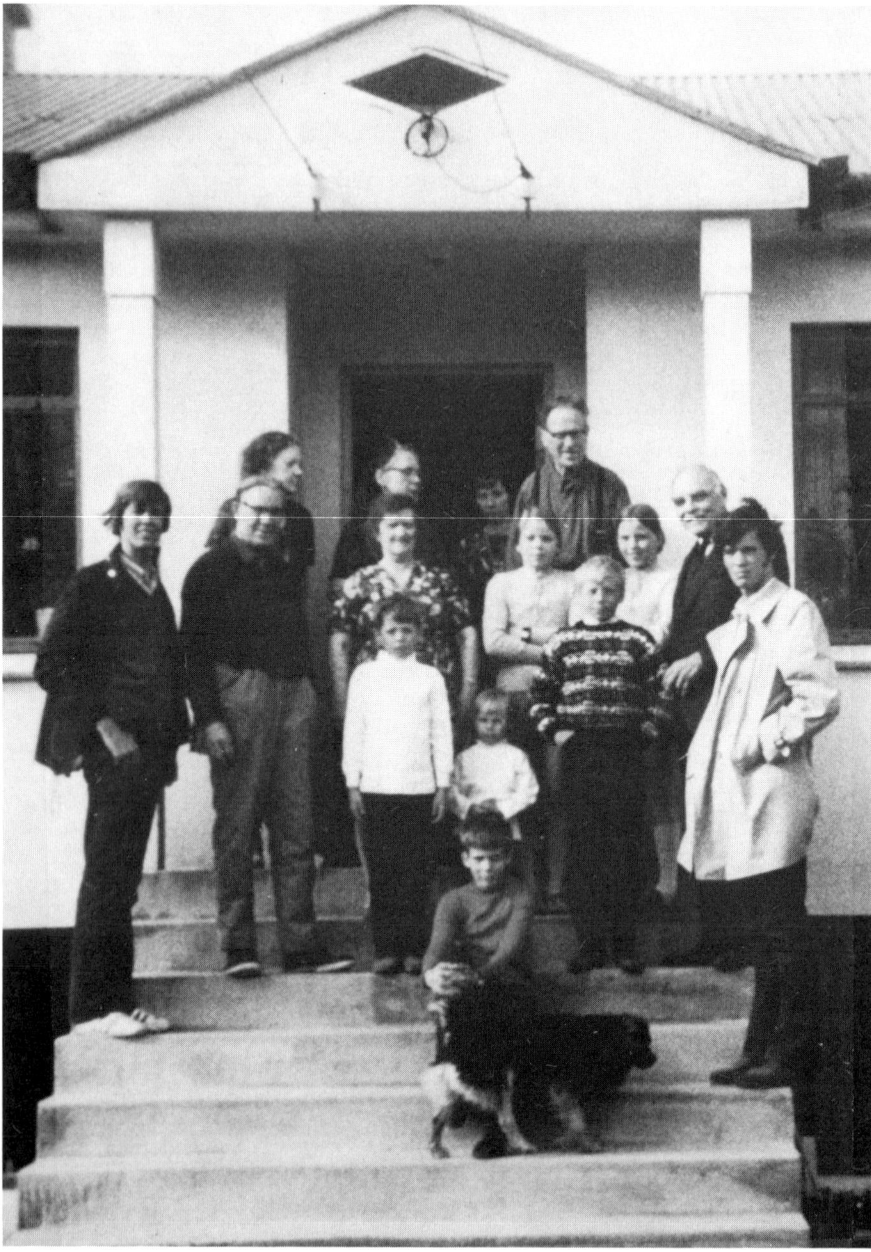

In 1971 Dr. Thorlakson took his three grandsons to Iceland to acquaint them with the land of their forefathers. Pictured here is a schoolhouse that stands on a farmstead at Storu-Tjarnir, which was the home of Dr. Thorlakson's grandfather. He lived there between 1851 and 1873, when he left for America with his wife, three daughters and six sons. In the summer the schoolhouse is used as a hostel for tourists – a common practice in Iceland, and Dr. Thor and his companions stayed there – a unique link with the past. On the extreme left is Hartley Richardson, age sixteen; on the extreme right are David Richardson, age eighteen; Dr. Thorlakson; and Derek Thorlakson, age twelve.

had fewer problems and no one has had better travelling companions. Like you, they are, all three, good troupers and always ready on time. They out-distance me in at least three major activities of the tour; in eating, walking and sleeping.

It is great fun to see the country again through the eyes of the young. The zest and vigour they display for each day's program has its rich rewards.

We have been in almost every corner of Reykjavik, by car or on foot. We have bought Icelandic sweaters, visited the Nordic Centre, built and supported by the five Scandinavian countries, visited art galleries, sat through two hours of mostly Icelandic speeches at the famous Saga Hotel. Our table companion and the chief speaker at the welcoming party or social event was the Grand Old Man of Iceland, the former President, Ásgeir Ásgeirsson. The food that was served was excellent, including thin Icelandic pancakes filled with whipped cream and laced with rum!

The next day being Sunday, we attended a special service at the Cathedral for the seamen of Iceland. Bishop Einarsson conducted the service. In part, it was a memorial service for the twenty-eight seamen who had perished during the previous year. . . . The church was packed to the doors. We met His Grace after the service and the boys had a few moments with him.

On Monday we travelled by car to Thingvellir, Gullfoss, the magnificent waterfall, to the site of the Geysir, from which all such recurrent explosions of steam and boiling water derive their name. The one we saw in 1930, which had erupted for untold centuries, is now unfortunately dormant, but several other small ones erupt frequently. They only rise, however, about 50 feet in the air.

On the same day we travelled to Skálholt, the site of the first bishopric in Iceland, founded in 1056 AD; to Hveragerdi, where we saw the many hothouses built over a large area from which steam rises steadily to provide warmth for the many varieties of flowering plants, tomatoes etc. produced there. . . .

This evening (three days later) we returned at 10:30 p.m. (in broad daylight) from a trip which covered 450 miles of southern Iceland. The distance, of course, included the return journey, which did not always follow the area seen on our way out east. This trip took us as far east as Vatnajökull, the largest glacier in Europe. It covers 3,000 square miles of the 40,000 square miles of Iceland. When we leave we will have seen all but one of the glaciers of Iceland, and that one is in the very centre of the island.

During the past three days we have traversed vast lava fields and have had their origins explained to us. We also passed over many miles of beautifully green pasture lands on which there are large, prosperous farms and large dairy herds. Wherever we travelled we saw sheep grazing on the hillsides. At this time of year practically every sheep is followed by one, two or even three lambs – fifty percent, I believe, have two lambs.

We travelled in a large, comfortable Mercedes-Benz bus, air-conditioned. Gisli Gudmundsson is a perfect guide. He speaks excellent English. He is, quite naturally, well-versed in the lore of the countryside. He is a good raconteur and tells us many interesting stories. Being a member of a male voice choir, he occasionally sings well-known Icelandic songs over the loudspeaker. He stands over six feet and in every way runs a "tight but good ship." The sleeping accomodation is comfortable and scrupulously clean, and the food is excellent. All four of us have a tremendous appetite.

The boys have climbed mountains, walked behind and under waterfalls. They have walked over ancient lava fields, now covered by a one- or two-foot carpet of moss. One of these areas, between Myrdalsjökull and the sea, was the site of a volcanic eruption 200 years ago. They have taken many pictures of some striking scenery. I do hope their pictures turn out.

Hartley's ambition at the moment is to buy an Icelandic farm. He also plans to persuade his father and mother to return with him to Iceland so that he can show them some of the sculpture which seems to fascinate him.

David inspects everything in sight very carefully and always has some interesting observation to make. He has an unerring eye for feminine beauty, which he comes by honestly on both sides of the house.

Derek is a good trouper and keeps up with the best of them. He has beaten all of us at one time or another at cribbage and eats everything in sight, including fish, smoked lamb, prune pudding, vegetables and skyr. After two plates of skyr for dessert at dinner this evening at Hveragerdi, he announced that he was going to have skyr every morning for breakfast (which they serve here at our hotel). Derek's only complaint is that his grandfather snores occasionally.

Tomorrow we go to the home of Dr. and Mrs. Ofeigur Ofeigsson for early dinner and then for a thirty-mile drive in their car to Krisuvik, where there are some unusual geological phenomena.

On Sunday we go fishing. The Eggert Steinthorssons are taking us out to their summer home. In addition to fishing, they have promised to show us some historic relics from the early days of settlement that have recently been uncovered under a lava flow that covered and buried farms and buildings.

This letter, which was to have been a short message telling you that "all was well with us," has now developed into a sizable travelogue of the first week of our journey over the land of the ancient sagas and the people who, over the centuries, have experienced and lived through devastating calamities and undergone every conceivable hardship, yet have somehow managed, through it all, to develop a high standard of living and have achieved much in the fields of democracy, responsible government, in education, in art and literature. Despite their small numbers and limited natural resources, they now enjoy most of the modern amenities.

I know that my three companions have the capacity to understand and appreciate what they hear and see. I am sure this trip will serve to enrich their minds and add something of value to their experiences.

By all accounts this has been the finest spring they have enjoyed for a century! The weather since we arrived has been most pleasant. Every day we have our share of sunshine and, of course, continuous daylight.

So many people have asked to be remembered to you and for that as well as for other reasons I wish you were here with us.

As ever,

Thor

The boys send you their love – me too!

LETTER TO CARLA

When this letter was written, Carla was on the staff of the Department of External Affairs, posted at the Canadian Embassy in Rome.

Oslo, Norway
Sunday, August 4, 1974.

Dear Carla:

After spending ten days in Iceland as the Canadian Government's official representative to the 1100th anniversary of the settlement of Iceland from Western Norway and also in part from the North of Scotland and Ireland, we are here in Oslo. Your mother and dad were in Reykjavik during the last part of their tour, so we were able to see each other during our stay. The weather was perfect, as it had been during the whole previous month. Just imagine 55,000 people coming together on Thingvellir on Sunday, July 28. The country never looked better. Thirty countries were represented. The official parties left Reykjavik at 8:45 a.m. in three large comfortable buses with a motorcycle escort. The arrangements for the sitting of Althing were excellent. A huge platform had been built on the site of the first session of the Althing in 930 A.D. and the speakers' podium was near or at the spot – Lögberg – the Law Rock on which the first speaker stood in 930 A.D. Loudspeakers were strategically placed at many points in the valley so that wherever the 55,000 people had settled themselves the voices could be heard.

Grandmother did not come out for the morning session but came out with Mr. and Mrs. Hallgrimur Hallgrimsson, the Icelandic Consul-General for Canada, and his wife Margaret in their chauffeur-driven car. Between 3 and 4 p.m. the official representatives of the Nordic countries, the USA and Canada were called to the podium to deliver the greetings from their respective governments. As each spokesman stepped up on the podium the band played the National Anthem of the country. You can imagine how pleased and proud I was to be representing the Government and people of Canada. I shall mail you a copy of my speech when I return home or probably ask Miss Banks to send you a copy before.

We have now decided to spend the next three weeks at the Park Hotel, at Bad Sandefjord, which is on the Oslofjord about eighty miles south of Oslo. The place has been highly recommended to us by the Canadian Ambassador to Norway and Iceland – Mr. Ken McIlwraith. We will send you a report from there. We leave here Wednesday August 7. We are due in Stockholm on August 31 to attend the World Medical Association Meeting which lasts for a week. (Our address there will be the Grand Hotel. S. Blaisie-Holmshamnen 8, 111-48 Stockholm.)

Yesterday noon Anna Holck and Anna Margrethe Waaler came to our hotel for lunch and last evening we went to Anna Holck's apartment for supper and a most enjoyable evening. Anna Margrethe and her brother Dr. Georg Waaler were also there. You surely made a great hit with our relatives in Norway. Anna Holck told us how much she enjoyed your visit with her and said you were the kind of guest she would like to have for a much, much longer visit.

As usual for her, Grandmother is a great trouper and makes a wonderful travelling companion. You will hear from us shortly. Grandmother sends her love.

Grandfather

LETTER FROM PATRICIA (AGED NINETEEN)

February 15, 1978.

Dear Grandmother and Grandfather:

Happy Valentine's Day. Sorry I'm a bit late with that greeting. The enclosed picture is sent expressly for Grandfather – a picture of his "No.

1 Valentine"! As I couldn't find any cardboard mounts for it, I had to make one myself – it even stands up! Not only is Grandmother's dress the perfect birthday gown – it's an even more perfect Valentine's Day gown!

Thank you for your letter, Grandmother, which I just received tonight and read to the family at the dinner table. This is the picture you were talking about in your letter – this is just where you were sitting down when Bunty [the family name for Mrs. Thorlakson's sister, Mrs. J.B. Shepherd] and I arrived in your room before our outing to the Royal Hawaiian! I didn't send it with my last letter, because, as I mentioned before, only Grandfather should have it – I think it's a perfect picture of you, and of course, my favorite of all the snaps I took in Hawaii!

And, Grandfather, I must thank you for the letter to Ian and I and the clippings you sent. Your letter arrived when Mom and Dad were in Vancouver, and so Ian and I read it at the dinner table, just the two of us (after all, it *was our* letter!) just as if Mom and Dad were home (of course, we did let them read it when they got home!). I found the clippings very interesting, especially after having read James Michener's book "Hawaii", and then getting a first-hand experience with the islands last February! This time last year, we had lunch at the Royal Hawaiian, did some shopping (remember the dresses you tried on, Grandmother? – and I bought a gold purse), and then Bunty and I had French toast, and Mrs. Oughton came over. Actually, it's not my memory that is so good – Bunty will tell you that I kept a diary, and I'm just referring to it!

By the time you get home, I will have started a new job. After an interview and some tests, I was accepted by the provincial government for the position of (Court) Reporter. This involves going to court and recording all the things that people say in the session. I will be using a stenomask – which is an apparatus that fits over the nose and mouth, and contains a microphone, which records what I say as I repeat what other people have been saying. I have been interested in this position for at least nine months now, and am quite excited about it. Not only is it a new career, and involves a substantial increase in wages, but it will be a great learning experience. The manual for Court Reporters which I have been given indicates that, in order to become more proficient, one should read all the material one can, not only every page of the newspaper, but also novels (classics), business journals, and the like. I will be starting on March 13, and training for about a month. I'm looking forward to telling you more about it.

I will be working at Tupper, Adams for 2 more weeks, and then will take a week off to visit Carla [her sister] in Ottawa (March 3–12). Needless to say, I am also looking forward to that!

I have attended a few lectures given by the YMCA on health and nutrition. A woman who worked at Tupper, Adams for a short time has invited me to them – she works for Richardson's; the lectures are given in one of the lecture rooms on the 27th floor of the Richardson Building. They are extremely interesting, and are given by a young girl who speaks with such skill that one hangs on every word. She is a school friend of David Richardson; her name is Pat McCarthy. I saw David at the last lecture, which was about heart attacks – the danger signals, what to do when someone is having a heart attack, and what a heart attack feels like so that you can detect it in yourself and get immediate treatment. Because of that lecture, I am hoping to fit in a St. John's Ambulance course sometime. Unfortunately, the course is not offered on Saturdays or Sundays.

Tonight, Mom and Dad are at the Health Sciences Centre, at the lecture given by Evelyn Shapiro on health care in Canada. Both Mom and Dad find the lectures extremely interesting. And Ian is at Scouts tonight, and will soon be taking canoeing lessons at the Pan-Am pool in anticipation of a canoeing camping trip this summer with the Scouts!

The weather has continued to be cold – today the temperature was −12° C, which is balmy for this time of year; however, there was a nasty wind which made it quite miserable. But I'm sure spring is just around the corner – at least, that's the thought that keeps all Winnipeggers going, isn't it?!

I know you will be reading this letter to Bunty, so – "Hi, Bunty! I certainly miss going down to the beach with you – hopefully, it won't be too long before I can do it again"!

All my love,

Patricia

LETTER FROM IAN (AGED TWELVE)

March 11, 1979.

Dear Grandfather, Grandmother, and Bunty:

Thank you for your last letter. The article was very interesting, and it reminded me of our CTBS tests that I had in grades 1, 3, and 6. I tried to work out all the questions on the article and found that I was successful.

Hasn't the time gone fast? I hear that you are coming back in a month. Carla is coming here to visit us in 2 weeks.

My piano playing is improving over the weeks, and I have learned to

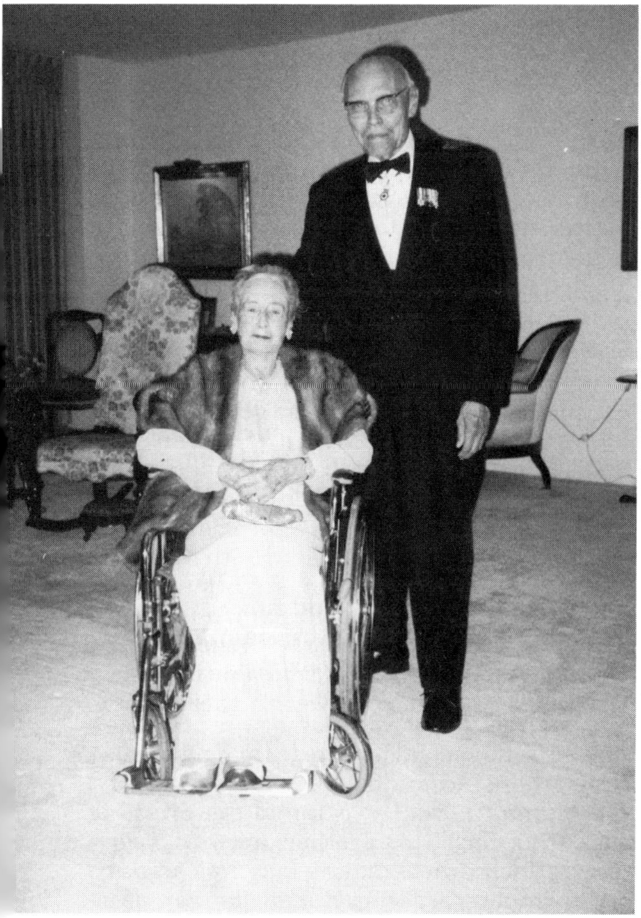

r. and Mrs. Thorlakson were invited by Prime inister Mulroney to be head-table guests at the nquet for Her Majesty Queen Elizabeth and ince Philip when they visited Winnipeg in tober, 1984. Prior to departure for the banquet is picture was taken in their apartment in linburgh House.

play "The Entertainer," and the "Maple Leaf Rag." The next time you visit us, I'll play these two Scott Joplin pieces for you.

I am wondering if you saw the eclipse in Hawaii. Brandon was in direct line with the sun as it (the sun) went into an eclipse. When the eclipse was in totality, we could look at the sun without any eye protection, and still not get any eye damage. It must have been darker in Brandon than in Winnipeg, (when the eclipse occurred) but it was still quite dark. We made many gadgets to view the eclipse when it wasn't in totality and we were quite successful. They were all ways to project the sun's image on cardboard through a telescope or pinhole. We also used a mirror to reflect the sun's image onto Dad's movie projector screen. It was very exciting when the sun was in totality, but quite boring when the sun was in a partial eclipse. Still, looking at those projection methods was a lot of fun, and it was especially exciting when the light outside got duller and grayer.

We haven't gone cross-country skiing as much as we'd like to, but the odd times that we have gone were relaxing and fun.

I am reading an excellent book called "The Sword of Shannara." It is an epic fantasy by Terry Brooks and is a 726-page book in paperback form. It has been so interesting that I have read about half of the book, starting Tuesday. It is about Dwarves, Elves and Man against Gnomes and a Druid warlock lord who uses his special powers for evil purposes. A great war is brewing between these races and all is lost unless Shea Olmsford, a true heir to the Shannara family, can find the Sword of Shannara to kill the warlock lord. Shea, his brother, a dwarf, two princes, a mystic druid and two elfin brothers make a long trek across the country to find the Sword of Shannara, going through dangerous forests, crossing dangerous valleys, climbing mountains, and experiencing members of the spirit world. The book is similar to J.R. Tolkien's books, and after I finish the Sword of Shannara, I might tackle "The Lord of the Rings" or "The Hobbit." I saw the movie "The Lord of the Rings" at a movie theatre. It was an excellent show. I also saw "The Hobbit" last year on television. It was also an excellent show. These two shows were animated.

I am looking forward to seeing you when you come home.

Love from,

Ian

Appendices

APPENDIX 1

The Future of Canadian Medicine

From 1962 until 1970 Dr. Thorlakson was a member of the Provincial Government agency now known as the Manitoba Health Services Commission, which funds hospitals, personal care homes, public and private diagnostic facilities, and the medical care plan. Due to his long and varied experience as a surgeon and as an organizer of medical service, his strength of purpose, and his stature in the community, he had a substantial influence in shaping Commission policies during his tenure of office. The following paper, published in the Winnipeg Clinic Quarterly in the fall of 1967, expressed his views when the approaching change in the funding of medical care was the subject of vigorous discussion. The Government-funded plan came into effect in 1968.

The Present Position

Now that Canada is celebrating the centenary of Confederation it is appropriate that we, as doctors of medicine, should survey the prospects of the future; seek out the many opportunities that now present themselves; and provide constructive leadership in medical education and practice. We must try to have a clear understanding of the relevant political, social, economic and medical forces which are causing changes in our way of life. We must compare the goals set for our own province with the aspirations of the others, and with those of countries overseas with comparable human and financial resources. Our obligations extend beyond our national boundaries to the peoples in the underdeveloped regions of the world, for, though Canada's foreign aid program is imaginative and constructive, it should be extended.

Long-term planning in medicine is a new development. On the present scale, it was not even being considered ten years ago. New plans in the field of medical education, practice, hospital services and economics should be based on a knowledge and an appreciation of our accomplishments, past failures and present shortcomings. Planning must always be a continuous process for nothing is static or unchangeable; it must not be confused with decision making. The first step is to determine needs and objectives; next, set out alternative recommendations and carefully study their possible consequences; finally comes the selection of priorities and the decisions. This is a slow and laborious process, it requires patience, a consensus of opinion and reasonable compromises.

Philosophy and technique in the health field are changing at an accelerating and almost incredible pace. It is worthy of note however that much of the change has been initiated by the physicians themselves. Many frustrating and complex problems face the medical profession in Canada. Out of the present period of debate and uncertainty, plans, policies and decisions will change in the present patterns of practice.

Changes, which appear to threaten a doctor's security or accepted mode of life, naturally create apprehension and meet with resistance. History records that progress has been interrupted by periods of dissension and conflict. To move forward requires understanding based on free discussion, tolerance for other people's rights and points of view, confidence in the future, and acceptance of the inevitability of change. These factors constitute the lubricant which alone can enable divergent groups to work together smoothly; these are the elements which lead to acceptable compromise and constructive progress.

The perfect answer eludes me. The very thought of ever-expanding bureaucratic controls evokes misgivings and apprehension, but it stimulates a desire to study the problem in depth on a provincial and on a national basis. Let us not fall into the error of blaming politicians for all our woes; their intelligence, judgment, dedication and integrity are equal to those of any other responsible group of citizens.

Economic and Social Change

The provision of adequate and reliable medical care has become a matter of great public concern. Canadian society has accepted the principle that every citizen is entitled to the best available medical care, irrespective of his individual resources.

It is a sobering fact that the conservative attitude of the medical profession and the general resistance to radical changes in methods of practice has contributed, in part, to the rising costs of medical care and to increasing government involvement.

In the foreseeable future many changes will influence and modify our view on the economics of practice. The majority of Canadians are now covered by some form of prepaid medical insurance; this may be on a voluntary basis, or by government subsidy. At the moment the two principles of compulsion and universality are being hotly debated; whatever the outcome, no hospital in future will need to organize a charity out-patient or in-patient service for the medically indigent. Out-patient departments for insured patients will be a new feature in all teaching hospitals and more clinical teaching will be done on ambulant patients. Clinical teaching facilities will be geared to, and their size will be limited by, the need to train increasing numbers of family doctors and other specialists. Interns or residents are unlikely to be available in hospitals other than university affiliated teaching institutions. The responsibility for providing medical services all day and every day in the service hospitals will fall on the private practitioners. In the future hospitals will have no financial responsibility for the physician component of their services, but all members of the medical staff will be expected to provide professional services on a rotating basis, day and night. This is already being done in rural hospitals and it will soon become a necessity in many metropolitan areas.

Modern medicine has so much to offer to the healthy as well as to the sick person. There is no limit, absolutely no limit, to the amount of medical service the public can and will expect; conversely, the physician will always provide whatever service lies within his power, for it is his duty to provide reassurance in the absence of serious illness and relief or cure when organic disease is present. This "new medicine" is costly. The doctor is constantly walking a tightrope between over- and under-utilization of the available diagnostic procedures, for the results of error, lack of foresight or clinical acumen, can be tragic for the patient.

Education and Training

The reorganization of the physician's education should and will remain in the hands of the universities; they must, however, ensure that the teacher remains with the patient and the student, and that he does not become cloistered in a research laboratory. This is no idle warning; it is a cause for serious concern. Some full time teachers find it inconvenient or tedious to leave their laboratories in order to teach and others have little interest in clinical practice. Following ward rounds in the surgical department of one of the more progressive medical schools on this continent, a professor said to me: "The sooner we get back to the patient and teach, the better for American medicine." This is not an isolated opinion. I do not imply criticism of research nor doubt its value – without research progress is impossible – but I do suggest that teaching, clinical practice and research all have their proper place. A good teacher of medicine is not necessarily a good administrator; a successful and dedicated research worker may not be the best teacher for the future practitioner of medicine; nor is a successful practitioner necessarily a skilled teacher or research worker. The art of pedagogy requires special aptitudes and training. The responsibilities of the instructor, be he full time or part time, do not cease after the graduation of his students, nor even when higher degrees are obtained; his is a continuing obligation, for the education of a physician ends only on his retirement from practice.

Modern hospital practice provides admirable opportunities for advancing the art of teaching and the continuing duty of learning. University affiliation is desirable, but not essential. In fact, affiliation should be governed by the needs of the Medical Faculty and not by the plans and ambitions of hospitals. A full time Director of Continuing Education could be assigned to a large hospital or a group of smaller hospitals; however, recognition of such a director by the university would not necessarily establish that hospital as a university-affiliated institution. It is neither necessary nor desirable that all education for practising physicians, all clinical investigation and all basic research should be initiated, planned and directed by a Faculty of Medicine. These activities, in the course of time, may receive the stamp of approval or 'come under the umbrella of the university', but over-centralization of authority and control may stifle initiative, freedom of thought and imaginative action, and consequently the progress of medical practice.

Methods of Practice

Another challenge confronting the profession is the organization and provision of primary contact medical care on a 24 hour, 7 days a week basis. John W. Gardner, Secretary of Health, Welfare and Education in the United States of America, recently said: "It is not known whether the country's health care system should be organized around hospitals, around groups of physicians or around organizations such as state health councils."

Should any large medical institution or clinic close its doors at 6 p.m. each day, and remain closed over weekends and public holidays? Is it not the profession's responsibility to organize and provide "out of hours" services, including emergency care? Are state-financed hospitals and clinics to be encouraged to take over an increasing share of the practice of medicine as a result of the default of private physicians? It is easy enough to ask these questions; to provide practical solutions is, however, quite another matter. The answers will inevitably have a profound effect on medical practice.

It is my conviction that the more we rely on the public treasury to develop and finance the facilities necessary for medical practice, the more circumscribed and regimented the private practitioner's role will become. On the other hand, it cannot be denied that government participation and financial support have been important factors contributing to progress in the fields of general medical and hospital care during the past ten years. The principle of government involvement is no longer a debatable point, it is an established fact. The question is: How far and how fast?

Twenty or thirty years from now probably no family doctor or specialist will be in solo practice; the increased volume of work, the result of the unlimited public demand for health services, will force physicians to work in groups. Furthermore, they will tend to congregate in those towns which have hospitals with at least 75 or 100 beds. Physicians will run the community medical services from these larger hospitals or primary health centres, where patients can obtain comprehensive investigation and care. The provinces will be organized into medical regions and the primary health centres will be affiliated with larger regional Base Hospitals of 350 to 500 bed capacity, located in larger towns and cities and staffed by teams of specialists and consultants. The health centres and the Base Hospitals will be connected to highly sophisticated diagnostic equipment in the Provincial Health Services Centre. Computers will enable diagnostic and therapeutic information to be relayed rapidly to and fro between the central and peripheral units.

The ten or twenty mile limit on travel of pioneer days, using oxen or horses, has been out-moded by the development of a sixty-miles-an-hour highway system. Specially designed, equipped and staffed ambulances will convey critically ill and severely injured patients quickly and safely to an appropriate hospital. These vehicles will become in effect compact travelling hospital rooms for acutely ill or injured patients who need emergency care at home, on the road-side, or during their journey to a hospital – a critical period when resuscitation is often vital.

It is inevitable that the medical and hospital organizations of the provinces will come to grips with the extraordinary advances in medical technology and the consequent changes in medical economics. While health care will continue to be the primary responsibility of the medical and allied health professions, and while university faculties of medicine, nursing, dentistry and pharmacy will continue to produce the professional personnel; the processes of learning must nevertheless be redesigned so as to produce practitioners who will be equipped to meet the requirements of the future. Further fragmentation into specialties and more intensive training will be necessary if we are to gain the knowledge and acquire the many special skills required to practice modern scientific medicine. This has been accepted by the Canadian College of General Practice which now advocates postgraduate training leading to a specialist status for the family practitioner.

The means and the methods of bringing high quality medical care to the greatest number of citizens will require great ingenuity and managerial skills such as are now being employed in our major industries. This does not mean that the important patient-doctor relationship will necessarily be lost; even today this relationship starts with a telephone operator, then involves a receptionist and a nurse; only after these encounters does the personality of the physician enter into the relationship. In all these matters, however, the physician should provide the incentive and the example!

We may not agree with all the methods that are being proposed to enable Canadian Medicine to achieve national goals. However, we cannot escape the fact that we are being thrust into a new era in which no doctor will be as sufficient unto himself as were the physicians of the past. The private practitioner of the future will realize his ideals and due rewards only by cooperating with his colleagues in national and provincial organizations and with private agencies working in the health field.

Research Requirements

It has become obvious that the products of research are outstripping our ability to apply them, except perhaps in large and fabulously expensive centres. We need to find effective and economical ways and means of applying our new knowledge if we are to meet the growing demands for more comprehensive medical care for an ever increasing number of citizens. High priority must therefore be given to research into methods of providing primary contact and emergency clinical service on a 24 hours a day and 7 days a week basis. We must learn to use expensive space, equipment, trained medical personnel and ancillary staff more efficiently for clearly the present system is imperfect and wasteful. I envisage a merging of private medical groups and a reorganization of health and welfare agencies in an endeavour to correct the present duplication and waste of both private and public resources. We must have the courage and the foresight to face the stern and compelling realities of our jet and space age existence.

Canada's Second Century

In contemplating all these new developments, it becomes obvious that the role of the physician will change, the role of the hospital will change, as will the habits of patients seeking medical care. In the future, the emphasis will be on the prevention of illness and maintenance of health rather than on the cure of advanced disease. This statement was frequently made thirty to forty years ago, but at that time it was just a hope; today the aspiration is about to be realized.

If we wish to survive as a free profession, we must understand and accept these new social and economic changes; we have no alternative but to adjust to essential and inevitable change. We should, however, strengthen our professional solidarity and co-operative endeavour, and we must accept the fact that the medical profession is rapidly moving into a working partnership with governments and with other agencies. Medicine should have no factions. The primary aim of doctors is to help the patient, not to secure an advantage over another member of the profession; excessive competition and rivalry should be as obsolete as the horse and buggy. Every effort must be made to weld the members of the medical profession together in order that we may speak effectively in our advocacy of sound, constructive and progressive legislation. Individually and collectively, we must continue to advance the legitimate aims and purposes of our honourable profession. We will never reach Sir Thomas More's 'Utopia' because changing circumstances and technological advances constantly create new horizons. To be an active participant in a team which is striving towards new and constructive objectives is however, a rewarding experience. Canadians are now stepping forward across the threshold of their second century as a nation. Coincidentally, Canadian doctors and their patients are moving into a new professional and financial relationship for which the past one hundred years of experiment and adjustment have been but a preparation. Ideas that only thirty years ago would have been incomprehensible to the physician and unworthy of serious thought, are now part of our way of life. Further anticipated changes are being faced and even accepted by the doctors of Canada with some misgivings, it is true, but without resentment or hostility.

Let no young student be discouraged by the future prospects from entering upon a physician's career. The opportunities that lie ahead cannot be over-estimated; this is surely the most exciting and challenging time in all the long history of medicine. Doctors now have greater opportunities than ever before to prepare themselves in our medical schools and teaching hospitals for a full and active life devoted to the prevention of illness, the cure or control of disease, and the rehabilitation of the disabled. Whatever benefits the patient, helps the family and society – what greater privilege can any Canadian doctor ask than to become a member of an efficient medical team supported by graduates of the allied health professions?

APPENDIX 2

A Centennial Gift

Dr. Thorlakson, as Chairman of the Canadian (Icelandic) Centennial Committee, gave a speech on the occasion of the presentation of a bronze plaque to the Government and people of Canada as a centennial gift from Canadians of Icelandic descent. The presentation took place in Ottawa on April 14, 1967. The Right Honourable Lester B. Pearson accepted the gift on behalf of the Government.

Mr. Minister, Mr. Prime Minister, your Excellencies, Honourable Senators and Members of the House of Commons, ladies and gentlemen: On the first day of July, our country will cross the threshold into the second century of confederation. In honour of this historic occasion, Canadians have extended the traditional one day birthday celebration to one year of commemoration.

Many Centennial projects, varied and inspired in their conception, will remain as permanent tributes to the imagination and resourcefulness of the Canadian people.

There is an unmistakable desire on the part of many groups of Canadians to examine their own position and accomplishments relative to the opportunities that have been available to them since their arrival in this land.

At the close of this memorable Centennial year, every person will know more about the history and achievements of Canada – the land of his birth or the land of his adoption – and will have a deeper appreciation of what it means to be a Canadian.

We have gathered here today, in this magnificent National Library and Archives Building, to honour the Centennial of Confederation and to commemorate the discovery of the Western Hemisphere by mariners from Iceland and Greenland in the late tenth century.

From the dawn of history, the Western Ocean – also called the Green Sea of Darkness – was a constant challenge and a mystery to the seafaring nations of Europe.

A period of great expansion – commonly known as the Viking Age – commenced towards the latter part of the eighth century and continued for over two hundred years. From the present Norway, Sweden and Denmark, this expansion took Norsemen to the east, to the south and to the west. They landed in Normandy, England, Scotland, and Ireland. In 874, they reached Iceland and established the old Icelandic Republic in 930. Towards the end of that century, they pushed on, first to Greenland and then further westward to the shores of a new continent which they called Vinland. Thus the North Atlantic Ocean – the dreaded Green Sea of Darkness – was successfully spanned for the first time.

Knowledge of these explorations was bound to come to the attention of navigators and scholars in other countries. Indeed, we find the record of this knowledge in the writings of European scholars of that era, notably Adam of Bremen, one of the most distinguished scholars of Europe in the eleventh century. In his book, published in Latin between the years 1072 and 1076, he gives an account of the discovery of Vinland as related to him by the King of Denmark.

The settlements of Iceland and Greenland depended on foreign trade, mainly with Norway and England, for their existence. Sheepskins, hides, wool, tallow, cheese, sulphur, and dried fish were exchanged for timber, tar, flour, honey, linen, and metals. The luxury items of this trade and commerce – in those days – were white polar bears, walrus tusks and the renowned falcons, the hunting birds of royalty.

In the year 1396, the son of the Duke of Burgundy was captured by the Saracens. The Prince was held ransom for twelve Greenland falcons and this demand was duly met. This exchange serves to corroborate the fact that the trade routes to the far north were widely known.

Special mention should be made of the "court poetry" and the language of Iceland. During these early centuries, learned men – especially the Skaldic Poets – were invited to visit the courts of many European countries. These gifted men brought back important information from these foreign lands regarding current events, much of which was later incorporated in the vast Saga literature of Iceland. This ancient, classic language of Northern Europe – Old Norse – preserved through the centuries and still spoken in Iceland today – has a close kinship with Anglo-Saxon which forms the basis of the most forceful and effective speech in modern English. Icelandic is one of the

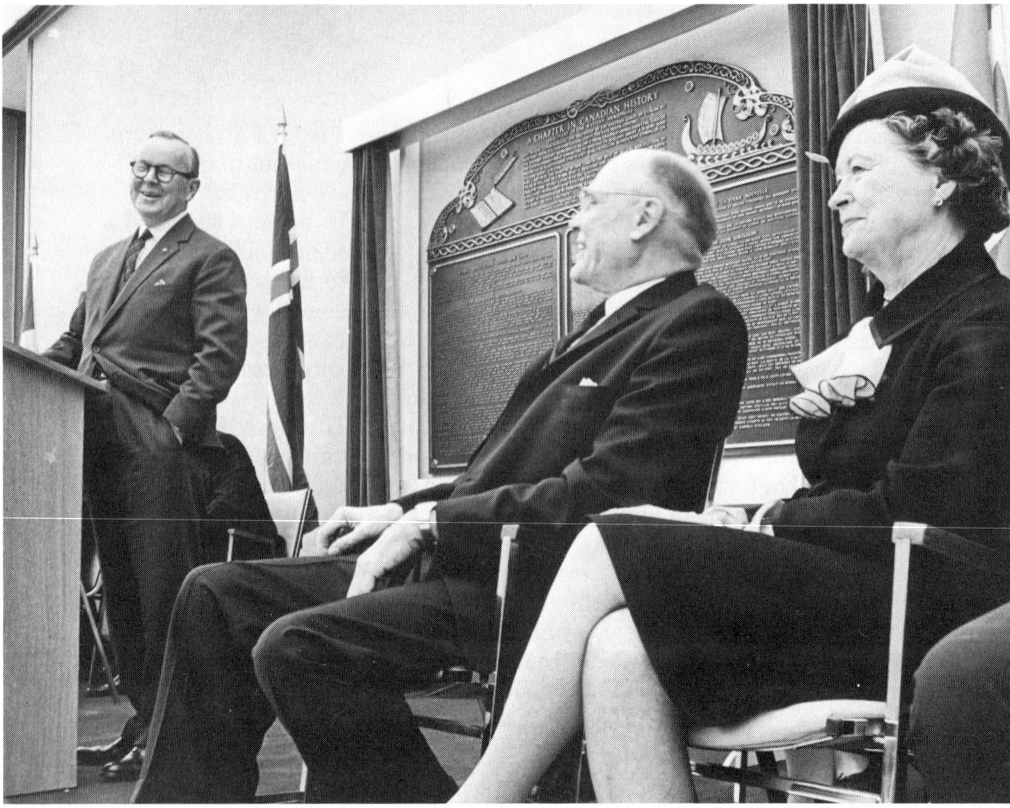

Prime Minister Lester B. Pearson jokes about the advantages of the economy of words necessary to convey the centennial message on this plaque in the Icelandic language compared with the versions in English and French. The bronze plaque had just been presented by Dr. Thorlakson on behalf of the Canadians of Iceland origin to the Government and the People of Canada in the year of their centenary Mrs. Pearson shares his amusement.

required subjects in advanced studies of English in the Universities of Great Britain, the older Universities of North America and in institutions of higher learning in other countries.

Trade and communication between Iceland and Greenland with the rest of Europe continued up to, and beyond, the period of active exploration and conquest of the new World by the Spanish, Portugese, English, French, and Dutch navigators and explorers.

During the years before and after AD 1470, there was a determined effort by experienced and seasoned navigators to explore the lands they knew existed beyond the western horizon. They were encouraged and supported by merchants of means and by people in high authority.

On August 3, 1492, Christopher Columbus sailed southwest from Palos, Spain. He had carefully calculated the latitude along which he intended to travel. From his earlier experience as a navigator, while exploring the west coast of Africa, he knew that the prevailing trade winds blew westward at that time of the year. When he finally reset his course due west, after reaching the Canary Islands, he full expected to reach the shores of Asia.

Thirty-two days later, he and his crew landed on the Island of San Salvador in the Bahamas – the first Europeans to sail that broad southern expanse of the Atlantic Ocean.

On some of the maps drawn in the fifteenth century, Vinland was shown as just another large island – "Vinlanda Insula" – in the North Atlantic, over twelve hundred miles north of the Caribbean Islands discovered by Columbus.

It is greatly to his credit that Columbus thoroughly informed himself before embarking upon his long and hazardous journey. By all reliable accounts that are available to us, he certainly did not just sail "out into the blue". If we can accept the biography written and published in 1521, by his own son Ferdinand, as a reliable source of information, then Columbus did visit Iceland in February 1477. His genius as a navigator and an explorer was enhanced because he had studied the scientific records of the time and thus, contrary to the popularly accepted theory of the day, he had sound reasons to believe that the world was round. By using the navigational information at his disposal, Columbus calculated that land could be reached by travelling seven hundred leagues westward from Spain. This estimate proved to be correct, even though he failed to reach the East Indies.

When Columbus was forced, at the Robida Convent, to give his reasons for his belief that land existed beyond the rim of the Western Ocean, he stated that he based this conviction " . . . first, on the nature of things, second, on the reports of navigators; and third, on the authority of learned writers. . . . "

In 1497, John Cabot sailed westward from Bristol, England, on a

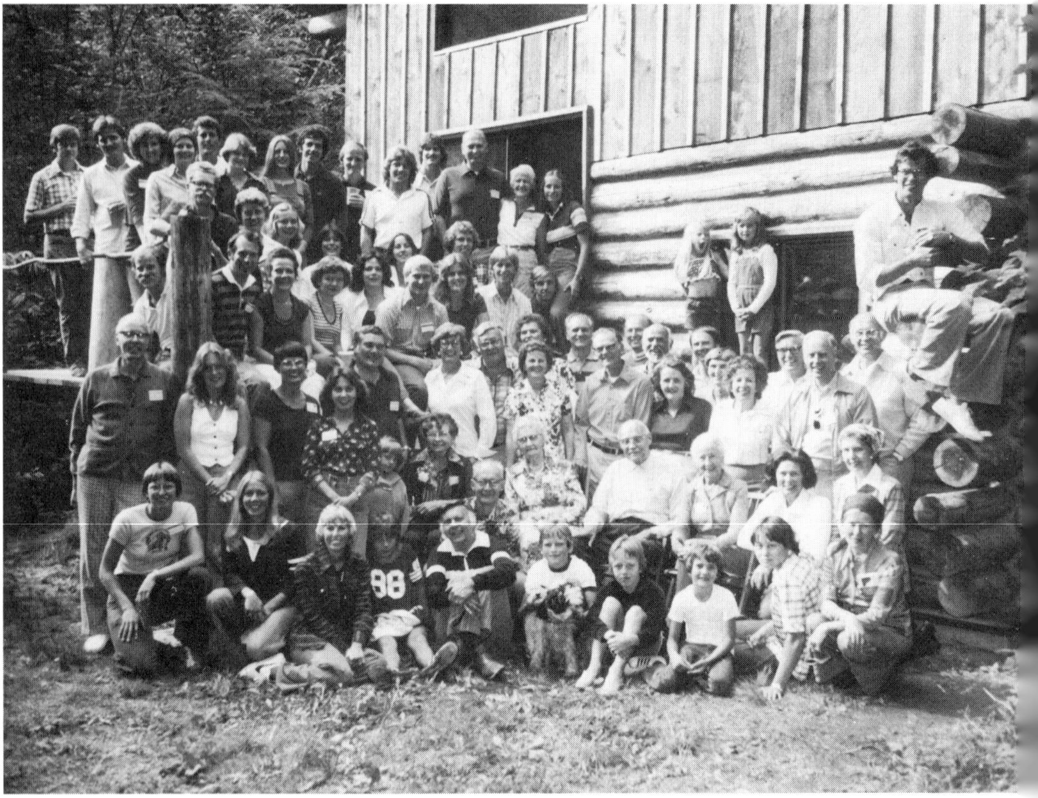

Thorlakson "Roots" reunion. Descendants of Niels Steingrimur Thorlaksson, from Iceland, and Erika Christopha Rynning Thorlaksson, from Norway, met on Labour Day weekend, in 1977, in Seattle, Washington.

voyage of discovery. According to the well-known Canadian historians, Lower and Chafe, " . . . the prosperity of Bristol was dependent on the cod fisheries of Iceland. The agreement under which these were open to Englishmen was about to run out and the merchants of Bristol were naturally anxious to find new fishing grounds. . . . "

Cabot explored and charted the coasts of Newfoundland and Nova Scotia. On his return to England, he reported – amongst other things – on the fabulous fishing grounds off the coast of Newfoundland. Subsequently, these fishing grounds provided an important source of food for the people of Europe.

In 1534 and 1535, Jacques Cartier sailed from France and explored the mighty St. Lawrence River as far as the Indian village of Hochelaga where the City of Montreal now stands. Cartier was the first person to apply the name Canada to this country.

Mr. Prime Minister, Ladies and Gentlemen – to become involved in a Centennial project of this kind has many compensations, one of which is that it adds to one's knowledge of the time and events described in the early Icelandic documents.

The ancient Icelandic Sagas are receiving increasing attention by modern scholars because of their great literary value and by historians because of the important information they shed on events that occurred in the early history of northern Europe.

Lord Tweedsmuir, a former governor-general of Canada, said: "For myself, I put the Icelandic Sagas among the chief works of the human genius. . . . "

In 1966, extensive use was made of the Sagas as the most authentic and complete source of information regarding the Battle of Hastings in 1066. These ancient records also have preserved a great deal of early Scandinavian history which would otherwise have been lost.

In 1965, the Yale University Press published a Pre-Columbian Vinland Map which provided further evidence to confirm the discovery of Vinland. This map was made about the year 1440 by a Swiss monk. At the top left hand corner of the map is inscribed the information that Vinland was discovered by Bjarni Herjolfsson and Leifr Eiriksson who found it a land of great fertility and many vines. The two inlets leading to the Hudson's Bay and the Gulf of St. Lawrence are clearly discernible on this map.

The recent archaeological discovery made at L'Anse-aux-Meadows, on the northern tip of Newfoundland, by Dr. Helgi Ingstad and his associates, has provided scientific proof of the existence of early Norse settlements in Newfoundland about the year A.D. 1000.

When the plaque is unveiled, it may come as a surprise to you, Mr. Prime Minister, and to others – as it did to me – to see how small a portion of the plaque is occupied by the original Icelandic version in the centre as compared with the English and the French translations which appear on either side. The reason, of course, is that some of the original Icelandic words – when inscribed on thin leather – were abbreviated to conserve space. One letter and a mark may stand for a word or even a phrase.

The upper section of the plaque shows, on the left, an open book and a quill which recalls the work of the Icelandic scholars who, in the eleventh and twelfth centuries, preserved the records of their time for posterity. On the right, is a replica of that sturdy Viking ship in which the ancient mariners sailed across the stormy North Atlantic to the eastern coast of North America and made the first attempt at settlement.

The introductory paragraph at the top of the plaque reads:

"This plaque commemorates the discovery of the eastern coast of Canada by mariners from Iceland and Greenland in the late tenth century.

"The historic excerpt reproduced below is from Graenlendinga Saga (the saga of the Greenlanders) first committed to writing in Iceland about A.D. 1200 and preserved in Flateyjarbok (the Flatey Book), a vellum manuscript compiled in Iceland about AD 1390.

"Part 1 records the sighting of new land in the west by Bjarni Herjolfsson, of Eyrarbakki in Iceland, in AD 986.

"Part 2 describes the voyage of discovery of Leifr Eiriksson some years later and his landings in Helluland (Flatstoneland), Markland (Woodland), and Vinland (Wineland). These explorations led to an attempt at colonization by Thorfinnr Karlsefni whose son, Snorri Thorfinnsson, was born on this continent.

"Archaeological research in western Greenland and eastern Canada supports these ancient Icelandic records of exploration and colonization."

The discoveries of Bjarni Herjolfsson and Leifr Eiriksson surely constitute one of the earliest chapters in Canadian history.

I have the honour, Mr. Prime Minister, to present this bronze plaque to the Government and to the people of Canada as a Centennial Gift from Canadians of Icelandic descent.

Mr. Prime Minister, may I now invite you to unveil the plaque.

APPENDIX 3

Notes from Moscow

Dr. Thorlakson attended the Twenty-fourth Congress of the International Society of Surgery in Moscow, USSR, from August 21 to 28, 1971. The following impressions were recorded during and immediately following his visit.

These are some of my impressions received during a recent visit to the USSR but which was limited to Moscow and Leningrad. I shall not attempt to pass any judgements, nor to make comparisons. For me, the journey was, in every respect, a happy and rewarding experience.

I was impressed by what I saw in magnificent buildings, both old and new. The Russian Government is now taking an increasing interest in renovating and preserving old buildings that possess historical interest. The old cathedrals within and outside the Kremlin walls and other priceless treasures that form part of the heritage of the Soviet people are being carefully preserved and are being shown freely to the foreign traveller. On the three occasions that I attended functions inside the Moscow Kremlin enclosure, the cameras were busy everywhere. Only an occasional guard, who appeared to be unarmed, was on duty.

The cities of Moscow and Leningrad are the cleanest and the least polluted cities I have seen in my travels at home and abroad.

Moscow has a population of about seven million people. Power, light and heat are provided by electricity and gas. No coal is burned in the city. The streets are tidy and clean. The women who "brush" the streets or cut the grass on the boulevards seem to take pride in their work. There must be no "litter bugs" in these cities. During my brief stay, I saw no "hippie" types anywhere.

In addition to attending meetings of the International Society of Surgery, I increased the length of my stay in order that I could learn, at first hand, more about their medicine, education and training, and their method of delivery of health services.

I was particularly interested in the training and functions of their feldschers. Contrary to my prior understanding, feldschers are not "doctors' assistants". They are, in their own right, "junior" doctors whose responsibilities are carefully spelled out in legislation. Their training takes three and a half to four years. The subject studies are Latin, Biology, Anatomy, Physiology and Microbiology in the first year for those who possess a Grade 10 standing. In their second year, they study pathological anatomy, psychology and pharmacology. They receive their clinical training in hospitals and in some polyclinics. When he or she has acquired three years of practical experience, the feldscher may serve in a small rural medical station, provided there is a doctor within telephone communication and who is available for consultations.

The feldscher is authorized to perform the following medical procedures:

1. Open a superficial abscess.

2. Extract foreign bodies which do not require complicated techniques and are not associated with marked disruption of tissues.

3. Skin suturing and ligation of bleeding vessels.

4. Veno-punctures.

5. Subcutaneous intra-muscular or intravenous injection of medications or fluids such as Ringer's or glucose solutions.

6. Blood grouping.

7. Application of a tourniquet to control haemorrhage.

8. Treat minor dislocations.

9. Apply splints for simple or compound fractures.

10. Apply plaster of Paris bandages.

11. Apply adhesive to the skin and apply weights to reduce fractures.

12. Use ethyl chloride or local injection of novocaine.

13. Tamponade in nasal or vaginal bleeding.

14. Extract teeth in uncomplicated cases.

These regulations are all laid down in special legislation authorized by the Ministry of Health and come under the authority of the local city or district department of health.

The present act was passed in 1965 and reaffirmed in July 1970. These regulations also stipulate that a diploma for a feldscher is issued on the basis of spending forty per cent of their training period in acquiring theoretical knowledge and sixty per cent in participating in the practice at a recognized medical institution. At the beginning of this course of training, they spend roughly three days on theory and three days in practice. Towards the end of their training, there is increased time spent in practice.

The student will spend some time in the hospital acting as an orderly. By the end of the second year, the feldscher student will devote time to carrying out, under supervision, those duties and procedures expected of him or her in actual practice. Finally, they sit for examinations but only if they have received good references from their teachers. The student takes four oral examinations: (a) internal medicine; (b) surgical diseases; (c) midwifery and gynecology; (d) pediatric diseases. The Board of Examiners are members of a large medical establishment.

The mid-medical school, where I obtained the above information from the Director – Dr. Nina Gruzinskaya – accepts 400 to 420 students a year of which 60 are taking the feldschers' course. Sixty students enter the school for training in midwifery and the rest are nurses in training. By careful selection of applicants and close supervision, the failure rate is only one percent.

Dr. Walter MacKenzie and I were able to team up for this visit. We were most impressed with the dedication and enthusiasm of the Director and members of her staff in their work. The Director, Dr. Gruzinskaya, was most gracious and generous and patient in first giving us a detailed description of the courses of training and then answering our questions through an excellent interpreter, Mr. Sanchehkin. Later, we were taken to every section of the school. It is admirably equipped for feldscher, midwife and nurses' training.

The large majority of feldschers in USSR are women. Their training was instituted early after the 1917 revolution because of the great shortage of qualified doctors. Now, apparently, the feldscher system is going to be gradually replaced by training more family physicians, supported by specially trained nurses at every level of service. It is acknowledged that, as nurses always work closely with doctors in the delivery of health care, they should be in an excellent position to acquire clinical sense and judgement.

At present, there are 675,000 doctors practising in the Soviet Union, up to seventy percent of whom are family physicians. The ratio of physicians to para-medical staff are one to two and a half. There are three physicians to each 1,000 people in the population. It is hoped to increase the supply of physicians to 800,000 in the near future. In order to raise the status of the family physician, he is now being included in some hospital establishments. Some doctors work in both a polyclinic and in a hospital. This change began ten years ago.

I asked many questions. Suffice it to say that, by our standards, the monthly pay for a doctor is low but there are additional substantial advantages and privileges provided to the individual who renders exemplary service. I am also convinced that it is unfair and stupid to simply take immediate financial returns as an accurate index of the standard of living and then compare these figures with our incomes.

Every graduate in medicine receives first a Diploma in Family Practice. Later on, after having served in this capacity, he may be permitted to enter the intern and resident system of training to become a specialist.

It is important to bear in mind that over eighty-five percent of all medical staff are women and, furthermore, a student may enter the educational process as a nurse in training and, if suitably motivated, may proceed on to become a feldscher and later a doctor. He or she always receives credits for prior training. In our Canadian system, a person must start at the beginning again whenever he or she decides to advance their qualifications in medicine. It is interesting that young women are *now* applying to become feldschers rather than midwives. They seek a degree of independence from direct supervision of the doctor.

Hospitals in Moscow have been increasing rapidly in numbers so that there is a shortage of 1,700 para-medical personnel. There are presently 12,000 hospital beds in Moscow. By 1976, this will be increased to 24,000 beds. In the whole of the Soviet Union, they plan to increase the number of hospital beds by three million during the next five years.

In conversation with delegates to the Congress of the International Society of Surgery, I have been given to understand that the feldscher system was adopted in other eastern European countries years ago because of an acute shortage of doctors. Now, the feldscher has been eliminated except for army establishments in these other eastern European countries.

During my visit I also had the opportunity to visit a polyclinic and to receive detailed information as to the organizational structure, including the composition of the administration of medical and para-medical personnel.

On Friday, August 20, I visited the Polyclinic No. 53 on Domitry Ulynor Street, serving thirty-eight to forty thousand citizens. This visit was arranged by the staff of the Medical Workers Union of Russia by courtesy of the General Secretary, Mr. Ivanov. I was accompanied by Youri Kozken, the Deputy Director of Foreign Relations and Nina Lazareva who acted as interpreter.

We were graciously received by the chief physician of the polyclinic. Dr. Nira Grigorevna Borisova, who first provided us with a description of the physical facilities, the administrative staff, the population covered, the professional staff and total medical services provided.

In District No. 53, there are ten polyclinics. Six of these medical clinics serve adults and four attend to the children of the area. There are five supportive units providing specialized consultative services and care in gynecology; major surgery; dermatology and venereal diseases; psychiatry; and tuberculosis. There is an outdoor dispensary attached to special institutions or hospitals.

The administrative and medical complement for Polyclinic No. 53 are:

1. Administrative

(a) chief physician (b) first deputy chief physician (diagnostic and treatment services) (c) second deputy chief physician (responsible for assessing the effects of various acute or chronic disabilities) (d) administrator (who acts as Comptroller of the group).

2. Medical staff (the Director, twenty generalists and fifty-five specialists), 76; nurses, 100; aides, orderlies, 33; total, 209.

The medical staff of Polyclinic No. 53 provides diagnostic and treatment services to ambulatory patients and home care. Emergency services are available twenty-four hours a day – seven days a week for 365 days a year. An ambulance service is available. A doctor and a nurse accompany the city ambulances.

By dialing the number 03 anywhere in the Soviet Union, the ambulance attendants or any person can contact the central emergency despatch centres for information regarding the nearest available hospital bed for the sick or injured person. This may be in the patient's own medical district or in a hospital in an adjacent district.

The area served by Polyclinic No. 53 is divided into nineteen sectors with about 2,000 people in each. One doctor and one nurse are responsible for the home care of the persons assigned to a sector and will also attend their patients at the Polyclinic. Provision, of course, is made to cover these services when members of the staff are off duty, on holidays or absent for any reason.

Six sectors (having a combined population of about 12,000 people) have assigned to them a medical team consisting of a surgeon, neurologist, urologist, oncologist, radiologist and a laboratory physician. Blood samples for the clinical laboratory are taken by the nurse.

Approximately 640 or more patients a day attend the Polyclinic. The medical staff make seventy to eighty house calls a day in summer. During epidemics in winter, this number has been as high as 300 a day. On one occasion only, the medical staff has been forced to call for sixth year medical students to assist.

The working hours for medical staff are six and a half hours a day, five days a week. Those who are on duty on Saturday have Monday off.

On Sundays there are two doctors and two nurses on twelve-hour duty. One doctor stays in the Clinic and the other makes house calls. On the average, on Sundays forty patients attend the clinic and 18 or 20 require house calls.

Annual "health check-ups" are apparently not a part of the Soviet health system. However, pre-employment examinations are routine and a thorough follow-up system is employed to keep check on patients with heart disease, hypertension, cancer, arthritis, diabetes, pernicious anaemia, tuberculosis, and other chronic conditions.

The medical staff of the Polyclinic send their patients for in-patient care to two hospitals in the district, one having 1000 beds and the other 1200 beds.

The Soviet system places great emphasis on ambulatory medical service at the polyclinic together with home care. Hospitalization is used with appropriate discretion as to need.

The sociological factors affecting each person's health receive special attention by the doctors and staff of the Soviet polyclinic. Public health also comes under their direct scrutiny and control. The medical team attached to the various polyclinics of a health district, accept the responsibility for all these problems – such as tuberculosis surveys; and the identification and treatment of all other infectious diseases. Careful records are maintained in these cases and statistics prepared for the city health department and the Ministry of Health.

The physicians of the polyclinic take part in health education campaigns. Information on personal hygiene and public sanitation are disseminated to the public through lectures given by the attending doctors. Specific rules governing the provision of health services and attendance at the local polyclinic are described to the individual or family by the home visiting nurse. The visitor cannot detect or assess the affectiveness of all these arrangements but there is no doubt in my mind that the doctors and their assistants are enthusiastic about the system of total health supervision and medical care, and carry out their duties with a high degree of dedication and purpose.

In the performance of these general supervisory and detection duties, the polyclinic is assisted by a Council consisting of interested local citizens and representatives from industrial plants of the district. Numerous visual aids serve to illustrate the benefits and importance of the available health services.

PAYMENT FOR PROFESSIONAL SERVICES OF PHYSICIANS

Doctors are all paid a salary. Starting income is about 100 roubles a month – this can increase in stages to two-hundred roubles a month. (Present exchange for tourists is ninety roubles for $100 American.) I do not know the real purchasing power of the rouble for the average Soviet citizen. Many luxuries that we now consider necessities for even a minimal standard of living are, I am certain, not essential in the USSR.

The standard of living in relation to income is a relative matter. For some people in Asia, Africa, Europe and even in North America, a certain standard of living for some individuals and families could be a luxury for others. Contentment or happiness is not necessarily related to income levels. In other words, to equate the average income in any other country to the standard of living in our country is totally irrational and meaningless.

I am also convinced that the Soviet social workers, sociologists and economists are more realistic and practical in their estimates of needs than their opposite numbers in Canada or the United States. I am also certain that the people of the USSR "spend their time meeting their needs whereas we spend our time increasing our desires".

There are monetary compensations in the Soviet Union in regard to pensions and retirement privileges that our economists and planners have not taken into consideration. The pensions average 60% of the doctor's annual salary on reaching the retirement age of 55 years for physicians and surgeons, whereas the retirement age for radiologists is forty-five. Dr. Borisova, the Chief Physician of the Polyclinic No. 53, says that she does not know of a case of a radiologist disabled because of radiation exposure.

Despite the early pension arrangements the doctor may continue to practice as long as he or she wishes or is able. I was introduced to a practising ENT specialist who is hale and hearty at seventy-three years and has no intention of retiring. His life's work is not finished.

When a doctor reaches the retirement age and decides to continue in active practice, he or she receives his pension plus full salary. These are useful incentives to continue to work and to be productive.

After lunch one day, Comrade Nina, who was the guide assigned to me, conducted me by motor cruise and on foot over a great part of the City of Moscow.

I shall simply jot down some impressions gained along the way. Moscow must have gone through a period of remarkable transformation since the Revolution of 1917. New areas have been developed to accommodate an impressive expansion and renovation. Many very large and remarkable new buildings have been constructed; e.g., the University of Moscow or the new building of "Lomosov," the state University, named after its original founder in 1755. Fourteen faculties are accommodated and 40,000 students are enrolled.

The spacious area surrounding the many buildings that comprise this University contains rows of beautiful trees, hedges, flower gardens and a large area of green grass. It must be a most unusual setting for a University built during a period when speed of construction was essential and the aesthetic needs too often neglected in our own country.

The new Palace of Congresses within the Kremlin walls is absolutely magnificent and spacious with a seating capacity of 6,000. Saw the ballet there – "The Three Musketeers" by Alexander Dumas – depicting the flashing duels of many swords, the courtly Prince and other gentlemen (nobles and ladies) in their exquisite finery; the Cardinal, the Christian Cross embroidered on the back of the blue cloaks of the young men, and the final meeting between the Prince and the beautiful "Cinderella." All was elaborately staged and artistically portrayed. A huge orchestra pit accommodates seventy-five to ninety instrumentalists. The music added greatly to the evening's pleasure.

The Hotel Russia cannot be described – 5,000 rooms, I believe. It, again, sits in a spacious setting surrounded by ancient churches and trees, flowers, shrubs and green grass and the tortuous river Moscva courses its way through the city, in front of the hotel.

Across and along the river from the Kremlin and the Hotel Russia is a long stretch of park land. One section is devoted to a large array of what we know as ferris wheels of varied design, carrying their excited passengers swiftly through the air. Beyond this area is park land with flower beds and fountains and shade trees and walks and beyond that again "nature forest" on both sides of the river. Car traffic moves along the river-side and motor boats ply up and down the stream carrying pleasure-seekers on holiday. There are many areas to disembark on either side. We took a river-boat trip to finish off our sight-seeing excursion.

We motored out to see the Ostankino TV tower. Elevators take guests up to the dining-rooms at different heights. One is a revolving restaurant.

We saw the obelisk built to commemorate the launching of the first earth satellite by the Soviet astronauts.

En route, we saw the Lenin Stadium. This sports arena seats 103,000 spectators. In this area and along the river front are over 130 sports installations of varying kinds.

The people one sees on the street, and today I saw many thousands of them, appear active and healthy; and certainly the ones at the amusement park – thousands of them – were having fun, but were not boisterous or jostling one another in the crowds or in the long queues waiting for their turn to get on the "wheels" and rides. There was a sense of joy permeating the whole scene.

The government is now actively engaged in re-constructing and restoring many old buildings, including monasteries and Cathedrals. At one time, there were 1,600 Cathedrals and Christian churches in Moscow. Now there are forty-one. Like many of our people at home, however, many non-believers still like to attend services at Easter and Christmas, or on other special religious occasions. There are now only three monasteries open and active, and these are in remote areas of Russia.

The vast riches of oil and gas, of gold and other metals, and diamonds are being explored and developed. One of the difficult problems in Russia as in Canada is that doctors and others do not choose readily to go into the developing north.

Before heading home, Dr. Thorlakson visited Leningrad, Finland and then Norway, where he visited his cousins in Oslo and Bergen. He then made a stop in Ottawa where he was given an opportunity to address the World Medical Association's meeting regarding the First International Congress of Group Medicine meeting, which was held in Winnipeg in April 1970. He had an opportunity to meet delegates from Brazil and other countries who would also be attending the meeting in Winnipeg as well as renewing his acquaintance with the president of the Medical Workers Union of Russia.

APPENDIX 4

Changing Concepts in Medical Care

Dr. Thorlakson presented a paper at the Western Conference on Prepaid Medical Service Plans, in Portland, Oregon, on November 10, 1971:

The subject we are concerned with today is the division of responsibility and labour between various members of the health team.

When I entered the practice of medicine over fifty years ago, the situation in most parts of North America was relatively uncomplicated. More than ninety per cent of all medical care was conducted in the patient's home. It was an intimate, private and largely confidential relationship between the patient and the doctor. Clinical records were rarely kept. The doctor carried the necessary equipment in his little black bag to deliver a child, to treat a fever or to mend an injury. Members of the family stood by to feed and comfort the patient.

The physician had five or six specific drugs available to him, plus castor oil and a host of placebos.

Clinical tests were rarely performed on patients confined to their homes except for an occasional urinalysis or hemoglobin estimation. There were few specialists or consultants. Eighty per cent of the population lived in farming areas. The physicians in these rural settings performed some minor surgery but referred the majority of surgical problems to a general surgeon in a nearby city. The general surgeon did all the surgery that was possible under the circumstances of that day. The doctor was then the sole arbiter on all health matters. There were no government departments of health and no private health agencies, as they exist today, except for a few citizens who sat on the boards of directors of general hospitals. Generous citizens kept the local hospital fairly solvent but always took for granted that the doctors would attend the many charity patients, both in and outside the hospital, without charge. This arrangement was, in fact, the origin of our present large university teaching complexes. In the home, the mother acted as the nurse. In the hospital, a *few* trained nurses but more often the nurses-in-training took the mother's place.

Nothing very dramatic occurred to disturb the personal relationship between the doctor and the patient until a short thirty years ago. Then began a fantastic increase in scientific medical knowledge and technology. Three striking phenomena have resulted: specialization of physicians, a steady proliferation of health workers, and replacement of the home environment by institutional care.

Conservatively speaking, we have now thirty or more categories of physicians and a large number – over two hundred categories – of other essential professional and technical members of the health team. Today, the patient, the physician and the nurse are supported by a veritable army of co-workers. Each category of this vast team is forming its own national organization and demanding recognition with special rights and privileges to set its own standards of work and pay. In addition, we have experts in medical engineering, medical sociology, medical economics and administration.

On top of all this, we are now faced with third party involvement by government and private agencies. Speaking specifically about prepaid medical and hospital insurance plans, there is a basic difference between the United States and Canada. Whereas your pre-payment plans are, for the most part, underwritten by private insurance corporations, in Canada, our Federal and Provincial governments have introduced – by law – compulsory hospital and medical insurance for *all* Canadians. Universality and transferability from one province to another formed the cornerstone of the Federal Government's plan. Our Federal Government practically forced the provinces into this scheme by offering to contribute approximately one-half of the cost of both services. But here, I would like to stress another difference in our two situations. In the United States, some private paying agencies have, I understand, a fee schedule under which physician's assistants are reimbursed for their services but, in Canada, no such provision has been established.

Another important factor is that, in the United States, there is available a large pool of corps-men who, during their military service, have acquired considerable experience in the care of the sick and injured. With some additional training, these people can be absorbed into the health team. In Canada, the main available source of supply at present is our registered nurses as they are eligible to enter the courses organized by our universities for physician's assistants.

In Canada, the term "nurse practitioner" or "clinical assistant" seems more appropriate. The first term more accurately indicates the basis of her training and her status in the health team. Speakers at the recent Assembly of the World Medical Association expressed the fear that the terms "physician's assistant" or "physician's associate" might mislead the public into thinking that the person was medically qualified.

Today, we are discussing the problems and benefits in the use of allied health personnel, particularly in the field of primary contact and continuing care. One reason for our present difficulties in this area is that, during the past thirty years, the medical faculties of our universities have supplied us with an increasing number of specialists but with very few family or primary contact practitioners. In Canada, this valuable member of the profession is diminishing at an alarming rate and there is no adequate replacement for him in sight. In some areas there has been a slight increase since 1967 due to the importation of graduates from other countries.

In North America, twenty years ago, we were told that the specialist in Internal Medicine would be the primary contact physician of the future but this specialty has now become as fragmented as the surgical specialties. By former standards, there are few general surgeons and general internists and a totally inadequate number of general or family practitioners. We have been assured, by the College of Family Physicians of Canada, that a specially trained family practitioner can attend to eighty-five percent of the common illnesses of mankind. But it now takes an additional two or three years to train a family physician as a specialist in his or her own right.

How then have we managed? If Canada and the United States had not been able to entice large numbers of foreign doctors and postgraduate students to join our ranks, our much vaunted North American system of medical care would now be in very serious difficulty. To walk into a large teaching hospital now is like walking through the corridors of the United Nations. In some respects this is marvellous but at what a sacrifice to other nations who cannot afford to lose any of their trained health workers and, consequently, are suffering more acutely while we – in our affluent society – reap the benefits.

I heard this complaint voiced strenuously by several speakers from the under-developed countries at The World Medical Association Assembly in Ottawa, Canada, in September of this year.

In effect, they pleaded with representatives of the "have" nations to stop raiding their medical manpower and said: "If you want to help us, come and train our specialists in our own country where they will remain to practice." In support of this plea, one needs only to state that, in 1967, the immigrant doctors registered to practice in Canada exceeded Canadian graduates for the year by 1213 to 923 and many of these immigrant doctors were from underdeveloped countries. Furthermore, in 1970, Canada produced 1094 doctors compared to 894 in 1955. This is surely a very meagre increase. I doubt very much if the United States of America is doing any better in relation to its total population.

In the United States and Canada, we train all our own doctors in large health sciences centres in large cities. As a result, most of the graduates now wish to become professors, medical scientists or specialists but not practitioners who normally would be expected to provide most of the comprehensive, continuing care of the patient and the family. The answer is obvious: a substantial part of clinical training should take place in institutions providing medical services to ambulatory and home-care patients and not entirely in highly specialized hospitals.

To try and compensate for the lack of family physicians, doctors have depended more and more on staff who have been trained "on the job" to relieve them of certain routine duties.

The duties and responsibilities of a physician's assistant will, of course, vary considerably depending on whether she works in a remote nursing station, a hospital or a doctor's office. For practical purposes, I will direct my remarks to this type of physician's assistant who is employed in a doctor's office.

Public focus is now centered mainly on first contact and continuing health care. With our present medical manpower shortage, this must be provided, in many instances, by a person who can appraise the situation and decide on the next step; but physicians are finding it difficult or impossible to meet the demand for primary health care.

Who can provide this essential service? An idea gaining ground was well expressed by John F. McCreary, Dean of Medicine, University of British Columbia, before the Canadian Public Health Association: "I had five years in a general practice of pediatrics. A great deal – perhaps a majority – of the work which I did could have been done as well or better by public health nurses, dietitians, clinical psychologists and others of the health group. It was a ridiculously costly arrangement for one who had taken a medical degree and six years of post-graduate training to be performing tasks which could be better done by less costly personnel."

Speaking on this subject, Dr. J. Wendell Macleod, the former Executive Director of the Association of Canadian Medical Colleges said: "I would assert that in most cities and countless scattered rural communities in Canada, a substantial proportion of the people will not receive appropriate care until the physician relinquishes to others some of his responsibility for diagnosis and treatment."

Reporting on examined health needs and services in some twenty countries around the world, John Bryant of the Rockefeller Foundation commented that the insistence of the medical profession that only physicians can evaluate and treat the sick, "has a paralysing effect on the design and implementation of health services and is one of the most serious obstacles to the effective use of limited health resources."

The precise role of the physician, nurse, medical assistant or others of the health team must, of course, be determined in relation to local needs and resources. We have a gross shortage of primary care physicians in Canada. Can we, and should we, learn to utilize nurses in primary health care? In a liaison role, could nurses also help to make health care more continuous and comprehensive?

Bryant suggests that the nurse act in a complementary relationship with the physician – "[the] two parts acting together complete a whole. Given appropriate educational background and adaptability, the nurse can range between working with the physician in planning and policy, on the one hand and implementation with other paramedical and auxiliary workers, on the other."

Before a significant move can be made in this direction – and, to this moment, we have accomplished very little in Canada – changes in medical and nursing education are required, but the public must also be educated as to what is and what is not possible in modern medicine. There must be broad acceptance by both the providers and the recipients in this new concept of primary health care.

The physician's assistant may be well qualified but the physician must delegate duties to her in accordance with his confidence in her ability and his particular need for her services. Her degree of involvement in the patient's initial investigation will be determined by the doctor or doctors with whom she is working. If this basic principle is not accepted by our planners or by the physician's assistants, then there is no point in proceeding further with this arrangement.

To gain the confidence of the doctor's patients, she must impress upon each one – at the outset – that what she is doing is at the request of, and under the direction of, the doctor. It should be incorporated in her record on the patient's chart that this fact is fully understood by the patient. In creating this additional member of our team, it must be realized and accepted that the physician's assistant is not replacing a doctor. The final responsibility for all aspects of the patient's medical care must, and will always, rest with the doctor. But surely there can be no question that we must rapidly train many more family physicians or else augment the training of, and increase the responsibilities of, other health workers. Even better still, we must do both. Time is of the essence if we are to meet the needs of society.

In preparation for this presentation, I wrote to twenty-eight of the larger clinics across Canada inquiring about their utilization of specially trained physician's assistants. Of this number, only three clinics presently employ physician's assistants. They perform the following duties:

1. Dealing with inquiries made by patients new to the Clinic and directing them to the appropriate doctor or doctors and arranging advance investigation according to instructions from the Clinic doctors.

2. Determining the urgency of appointments.

3. Assisting new patients to complete questionnaires prior to consultations.

4. Seeing patients referred for screening prior to attending their regular doctor. This service applies to routine cases where the index of suspicion of disease is low. The nurse performs a standard series of examinations based on the patient's sex and age and arranges a standard group of tests. The patient sees his or her own doctor subsequently but much time is saved because of the preliminary "work-up."

5. Performing cervical smears.

6. Post-operative wound dressings.

7. Removal of sutures.

8. Vaccinations.

9. Contact patients by telephone or makes house calls.

10. Skin testing for allergy.

The remainder of the clinics I contacted use members of their non-medical staff in the traditional manner to assist the doctor after he has written the patient's history and performed a physical examination. These para-medical personnel have usually been trained "on the job" for the specific duties assigned to them.

[Here Dr. Thorlakson described the services provided by feldschers in the USSR (see Appendix 3).]

In attempting to establish the physician's assistant as a member of the health team, we are liable to meet with resistance from some doctors who may argue that the doctor-patient relationship is in jeopardy.

Fears likely will be expressed about professional and legal responsibilities, and the anticipated increase in over-head expenses. The economic consideration will probably apply chiefly when a doctor is working on a fee-for-service basis because salary for the nurse associate will be charged against his income. The doctor-patient relationship must be maintained and could be substantially improved by making it easier for the patient to enter the health care system. This can be achieved if the doctor is willing to relinquish part of his traditional role and assign certain duties to a physician's assistant. Relief from some of his present routine procedures would give the doctor additional time for more complex procedures for which his particular knowledge and skill are essential.

The employment of para-medical personnel in Canada and the United States is, of course, a matter of personal necessity and choice for the individual doctor to decide. However, from experience, I wish to state that – at the Winnipeg Clinic – we have found the services of a physician's assistant most useful in performing a number of routine duties which, while necessary, were time-consuming for busy doctors and consequently proved to be rather tedious for them when they knew their time could be utilized to better advantage by attending to more urgent medical or surgical problems.

The majority of patients seem to accept the services rendered by a physician's assistant more readily than some members of the medical profession. This is particularly true when a patient has had an initial interview with the physician's assistant and then requires information or advice about the investigation ordered by the doctor or concerning the medication or treatment he has prescribed. The patient needs answers to certain questions and often hesitates to bother a busy doctor but feels differently about a call to the physician's assistant.

No health system in the world can ever be perfect or ideal but we should continue to strive towards improving and adding to our services. The establishment of so many types of para-medical personnel carries with it numerous problems, such as the status of each category in the health team; licensing or registration; legal responsibility for services performed in their line of duty; the limitations to be placed on their respective capacities; the possible formation of many more technical or professional associations or organizations, which will eventually want to be recognized as the authority to set acceptable working conditions and scale of remuneration for their members.

In the July 24 issue of The Canadian Medical Association Journal, it was reported that "The Canadian Medical Association is presently engaged actively with only about thirty allied health professions; potentially as many as two hundred of these organizations could conceivably solicit Association involvement in their training programs –

at a cost to the CMA currently averaging between $4,000 and $5,000 each. The Council on Medical Education will, in the coming year, study methods of coping with proliferation in anticipation of preparing a policy on allied health profession training and the extent of CMA participation and financial support of approval programs for emerging health professions."

Opinions differ as to how to train physician's assistants. In Canada, two opposing views are held by Dr. J.B. Ralph McKendry, Assistant Professor of Medicine at the University of Ottawa, and by Dr. Helen K. Mussallem, Executive Director of the Canadian Nurses' Association. Dr. McKendry believes that the best way to prepare this "new breed of health professional" is to devise a four-year course of studies which would train individuals to take a position somewhere between the doctor and the nurse. Dr. Mussallem, on the other hand, insists that graduate nurses could be specially trained and utilized to function in this area. She points out that there is a surplus of nurses in some urban areas. In any event, in this context, we are not training the traditional assistant who carries out procedures after the doctor has written a history and completed his physical examination. We are training people who can assist patients, and ultimately the doctor, by initially interviewing them and assisting them to enter the health care system, which is rapidly becoming too complicated for many of them to understand. . . .

There are two sides to every coin and, if the doctor hopes to utilize the skills and services of trained para-medical personnel to the best advantage, then he must be prepared and willing to delegate certain responsibilities to competent assistants and associates in whom he has confidence.

Emphasis is placed now on the "health team" but the team will only function efficiently and effectively if each member shows respect and consideration for the positions allocated to their team-mates.

While some doctors and some patients may be reluctant to admit that new trends in medical practice are necessary, I believe the great majority recognize that our system of delivering health services requires re-organization. Both the patient and the doctor will benefit by utilizing all the skills available for providing comprehensive and continuing health care.

The pivot around which this concerted team effort is centered is the patient. Most patients are accustomed to the traditional form of medical practice and they must be carefully alerted to the new trends in the delivery of health services. The health team needs the complete cooperation of the doctor, the para-medical personnel and the patient.

APPENDIX 5

The Challenge of Sir Frederick Banting

This address was delivered to the annual meeting of the White Cross Guild of the Winnipeg General Hospital in 1952, and subsequently published in the *Manitoba Medical Review* (Vol. 32 No. 7: 436–438, August–September, 1952).

The discovery of insulin for the control of diabetes by the late Sir Frederick Banting in 1921 has been hailed as the beginning of an active programme of medical research in Canada. In addition to his own special contribution and discovery, he encouraged and influenced medical research in all parts of Canada. Young scientists were attracted to him and applied for permission to work in his laboratory. Wherever he travelled, young men and women were eager to hear him speak and were encouraged when he told them about the opportunities that were being created in order that they might pursue a particular research problem. It is not generally known that during the last fifteen years of his life he conducted research in cancer.

In 1936, President McNaughton of the National Research Council submitted proposals concerning the organization of medical research in Canada to the Canadian Medical Association, the Royal College of Physicians and Surgeons of Canada and the Departments of Pensions and National Health. As a result of these discussions, the National Research Council in Ottawa created the Associate Committee on Medical Research in 1938, with Sir Frederick Banting as Chairman. Beginning in October of that year, he set out to make a survey of research facilities in Canadian medical schools. In his travels he found many medical scientists eager to carry out research. In his speeches that year, he urged Canadians generally and the Universities in particular to do whatever lay in their power to stop the annual loss of many of our young trained scientists. These young men and women were leaving Canada because of the lack of research facilities and financial support. How far has Canada progressed in the last fourteen years in meeting the challenge presented in 1938 by Sir Frederick Banting?

The Associate Committee in 1938 was given in its first year a budget of $53,000. Medical scientists in the Universities were invited to make application for research assistance. More requests came than could be satisfied and preference was given to investigations bearing on chronic diseases.

The program of medical research had hardly begun when suddenly we were at war. Canada's medical research efforts had to be turned to the solution of problems associated with aviation, naval and army medical research. The problems investigated related to the comfort, safety, protection, clothing, and nutrition of the particular service for which special committees were established. During a five-year period much was accomplished in the practical application of fundamental knowledge previously learned. Subjects receiving special attention were the prevention and treatment of shock, storage of blood, the preparation and storage of blood derivatives, treatment of infection of wounds and the treatment of burns and injuries. Much was also accomplished in problems of special interest to aviation medicine, especially those related to the physiological reactions of pilots at high altitudes and sudden changes in gravitational forces. In the Navy, Canada had a specific contribution to make in the treatment of what is called "immersion foot." Important contributions were made on the subject of motion sickness by Dr. Best and his associates. In matters related to army problems, the work done at Suffield in Alberta was outstanding for the contributions made to the allied cause in the subject of gas warfare.

And what of the post-war period? Very briefly, it might be stated that there has taken place, since the end of the war, a vast acceleration of medical research across our country. Due largely to public interest in the problem of cancer created by the active Divisions of the Canadian Cancer Society, definite steps were taken to ensure a more concerted effort in the field of medical research related to cancer. In January, 1947, the Honourable Paul Martin, Minister of National Health and Welfare, called a conference of representatives of all those organizations which might be interested in cancer research and treatment. Out of this came the organization of the National Cancer Institute, which undertook to co-ordinate cancer research in Canada and to support graduate training in cancer research and treatment.

The National Cancer Institute required funds. The trustees of the King George V Jubilee Cancer Fund offered its capital sum of $450,000 to the National Cancer Institute in three annual installments as a nucleus for its programme. Additional funds were subscribed by the

Canadian Cancer Society. The new organization was then in a position to invite applications for assisted research grants and fellowships in the problem of cancer. The Institute decided that any investigation involving problems of growth and metabolism would be acceptable in its research program. This opened the field to botanists, zoologists and biochemists, as well as to experimental pathologists, physiologists, physicists, cytologists and virologists. In 1947 the Institute made twenty-eight awards amounting to $84,000. In 1949 it made fifty-seven awards and appointed research fellows. As soon as the National Cancer Institute was able to give grants for cancer research, the National Research Council withdrew from the field. The most remarkable feature of this change, however, was that whereas the National Research Council had received very few applications for research in cancer and made only two awards in 1946, the National Cancer Institute within a year of its establishment received 48 applications amounting to $360,000. This was due partly to the liberal interpretation of what constitutes research in cancer, partly due to the interest awakened by the great publicity attending the new organization, and partly due to the expansion in research facilities in the Universities. The National Cancer Institute has now been in existence for almost five years and during that period has assisted cancer research in our Canadian medical schools and hospitals to the extent of over $1,000,000. Over seventy research projects are currently being supported in our medical schools, and up to as many as fifteen men per year are assisted in their research training. That the public has whole-heartedly supported the efforts of the National Cancer Institute is made evident by the fact that the Canadian Cancer Society, through its Provincial Chapters, has contributed over one-half of the funds available for its work. The remainder of the funds have come from federal and provincial grants for the control of cancer.

But interest in our various health problems has not been confined to the subject of cancer alone. The Canadian Arthritis and Rheumatism Society is now active in the diagnostic and treatment field and also in the support of research relating to the peculiar problems of arthritis and rheumatism. The federal health grants announced in 1948 have made available several hundred thousand dollars per year for public health research. The Defense Research Board is supporting investigation on problems of particular interest to its work. Other amounts are available for mental health research and public-spirited groups, such as the Canadian Life Insurance Officers' Association and several pharmaceutical companies, have contributed munificently to the support of medical research in Canada. That Canadian scientists are capable of making an important contribution in medical research is also shown by the fact that American fund-granting bodies give approximately $200,000.00 per year towards the support of the medical research in Canada. In 1947 and 1948 Canadian Universities were receiving, for medical research purposes, more than $1,250,000 per year. At the present time, the figure is $2,355,000 and the total number of Canadians actively engaged in medical research in Canada now probably exceeds 1,200. I am sure that Sir Frederick Banting would have been pleased with this evidence of progress. The fact that young Canadians are able to carry out research to this extent in our Canadian Universities is, in part, a tribute to his leadership.

Having reviewed briefly the story of the growth of medical research in Canada or, what we might better call, our coming of age in the field of medical research, I would like to turn for a few minutes to the story of cancer.[1]

One of the greatest figures in the history of medicine, Galen, developed a remarkable clinical classification of tumors about 150 A.D. This classification has stood well the test of time and requires no alteration to bring it within the scope of what we know today. He spoke of "tumors according to nature," which would include the enlargement of the breasts during pregnancy and lactation and the increase in the size of the uterus during pregnancy. He referred also to "tumors exceeding nature," an example of which was the callous formation seen in the healing of broken bones. Then again, he referred to the "tumors contrary to nature" and within this group he placed the benign and malignant tumors which we know today.

The microscope was invented by a Dutchman in the seventeenth century AD but almost two centuries were to pass before it was recognized that the cell was the fundamental unit of all living matter. It was then just one short step before it was shown that cancer tissue is but an aggregate of individual cells. Some clarification of the nature of cancer thus became possible and the idea that cancer represented an abnormal proliferation of cells seemed to evolve naturally. Side by side with the careful classification of tumors under the microscope, clinicians were also carefully recording the clinical nature of cancer. That is to say, how it behaved in humans and the various forms in which cancer manifests itself.

In 1911, Dr. Peyton Rous, working at the Rockefeller Institute in New York, visited a marketplace and offered $5 for every live bird brought to his laboratory with a tumor. Many birds had abscesses and other swellings but eventually a Plymouth Rock hen was brought in with an unusual tumor. It was a sarcoma known since as Rous' Sarcoma. He was able to transplant this tumor into other birds. Furthermore, the fluid from the tumor could be passed through a Berkefeld filter and when the solution was injected into the tissue of a bird, the same type of tumor developed. This observation created quite a furore in scientific circles. Was cancer in the human caused by a certain virus infection? The evidence is against such a theory. However, this particular tumor has been investigated in research laboratories in many parts of the world. All of them, however, trace their original source to the same tumor found in this one Plymouth Rock hen in New York City in 1911. No other example of a similar spontaneous tumor in fowl has been discovered. However, the investigation of this particular tumor has contributed to our knowledge of the behaviour of malignant tumors.

In 1915 two Japanese produced cancer on the ear of the rabbit by painting it for long periods with tar. One of the finest stories in medical research was to take place over the next fifteen years. It is the story of Kennaway and his colleagues in London who persevered for fifteen years in attempting to islolate from tar the agent responsible for producing cancer. They were successful. Since then some 300 cancer-producing chemical compounds have been described and our experimentalists today are able to produce cancer at will and study the nature of the changes which take place.

Progress in medical research related to cancer cannot be measured in terms of what is accomplished from year to year, but in terms of what is accomplished in ten and twenty-year periods. Our research workers are making their individual contributions to the total sum of knowledge concerning the nature of cancer and it can be said, in all fairness, that Canada is now making its proportionate contribution to the international effort devoted to finding the cause and the cure of this disease.

A few examples of work now being supported in Canada will serve to illustrate this fact. In British Columbia, a botanist is devoting his time to a study of tumors which occur in plants where the phenomena of cell division can be more easily observed and interpreted than is possible in the complex animal organism. In Edmonton, the anaemia characteristic of some forms of cancer is being studied in tissue culture and an anatomist is extending an observation, made by him several years ago, that there is a great concentration of iron in the breast tissue of mice which have a tendency to develop cancer in this organ. In Saskatoon, a young and most capable physicist, working in collaboration with his medical colleagues, has made possible the treatment of patients with the high energy x-rays produced by the betatron and the tremendous energy in the form of gamma rays produced with radioactive cobalt. We may take some pride in the fact that this is the only country in the world at the present time in which this latter form of treatment is being use.

In Winnipeg and several other centres, doctors are studying the effects of radioactive iodine in the treatment of cancer of the thyroid gland. At the University of Western Ontario in London, benign and malignant tumors of the breast (in rats) are being intensively studied by the Department of Medical Research under Dr. J.B. Collip, who played so significant a role in the development and purification of insulin. In Toronto, animal tumors are being grown in the yolk sac of fertilized eggs and their reaction to a variety of growth inhibitors is being observed. A biologist, using the technique of tissue culture, is endeavouring to establish exactly which chemical substances are necessary for the growth and division of normal and cancer cells.

At McGill University, the man who was responsible for the discovery of 2,4–D, the now well-known weed killer, is devoting his efforts to a study of the differences in biochemical behaviour of normal and cancerous cells.

Many more examples might be quoted but these few will serve to demonstrate that an active and earnest effort in cancer research is being made in Canada at the present time. This effort will continue and expand and there is no doubt in my mind that the young men and women who are being supported in their research training by the National Cancer Institute of Canada will have many and useful contributions to make in the years to come.

Sir Heneage Ogilvie, one of Britain's leading surgeons, summarized the situation with regard to cancer research in an address delivered at the last annual meeting of the British Empire Cancer Campaign: "The progress of the Cancer Campaign can be compared with the progress of a ship across the ocean. Each day those on board wake up to look over an unbroken expanse of sea, – bright and calm one day, dull and stormy the next. They have no visible evidence of progress towards their destination, but only of movement through the restless waves which billow in all directions as far as the eye can see. Those responsible for the ship's navigation have, perhaps, a greater conscious appreciation of the advance, although even to them it appears as no more than a change in the position of a pencilled dot on a chart. But in the fullness of time land appears over the horizon; the harbour is reached; and those on board are brought to a conscious realization that they have come some great distance across the world. So it is with the Cancer Campaign. Day by day the work goes patiently on, sometimes easy and satisfying, more often difficult and perplexing. The distant harbour still lies somewhere below the horizon, and it is at times difficult to appreciate that the ever-increasing store of knowledge being produced is, like the unseen propeller of the ship, steadily but surely driving the Campaign onward to that harbour."

APPENDIX 6

Address to Cancer Chemotherapy Symposium, Montreal, June 22, 1967

It has been a rewarding and stimulating experience for me to attend the scientific sessions of the Cancer Chemotherapy Symposium today and I deem it a distinct honour to have been invited to speak at this dinner.

In 1919, I established myself in the practice of medicine in the town of Shoal Lake, situated two hundred miles west of Winnipeg. . . .

When I recall my five decades of active practice, I am reminded of the story told about the late Somerset Maugham. His friends gave a dinner in honour of his ninetieth birthday. When the congratulatory speeches were over, Somerset Maugham rose slowly to his feet, surveyed his audience and said: "Ladies and Gentlemen, there are distinct advantages to growing old." Then he looked down at the table and stood silent for so long that his friends became somewhat alarmed. Finally, however, he raised his head and said: "I have been standing here trying to think just what the advantages could possibly be."

For a professional man who has been involved in the study and practice of medicine for over fifty years – first as a student and a resident in training and then as a surgeon and a teacher – there are strong temptations to reminisce, to draw comparisons and even to admonish and to advise. I have no special right nor desire to admonish or to advise but I shall succumb to the temptation to reminisce and to compare because the comparisons that I shall make will be in favour of the present and not of the past.

Half a century ago, when I began my training at the Winnipeg General Hospital, we were able to order only five or six routine laboratory tests apart from microscopic diagnosis. The common tests were: blood counts, urinalyses, blood Wassermann, blood sugar, blood urea nitrogen, and blood creatinine. This compares to the many hundreds of clinical laboratory tests available to us in the same hospital today. The famous Professor William Boyd was the pathologist of the Winnipeg General Hospital and Professor of Pathology at the Manitoba Medical College at that time. I believe he had two microscopes in his laboratory and one part-time assistant.

The X-Ray Department in the hospital had one machine and the plates were poor by comparison to present day standards – in fact, we had only recently graduated, I believe, from glass x-ray plates. Routine chest x-rays, of course, were not taken. Patients with unrecognized active tuberculosis lay in the beds of our hospitals in this country spreading the infection to both interns and nurses.

We had a few specific drugs: digitalis for heart disease; quinine for malaria; salvarson (606) for syphilis; iron for anemia; and emetine for amebiasis. In addition, potassium iodide was added to many mixtures. Arsenic, in minute doses, was prescribed for a variety of diseases, as were a host of cathartics, stimulants, digestants and sedatives of variable or doubtful benefit.

Acute or recurrent abdominal pain was treated by appendectomy through a small McBurney incision. Before the discovery and introduction of the Graham-Cole technique in 1924 to visualize the gall bladder, forty per cent of cholecystectomies were performed for so-called "chronic acalculous cholecystitis". Tonsillectomies and teeth extractions were done for removal of suspected foci of infection. Excision of tuberculous glands in the neck was common before the testing of cows and pasteurization of milk.

Occlusive vascular disease of the lower extremities was treated by amputation of the leg above the knee. Now our vascular surgeons short-circuit the block by a nylon tube which allows the patient to carry on with comfort with his own leg.

Brain surgery consisted of raising a flap of skull to relieve intracranial pressure due to expanding malignant tumors and the raising of depressed fractures of the skull.

Thoracic surgery consisted almost exclusively of removal of a small segment of one rib under local anaesthesia to drain a post-pneumonic pleural abscess.

Internists had little to offer or advise except bed-rest, vile-tasting concoctions, placebos and a trip to a spa or to the sea-shore!

Today, thanks to the energetic pursuit of knowledge, basic and clinic research, and the development of a multitude of specific drugs, progress has been substantial during the past few decades. For instance, lobar pneumonia, formerly called "the old man's friend" – or kidney infections with terminal uremia, do not destroy the aged and infirm at their allotted time. Instead, these unfortunate souls now, by the tens of thousands, languish in beds in our chronic hospitals and nursing homes in a state of utter helplessness, forgetfulness and creeping senility, waiting and praying for that old-age privilege of dying without medical restraint, without repeated intravenous infusion, indwelling catheters and recurrent faecal impaction of the rectum. Many of them pray fervently for the time when they will be allowed to pass into that happier land beyond the sunset. We have managed to create the new specialty of Geriatrics – a rapidly increasing challenge to modern medicine. It is obvious that while our miracle drugs, new inventions and other discoveries are a blessing in many cases, they do not always serve the best interests of all our patients.

Some months ago, a writer for one of our national magazines called to say that the Dean of one of our Canadian Universities had advised him to interview me because he was certain that I would be able to inform this journalist about many of the changes which have occured in medical practice, especially in group practice, during the past few decades.

The greatest changes, I explained, are the results of the rapid advances in knowledge that have become available to the practitioner of medicine. The complexity of modern medicine, I added, is responsible for limiting fields of practice to an ever increasing degree and that eventually, all doctors – including the family practitioner – will have to be specialists.

I told him that my surgical practice, as a "general surgeon", had become more and more restricted – in an anatomical sense – even though we are now able to perform a greater number of major operations, in a localized area of the body, with safety and confidence. I explained that many of the operations which a "general surgeon" was expected to do twenty-five or forty years ago, are now performed by surgeons limiting their practice to urology, gynaecology, orthopaedic surgery, chest surgery and so forth. The tremendous increase in knowledge of diseases in these areas and the special surgical skills required to deal with them, have created new and more effective approaches to many of the problems. I observed that no "general surgeon" could be expected to keep completely informed in all these fields of surgical work.

I also said that the role of the general practitioner had likewise undergone a radical change during this period. Only a few short decades ago, the general practitioner devoted his entire time to visiting and treating sick people in their homes. He made his rounds on a bicycle or with a horse and buggy. He knew and treated every individual member of the family and understood the family background, the financial circumstances and the home surroundings. Now this has changed. The present day general practitioner does the greater part of his professional work in his office and in the hospital, as do the specialists.

Today, the doctor can no longer transport the necessary diagnostic tools and facilities from his modern office or from the hospital, in a little black bag, as did the physician of thirty-five or forty years ago. His bag contained a stethoscope, a blood pressure machine, an obstetrical forceps, a scalpel and a few forceps, a bottle of codeine and morphine tablets, some bandages and adhesive tape. House calls now are largely a matter of professional sociability rather than for purposes of expert diagnosis and medical treatment. Furthermore, with the trend towards unlimited demands for medical services by the public, but with our limited human and financial resources, a concentration of the physician's work has become mandatory.

In other words, I told the representative of the magazine, this all means that the terms "general surgeon" and "general practitioner" are now, to a large extent obsolete. At this time, the interview was interrupted and terminated by an urgent professional call. Sometime later, I read his article. He obviously had taken note of my comments and described me as an "obsolete" general surgeon. It takes a frank and honest opinion like this to force a man to take serious stock of himself and to re-appraise his place in the society of professional men.

This brings up the question of obsolescence. Much of the expensive medical equipment that we are purchasing now will be obsolete in five to ten years. Doctors, themselves, can rapidly become obsolete unless they read and study more after graduation than they did before. Some are running a race with scientific progress and finding the pace almost beyond their capabilities, except in some restricted fields of medicine. As Dr. Wilder Penfield observed recently, in an address on the Vanier Institute of the Family, and I quote: "The time has now arrived when practically all bread earners in our land will be specialists."

While I am reminiscing, may I make one more observation which I believe to be significant. Thirty years ago, most patients who entered my consulting-room were obviously sick people. This is in sharp contrast to the healthy-looking people who now come for a routine medical check-up with early symptoms but few physical signs of serious organic disease. In those so-called "good old days" of medicine – which, in retrospect, were really bad days – a history and physical examination too often revealed that the patient was suffering from advanced or hopeless disease. Symptoms and signs were localized. Intensive investigation was neither available nor necessary. It was the era of inexpensive medicine when very little could actually be done for many patients. Too often they went to hospital to die, not to be cured. The mention of a hospital to the patient's relatives, around the turn of the last century, struck fear into the whole household.

One hardly walked down a street without seeing a "quarantine" sign on some door. In 1906, when Winnipeg was a small city, there were three thousand patients admitted to the Winnipeg General Hospital with typhoid fever alone and yet another three thousand or more were treated in their homes after drinking contaminated water from the wells along the Red and Assiniboine Rivers.

Family planning was not necessary, in those days, because diphtheria, scarlet fever, typhoid fever, pneumonia, tuberculosis, poliomyelitis, infantile diarrhoea, gonorrhoea, and syphilis – some of which are preventable and all of which are curable by modern means – decimated the population.

Now is certainly the most rewarding time in the history of mankind to be a doctor of medicine. The medicine of 1967 has so much to offer the sick and the depressed and the injured. Methods of prevention, diagnosis and treatment of disease – not even dreamed of fifty or thirty years ago – are now available to the physician.

At the Cancer Chemotherapy Symposium today, and at this dinner tonight, we have with us a group of medical scientists who are involved in one of the most important fields of medical research – the chemotherapy of malignant disease.

This group of scientists are the inheritors of the basic research work performed by a great number of scientists working in the laboratories of the universities and in the chemical and pharmaceutical industries of Germany, France, England, Switzerland, the United States, Canada and other countries. This effective collaboration between academically-based and industry-based scientists had its beginning with the work of Paul Ehrlich during his medical undergraduate years in Breslau and Leipzig from 1872 until 1878. His thesis at graduation was entitled "Contributions to the Theory and Practice of Histological Staining." He was able to enunciate the basic principle "that pharmacological activity was based on an affinity of the molecules in living matter for certain chemical substances." After many years of painstaking and fruitful work in the fields of bacteriology, immunology and chemotherapy, this eminent medical scientist, Professor Ehrlich, and his Japanese assistant, Dr. Sahachiro Hata, reported to the Congress of Internal Medicine at Wiesbaden, Germany, on April 19, 1910, that the chemical compound labelled 606 in their series – Hydrochloride of dioxy-diamino-arseno-benzine or Salvarsan – was effective in the treatment of syphilis, a disease which had destroyed countless millions of the human race. This achievement in chemical synthesis and testing against the specific spirochete of syphilis set the stage for intensive activity in a new branch of medical science-chemotherapy.

By intensive, painstaking laboratory work and extensive clinical trials, our special guests of honour are today applying the knowledge and techniques developed during the past century to combat that devastating and fatal parasite – the cancer cell. In their work, they are following the admonition of Professor Ehrlich when he said: "We must search for magic bullets. We must strike the parasite only, if possible, and, to do this, we must learn to aim with chemical bullets."

The inter-dependence of the University-based and industrially-based laboratories in the synthesis and application of new drugs was forcefully expressed by Professor Ernst B. Chain of the Imperial College of Science and Technology in a lecture delivered to the Royal Society of Arts in London in 1963, and I quote from his address:

"I hope to have made it quite clear that notwithstanding the many important contributions from University laboratories, drug research and development without the active participation of the pharmaceutical industry is impossible.... I, for one, prefer to have an active pharmaceutical industry and life-saving drugs, accepting in the bargain a few abuses, than to have a system in which theoretically no abuses are possible, but which produces no drugs ... Let us, once and for all, accept the indisputable fact which the history of drug research teaches us through innumerable examples ... that the best results in the field have been obtained by close collaboration between industrial and academic laboratories. This collaboration is, in my view, of the utmost importance for the future ... Let us be sure to deploy all our available resources ... so that we can give the scientists, concerned with drug research, both in the university and in industry, the most favourable conditions in which they can advance ... their one great aim ... to combat and conquer pain and an ever-increasing range of diseases through the discovery of new and more effective drugs."

Professor Chain is one of the Nobel Laureates who, together with Sir Alexander Fleming and Sir Howard Florey, were honoured for their discovery and practical application of penicillin.

The medical scientists, who we have listened to today, have given us a clearer insight into their particular approach to the problems of abnormal growth and the manner in which they are attempting to break the vicious cycle of uncontrolled malignant proliferation of the cancer cell in the human body by using new chemical compounds. As we heard them present their experiences, we were surely impressed with the fact that modern scientific research workers, as well as modern medical practitioners, are demonstrating the vital importance of good team work. Multi-discipline approach is rapidly replacing the solo research worker and the lone medical practitioner of the past.

Ladies and gentlemen, we Canadians are now celebrating the Centennial of Confederation. In honour of this historic occasion, Canadians have extended the traditional one day birthday celebration to one year of commemoration. Many Centennial projects, varied and inspired in their conception, will remain as permanent tributes to the imagination and resourcefulness of the Canadian people. At the close of this memorable Centennial year, every person will know more about the history and achievements of Canada – the land of his birth or the land of his adoption – and will have a deeper appreciation of what it means to be a Canadian.

As visitors to this great city of Montreal, we have had the opportunity to witness the ingenuity and the handywork of man. Expo 67 is this year's show-place and meeting-place of the nations of the world. Progress is depicted in its most attractive and awe-inspiring attire. This is the background against which we have held the scientific meetings today and been entertained at dinner tonight.

This evening, we look back one hundred years with wonderment and thanksgiving for the remarkable progress in medical science and in human understanding. Canadian medical scientists have made noteworthy contributions to the advancement of knowledge. We cannot help but wonder what lies ahead for our grandchildren and great-grandchildren during the next one hundred years.

"It is an extraordinary era in which we live. Everybody knows that the age is remarkable for scientific research into the heavens, the earth, what is beneath the earth; and perhaps more remarkable still is the application of this scientific research to the pursuit of life. The ancients saw nothing like it. The moderns have seen nothing like it until the present generation. The progress of the age has almost outstripped human belief." Ladies and gentlemen, these words were spoken one hundred and twenty years ago by Daniel Webster.

APPENDIX 7

Colleagues Remembered

DR. BRANDUR JONSSON BRANDSON

The following appreciation of the late Brandur Jonsson Brandson was published in the *Manitoba Medical Review* in August 1944. Besides his BA, MD and MS degrees, Dr. Brandson was awarded the FRCS (Can.), the FACS, an MD Honoris Causa (Iceland), the Grand Knight Commander of the Royal Icelandic Order of the Falcon, and the LL D Honoris Causa (Man.).

A request to write a brief appreciation of the life and work of the late Dr. B.J. Brandson, Professor Emeritus of Surgery of the Medical Faculty of the University of Manitoba, imposes a responsibility to present a concise but adequate appraisal of his character and achievements. His friends will agree that Dr. Brandson's contribution to the community he served so generously and with such distinction for nearly forty years is beyond calculation. His great qualities as a Canadian citizen, as a leader, as a surgeon and teacher have been given wide recognition. To write about him with moderation and restraint, as he would have wished, is difficult for anyone who knew him well.

Outside his professional work as a surgeon, he sought and found constant delight and companionship in his family, his friends, his books and his Church. He lived a full and useful life. Intellectually, he had a clear, logical mind, tinctured by a wholesome sense of humor. He was intensely sympathetic in his human relationships. His friends and many patients will long remember his words of assurance and comfort, his gentle but firm touch, the slow wave of his hand, his friendly smile with the knowing twinkle in his eye and his characteristic chuckle. He was intensely human – a priceless quality in his profession.

In limited space, one can only enumerate his many excellent qualities. He possessed great strength of character, unusual capacity for service, good judgment, loyalty and constancy in friendship, generosity and steadfastness. These attributes of his character are illustrated by his fidelity and constant devotion to the four institutions with which he was prominently affiliated, the Medical Faculty of the University of Manitoba, the Winnipeg General Hospital, the First Lutheran Church of Winnipeg and the Icelandic Old Folks' Home, Betel.

The Church

The Church had a large place in Dr. Brandson's life, and he gave to it the best that was in him. He was a member of the First Lutheran Church in Winnipeg almost from the day of his arrival in the city and was one of its most regular attendants. In periods of difficulty and transition he was a staunch supporter and bulwark of strength. At the time of his death he was Honorary President of the congregation. He has been repeatedly proclaimed the outstanding layman of the Icelandic Lutheran Church of North America.

Betel

Betel is an institution located at Gimli, the home of the earliest Icelandic pioneers of Manitoba. Here the homelike atmosphere of congeniality and genuine solicitude for their comfort have permitted many to spend their sunset days in peace and contentment. In a large measure the success of this enterprise was due to Dr. Brandson's personal effort and good judgment. It stands today as a monument to his steadfastness of purpose and his generous spirit.

The Hospital

Dr. Brandson was on the surgical staff of the Winnipeg General Hospital from 1912 to 1934. During the last eight years of this period he was Surgeon-in-Chief. In 1934 he was appointed Consultant in Surgery to the hospital. The Hospital was his second home. During the latter half of his professional life he spent his entire mornings in the operating room, on ward rounds and in teaching. He was conservative but examined all new methods critically. His work as a surgeon was on a high plane of excellence. The enviable record of the Winnipeg General Hospital in the management of acute appendicitis is due in a noteworthy degree to his early insistence on the conservative non-surgical management of late appendicitis.

His last visit to the hospital was on Tuesday, June 16th, at 2 p.m. He came to have one of the interns give him an injection of Salyrgan.

Though obviously tired and ill he nevertheless maintained his delightful humor and also his professional interest in the drug and its effectiveness. Two or three of the interns were privileged to discuss this matter with him on that last visit.

THE UNIVERSITY OF MANITOBA

Dr. Brandson was appointed to the surgical staff of the Medical Faculty of the University in 1910. His aptitude for teaching quickly became recognized and he was greatly admired and respected by all interns and nurses. In 1927 he became Professor of Surgery, a post which he held until his retirement from active teaching in 1934. During this period he did not publish his surgical lectures in the medical or surgical journals. This is regrettable in view of his rare gifts of clear expression. It is to be hoped that his paper on Hydatid Cysts will sometime be published. His knowledge and experience of this subject was unique. No surgeon in this hemisphere has seen or operated on as many patients with this condition, nor will this experience ever come again to another surgeon. At convocation on May 12th, 1944, the University of Manitoba befittingly conferred on Dr. Brandson the degree of Doctor of Laws honoris causa.

It is with regret that I bring to a close this brief review of the life of an exceptional man. It was a great privilege to have known him. I deeply appreciate the opportunity of recording something of his interests and his achievements. The memories evoked in so doing will remain with me, a happy and cherished possession.

DR. NEIL JOHN MACLEAN

"There are four people," Dr. Thorlakson says, "who have had an immense influence on my life: my parents, my wife and Dr. Neil John Maclean." Dr. Maclean was an eminent member of his profession, highly respected by his colleagues, and esteemed by his friends and patients. The inaugural issue of the *Winnipeg Clinic Quarterly* in September 1948 was dedicated to the memory of Dr. Maclean, who died in 1946. Dr. W.A. Gardner, an orthopedic surgeon and a contemporary of Dr. Maclean, described his life and work:

For almost half a century Dr. Neil John Maclean was a medical practitioner and surgeon in our city of Winnipeg. For a great part of that period he was recognized throughout Canada as one of the leading surgeons of this Dominion.

In 1883 Winnipeg was a city of seventeen thousand. The young Maclean was working in the office of Dr. J.R. Jones. . . . Doubtless his association with Dr. Jones [and other medical men] contributed largely to Neil John Maclean's determination to study medicine. He certainly never lost interest in these pioneers. He was particularly interested in the surgery of the late Alexander Hugh Ferguson, Winnipeg's first surgeon, and later one of the three leading surgeons of Chicago: J.B. Murphy, Oschner and Ferguson. Dr. Maclean wrote Dr. Ferguson's biography for the Master of Surgery series, published in 1926 in the Journal of Surgery, Gynaecology and Obstetrics.

Neil John's ambition to study medicine could not be accomplished without delay. Before entering Medical School in 1894, he worked in several positions to meet the expenses of the education he planned. It was during this period that he became the first school teacher in the Shoal Lake district at the Wolfe Creek School (No. 817).

After graduation he elected to see some of the world as a ship's surgeon. Postgraduate work followed in 1904 and 1905. He obtained his membership in the Royal College of Surgeons of England and studied in Berlin and Vienna.

When our doctor returned to Winnipeg he opened an office at Main Street and Logan Avenue and soon had one of the largest practices in the city. This was the period when this city was transformed from a frontier town to the foremost industrial and distributing centre in Western Canada. It was also the horse-and-buggy period, when Doctors carried drugs and instruments with them in their medical bags and much of their surgery was done on the kitchen table. It seemed to me that wherever I went, I saw Dr. Maclean driving his horse on his round of visits. One wondered when he did his office and hospital work, but that was done late into the night. Time was never one of his serious or disturbing considerations.

The era Dr. Maclean entered was outstanding in the history of medicine. Modern surgery was in its infancy. Illustrious figures dominated its ranks. Their achievements were made possible by the great discoveries of Pasteur and Lister. Nevertheless their reputations were formed by their own extraordinary capacities to devise new methods in man's struggle against disease. Halstead, Bergman, Mayo-Robson and Robert Jones, among others, were leaders in the surgical field. They were capable and resourceful, directing their newly acquired techniques to explore and control the vast unknown which had hitherto resisted mankind's efforts to conquer it. After these came a younger group, including Moyniham, the Mayos and Crile, who were destined to bring fame to themselves and to their profession. It was during this period that Dr. Maclean established his own reputation in Western Canada.

From the beginning he did his own surgery; then followed the surgery of many of his fellow practitioners, until surgery took all his time and attention. The preparation of his patients for operation, the technique of his surgery and the post-operative care were performed with meticulous attention to detail. Because of this the results of his work were extraordinary. Particularly so considering that many of the more recent advances in surgery had not become available. As he developed his surgical skill, he developed sovereign qualities which were so important in the results he achieved. He was endowed with a liking for hard work, and no trifling demand was too unimportant for his attention. In addition to thoroughness, he possessed patience, sympathy and kindness. It can be said that his habits were beyond reproach. This combination of splendid virtues inspired great public confidence in Dr. Maclean; a confidence which endured until his death.

Dr. Maclean loved to teach. He was appointed to the Medical Faculty of the University of Manitoba in 1910 . . . . He was at his best when he discussed a surgical subject. His interest remained equally keen whether it was with a young student or a group of his associates. Throughout his long life he kept abreast of the times, visiting medical centres and taking an active part in surgical meetings in Canada and the United States. He contributed papers on subjects in which he was interested and always took a very active part in the scientific discussions. . . .

Apart from his work among patients, Dr. Maclean enjoyed the company of his fellow men. He was a staunch supporter of the Church. During the first World War he was interested in the militia and did much work in the Military Hospital in Tuxedo. He was an active member of the Board of Trade. He was responsible for the formation of the Maclean Clan, of which he was Chieftain for several years.

Nature bestowed on Dr. Maclean fine physical attributes, and in later years his calm, handsome features and silver hair were a pleasing and striking picture to patients and colleagues alike. As his life drew to a close, he gradually gave up the technical part of his specialty. He never yielded, however, his keen interest in the solution of the problems of the sick. He changed so little that his patients continued to turn to him in their need and he did not fail them.

Dr. Maclean died on November 13th, 1946, in his seventy-seventh year. He was survived by his wife [Mary Taylor Maclean]; three sons, all of whom are doctors; and three daughters. One son, Captain D.S. Maclean, was killed while landing in Normandy on D-day, June 6, 1944, with the First Canadian Paratroop Battalion.

Dr. Maclean was mourned by the whole community which he so enriched by his example and devotion to duty. He could have said "for myself I am unconscious of ever having done any man an injury or omitting any fair opportunity of doing any man a benefit."

APPENDIX 8

Three Letters

FROM DR. BRIAN BEST

Dr. Brian D. Best was a longtime member of the Winnipeg Clinic and Head of its Section of Obstetrics and Gynecology. This letter was written at midnight on September 24, 1963, after a meeting of the members of the clinic:

Dear Thor:

Just a note (not a "memo") to tell you how much I admire your ability to accept criticism good naturedly and to end up laughing it off in good humour. I do hope you will not consider these remarks flippant or presumptuous – I am sincere in saying them, and I believe this great virtue has been one of your many talents which has led to your great success in medicine and community life. I felt impelled to write this down before turning in after another Administrative Board meeting – one of hundreds of clinic meetings I have attended and that have always found you equal to the occasion, however troublesome, critical or contentious.

May I also add my sincere congratulations to you, personally, on the completion of the terribly complex, tedious and sometimes thankless job of re-building The Clinic, a magnificent monument to a great director. Too often encomiums are withheld from those who deserve them, sometimes until it is too late. I was determined I would not make this error.

Sincerely,

Brian

FROM DR. ALAN DOWNS

Dr. Alan R. Downs was Professor and Head of the Department of Surgery, University of Manitoba and the Health Sciences Centre. This letter was written on May 1, 1980:

Dear Dr. Thorlakson:

Thank you very much for the copy of the letter which you received from Dr. Harkins [see Chapter 26 note 4]. Many of the points which you have made are applicable to 1980. This observation in itself, interests me, but it does not surprise me.

If it were at all possible, I would really like to have the submission which you made to Dr. Harkins to which he has responded. Reading his letter provides some of the information, but it doesn't give the total insight into some of the recommendations that you had obviously made. I think that it would be very useful for the Department to have this in its archives, and it would also probably be very useful for me to have access to it for my own edification at the present time.

For many years I have said that "if Thor had been the Professor of Surgery when I was a medical student, the Department of Surgery would be much further advanced at this time." It is almost incredible to me that this letter is 32 years old, and it certainly supports my contention. There is no doubt in my mind that if you had been the Full Time Professor of Surgery here 30 years ago, many of the things that I have been trying to accomplish over the last seven years would have long been accepted as the norm. It proves the old adage that not only must the ideas be right, but the timing must also be right.

I appreciate your continued interest in our Department.

With kindest personal regards to you and Mrs. Thorlakson,

Yours sincerely,

A.R. Downs, M.D.

TO THE HONOURABLE RENE E. TOUPIN

Following his retirement from an eight-year appointment as a member of the Manitoba Hospital Commission, Dr. Thorlakson addressed the following letter to the Hon. Rene E. Toupin, the Minister of Health and Social Development. The letter was dated November 7, 1970.

Dear Mr. Minister:

I wish to thank you again for the invitation to attend the dinner at the Fort Garry Hotel on October 26th. It was a most pleasant and appropriate way to bring together all the individuals who have worked to launch the Provincial hospital and medical insurance plans.

You and your colleagues in the Department and the members of the Commission are facing challenging times. The whole organization and structure of all hospital and medical services are being critically examined by Government and other organizations, in order that the public may receive the fullest benefits of modern medical science and technology.

In 1952, as President of the National Cancer Institute of Canada, I hosted a luncheon for the noted Canadian pathologist Professor William Boyd, who had preceded me in office. By that time I had already served eight years as a member of the first Associate Committee on Medical Research of the National Research Council of Canada under the Chairmanship first of Sir Frederick Banting and then of Dr. J.B. Collip – both great men of medical science.

My experience and observations during the years of service on these two national committees prompted me to make the following statement at the luncheon for Professor Boyd: "... in the foreseeable future we in Canada will witness a close partnership established between the medical profession and the government." After the luncheon professor Boyd said that he was intrigued and surprised that I should make this prediction.

Now it is the responsibility of government, the medical profession and the public to make the plans work effectively within the limited resources of personnel and money. I am sure that, given the opportunity, the Manitoba Medical Association will strive to make a contribution worthy of its responsibilities. After all, it was the Manitoba Medical Association which initiated an excellent prepaid medical plan in Manitoba.

The responsibilities and contributions of the members of the many allied health groups must be re-assessed and directed into channels related to their special training and competence. Specially trained nurses can perform many of the duties now carried out by physicians. In the interests of the patients, these para-medical or first contact health services must be carried out under the supervision of a medical team; in other words, these members of the health personnel must be part of a well-coordinated medical team. We, in the Winnipeg Clinic, are now working on a project which we hope will assist in development of this type of work. In several departments we already have some trained and very efficient doctors' assistants.

Again let me say how much I have enjoyed my work on the Manitoba Hospital Commission during the past eight years, and how much I have appreciated the opportunity to meet large numbers of Manitobans who, as a result of this contact, I can now number among my personal friends.

Yours sincerely,

Paul H.T. Thorlakson, M.D.

Chronology

1895 Born on October 5 at Park River, North Dakota, USA, son of the Rev. and Mrs. Niels Steingrimur Thorlaksson. His father was born at Storu-Tjarnir, Ljosavatnsskard, Thingeyjarsyslu, Iceland. His mother (née Erika Rynning) was born at Eidsvold, Norway.

1900 Family moved to Selkirk, Manitoba, Canada, where his father was appointed Pastor of the Lutheran Church.

1914 Entered Manitoba Medical College, after attending Selkirk grade and high schools and taking arts and science course at Gustavus Adolphus College, St. Peter's, Minnesota, USA.

1916 In the spring, enlisted in the Canadian Army, after completing second-year examinations in medicine.

1917 Service overseas with Canadian Expeditionary Force (medical sergeant).

1919 Graduated with M.D., C.M., from the University of Manitoba having served as undergraduate intern for one year at the Children's Hospital of Winnipeg and also at the Winnipeg General Hospital on the surgical service of Dr. Neil John Maclean.

First practised in Shoal Lake, Manitoba, in partnership with Dr. W.H. Brothers.

1920 Married on November 10 in Calgary, Alberta, to Miss Gladys Maree Henry, a graduate in home economics of the University of Manitoba.

Postgraduate training in surgery in London, England, and on the Continent.

1922 Received MRCS (England) and LRCP (London).

1923 Returned to Winnipeg; joined the Maclean-Gunn Clinic.

Was guest speaker at meeting of Winnipeg Medical Society: "Primary Ulcerative Colitis."

1926 Maclean-Thorlakson Clinic organized.

Appointed demonstrator in clinical surgery, Faculty of Medicine, University of Manitoba.

1928 Was guest speaker at meeting of Canadian Medical Association in Charlottetown: "Ulcerative Colitis."

Appointed lecturer in clinical surgery, Faculty of Medicine, University of Manitoba.

1929 Was guest speaker at Thirtieth Annual Session of the American Proctologic Society in Detroit: "Ulcerative Colitis."

1930 First trip to Iceland (1000th-year celebration of the Icelandic Parliament).

1931 Gave radio broadcast under auspices of Winnipeg Health League (local branch of the Social Hygiene Council of Canada): "Appendicitis."

Received Specialty Certificate (dated June 12) granting Fellowship in Royal College of Physicians and Surgeons of Canada.

1932 Was guest speaker, postgraduate tour, Alberta Medical Societies: "The Management of Some Common Ano-Rectal Disorders."

1933 Was guest speaker, The Surgeons' Club of Winnipeg: "The Practice of Medicine and Surgery in Ancient India."

1934 Was guest speaker, Pan American Medical Association Congress (South America): "Common Duct Obstruction."

Was guest speaker at meeting of Brandon and District Medical Society at Ninette Santorium: "Ano-Rectal Tuberculosis."

1935 Appointed assistant professor of surgery, Faculty of Medicine, University of Manitoba.

1936 Delivered address to the graduates, Selkirk Hospital School of Nursing.

Was guest speaker at meeting of Royal College of Physicians and Surgeons of Canada in Ottawa: "Gastroscopy – its Indications and Value."

1938 Winnipeg Clinic founded. On March 15, the new name was placed above that of Maclean-Thorlakson Clinic on the door of the offices in the Medical Arts Building.

Appointed a member of the First Associate Committee on Medical Research of the National Research Council of Canada under the chairmanship of Sir Frederick Banting. Served in this capacity until 1945.

Was guest speaker at annual meeting of Ontario Medical Association in Toronto in May and at meeting of Manitoba Medical Association in Winnipeg in September: "Diagnosis of Gastric Lesions Aided by Gastroscopy."

1939 Made a Knight of the Order of the Falcon by the Government of Iceland.

Was guest speaker, postgraduate course, Saskatoon and Regina: "The Diagnosis and Surgical Aspects of Jaundice."

Took canoe trip with family to Churchill, Manitoba; returned by train via The Pas and Flin Flon.

Was guest speaker at the Inaugural Meeting of the North of '53 Medical Society in Flin Flon: "Surgical Significance of Jaundice."

Was guest speaker at meeting of Canadian Medical Association in Montreal: "Intractable Gastric Ulcer with Final Malignant Change associated with a Benign Tumour of the Brain."

1940 Was guest speaker at postgraduate course, University of Alberta, Edmonton: "Present-Day Views on the Surgical Treatment of Duodenal Ulcer."

1941 Elected a Fellow of the American Surgical Association.

Appointed member of the Board of Trustees of the Manitoba Cancer Relief and Research Foundation and served subsequent appointments in this capacity until 1954.

1942 First building of Winnipeg Clinic completed.

As a postwar project, he proposed the creation of the Manitoba Medical Centre (now known as the Health Sciences Centre).

1943 First president of the Manitoba Institute for the Advancement of Medical Education and Research, which was incorporated by an act of the provincial legislature. The name of the institute was changed by Chapter 108 of the Statutes of Manitoba in 1957 to the Winnipeg Clinic Research Institute.

Was organizer of the Manitoba Medical Centre Corporation.

1944 Presented submission to the annual meeting of the National Research Council of Canada recommending the establishment of a Western Regional Committee and plans for postwar medical research.

Elected a Fellow of the American College of Surgeons.

Was guest speaker, Civic Bureau, Winnipeg Board of Trade: "Plans for the Manitoba Medical Centre."

Delivered Presidential Report at annual meeting of the Columbia Press.

Was guest speaker at annual meeting of the Canadian Medical Association in Toronto: "Carcinoma of the Stomach."

1945 Gave address to Winnipeg Medical Society: "Basic Health Proposals of the Province of Manitoba."

Manitoba Medical Centre incorporated; appointed Chairman and served in this capacity until 1962.

Responsible for the formation of the Western Regional Committee of the National Research Council of Canada and appointed its first chairman.

Was guest speaker at meeting of Regina and District Medical Society in Regina: "Some Problems in the Management of Thyroid Disease."

Was guest speaker at annual Icelandic Celebration at Gimli, Manitoba: "A Toast to Canada."

1946 Winnipeg Clinic building enlarged to five floors.

Was guest speaker, Young Men's Section, Winnipeg Board of Trade: "The Manitoba Medical Centre."

Was guest speaker, Civic Bureau of the Winnipeg Board of Trade: "The Manitoba Medical Centre."

Was guest speaker, Manitoba Music Teachers' Association: "The Manitoba Medical Centre."

Was guest speaker at joint meeting of the Winnipeg Medical Society and the Canadian Anaesthetists' Society (Manitoba, Saskatchewan and Alberta Divisions): "The Surgeon-Anaesthetist Relationship."

Accepted invitation to attend a three-day meeting at Massachusetts General Hospital in Boston commemorating the hundredth anniversary of the first public demonstration of the anaesthetic properties of ether.

Was guest speaker at sectional meeting of American College of Surgeons in Minneapolis: "Injuries to the Bile Ducts – Their Prevention and Repair."

Elected a member of the Western Surgical Association.

Appointed Professor of Surgery, Faculty of Medicine, University of Manitoba.

1947 Was guest speaker at annual meeting of the American Surgical Association: "Report on Experience with Vagotomy."

Was guest speaker at meeting of Grand Forks and District Medical Society in Grand Forks, North Dakota: "Lesions of the Abdominal Wall."

Was moderator of panel discussion at sectional meeting of American College of Surgeons in Winnipeg: "Gastric Surgery."

Attended annual meeting of Canadian Medical Association in Winnipeg; made member of panel, Round Table Conference: "The Management of Peptic Ulcer."

Gave the Founders' Lecture, Thirty-Fourth Meeting of North Pacific Surgical Association in Victoria, BC: "Chronic Ulcerative Colitis";

"Injuries to the Bile Ducts – Their Prevention and Repair"; "Observations on the Surgical Management of Chronic Duodenal Ulcer with Special Reference to the Role of Vagotomy."

Received second Fellowship Certificate from the Royal College of Physicians and Surgeons of Canada (the record of former one not located in office at Ottawa).

Appointed Chairman of Campaign Committee to establish a chair of Icelandic Language and Literature at the University of Manitoba; served in this capacity until 1951.

1948 Was guest speaker at sectional meeting of American College of Surgeons in Minneapolis: "Intestinal Obstruction of Malignant Origin."

Second trip to Iceland (guest of Icelandic Medical Society and Government of Iceland). Guest speaker at meeting of the Icelandic Medical Society in Reykjavik: "Carcinoma of the Colon."

1949 Was guest speaker at meeting of Ontario Medical Association in Port Arthur: "Clinical Significance of Chronic Dyspepsia."

Was guest speaker at sectional meeting of American College of Surgeons in Edmonton: "The Management of Acute Diverticulitis and its Complications."

Was guest speaker at Sixtieth Anniversary Service, Selkirk Lutheran Church, Selkirk, Manitoba.

Participated in Round Table Conference at annual meeting of Canadian Medical Association in Saskatoon.

Was guest speaker at meeting of Medico-Chirurgical Society in Montreal: "Group Practice and its Contribution to Medical Education."

Was Vice-President, National Cancer Institute of Canada.

1950 Appointed member, Canadian Committee for Manitoba Flood Relief Fund.

Was collaborator on panel at sectional meeting of American College of Surgeons in Winnipeg: "Surgical Lesions of the Stomach."

Gave broadcast over Canadian Broadcasting Corporation Dominion Network in Canadian Cancer Society Series: "Cancer in a Century of Progress."

Elected President, Western Division, Canadian Association of Clinical Surgeons.

Was guest speaker on occasion of Thirty-Second Anniversary of the Icelandic National League: "The Challenge of the Future."

Was guest speaker at meeting of Canadian Medical Association in Halifax: "Diverticulitis of the Sigmoid."

Was guest speaker at meeting of International College of Surgeons in Cleveland: "Multiple Primary Foci of Carcinoma of the Colon."

Was re-elected Vice-President, National Cancer Institute of Canada.

1951 The Chair of Icelandic Language and Literature was founded at the University of Manitoba – the first endowed chair in a University in Western Canada – and so completed chairmanship of Campaign Committee.

Made a Commander of the Order of the Falcon by the Government of Iceland.

Elected President, National Cancer Institute of Canada.

1952 Received honorary Doctor of Laws, University of Manitoba.

Was guest speaker at annual meeting of White Cross Guild of Winnipeg General Hospital: "The Challenge of Sir Frederick Banting."

Was guest speaker at meeting of St. Paul Clinical Club in St. Paul, Minnesota: "Multiple Primary Foci of Carcinoma of the Colon."

Appointed member of Committee on Cancer, American College of Surgeons and served on this committee until 1962.

Was guest of honour at dinner given by members of Winnipeg Clinic to celebrate award of honorary degree of Doctor of Laws by the University of Manitoba on the occasion of the seventy-fifth anniversary of the founding of the University.

1953 Was guest of honour at testimonial dinner given by the Icelandic National League.

Chaired Round Table Conference at annual meeting of the Canadian Medical Association held in Winnipeg: "The Treatment of Thyroid Disease."

Accompanied Dr. C.W. Burns, President of the Canadian Medical Association, on presidential tour of the maritime provinces and Newfoundland. Guest speaker at meetings in Saint John, Charlottetown, and St. John's: "Indications and Contraindications for Cholecystectomy and Multiple Primary Carcinoma of the Colon."

Chaired panel discussion at annual meeting of New Brunswick Medical Society: "Thyroid Disease."

1954 Was appointed Surgeon-in-Chief, Winnipeg General Hospital.

Attended joint meeting of American College of Surgeons and the Association of Surgeons of Great Britain and Ireland held in Leeds and London, England. Participated in discussion on ulcerative colitis in Leeds and was collaborator on panel discussion in London: "Intestinal Obstruction."

Appointed Professor in the Department of Surgery, Faculty of Medicine, University of Manitoba.

Invited to write guest editorial for Surgery, Gynecology and Obstetrics: "Diagnostic Laparotomy in Chronic Abdominal Disease."

Invited to be a collaborator on panel discussion at meeting of American College of Surgeons in Atlantic City: "Obstructing Diverticulitis."

1954 to 1956 Was chairman, Manitoba Medical Services.

1954 to 1963 Was member of Committee on Cancer, Manitoba Medical Association; acted as chairman of this committee from 1956 to 1962.

1955 Chaired Building Fund Campaign, The Betel Home of Gimli.

Appointed member of Medical Advisory Committee to the Rehabilitation Commission of Province of Manitoba and served in this capacity until 1961.

Chaired Advisory Committee on Arrangements for Sectional Meeting of American College of Surgeons in Winnipeg; presided at morning session on April 25.

Appointed by Royal College of Physicians and Surgeons of Canada to a Committee: "Considering the Problem of Utilization of Private Patients for Graduate Training in Hospitals."

Made Honorary President, University of Manitoba Alumni Association.

1955 to 1958 Was Governor of the American College of Surgeons.

1957 Inaugural meeting, Manitoba Chapter, American College of Surgeons; As Governor of the College, presented Charter No. 62 to Chapter on January 19.

Attended sectional meeting, American College of Surgeons in St. Paul, Minnesota; presided at morning session on April 9.

Attended annual meeting, Canadian Medical Association in Edmonton; participated in television panel discussion: "The Diagnosis and Treatment of Thyroid Disease."

Served as chairman, Board of Directors, Betel Old Folks' Home, Gimli.

Elected member, Board of Directors, Manitoba Heart Foundation.

Appointed Professor Emeritus of Surgery, Faculty of Medicine, University of Manitoba.

1957–58 Was member of Advisory Medical Board of Manitoba Cancer Relief and Research Foundation.

1958 Was visiting Professor of Surgery, University of Saskatchewan, Saskatoon: "Carcinoma of the Colon"; "Gall Stone Disease"; and "Surgical Treatment of Peptic Ulcer."

As Director of Winnipeg Clinic, presented report to Winnipeg Clinic Research Institute on occasion of the fifteenth anniversary of the Institute.

Was guest speaker at annual meeting of Canadian Medical Association in Halifax: "Carcinoma of the Stomach."

Served as chairman of editorial board, Lögberg-Heimskringla (Icelandic weekly newspaper); held this office until 1967.

Was guest speaker, Manitoba Chapter, American College of Surgeons in Winnipeg: "Colon surgery."

Elected President, Medical Alumni Association of Winnipeg General Hospital.

1959 Elected President, Manitoba Division, Canadian Conference on Education.

Presented with life membership in Winnipeg Medical Society.

Was guest speaker at meeting of Park Region District and Ottertail County Medical Societies in Fergus Falls, Minnesota: "Problems of Gall Bladder Disease."

Was guest speaker, Saskatchewan Chapter, College of General Practice of Canada: "Diverticulitis of the Colon."

Moderated panel discussion at meeting of American Association of Medical Clinics in Chicago: "How Can Group Practice Aid in the Care of the Aged?"

1960 Was president of First Manitoba Conference on Education held in Winnipeg. Dr. Wilder G. Penfield of Montreal was guest speaker: "Education in Long Perspective."

Was guest speaker at Sectional Meeting of American College of Surgeons in Minneapolis: "Regional Enteritis."

Was guest speaker at Fifth Annual Cancer Symposium in Regina: "Diagnosis and Management of Rectal Polypi."

Was guest speaker at meeting of American Association of Medical Clinics in New Orleans: "The History of Prepaid Hospital and Medical Care Plans in Manitoba."

Collaborated on panel discussion at meeting of American Association of Medical Clinics in New Orleans: "Problems in Graduate and Postgraduate Medical Education."

Appointed as chairman, United Health Insurance Corporation Limited.

1961 Was guest speaker, Icelandic Canadian Club: "The Shaping of the New Canada."

Served as President of Second Manitoba Conference of Education held in Brandon; guest speaker was Dr. Malcolm G. Taylor, Principal, University of Alberta (Calgary): "The Horizons of Education."

Was guest speaker, sectional meeting, American College of Surgeons in Winnipeg: "Surgical Treatment of Hemorrhoids."

Extended greetings to His Excellency, the President of the Republic of Iceland, and Mrs. Asgeir Asgeirsson on occasion of their visit to the Betel Home at Gimli on Icelandic Day.

Made third trip to Iceland; received honorary M.D. degree from University of Iceland. University of Iceland then was celebrating its fiftieth anniversary.

Appointed corresponding member, Committee on Cancer of Canadian Medical Association.

1962 Invited to write guest editorial for *The Manitoba Teacher,* (January-February): "Learning a Second Language."

Served as chairman of Forum F at the Second Canadian Conference on Education held in Montreal: "The Citizen in Education."

Invited by the Chairman, Mr. Justice Emmett M. Hall, to prepare a brief on group practice and present it to the Royal Commission on Health Services; appeared before the Commission in Montreal on April 16.

Was guest speaker at the Rotary Club of Winnipeg; "The Role of the Citizen in Education."

Appointed to the Manitoba Hospital Commission.

Was guest speaker at Twelfth Middle East Medical Assembly at the American University, Beirut, Lebanon: "Regional Enteritis."

Was a guest speaker at the official opening of the Manitoba Rehabilitation Hospital.

Was guest speaker at the Canadian session held in collaboration with the annual meeting of the American Association of Medical Clinics in Portland, Oregon: "What is Group Practice."

1962 to 1964 Was member of Advisory Medical Board of the Manitoba Cancer Relief and Research Foundation.

1962 to 1965 Was member of Board of Directors, United Health Insurance Corporation Limited.

1963 Winnipeg Clinic building enlarged to twelve floors.

Appointed member of Board of Civic Development Corporation.

Was guest speaker at annual meeting of Victoria General Hospital: "Your hospital – a Community Partnership."

Appointed member of an informal committee for Manitoba on bilingualism and biculturalism.

Was guest speaker at meeting of Pan Pacific Surgical Association in Honolulu, Hawaii: "Carcinoma of the Colon and Recto-Sigmoid."

Received Community Service Award, City of Winnipeg.

Was guest speaker at Seminar on French-English Relations sponsored by the Canadian Council of Christians and Jews, Winnipeg: "Canada – a Multi-Cultural Nation."

Was a guest speaker at the dedication and official opening of the Elizabeth M. Crowe Memorial Hospital at Eriksdale, Manitoba.

Appointed member of National Executive Council, Pan-American Games (1967) Society.

Appointed member, Advisory Board of *Quest,* publication of the Canadian Home and School and Parent-Teacher Federation.

1964 Appointed director of the Great-West Life Assurance Company.

Was guest speaker at Seventy-fifth Anniversary Service of Selkirk Lutheran Church, Selkirk, Manitoba.

Appointed Ex-Officio Member, Organizational Board, Pan-American Games (1967) Society.

Extended greetings on behalf of the Canada Iceland Foundation at dinner in honour of Dr. Bjarni Benediktsson, Prime Minister of Iceland, and Mrs. Benediktsson.

Received Golden Boys' Good Citizenship Award of the Manitoba Travel and Convention Association.

1965 Served as Chairman of the Editorial Board, Lögberg-Heimskringla, the Icelandic weekly newspaper, which published the English Literary Supplement.

Invited to write Foreword, *Winnipeg General Hospital Nurses' Alumnae Journal.*

Invited to write brief statement called "Books" for Canadian Home and School and Parent-Teacher Federation.

Appointed member, Board of Trustees, United Way of Greater Winnipeg.

1966 Was guest speaker at meeting of Manitoba Chapter of the International College of Surgeons in Winnipeg: "Trends in Management of Diverticulitis."

Attended Pan Pacific Surgical Association Meeting in Honolulu, Hawaii; Dr. Kenneth Thorlakson and Dr. Robert Thorlakson showed their coloured film, "The Complete and Synchronous Excision of the Rectum for Cancer."

Appointed President of the Winnipeg Clinic.

Was guest speaker at meeting of Manitoba Medical Alumni of Alberta in Edmonton: "Biliary Tract Surgery"; and "A Century of Medicine in Manitoba."

Was guest speaker at meeting of Catholic Physicians' Guild of Manitoba in Winnipeg: "One Hundred Years of Medicine in Manitoba."

Was guest speaker at official opening of The Betel Home, Selkirk, Manitoba.

1967 Was guest speaker at meeting of Dietetic Association of Manitoba and Manitoba Home Economics Association in Winnipeg: "One Hundred Years of Medicine in Manitoba."

Chaired Canadian (Icelandic) Centennial Committee; delivered presentation speech in Ottawa when the Prime Minister, the Right Honourable Lester B. Pearson, accepted the gift of a commemorative bronze plaque on behalf of the Government of Canada.

Introduced Dr. Wilder G. Penfield, the guest speaker, at the inaugural meeting of the Manitoba Chapter of The Vanier Institute of the Family.

Chaired Panel Discussion at meeting of Canadian Association of Medical Clinics in Toronto: "Group Practice in University Affiliated Hospitals."

Invited to write Foreword to *Report on Group Practice in Canada,* published by The Canadian Medical Association.

Was guest speaker at dinner for delegates to Cancer Chemotherapy Symposium in Montreal: "A Century of Medical Progress."

Delivered address to His Excellency, Asgeir Asgeirsson, President of the Republic of Iceland, at dinner given in his honour by the Icelandic Community in Manitoba.

Introduced Dr. Lennox G. Bell, guest speaker at the Joseph Doupe Memorial Symposium luncheon at the Winnipeg General Hospital.

Was guest speaker at Ninth Western Medical Meeting of Mexico held at the University of Guadalajara, Guadalajara, Mexico: "Gall Stone Disease."

1968 Submitted report to the Winnipeg Clinic Research Institute on occasion of the twenty-fifth anniversary of the Institute.

Appointed member of Advisory Committee, United Way of Greater Winnipeg.

Elected Second Vice-President, Canadian Association of Medical Clinics and Program Chairman for annual meeting in Vancouver.

Elected senior member in the Canadian Medical Association; investiture took place at the 101st Annual Meeting of the Association in Regina on June 19.

Elected Honorary Fellow, International College of Surgeons; fellowship conferred at Sixteenth Biennial International Congress held in Tokyo and Kyoto, Japan, October 6 to 11.

Appointed president and General Chairman of the First International Congress of Group Medicine held in Winnipeg April 26 to 30, 1970.

1969 Elected Chancellor of the University of Winnipeg.

Appointed President, Canadian Association of Medical Clinics.

1969 Was guest speaker at meeting of University of Winnipeg Alumnae Association: "The Universities of the Province of Manitoba – Their Origin and Growth."

Invited to deliver address to the graduates at the Eighty-first Annual Commencement Exercises of the Winnipeg General Hospital School of Nursing.

Guest speaker at meeting of North of '53 Medical Association at The Pas, Manitoba: "Our Provincial Universities, Faculty of Medicine and Teaching Hospitals – 100 Years of Progress."

Appointed member, Board of Directors, Central Region of the Canadian Council of Christians and Jews.

1970 Travelled to the United Kingdom, Norway, France and the Federal Republic of Germany to promote interest in the First International Congress on Group Medicine.

Organized the First International Congress of Group Medicine held in Winnipeg April 26 to 30 at the Manitoba Centennial Concert Hall. As President and General Chairman, presided at the welcoming ceremony when the Congress was officially opened on April 26 by the Honorary President, His Excellency, The Right Honourable Roland Michener, CC., C.D., Governor-General of Canada; presided at the closing ceremony on April 30 and accepted the invitation from the Brazilian delegation to hold the Second Congress in Rio de Janeiro in 1973.

Was given Honorary Doctor of Science, Brandon University.

Was guest speaker at testimonial dinner held at Shoal Lake, Manitoba, on May 23 in honour of Dr. S. Bardal.

Attended luncheon with The Queen on July 15 – Manitoba's hundredth birthday.

Was guest speaker at annual banquet on September 1 of the Canadian Association of Medical Record Librarians: "The Development of Medical, Educational and Hospital Facilities in Manitoba."

Retired in October from the Manitoba Hospital Commission.

Term of office expired as member of Board of Trustees, United Way of Greater Winnipeg.

Celebrated fiftieth wedding anniversary on November 10.

Was guest speaker at testimonial dinner held at Eriksdale, Manitoba, on November 26 in honour of Dr. G. Paulson of Lundar.

The members of the Winnipeg Clinic gave a reception and dinner in honour of Dr. and Mrs. Thorlakson on December 15. The bronze bust of Dr. Thorlakson, done by Mr. Leo Mol, was unveiled on this occasion.

Appointed a Companion of the Order of Canada in the list of honours announced in Ottawa on December 18.

1971 Retired as a Director of the Great-West Life Assurance Company on March 17.

Installed as a Companion of the Order of Canada by His Excellency, The Governor-General, at investiture held at Government House in Ottawa on March 31.

Presented with Fifty-Year Jewel by Ionic Lodge, A.F. and A.M., No. 25 G.R.M. on May 3.

Was guest speaker on May 13 at presentation by Mr. Clarence Tillenius of one of his paintings to the Museum of Man and Nature in memory of the late Dr. Walter F. Tisdale.

Presented report to Winnipeg Clinic Research Institute at annual meeting on May 20.

Fourth trip to Iceland, accompanied by three grandsons: David and Hartley Richardson and Derek Thorlakson.

Appointed in July to the Board of Directors of the Traffic Injury Research Foundation of Canada.

Attended the twenty-fourth Congress of the International Society of Surgery in Moscow, USSR August 21 to 28.

Extended greetings on behalf of the University of Winnipeg to Her Royal Highness, The Princess Margaret, and the Earl of Snowdon at a luncheon held at the University on September 25.

Re-appointed in October to the Manitoba Health Services Commission (formerly the Manitoba Hospital Commission).

Elected to titular membership in the International Society of Surgery.

Was guest speaker at Western Conference on Prepaid Medical Service Plans in Portland, Oregon: "Some Observations on Changing Concepts in the Provision of Medical Care."

Was guest speaker at Centennial Seminar at St. Boniface General

Hospital: "Medical Education at St. Boniface Hospital – The First Fifty Years."

Received Centennial Commemorative Medal of the Manitoba Historical Society.

1972 Was guest speaker at farewell dinner in honour of Dr. S.S. Peikoff given by the medical staff of Victoria General Hospital.

Invited to attend Brazilian Symposium on Group Medicine in Sao Paulo and extend greetings at the opening session.

Appointed Executive Vice-President for North America for the Second International Congress on Group Medicine held in Rio de Janeiro March 10 to 15, 1973.

Appointed a Director of the Manitoba Medical Service Foundation, Incorporated.

Appointed Chairman of the Centenaries Celebration Committee (Icelandic).

Awarded Honorary Fellowship in the American College of Hospital Administrators at the Thirty-eighth Convocation Ceremony in Chicago on August 6.

Invited to attend the Fifth World Conference on General Practice in Melbourne, Australia, and to officially open the exhibit, "Our World of Tomorrow," and to be a guest speaker: "The Expanded Health Team."

1973 Received National Human Relations Award of the Canadian Council of Christians and Jews at a banquet on February 22.

Attended Second International Congress on Group Medicine in Rio de Janeiro and was invited, as Vice-President for North America, to extend greetings at Opening Session on March 10.

Was guest speaker, Bruin Chapter of the Icelandic National League at Selkirk, Manitoba: "Sumardagurinn Fyrsti (The First Day of Summer)."

Was guest speaker at luncheon meeting of the Canadian Association of Medical Clinics in Regina on May 25: "The Second International Congress on Group Medicine."

Appointed a member of the Canadian Consultative Council on Multiculturalism.

Was guest speaker at meeting on Multiculturalism in Arborg, Manitoba, on November 30: "The Significance of the New Canadian Policy on Multiculturalism."

1974 Received the Hall of Fame Award of The Red River Valley Historical Society at a banquet held in Fargo, North Dakota, on April 19.

Invited to write article, "The Organization and Administration of

Group Practice," for the *World Medical Journal* which was published in the May-June issue.

Was guest speaker at the Eighty-fifth Anniversary Service on June 9 of the Selkirk Evangelical Lutheran Congregation at Selkirk, Manitoba.

Took fifth trip to Iceland – official representative of the Government of Canada at the celebrations marking the 1100th anniversary of the settlement of Iceland on July 28 and 29.

Invited to write article for publication in program for the Icelandic Festival of Manitoba: "A Tribute to the Pioneer Icelandic Settlers in Canada."

Received Winnipeg Centennial Medal commemorating the centenary of the City of Winnipeg and the sixtieth anniversary of the Winnipeg Medical Society.

Invited to address the associate members at the Twenty-eighth World Medical Assembly on September 3 in Stockholm, Sweden: "What Associate Membership in the World Medical Association has Meant to Me.

Elected Co-Chairman for the Central Region of the Canadian Council of Christians and Jews.

Resigned from the Manitoba Health Services Commission.

Re-elected Chancellor of the University of Winnipeg.

1975 Presented report on behalf of the Manitoba members to the prairie regional meeting of the Canadian Consultative Council on Multiculturalism on February 15.

Was guest speaker at Annual Samkoma of the Twin Cities Hekla Club in Minneapolis: "The Canada-Iceland Centennial Conference."

Retired from Board of Directors of the Traffic Injury Research Foundation of Canada.

Invited to write Foreword for *The Gimli Saga,* the Gimli Women's Institute prize-winning community history which received the Lady Tweedsmuir Trophy in 1973, in a Federated Women's Institute of Canada triennial competition.

Was guest speaker at concert given by Icelandic Centennial Children's Choir.

Chaired the Canada Iceland Centennial Conference held in October to commemorate the hundredth anniversary of the arrival of the first 285 Icelandic settlers to Manitoba.

Was guest of honour at dinner given by the Manitoba Health Services Commission.

1976 Received the Manitoba Medical Association Distinguished Service Award.

Was made Honorary President, Third International Congress on Group Medicine held in Paris, France, June 21 to 26 and a guest speaker at the inauguration ceremony.

Was guest speaker at the centennial celebration at Riverton, Manitoba.

1977 Appointed Chairman, Manitoba Chapter of Canadians for Health Research.

Was made a member, Advisory Committee, United Nations Association, Winnipeg Branch.

Completed term as member of the Canadian Consultative Council on Multiculturalism.

Attended family reunion of descendants of Niels Steingrimur Thorlaksson and Erika Rynning Thorlaksson held at Seattle, Washington, September 2 to 4. At family banquet, told the love story of the Rev. and Mrs. N.S. Thorlaksson.

Awarded the Canadian Silver Jubilee Medal commemorating the twenty-fifth anniversary of the accession of Her Majesty The Queen to the Throne.

In the presence of Her Majesty, attended a luncheon given in Ottawa on October 17 by the Secretary of State of Canada and the Minister of State (Multiculturalism) to honour the Queen's Silver Jubilee visit to Canada.

Resigned as Protestant Co-Chairman for the Central Region of the Canadian Council of Christians and Jews and appointed Honorary Co-Chairman.

Organized James Ross Jenkins Memorial Symposium, "Provision of Health Care to Remote Areas and Medical Education," held at the Medical College on October 22. Two of the guest speakers were: Dr. Moshe Prywes, Dean, University Centre for Health Sciences, Ben Gurion University of the Negev, Israel; and Dr. Arne Nordoy, Professor of Medicine, Medical School, Tromsø, Norway. Following the symposium, Dr. Thorlakson accompanied Dr. Prywes and Dr. Nordoy to Churchill, Manitoba, where they received information regarding northern medical services at the Churchill Health Centre.

Attended First Conference of Canadians for Health Research in Ottawa, October 24 and 25.

Was guest speaker on November 18 at luncheon meeting of the National Club of Winnipeg: "Medical Research."

Attended reception and dinner at the University of Winnipeg on December 9 in honour of Dr. and Mrs. Thorlakson. The evening's program included the unveiling of the portrait of Dr. Thorlakson – in his Chancellor's gown – painted by Canadian artist Thomas R. McDonald.

1978 In February, stepped down as Chancellor of the University of Winnipeg after serving in this capacity for nine years.

Became associated with Manitoba Citizens Bursary Fund for Native Peoples.

Was guest of honour at the thirty-fifth anniversary dinner of the Winnipeg Clinic Research Institute on May 18 at the Winnipeg Inn. During the annual meeting which followed, the President, Mr. Albert D. Cohen, announced that in recognition of Dr. Thorlakson's many notable contributions to Winnipeg, Manitoba and Canada, a Paul H.T. Thorlakson Research Foundation Incorporated was to be created by the Board of Directors and members of the Institute to demonstrate their admiration for his vision and generosity. Dr. Arnold Naimark, Dean of Medicine, presented Dr. Thorlakson with a bronze plaque in recognition of his outstanding contribution to the advancement of medical research.

Was guest speaker at the National Conference on Nursing Research held in Winnipeg: "Canadians for Health Research."

Introduced Dr. William A. Altemeier, President of the American College of Surgeons, at meeting of the Manitoba Chapter held in Winnipeg on December 2.

1979 Was given honorary life membership, Manitoba Medical Association, received at annual business meeting in Brandon on May 5.

Was given Honorary Doctor of Laws, University of Winnipeg, conferred at Convocation on May 27.

Resigned as Chairman of Manitoba Chapter, Canadians for Health Research.

1980 Presented with Sixty-Year Bar by Ionic Lodge, A.F. and A.M., No. 25 G.R.M.

Was guest of honour at reception and dinner given by the Winnipeg Clinic Research Institute and the Paul H.T. Thorlakson Research Foundation Incorporated at the Fort Garry Hotel on October 20. On this occasion, Dr. Thorlakson was presented with an illustrated scroll depicting the History of Government House in Winnipeg by His Honour F.L. Jobin, Lieutenant-Governor of Manitoba, and signed by him and two former Lieutenant-governors: The Honourable W.J. McKeag and the Honourable R.S. Bowles.

Elected to the office of Chief Hunter of The Order of the Buffalo Hunt and presented with a bronze buffalo on a marble stand on behalf of the Province of Manitoba by the Premier, The Honourable Sterling R. Lyon.

Presented with a bronze plaque by His Worship, Mayor William Norrie, Q.C., on behalf of the City of Winnipeg for "selfless dedication to the medical profession and to medical research in Manitoba. An exemplary citizen whose contribution to our community is immeasurable."

Celebrated sixtieth wedding anniversary on November 10.

1981 Resigned from Board of Directors of the Manitoba Medical Service Foundation Incorporated.

1982 Invited by Canada-Iceland Foundation to be guest speaker at reception in Arborg, Manitoba, in honour of Mr. Edward Gislason.

1983 Was host at Icelandic Dinner at Manitoba Club on February 3.

Celebrated the hundredth anniversary of the Faculty of Medicine of the University of Manitoba May 24 to 27; attended senior grads dinner and centennial dinner.

1984 Dr. and Mrs. Thorlakson were invited by the Prime Minister and Mrs. Mulroney to be head table guests at dinner – in the presence of Her Majesty The Queen – on October 6 in the Winnipeg Convention Centre.

Invited to speak at the official opening on November 6 of the new Surgical Intensive Care Unit at the Health Sciences Centre in Winnipeg.

1985 Invited to address the Sixth International Congress on Group Medicine held in Dallas, Texas, April 21 to 25. Informed that the Seventh Congress will take place in Vienna, Austria, in 1988, and the Eighth Congress is scheduled for 1991 in Helsinki, Finland. (The Fourth Congress was held in West Berlin, Federal Republic of Germany, and the Fifth Congress was held in Tokyo, Japan.)

Attended dedication ceremony on June 26 when the new Medical Support Services Building of the Health Sciences Centre in Winnipeg was named the Paul H.T. Thorlakson Building. Dr. Thorlakson was presented with a commemorative scroll by the Lieutenant-Governor of Manitoba, Her Honour Pearl McGonigal, on behalf of the Centre.

Hosted special dinner at the Manitoba Club in celebration of Dr. Thorlakson's ninetieth birthday and honouring physicians and surgeons. The family luncheon was held on October 5.

Was guest speaker at symposium held at the University of Manitoba October 24 to 26 to mark the twenty-fifth anniversary of the Medical Research Council of Canada: "Banting, Early Medical Research and the West."

Celebrated sixty-fifth wedding anniversary on November 10.

1986 Received the 1986 Award of Canadians for Health Research "for outstanding services in the promotion of health research in Canada."

Appointed Honorary Life Member of the Manitoba Club on March 20.

Invited by the White Cross Guild of the Health Sciences Centre in Winnipeg to officially open their new gift shop on May 1.

Participated in the burning of the mortgage on Winnipeg Clinic Building at meeting of the Board of Directors of the Winnipeg Clinic Research Institute held on May 12 at the Manitoba Club.

Was given bronze plaque on May 14 at the Westin Hotel by Manitoba Blue Cross "in recognition and appreciation for dedication and valuable contribution as Chairman of the Board of Directors of the United Health Insurance Corporation Limited during 1959 to 1961."

Publications

"Primary Ulcerative Colitis." *Canadian Medical Association Journal* 24 (December 1924): 1173.

"Ulcerative Colitis." *Canadian Medical Association Journal* 19 (1928): 656–659.

"Ulcerative Colitis." *Transactions of the American Proctologic Society, Thirtieth Annual Session, Detroit, Michigan* (May 1929).

"Rupture of the Liver." *Canadian Medical Association Journal* 20 (1929): 593–598 [with A.W.S. Hay].

"The Management of Some Common Ano-Rectal Disorders." *International Clinics* Vol. 4, Series 42 (1932): 123–138.

"The Practice of Medicine and Surgery in Ancient India." *The University of Manitoba Medical Journal* (April 1933) [with J.T. Lawson].

"Common Duct Obstruction." *Canadian Medical Association Journal* 31 (1934): 265–269 [with J.C. McMillan].

"Ano-Rectal Tuberculosis." *Manitoba Medical Association Review* 15 (1935): 5–9.

"Gastroscopy – its Indications and Value." *Canadian Medical Association Journal* 36 (1937): 345–354 [with C.B. Stewart].

"A Case of Strangulated Ovarian Dermoid Cyst in a Child of Six and a Half Years of Age." *Canadian Medical Association Journal* 38 (January 1938): 58.

"Carcinoma of the Rectum and Recto-Sigmoid." *Canadian Medical Association Journal* 38 (February 1938): 107–119 [with A.W.S. Hay].

"Recurrent Biliary Colic Associated with Four Months Pregnancy." *Review of Gastroenterology* Vol. 5, No. 3 (1938): 283–287.

"Diagnosis of Gastric Lesions Aided by Gastroscopy." *Manitoba Medical Association Review* 19 (April 1939): 68–72.

"The Diagnosis and Surgical Aspects of Jaundice." *Manitoba Medical*

Association Review 20 (January 1940): 5–10.
"Present-Day Views on the Surgical Treatment of Duodenal Ulcer." *Manitoba Medical Association Review* 21 (January 1941): 235–237.
"Intractable Gastric Ulcer with Final Malignant Change Associated with a Benign Tumor of the Brain." *Annals of Surgery* Vol. 113, No. 4 (April 1941): 521–527 [with Sarah Meltzer].
"Surgical Management of Gastric and Duodenal Ulcers." *Canadian Medical Association Journal* 45 (October 1941): 298–307 [with A.W.S. Hay].
"The Late Brandur Jonsson Brandson, M.D." *Manitoba Medical Review* 24 (August 1944): 233.
"Trends in Medical Practice." *Manitoba Medical Review* 24 (September 1944): 243–246.
"The Manitoba Medical Service (A Criticism and a Recommendation)." *Manitoba Medical Review* 24 (November 1944): 326–328.
"Report on a Case of Congenital Valvular Obstruction of the Upper Jejunum." *Manitoba Medical Review* 24 (December 1944): 354.
"Hazards of Surgery of the Biliary Tract." *Manitoba Medical Review* 25 (September 1945): 372–376.
"To Canada." *Icelandic-Canadian Magazine* (September 1945).
"Manitoba Medical Centre (Address to Young Men's Section, Board of Trade)." *Manitoba Medical Review* Vol. 26, No. 6 (June 1946): 351–354.
"The Surgeon-Anaesthetist Relationship." *Canadian Medical Association Journal* 55 (August 1946): 489–493.
"The Surgical Management of Chronic Duodenal Ulcer with Special Reference to the Role of Vagotomy." *Canadian Medical Association Journal* 58 (1948): 561–567.
"Intestinal Obstruction of Malignant Origin." *Winnipeg Clinic Quarterly* Vol. 1, No. 1 (September 1948): 9–23.
"Foreword – Dr. Neil John Maclean." *Winnipeg Clinic Quarterly* Vol. 1, No. 1 (September 1948): 8.
"Injuries to the Bile Ducts – Their Prevention and Repair." *Canadian Medical Association Journal* 60 (1949): 119–125.
"Toothpick Perforation of the Intestinal Wall – a Report of Four Cases." *Winnipeg Clinic Quarterly* Vol. 2, No. 2 (June 1949): 53–60 [with Ian S. Maclean].
"Chronic Ulcerative Colitis." *The Journal of the International College of Surgeons* Vol. 12, No. 4 (July-August 1949): 439–450.
"Occult Carcinoma of the Colon – Report of Two Cases." *Winnipeg Clinic Quarterly* Vol. 3, No. 1 (March 1950): 26–33 [with C.R. Gilmour and D.C. Brereton].
"Volvulus of the Stomach." *Winnipeg Clinic Quarterly* Vol. 3, No. 3 (September 1950): 101–104 [with P.J. Gouthro].

"Group Practice and Medical Education." *Canadian Medical Association Journal* 63 (October 1950): 336–339.
"Professional and Public Education on Cancer." *Canadian Medical Association Journal* 64 (April 1951): 344–345.
"Cancer in a Century of Progress (1850–1950)." *Manitoba Medical Review* 31 (April 1951): 235 [reprinted from *Canadian Cancer Society Newsletter*, February 1951].
"Multiple Primary Carcinoma of the Colon and Rectum – Report of Two Illustrative Case Histories." *Winnipeg Clinic Quarterly* Vol. 4, No. 2 (June 1951): 76–83.
"The Incidence of Multiple Malignant Growths of the Large Bowel." *Manitoba Medical Review* Vol. 32, No. 3 (March 1952): 158–159.
"Carcinoma of the Gallbladder (Present Concepts Regarding Prevention and Cure)." *Winnipeg Clinic Quarterly* Vol. 5, No. 1 (March 1952): 9–13.
"The Challenge of Sir Frederick Banting." *Manitoba Medical Review* Vol. 32, No. 7 (August-September 1952): 436–438.
"The Clinical Importance of Sigmoidoscopy." *Winnipeg Clinic Quarterly* Vol. 5, No. 3 (September 1952): 99–102.
"In Memoriam – Clifford R. Gilmour, M.D." *Winnipeg Clinic Quarterly* Vol. 6, No. 1 (March 1953): 5–7.
"Anomalour Peritoneal Encapsulation of the Small Intestine – A Report of Three Cases." *British Journal of Surgery* Vol. 40, No. 163 (March 1953): 490–493 [with I.W. Monie and T.K. Thorlakson].
"Sigmoid Diverticulitis and Carcinoma Without Bowel Symptoms." *Winnipeg Clinic Quarterly* Vol. 6, No. 3:113–115, (September 1953): 113–115 [with Dallas Medd].
"Diverticulitis of the Sigmoid." *Manitoba Medical Review* Vol. 33, No. 10 (December 1953): 545–547.
"Symposium on Hyperthyroidism." *Winnipeg Clinic Quarterly* Vol. 7, No. 1 (March 1954): 1–24 [with J.E. Isaac, J.M. Kilgour and J.E. Morris].
"Diagnostic Laparotomy in Chronic Abdominal Disease." *Surgery, Gynecology and Obstetrics* 98 (May 1954): 629–631.
"Symposium on Medical and Surgical Aspects of Chronic Gallbladder Disease." *Winnipeg Clinic Quarterly* Vol. 7, No. 4 (December 1954): 125–147 [with John Farr, D.L. Kippen and K.R. Trueman].
"The Indications and Contra-Indications for Cholecystectomy." *Canadian Medical Association Journal* 72 (March 15, 1955): 415–418.
"Some Problems in the Diagnosis of Rectal Bleeding." *Winnipeg Clinic Quarterly* Vol. 8, No. 1 [March 1955]: 35–37 [with Dallas Medd].
"The Etiology and Technique of Surgical Management of Pancreatic Fistula." *Surgery, Gynecology and Obstetrics* Vol. 102 (April 1956): 413–419 [with L.C. Bartlett].

"Surgical Treatment of Peptic Ulcer." *Winnipeg Clinic Quarterly* Vol. 2, No. 2 (June 1958): 33–41 [with T.K. Thorlakson].
"The Indications and Technique of Sigmoidoscopy." *Manitoba Medical Review* Vol. 38, No. 9 (November 1958): 606–608.
"Carcinoma of the Stomach." *Canadian Medical Association Journal* 79 (November 15, 1958): 857–859.
"Gallstone Disease." *Winnipeg Clinic Quarterly* Vol. 12, No. 3 (September 1959): 85–99.
"Problems of Gallbladder Disease." *The Journal-Lancet, Minneapolis* Vol. 80, No. 6 (June, 1960): 298.
"The Shaping of the New Canada." *The Icelandic-Canadian Magazine* (Spring 1961).
"The History of Prepaid Hospital and Medical Care Plans in Manitoba." *Canadian Medical Association Journal* 84 (April 22, 1961): 896–899.
"Trends in Medical Practice." *Winnipeg Clinic Quarterly* Vol. 14, No. 2 (June 1961): 62–79.
"The Shaping of the New Canada." *Eimreidin (Reykjavik, Iceland),* printed in Icelandic, 67. Ar. 111 Hefti: 195211 (September-December 1961).
"Learning a Second Language." *The Manitoba Teacher – Guest Editorial* (January-February 1962).
"Obstructive Diverticulitis of the Sigmoid Colon." *Winnipeg Clinic Quarterly* Vol. 15, No. 2 (June 1962): 37–43.
"Provision of Medical Services Through Group Practice." *Group Practice* Vol. 2, No. 8 (August 1962) 485–495 [portion of Brief submitted to Royal Commission on Health Services in Montreal on April 16, 1962].
"Some Recollections of Visits to Iceland." *Logberg-Heimskringla,* an Icelandic weekly newspaper, 77. Ar. No. 17 (April 25, 1963): 4–6.
"A Tour of Eastern Mediterranean Countries." *Manitoba Medical Review* Vol. 43, No. 5 (May 1963): 262–265.
"'The Egyptian Disease' – Schistosomiasis." *Winnipeg Clinic Quarterly* Vol. 16, No. 2 (June 1963): 68–71.
"Your Hospital – A Community Partnership." *Manitoba Medical Review* Vol. 43, No. 7 (August-September 1963): 403–411.
"Medical Authorship." *Manitoba Medical Review* Vol. 43, No. 9 (November 1963): 524–525.
"The Selkirk Lutheran Church – 1889–1964" (May 1964).
"Cancer of the Colon and Recto-Sigmoid." *Pacific Medicine and Surgery* 72 (September-October, 1964): 269–273.
"Principles and Policies of the Manitoba Medical Service." *Manitoba Medical Review* Vol. 44, No. 8 (October 1964): 473–477.
"Cancer of the Colon and Recto-Sigmoid Junction." *Winnipeg Clinic*

Quarterly Vol. 18, No. 1 (March 1965): 22–31.

"The Medicine of Yesterday and That of Today" dinner address given to Cancer Chemotherapy Symposium in Montreal, June 22, 1947 (from the proceedings published by the sponsors, Frank W. Horner Limited of Montreal).

"The Future of Canadian Medicine." *Winnipeg Clinic Quarterly* Vol. 20, Nos. 3 and 4 (Fall 1967): 92–101.

"The Organization and Provision of Community Medical Services," introductory remarks to symposium. *Winnipeg Clinic Quarterly* Vol. 21, No. 2 (Summer 1968).

"A Century of Medical Progress." *Manitoba Medical Review* Vol. 48, No. 7 (August-September 1968): 314–316.

"La médécine d'hier et celle d'aujourd'hui," after-dinner speech delivered at Cancer Chemotherapy Symposium in Montreal on June 22, 1967) *Laval Medical* Vol. 39, 766–771, October, 1968.

"Medicare in Manitoba – Reasons for 'Opting in.'" *Winnipeg Clinic Quarterly* Vol. 22, No. 1 (Spring 1969): 4–9.

"Gallstone Disease." *Winnipeg Clinic Quarterly* Vol. 22, No. 1 (Spring 1969): 15–31 [with Robert H. Thorlakson and T. Kenneth Thorlakson].

"Symposium on the surgical Management of Duodenal Ulcers" introductory remarks. *Winnipeg Clinic Quarterly* Vol. 22, No. 3 (Fall 1969) [with Kenneth R. Trueman, T. Kenneth Thorlakson and Robert H. Thorlakson].

"A Chapter of Manitoba's History – A Pictorial Essay." *Winnipeg Clinic Quarterly* Vol. 23, Nos. 1 and 2 (1970).

"A Tribute to Dr. Ross B. Mitchell." *Winnipeg Clinic Quarterly* Vol. 23, Nos. 3 and 4 (1970): 65–68.

"Dr. Thomas A. Lebbetter – An Appreciation." *Winnipeg Clinic Quarterly* Vol. 25, No. 1 (February 1972): 3–5.

"The Canada Iceland Foundation." *The Icelandic Canadian Magazine* (Autumn 1973).

"The Significance of the New Canadian Policy on Multiculturalism." *Lögberg-Heimskringla*, an Icelandic weekly newspaper (January 10, 1974).

"The Organization and Administration of Group Practice." *World Medical Journal* Vol. 21, No. 3 (May-June 1974): 44–46.

"A Tribute to the Pioneer Icelandic Settlers in Canada." *The Icelandic Festival of Manitoba Programme* (August 1974).

"A Love Story," presented at the family reunion of the descendants of Niels Steingriumur and Erika Rynning Thorlaksson, held in Seattle, Washington, on September 2, 3 and 4, 1977. *Lögberg-Heimskringla* No. 40 (November 24, 1977), No. 41 (December 1, 1977), No. 42 (December 8, 1977), No. 43 (December 15) 1977.

Notes

CHAPTER 2

1 Dr. Ross Mitchell, BA, MD, FACS, FRCP (Can.), Hon. LL D (Man.) was born in Winnipeg on October 13, 1880. After graduating from Winnipeg Collegiate with an Isbister Scholarship in 1896, he attended Manitoba College from 1896 to 1899 and gained the degree of Bachelor of Arts in modern languages. For two and a half years he taught school near Morden, Manitoba, and in September, 1902, he enrolled at Manitoba Medical College. After graduation in 1908, he began the general practice of medicine.

Dr. Mitchell served overseas with the No. 4 Casualty Clearing Station from 1916 to 1918. After the War he took postgraduate studies at Harvard University, and later at the Chicago Lying-In Hospital. He was appointed a Governor of the American College of Surgeons (1949–55); Associate Professor of Obstetrics and Gynecology at the University of Manitoba (1934) and Professor (1948); editor of the *Manitoba Medical Journal* (1949). He was an active member of the Manitoba Historical Society for more than sixty years; was elected its president in 1951; and in later years was honorary president. His book, *Medicine in Manitoba,* is a prolific reference for anyone interested in the history of the profession in this province. He was appointed archivist for the Winnipeg Clinic in May, 1964.

2 The official discharge certificate of Paul H.T. Thorlakson states that he enlisted in the 223rd Battalion of the Canadian Overseas Expeditionary Force on May 9, 1916, accompanied the Unit overseas, was returned to Canada, and discharged from the service at the discharge depot in Quebec on September 6, 1917, to complete medical studies.

While waiting for his passage home from Liverpool, the youthful medic was able to get a one-week leave to visit Edinburgh. Most of the time there was spent as a guest in the home of famous Icelandic composer and musician Sveinbjorn Sveinbjornsson.

3 Miss Sarah Lewis (known to her friends as Sally) was born in Wales, took her training as a nurse in London, and came to Canada prior to World War I. She joined the nursing staff of the Winnipeg General Hospital to take charge of what was quaintly named "the outdoor service." Miss Lewis left the Winnipeg General Hospital staff after some years, and moved to Banff, Alberta. There she married a gentleman who also bore the surname Lewis. Her husband became ill, and after his death, Mrs. Lewis returned to nursing and continued actively until she was nearly eighty years old. In this period she was the matron of hospitals at Weyburn, Saskatchewan, Salmon Arm, B.C., and Selkirk, Manitoba, followed by a number of years as a private-duty nurse in Winnipeg. She died in Winnipeg at the age of ninety-four.

4 *Medicine in Manitoba*, p. 86.

5 Dr. H.H. Chown was Professor of Anatomy, Manitoba Medical College, from 1885 to 1892. He was Professor of Surgery, University of Manitoba, from 1892 to 1917; and Dean of the Medical College from 1900 until 1917. Dr. Jamieson's father was Edward Bald Jamieson, Anatomist Emeritus at the University of Edinburgh, author of the seven-volume *Illustrations of Regional Anatomy* (Edinburgh: Livingstone, 1959–1961) and many published papers on this subject.

6 Among the staff on the Better Farm Train was a young man named John Bracken, who was destined to become President of the Manitoba Agricultural College (later to become part of the University of Manitoba), Premier of Manitoba (1922–43) and federal leader of the Progressive Conservative Party (1943–49).

CHAPTER 3

1 The late Dr. C.E. Corrigan, a student and colleague of Dr. Gunn, recalls his surgical skill: "Dr. Gunn was brought up in the old school of surgical theory that believed that operative speed was the best safeguard against the (then) otherwise inevitable perils of wound infections and anaesthetic complications. To watch him work in the theatre was to witness a delightful display of coordinated and strictly purposeful manoeuvres. His scalpel and scissors seemed to miss every arterial twig – even the most minor ones. Quite frequently a house-surgeon assistant who happened to arrive just a few minutes after the scheduled starting time of the operation, would find the closure of a colostomy completed before

the unhappy young man was properly gloved. On the day of his official retirement from active surgical work, at age seventy, he completed a partial gastrectomy with only a surgical nurse assisting him in an elapsed operating time of fifty-five minutes."

2 Warfield M. Firor, "The Practicing Surgeon," *Leaders in Medicine* (New York, Holt Rinehart and Winston, 1963).

3 This was the original Medical Arts Building, erected in 1923–24. It was replaced by a new structure in 1974.

4 Dr. A.W.S. Hay was the gold medallist in the Manitoba Medical College Class of 1928. He joined the Maclean-Thorlakson Clinic immediately after graduation. He was an exemplary surgeon and an excellent teacher. At the outbreak of World War II, he joined the Royal Canadian Army Medical Corps, and in 1944 was chief of surgery stationed in a large military hospital just outside London. Late in December of that year the hospital had to deal with a disturbing number of cases of infectious hepatitis. Col. Hay was active in the management of these cases and the efforts to control the disease. One day during the latter part of the month, after lecturing to the professional staff on the subject, he happened to look in a mirror and noticed the telltale yellowing of the eyes that marks the onset of hepatitis. He died on December 31, 1944, a tragic loss to his family and colleagues, and to the profession of Medicine.

Dr. C. Burton Stewart was also a Manitoba graduate in the Class of 1928. Immediately after graduation he took an appointment as medical officer for the construction crews who were building the Hudson's Bay Railway, which provided him with a year of unusual experience. He ultimately became a specialist in urology, and continued with the Group when the Maclean-Thorlakson Clinic evolved into the Winnipeg Clinic, where he practiced until his retirement.

CHAPTER 4

1 Rufus C. Rorem, *Private Group Clinics* (Chicago: University of Chicago Press, 1931). In the 1930s, when Dr. Thorlakson was seriously considering the possibility of establishing a group practice clinic, the Mayo Clinic staff consisted of more than 200 "permanent" specialists, about 175 Fellows in postgraduate training, and 900 lay employees. Only about one-third of its patients were resident in Minnesota; two-thirds came from other states and foreign countries.

2 *Group Practice in Canada: The Report of the Special Committee on Group Practice* (Toronto: The Canadian Medical Association, 1967), p. 3–10.

3 Dr. Thorlakson was not without some prowess – and luck – on the golf course, and it took self-discipline to give up playing. Early in May 1936, at the Niakwa Country Club, he became the first local golfer of the season to score a hole-in-one.

4 C.S. Gunn was President of C.S. Gunn and Company Limited, Real Estate, Insurance, Loans, Stocks and Bonds, Winnipeg.

5 It is of interest to note that a year after Dr. Hay and Dr. Stewart joined the Maclean-Thorlakson Clinic, provision was made to grant them leave (a sort of informal sabbatical) to take postgraduate study in Edinburgh, Dr. Hay in general surgery, and Dr. Stewart in urology. On their return, interest-free loans were extended to permit each of them to acquire a house and a car. Similar advantages of participating in a group continued, when appropriate, to be made available during the early years of development of the Winnipeg Clinic.

With reference to the influence of the Mayo Clinic on the organization of private group practice clinics, Rorem noted in his 1930 study of these clinics in USA (then about 155 in number), "Nearly every one studied includes at least one physician who, at some time during his training or practice, was associated with this organization." The tradition was upheld at the Winnipeg Clinic: three of the original members had received postgraduate training at the Mayo Clinic: Dr. Morse, Dr. Thorson and Dr. Trueman.

6 Mr. Kneeland died suddenly on the train while en route to a business meeting in eastern Canada.

7 *Canada Year Book* (1941), p. xlvii.

8 The following is the first written directive issued to the staff when the Winnipeg Clinic commenced operation in the new building at the corner of St. Mary Avenue and Vaughan Street:

Winnipeg Clinic
Memorandum October 27, 1942

In order that those connected with the Clinic are advised of the general facts of this Clinic, this memorandum has been prepared and is handed to you for your information.

1. The Winnipeg Clinic is an association of Physicians and Surgeons in the practice of their profession.

2. The Winnipeg Clinic comprises the following professional staff: Dr. Neil John Maclean, consultant in surgery; Dr. P.H.T.Thorlakson, Director of the Clinic and senior surgeon; Dr. Harry D. Morse, urologist; Dr. C. Burton Stewart, urologist; Dr. Lennox G. Bell, internal medicine; Dr. Kenneth R. Trueman, surgeon; Dr. Steven B. Thorson, internist; Dr.

Jacob E. Isaac, assistant surgeon; Dr. A. Douglas Bracken, assistant physician; Dr. Dorothea M. Wardrop, assistant physician; Dr. J. Currie McMillan and Dr. Robert A. Macpherson, radiologists; Dr. W. George Brock, dermatologist.

The following departments are established and are to be supervised as follows: Surgical Department, Dr. P.H.T. Thorlakson; Urological Department, Dr. H.D. Morse and Dr. C.B. Stewart; Medical Department, Dr. Lennox G. Bell and Dr. S.B. Thorson; X-Ray Department, Dr. J.C. McMillan and Dr. R.A. Macpherson; Laboratory, Dr. S.B. Thorson; Business Manager, Mrs. J.B. Shepherd; Drug Department and General Purchasing Agent, Mr. C. Wintrup; General Office, Miss E. Scott.

The following staff of the Clinic have been assigned duties as follows: Miss Edith Banks, Private Secretary to Dr. Thorlakson; Mrs. R.E. Ward, R.N., Senior Nurse of Clinic; Mrs. H. Henry, Receptionist – Second Floor; Miss Joan Faiers, R.N., Nursing staff – Second Floor; Mrs. A.R. Harris, R.N., Nursing staff – First Floor; Miss A. Sloan, R.N., Nursing staff – General; Miss P. McAllister, Laboratory and X-Ray Technician; Miss F. Rold, Laboratory and X-Ray Technician; Miss E.G. Clint, Laboratory Technician and Recorder.

General office: Miss E. Scott, Supervisor; Mr. H. Lewis, Auditor and Chief Accountant; Miss Audry Scott and Miss Ruth Raven, Receptionists and Registration of Patients; Mrs. Mary Garrod, Cashier; Miss E. Jones, Telephone Operator; Miss Irene Petrie, Stenographer; Miss Sigmar, Supplies and Lunch Room; Mr. Patrick Garrity, Janitor.

The purchase of all supplies necessary for the various departments are to be made under written requisition forms that will be supplied to the various departments. These requisitions must be approved by the head of the department and handed to Mr. C. Wintrup, who will act as purchasing agent as well as dispensing pharmacist. He will check the receipts of all purchases before delivering and charging same to the various departments. It is suggested that requisitions be made up not oftener than once a week, unless in the case of an emergency. It is proposed that the Drug Department make all purchases except in connection with items classified as Capital Expenditures, Office Supplies and Building Operation Supplies. The Drug Department will invoice by counter check book, or otherwise, each department with all departmental purchases.

All sales of prescriptions or otherwise to the public are to be *for cash only* and are in no event to be charged to patient's account. The Drug Department is established and operated entirely separate from the Clinic.

General: You will frequently be confronted with the question as to charges to patients obtaining treatments, etc., and we wish to impress upon you that this question should be answered in all cases as follows: "The charge or charges of the Winnipeg Clinic will depend entirely upon the service rendered and the tests required to arrive at an accurate diagnosis but the fee will be reasonable."

The office hours of the Clinic will be from 9:00 a.m. to 6:00 p.m. on weekdays and from 9:00 a.m. to 1:00 p.m. on Saturdays. The telephone system will be in operation from 8:30 a.m. to 6:00 p.m.

It will be the object of all those connected with the Clinic to see that the building throughout be kept immaculate, this applying also to uniforms and personal appearance of all engaged.

Suggestions as to the operation of the Clinic, conduct of employees and any other matters of importance pertaining to the Clinic are gladly welcomed and should be handed to Mrs. Shepherd.

It is to be hoped that all will give their complete cooperation, and should there be any dispute or difficulty arise in connection with the operation of the Clinic, kindly see that these matters are discussed with the heads of the departments who will bring them before those in authority for discussion and settlement.

These memoranda will be issued from time to time, and you are earnestly requested to read and study them carefully so that at all times the Clinic may run with as little interruption as possible.

Let it be remembered that the patients attending the Clinic must be the first consideration of all concerned.

P.H.T. Thorlakson,
Director of Clinic

R.J. McGuckin,
Secretary of the Board

9 The Winnipeg Clinic Holding Company Limited. The land on which the first two-storey Winnipeg Clinic building was erected was purchased by Dr. Thorlakson for a net price of $13,800. Actually, the property cost was $14,000, but Billinkoff and Company, who removed the house then on the site, allowed $200 as salvage value of the material, leaving a book value in the accounts of $13,800. This property was registered in the name of Dr. Thorlakson.

In 1942 the original furnishings and equipment for the Clinic were purchased by Dr. Thorlakson to permit the building to be utilized for the practise of the medical clinic partners. He was to recover these costs through rental payments from the partnership, in their capacity as tenants in the building.

However, it was clear to Dr. Thorlakson that to combine into a single set of financial statements transactions related to his personal or professional affairs and expenditures related to the Clinic building would result in accounting, legal and tax problems, and appropriate arrangements needed to be made. He was advised to form a holding company to encompass all the financial operations he had undertaken related to the Winnipeg Clinic building, so that they would be completely separated from his professional and private financial affairs.

Consequently, the Winnipeg Clinic Holding Company Limited

was organized, with Dr. Thorlakson as the sole owner. The necessary accounting and legal preparations were completed in the fall of 1942, and the Winnipeg Clinic Holding Company was registered under the Manitoba Companies Act on February 11, 1943.

Dr. Thorlakson immediately transferred the assets and liabilities related to the furnishings and equipment already in the Clinic building, and the property registered until then in his name was transferred to the new company.

Following a practice commonly applied in the case of incorporation of private companies, to comply with the requirement that there must be at least three directors who are shareholders, one share in the Winnipeg Clinic Holding Company Limited was assigned to Dr. C.B. Stewart and to Dr. Harry Morse, respectively, so that they, along with Dr. Thorlakson, as President, were directors of the Company. Dr. Morse was appointed Secretary. Thus, three senior members of the Group Practice, who were also members of the Executive Committee of the doctors associated with the Clinic, were responsible for the operations of the Winnipeg Clinic Holding Company Limited.

In March 1943, the Manitoba Institute for the Advancement of Medical Education and Research was incorporated, and title to the land on which the Clinic building stood was transferred by Dr. Thorlakson to the Institute as a gift, at the original net value of $13,800. At the same time the building itself became the property of the Institute. These transfers were subject to a ten-year lease back to the Winnipeg Clinic Holding Company Limited, which became the corporate manager of the property.

The corporate structures then in place, consequently provided that the medical associates of the Winnipeg Clinic carried on the business affairs related to their professional practice, and paid rent to the Winnipeg Clinic Holding Company Limited for the furnished, equipped and maintained clinical facilities. The Holding Company in turn paid rent to the Research Institute at an agreed rate for the building. The initial rent for the two-storey building was at the rate of $1,500 a month, effective August 1, 1942, subject to review at the end of three years, and at regular intervals thereafter.

Winnipeg Clinic Pharmacy Limited: what began in 1942 as the Drug Department in the new Winnipeg Clinic building was established as an independent entity by Dr. Thorlakson, both as a convenience for patients, and as a potential source of revenue for research and education. He personally funded the original stock. This dispensary operated as a self-supporting, rent-paying unit, with no withdrawal of profits until it was incorporated as the Winnipeg

Clinic Pharmacy Limited on December 18, 1945. At that time, Dr. Thorlakson stipulated that all the profits of the Winnipeg Clinic Pharmacy Limited should be transferred, in perpetuity, to the Manitoba Institute for the Advancement of Medical Education and Research, for the support of its objectives. "In my opinion," he said, "it is somewhat improper, and probably unethical, for doctors to profit from the sale of prescriptions."

Actually, the nominal directors named in the pharmacy incorporating documents (D.A. Thompson, president, and O.W. Struthers and Grace M. Lawson, directors – all associated with Mr. MacAulay's legal office) remained in place until January 7, 1950. At that time, Miss Lawson's share was transferred to Dr. Thorlakson, and for the first time he became a director on the Pharmacy Board.

On the same date, the share held by Mr. Struthers was transferred to Dr. H.D. Morse, and he became a director and the Secretary of the Company.

Mr. Thompson continued to hold the third director's share, and continued as President. The remaining 497 shares of the capital stock of the Winnipeg Clinic Pharmacy Limited were transferred to the Winnipeg Clinic (Incorporated) at the Directors' meeting on January 7, 1950. (The Clinic had been incorporated by an act of the Manitoba Legislature in 1949.)

It was not until March 14, 1951, that Mr. Thompson resigned as President of the Pharmacy, and transferred his shares to Dr. C.B. Stewart, who became a director. The directors then elected Dr. Thorlakson President of the Winnipeg Pharmacy Limited, Dr. Morse and Dr. Stewart being the remaining directors.

In a report dated February 4, 1966, Dr. Thorlakson confirmed that "not one cent of the earnings of the Pharmacy has been paid out directly to me or to any other doctor of this clinic. Over the years, the Manitoba Institute for the Advancement of Medical Education and Research, or, as it is now known, the Winnipeg Clinic Research Institute, has received substantial donations from the Winnipeg Clinic Pharmacy Limited and is continuing to do so."

10 Audrey Peterkin and Margaret Shaw (Winnipeg: Prairie Publishers, 1976), quoted with permission.

CHAPTER 5

1 The Institute did not have cash in hand for this payment, and the funds were provided for its share of the cost of the alterations through a donation totalling $10,500 from Dr. Thorlakson and Dr. C.B. Stewart.

CHAPTER 6

1 In 1950, the following doctors were members or associates of the Winnipeg Clinic: Dr. G.L. Adamson; Dr. A.W. Andison; Dr. L.G. Bell; Dr. B.D. Best; Dr. E.G. Brownell; Dr. H.W. Bottomley; Dr. J.E. Burch; Dr. L. Cherniack; Dr. O.S. Day; Dr. J. Farr; Dr. J.E. Isaac; Dr. J.M. Kilgour; Dr. D.L. Kippen; Dr. T.A. Lebbetter; Dr. B.E. Loadman; Dr. I.S. Maclean; Dr. J.W. MacLeod; Dr. J. McGeachy; Dr. M. McLandress; Dr. J.K. Martin; Dr. D. Medd; Dr. J.E. Morris; Dr. H.D. Morse; Dr. M.B. Perrin; Dr. G.H. Ryan; Dr. F.A. Sheppard; Dr. C.B. Stewart; Dr. J.R. Taylor; Dr. P.H.T. Thorlakson; Dr. K.R. Trueman; Dr. C.H.A. Walton.

2 Articles in the *Winnipeg Clinic Quarterly* were not confined to scientific matters. The first issue was dedicated to the memory of Dr. Neil John Maclean. Other issues focussed on timely events, or recognized the professional work of individual doctors. A concise, but remarkably informative and well-illustrated centennial edition was published in 1970 to honour the hundredth birthday of the Province of Manitoba. It provided a capsule account of the history of the Province, the City of Winnipeg, the Universities, the Medical College, and the two major teaching hospitals, Winnipeg General Hospital and St. Boniface General Hospital.

3 Part of a presentation given to the American Association of Medical Clinics in New Orleans on October 8, 1960, is given here:

PRIVATE CLINICS AND MEDICAL EDUCATION
In many clinics of moderate size, some departments are well equipped to offer excellent opportunities to the graduate. In these he will be able to enlarge his clinical experience and to receive some basic training; radiology and dermatology are probably the best examples, if the head of the department concerned is seriously interested in graduate education. The graduate trainee in internal medicine would also have excellent opportunities in many clinics. He could participate in the work-up and treatment and final disposal of many medical problems. According to the replies received to a questionnaire on postgraduate training in clinics circulated in 1959, only nine clinics reported they had a training program in internal medicine, four in radiology and one in dermatology. Thirteen clinics reported training programs in general surgery, and I suspect that some of these provided opportunity for surgeons to "fill their required practice time" after completing their formal residency.

The chief responsibility of the private clinics in the field of postgraduate education is, in my opinion, the continuous education of its own members. Graduate medical education should begin the day following graduation and should be continuous throughout the doctor's professional life. Herein lies one of the great functions and opportunities of group practice. One of the essential differences between solo practice and group practice is the constant and added challenge to study and to improve clinical knowledge and techniques in close association with medical colleagues. I first became actively involved in the organization of group practice in 1926, and one of the compelling reasons for my interest was the conviction that the stimulus of the University hospital group on the public charity wards could also be made to function in private group practice. The method by which this type of postgraduate education or continuing education is achieved in a private group is by developing a readily accessible reference library, by studying medical records, by frequently presenting and recording interesting and unusual case histories, by having spot consultations and corridor discussions, by frankly criticizing methods and results, and by participating in short courses of study at other medical centres which provide opportunities for young aspirants to improve their knowledge. This should be the extent and the goal of group effort in graduate training in the majority of private medical clinics in the United States and Canada.

There are two other situations in which a clinic organization can participate and contribute to undergraduate and graduate education.

(1) If the group is practising in a university centre, the individual members of the clinic should be encouraged to apply for active membership on the staff of teaching hospitals. They will make their contribution to the regular teaching programs as individual practising physicians or surgeons. They will have a dual loyalty, one to the university and teaching hospital and one to their private group. This will in no way differ from the contribution made by non-Clinic members of the teaching staff who are practising alone. In the University of Manitoba Faculty of Medicine, 26.7% of the clinical teachers belong to various private groups. In our clinic of fifty doctors [1960], thirty-eight are on the active staff of teaching hospitals and are members of the Faculty of Medicine. In addition, four of our senior members are former professors or associate professors and heads of departments in the Faculty of Medicine at the University of Manitoba.

From the beginning of our clinic, we have recruited our medical colleagues partly on the basis of their interest in the medical teaching and partly from those who have a concern for medical research or clinical investigation by either active participation or providing financial support to these activities. As a result of this type of selection it is probably worth noting that our former Chief of Medicine in the Winnipeg Clinic is the Dean and Professor of Medicine of the University of Manitoba; that our former Head of Gastroenterology is Dean of the Faculty of Medicine of the University of Saskatchewan and that one of our former paediatricians is the Head of the Paediatric Department of the University of Alberta.

(2) If a clinic is large and has complete control of adequate hospital beds it might be encouraged to organize an active graduate teaching program and

obtain approval of the American Specialty Boards or the Royal Colleges in Canada.

4 When Dr. Thorlakson transferred the ownership of the Pharmacy and the Winnipeg Clinic Holding Co. Ltd. to the new Corporation, he believed that he was providing a firm basis for the continuing development of a progressive, downtown Winnipeg medical diagnostic and treatment centre founded on the tripod of: (a) A high standard of comprehensive medical and surgical service; (b) Participation in medical education; (c) An effective interest and involvement in supporting scientific medical research; and free from recurring divisive discussions on individual ownership of land, buildings, furnishings, and expensive diagnostic equipment.

5 Following are extracts from Cap. 100 S.M. 1949 – An Act to Incorporate "Winnipeg Clinic":

Sec. 1. [The following persons, namely:] Gilbert L. Adamson; A. Wilson Andison; Lennox G. Bell; Brian D. Best; Louis Cherniak; Oswald J. Day; John Farr; Jacob E. Isaac; John M. Kilgour; Thomas A. Lebbetter; Ian S. MacLean; J. Wendell MacLeod; Harry D. Morse; Maitland B. Perrin; George H. Ryan; Frederick A.B. Sheppard; C. Burton Stewart; Paul H.T. Thorlakson; Kenneth R. Trueman; Charles H.A. Walton; together with such other persons as may from time to time become members of the corporation . . . as herein provided, are hereby constituted a body politic and corporate, under the name "Winnipeg Clinic", hereinafter referred to as "the clinic."

Sec. 2. The purposes and objectives of the clinic shall be to provide diagnostic, consultative, treatment and administrative facilities for the physicians and surgeons who are or may become members of the clinic, and others, and who are practising their profession of medicine and surgery in cooperation and association with each other.

Sec. 3. (1) In addition [to other] powers vested in the clinic, the clinic may

(a) acquire, establish, provide, operate, maintain and make available to its members and others, diagnostic, consultative, treatment and hospital facilities, or any of them, and buildings, premises and equipment, its organization and administrative staff and facilities, and engage, utilize and make available to its members and others, the services of duly qualified medical practitioners, pharmacists, technicians and staff members;

(b) enter into agreements with duly qualified medical practitioners whereby the practitioners agree to conduct the practice of medicine and surgery in association with each other and in so doing to make use of the facilities provided by the clinic . . . and to assign to the clinic all fees earned by them in the conduct of their practices, and whereby the clinic agrees to pay such practitioners' salary and other payments and benefits;

(c) with a view to furthering the purposes and objectives of the clinic, purchase, take on lease, acquire . . . by purchase, grant, donation, gift . . . and own . . . and administer . . . or deal in property of every kind . . . including the properties and assets of the association of physicians and surgeons now conducting a medical and surgical practice in the City of Winnipeg under the name: "The Winnipeg Clinic";

(d) establish, assist by grant or otherwise . . . and operate medical and surgical research laboratories;

(e) . . . carry on the business of a pharmacy;

(h) establish or support . . . funds calculated to benefit employees . . . or their dependents [such as] group insurance and pension plans . . .

(2) Notwithstanding anything expressed or implied herein, the clinic, as distinct from its members, shall not for hire, gain, or hope of reward practise medicine or surgery and shall in the conduct of its affairs observe the provisions of the Medical Act and every other Act of the Legislature.

Sec. 10. In the event of and upon the clinic ceasing to carry on, and winding up, its affairs, all the properties and assets of the clinic remaining after payment of its debts and liabilities shall go or be paid to the Manitoba Institute for the Advancement of Medical Education and Research.

6 The Partnership Agreement is a lengthy document, which includes, in part, the following sections:

Section 1. The objects of the Clinic shall be to enable the giving of better aid to the sick through the association of the physicians and surgeons created by this agreement, and to encourage scientific study, investigation and research. . . .

Section 3. Control of and decision concerning all affairs of the Clinic shall be exercised and made by members of the Clinic at meetings of the members of the Clinic to be held from time to time pursuant to notice and at any such meeting the decision of the majority of such members shall be final and binding upon members. . . .

[It seems that there may be two different uses of the word "Clinic" in this and subsequent sections of the Agreement; in the first case, "all the affairs of the Clinic" is a reference to the Clinic operated by the partnership of Thorlakson, Stewart and Morse, which carried on a medical and surgical practice and employed other doctors to assist them in this practice; the reference to "members of the Clinic" seems to refer to the members of the Winnipeg Clinic (Incorporated) as defined in Corporation By-law No. 1. The word "member" is not defined in the Partnership Agreement itself, and it may be that it is intended to designate a member of the partnership. It seems likely that the doctors in the Clinic found differentiation of these roles difficult.]

Section 5. The members may . . . appoint an Advisory Council consisting of not less than two nor in excess of seven physicians and/or surgeons associated with the members in the said practice of medicine and surgery, who shall act with such members in an advisory capacity. . . .

Section 6. Each member shall devote all his professional and business time, and all his skill and attention to the Clinic, and to the affairs of the incorporated Winnipeg Clinic . . . [unless he has the consent of the members].

The remaining eighteen sections of the Agreement set out management policies on a variety of topics.

7 The Act of Incorporation of the Winnipeg Clinic provided that its affairs would be managed by a Council consisting of not less than five and not more than nine members of the clinic, the composition of the initial council being eight members named as follows: Brian D. Best, John M. Kilgour, Thomas A. Lebbetter, George H. Ryan, C. Burton Stewart, Paul H.T. Thorlakson, Kenneth R. Trueman, and Charles A. Walton.

At the first meeting of the *members* of the Corporation, held on June 29, 1950, the number of council members was increased to nine, and Dr. Harry Morse was added.

8 By-law No. 1 of the Winnipeg Clinic (Incorporated) included, in part, the following sections:

Section 17. [At meetings of members or of the Council] every member personally present shall have one vote only. An associate member may not vote. A member may not be represented at a meeting by proxy.

Section 18(b). Drs. Harry D. Morse, C. Burton Stewart and P.H.T. Thorlakson shall be deemed to be elected members of the Council for a five-year term ending December 31, 1954, without the necessity of election, and, thereafter, if they are respectively members of the Clinic, shall be eligible for re-election.

Section 20. No person shall be elected or appointed a Council member to fill any vacancy unless he is a member of the Clinic in good standing.

Section 30. The officers of the Clinic shall be a Director and one or more

Vice Directors [later named Assistant Directors], as the Council deems desirable, and a Secretary, a Business Manager, and such other officers as may be provided for by resolution of the Council. . . . The Secretary and the Business Manager need not be members of the Clinic.

Section 32. The Director shall be the chief executive officer of the Clinic. He shall preside at all meetings of the members and the Council at which he may be present. He shall have executive authority to see that all orders and resolutions of the council are carried into effect, and shall perform all duties that shall pertain to his office or that of President of a Corporation, and such other duties as may be from time-to-time prescribed by Council or by-law. . . . The Director shall have the authority to make all appointments to positions other than those by by-law or resolution designated to be made by the Council.

CHAPTER 7

1 The statement may require some explanation for the modern reader, when 100% payment of the fee schedule is made by Manitoba Health Services Commission. At the time Dr. Thorlakson was writing, a majority of patients in Winnipeg, and a growing number in rural Manitoba, were members of the doctor-operated prepayment plan for medical care known as the Manitoba Medical Services Plan, or MMS. Doctors participating in the Plan agreed to accept as full settlement of their accounts the payment provided by the Plan, which was usually less than the billing. For services to patients without prepayment or insurance cover, some accounts were uncollectable. At the Winnipeg Clinic these factors reduced revenue from professional services by about eighteen percent.

2 Dr. T.A. Lebbetter came to the Winnipeg Clinic in 1946. He had been recommended to Dr. Thorlakson by Col. J.L. Ralston, Minister of National Defense during World War II. He had been the Ralston family physician at their home in Nova Scotia, and he had expressed an interest in coming to western Canada after the War. He was also recommended by Dr. Clarence Routley, long-time Executive Officer of the Canadian Medical Association. Although Dr. Lebbetter carried on a medical practice at the Winnipeg Clinic, he had a number of administrative assignments. For a time he was Secretary of the Winnipeg Clinic (Incorporated), as well as the Manitoba Institute for the Advancement of Medical Education and Research.

3 Membership of the Buildings, Properties and Investments Committee during the construction of the 1959–60 addition was: Mr. C. Gordon Smith, Chairman; Mr. H.C. Ashdown; Mr. P.A. Chester; Mr. Frank B. Lount; Mr. John A. MacAulay; Dr. C.B. Stewart; Mr. J. Elmer Woods; and Dr. P.H.T. Thorlakson.

4 The credit rating of the Winnipeg Clinic was well established by the time the 1960 construction took place, so that capital financing was readily available through regular commercial channels. Dr. Thorlakson arranged bridge financing (i.e., funds borrowed temporarily for contract payments during the course of construction) from the Royal Bank of Canada, for up to $600,00 at six percent interest.

5 In his address prior to the unveiling of the bronze bust of Dr. Thorlakson, Dr. Walton referred to some of Mr. Leo Mol's achievements:

> . . . Here in Winnipeg we found a distinguished sculptor who is perhaps better known abroad than here at home. Mr. Mol has been a resident of this area for many years and is deeply devoted to Manitoba and the West. He has done much to beautify our city and he is the creator of many of the stained glass windows in Winnipeg churches. He recently completed a superb bronze statue of the Queen which stands in one of the courtyards of the Centennial Centre. . . . He was commissioned to do a bronze sculpture of Pope Paul [by] a religious order in Germany. He was also commissioned to do a sculpture of Taras Shevchenko [for a site] in Washington, D.C. This brought him to the attention of President Eisenhower. Shortly afterwards, friends of the President commissioned him to do a bronze sculpture of that great soldier-statesman. He is presently working on a large statue which will be erected in Buenos Aires. . . .

CHAPTER 8

1 Letter of appointment to the National Research Council's Associate Committee on Medical Research written March 21, 1938:

> Dear Dr. Thorlakson:
>
> In accordance with the recommendations of the conference on the organization of medical research in Canada held in Ottawa on 18 February, 1938, the National Research Council at its meeting on 18 March 1938, established an associate committee on medical research and approved the personnel suggested by the nominating committee appointed by the conference.
>
> I have much pleasure in advising you that your name was among those proposed for membership on the associate committee, and on behalf of the National Research Council I extend to you a very cordial invitation to accept appointment to this committee for a period of four years. I would very much appreciate your acceptance of this appointment. As soon as we have heard from all of those to whom invitations are being extended it is proposed to hold a meeting of the committee to organize the work and to plan its activities.
>
> There are enclosed for your information a copy of the proceedings of the

conference and also of the memorandum submitted to Council regarding the formation of the committee.

Yours faithfully,

A.G.L. McNaughton, President

2 The committee comprised: Chairman, Sir Frederick Banting; ex-officio members, Major-General A.G.L. McNaughton, President of the National Research Council and Dr. R.E. Wodehouse, Deputy Minister of the Department of Pensions and National Health; Dr. Donald Mainland, Professor of Anatomy, Dalhousie University, Halifax; Dr. J.E. Gendreau, Director, Radium Institute, University of Montreal; Dr. A. Grant Fleming, Dean of the Faculty of Medicine and Professor of Public Health, McGill University, Montreal; Dr. J.B. Collip, Professor of Biochemistry, McGill University, Montreal; Dr. W.G. Penfield, Professor of Neurology and Neurosurgery, McGill University, Montreal; Dr. G.H. Ettinger, Professor, Department of Physiology and Embryology, Queen's University, Kingston; Dr. T.H. Leggett, President of the Canadian Medical Association (1937) Ottawa; Dr. J.C. Paterson, Director of Pathology, Civic Hospital, Ottawa; Dr. Duncan Graham, Head, Department of Medicine, University of Toronto, Toronto; Professor V.E. Henderson, Secretary Treasurer, The Banting Research Foundation, Toronto; Dr. P.H.T. Thorlakson, Assistant Professor of Surgery, University of Manitoba, Winnipeg.

When the decision was taken to survey the existing medical research resources in Canada, an able young man was recruited to do the necessary staff work: Dr. Chester B. Stewart. He was named assistant secretary of the Committee, and in this capacity he established Dr. Banting's itinerary, arranged the details with the local hosts and medical scientists, recorded observations, and drafted the report – all, of course in consultation with Dr. Banting. In the western section of the survey, the planning was shared with Dr. Thorlakson.

Dr. Stewart had graduated in medicine at Dalhousie University in the spring of 1938. His association with Dr. Banting, and his introduction to leaders in the medical schools across Canada, must have been a rewarding experience, strengthening his interest in academic affairs. After completion of his term with the Committee on Research, he returned to Halifax to spend most of his professional life in distinguished service with his alma mater. He took time to earn a master's degree in public health at Johns Hopkins, followed by a Ph.D. and an FRCP(C).

3 With the help of Charles H. Best, a graduate medical assistant, Dr.

Frederick Grant Banting in 1922 discovered insulin following long and persistent research in the Department of Physiology at the University of Toronto. No other Canadian medical scientist has been accorded as much acclaim for his achievements as that granted to Dr. Banting, both at home and abroad. In 1923 he was awarded the Nobel Prize in Medicine, to be shared with his department head, Dr. J.J.R. McLeod. Dr. Banting was disappointed that the Nobel trustees had failed to recognize the work of Dr. Best, and insisted on sharing the financial part of the award with him. It is one measure of the man, who once sold his furniture, his car, and some of his instruments to enable him to continue his insulin research, that he assigned all financial interests in his discovery to the University of Toronto. The House of Commons voted Banting a lifetime pension of $7,000 a year. He was created a Knight in the King's Honours List in 1934.

4 Dr. Alvin T. Mathers was born in Neepawa, Manitoba. He graduated in Medicine from the University of Manitoba in 1912. Subsequently he did postgraduate work in Boston, Massachusetts, and in England, France and Germany.

In 1916 he cut short his studies in Boston to enlist in the Royal Canadian Army Medical Corps. He was posted to Fort Osborne (Winnipeg) with the rank of Captain, and for the rest of World War I supervised the care of military patients in the Winnipeg hospitals. In 1918 he was appointed Provincial Psychiatrist, a position he held until 1942. During this time he was responsible for development of the Manitoba Government's program in mental health. For a number of the earlier years he was the only psychiatrist in Manitoba in private practice.

In 1931 he was appointed Dean of the Faculty of Medicine, University of Manitoba, a position from which he retired in 1949. He was appointed Professor Emeritus in Psychiatry in 1954.

Dr. Mathers was honoured by his colleagues in many ways, among others by his election as President of the Winnipeg Medical Association; President of the Royal College of Physicians and Surgeons of Canada; President of the Medical Council of Canada; and President of the Association of Canadian Medical Colleges. He was granted an LL.D., *honouris causa*, by the University of Manitoba in 1949.

Dr. Mathers died in Deer Lodge Hospital, Winnipeg, on January 4, 1960, at the age of seventy-one.

5 Dr. Ian MacLaren Thompson, B.Sc., M.B. Ch.B. (Edin.), D.Sc. (Man.), FRSC, FRSE, Professor Emeritus of Anatomy, University of Manitoba, died in Winnipeg on December 26, 1981. Dr. Thompson was born in Newfoundland in 1896. He was a student in medicine

and science at the University of Edinburgh from 1914 to 1920, with leave in 1917 and 1918 to serve as a surgeon probationer in the navy. He was lecturer in anatomy at McGill University (1920 to 1924); Assistant Professor (1924 to 1927); Associate Professor of Anatomy, University of California – Berkeley (1927 to 1932); Professor (1932 to 1936); and Chairman of the Division of Anatomy of Berkeley (1930–31, 1932–33 and 1934 to 1936). He came to Winnipeg in 1937 as Professor of Anatomy and Head of the Department, University of Manitoba. He held consultative appointments in major hospitals in Montreal, San Francisco and Winnipeg.

He published many scholarly papers, and his researches gained him Fellowship in the Royal Society of Canada (1947) and in the Royal Society of Edinburgh (1952). He authored a number of textbooks in anatomy. His memberships in scientific and medical societies, and the honours bestowed upon him by his colleagues, demonstrated the esteem in which he was held.

Dr. Thompson had a keen interest in the potential of the Manitoba Institute for the Advancement of Medical Education and Research to give useful support to scientific investigation in the Faculty of Medicine. He served on its Advisory Committee, and for a time was Honorary Secretary of the Institute.

6 Probably because the Report of the Western Survey of Research Facilities contained the candid views of the survey team, the Report was never published, nor was it tabled at a meeting of the Associate Committee. It may be of some historic interest, however, to quote the concise statement of "Impressions" inserted in the Report following the narrative account of the visit at each centre:

WINNIPEG (SEE P. 119).

SASKATOON

Lack of funds and a small staff have prevented much medical research from being carried out in the University of Saskatchewan. A very fine spirit of cooperation between the various groups and the excellent character of the students are the two outstanding features.

Dr. Ferguson's research work and system of control of tuberculosis are also outstanding.

EDMONTON

The Medical School of the University of Alberta is in a more fortunate position than others visited to date in the larger number of full-time professional members on the staff of each pre-medical department: anatomy, three; bacteriology, three; biochemistry, three; pathology, two; and physiology, three.

Laboratory space and other facilities are very good, and those of the De partment of Biochemistry are outstanding.

There is a marked lack of means for encouragement of students to enter research. The few who are so engaged are paying for their supplies and paying tuition to the University besides.

The number of hospital beds available for teaching and clinical research is relatively small.

VANCOUVER

Vancouver has an extremely active group in the Public Health Department and in the Connaught Laboratories, under Dr. C.E. Dolman; the cooperation between these two organizations and the University is very valuable.

Of the University Departments visited besides the Connaught Laboratories, the Department of Chemistry is outstanding as a research unit.

There is a very active group in the tuberculosis and venereal disease prevention departments, and excellent clinical facilities available at the General Hospital, but little research is being done.

There is a desire on the part of many members of the medical profession for the establishment of a medical school.

CALGARY

There is very little interest in, and limited facilities for, medical research at Calgary.

REGINA

While there is practically no research being carried out at Regina, there is a greater interest in it and greater spirit of cooperation than at Calgary. Dr. Moore and Dr. Riddell, two newcomers, are both trained in research methods and would be able to carry out some researches after they are thoroughly established in their new positions.

BRANDON

There is no research work being conducted at Brandon College, and not many facilities are available, but both Professor Cragg and Professor Johns have the ability to do research and are planning to do some work.

The Mental Hospital has very good clinical and laboratory facilities for research on mental diseases, and a keenly interested and cooperative staff.

7 We include extracts from two letters to Dr. Thorlakson regarding his brief on the establishment of a division of medical science at the National Research Council. The first is from Dr. J.B. Collip, Montreal, and is dated December 19, 1945:

Re: Division of Medical Science National Research Council

In general I am in agreement with the suggestions you have made irrespective of whether we can hope to have implementation of all of these at once. There is only one criticism I would make at this time; namely, in connection with the proposed Executive Committee (bottom of page 5).

1. Dentistry should be left out as they now have an Associate Committee of their own, and would no doubt resent any approach from us.

2. Military Medicine should be given a place, if, as and when the Military Authorities request it.

3. Since it is to be expected that by far the greater amount of work supported in the field of Medical Research will be of a fundamental nature in the basic sciences, there should be greater representation on the Executive Committee of these sciences than for Medicine, Surgery, and Industrial Hygiene. True, the size of the committee should be kept as small as possible, but one would like to see Physiology, Biochemistry, Pharmacology, and Pathology all adequately represented, as you will agree these subjects are basic.

The second letter is from Professor G.H. Ettinger, Queen's University, and is dated December 20, 1945:

Re: Division of Medical Science National Research Council

I agree in principle that the Associate Committee on Dental Research should come under the Division of Medical Sciences, although it is going to be difficult to prepare an agreeable formula for that.

I am not sure that I should like the Advisory Committee to include a rotating representation from the Deans of Medical Schools and from the Association of Provincial Deputy Ministers of Health, nor from the Department of National Health and Welfare. I think the more the Advisory Committee included automatic representatives, the more unwieldy it would become. In place of giving automatic membership to these bodies, I would favour occasional conferences to which they would be invited, or giving them invitations to attend meetings according to circumstances. I should make the Advisory Committee as small as possible, consistent with adequate representation of the specialties. We have had too many meetings of large committees, distinguished by verbosity rather than by wise decisions. The only bodies to which I would give automatic membership would be the Royal College and the Canadian Medical Association. The Medical Schools will have a voice through members of the Advisory Committee, who are bound to come from them, and through Chairmen or members of committees.

I approve your suggestion with respect to consideration of grants-in-aid. I think we should be advised by Panels of experts in any field, and I think that the committees which we may appoint in the various fields should arrange for these Panels.

I am glad to have your ideas about the placing of research persons, whom you designate as assistant directors. We are bound to be influenced in this respect by two considerations. (1) The need of offering employment to competent and enthusiastic research workers. (2) The most profitable places to have these men work. The profit can be in terms of (a) the immediate fruit of investigation, or (b) the spirit and enthusiasm which such people can create in the centres in which they are placed. Both of these would depend to a certain degree on the person selected, but we must also consider the facilities available at the different universities, and the need for the *stimulus to research*. As a guide to the latter, we may consider the present research output.

CHAPTER 9

1 The Winnipeg Foundation is a long-established and highly respected non-profit corporation established for the purpose of accepting gifts and bequests, administering them in the public interest, and making appropriate grants in aid of beneficial community projects. In considering how his purpose could be achieved, Dr. Thorlakson instinctively turned first to the Foundation as the agency that might accept the gift of title to the Clinic building, administer the rental income, and make grants in support of medical education and research in accordance with the direction of an advisory committee. A formal proposal to this end was submitted to the Winnipeg Foundation in August 1942; but after consideration, the trustees decided that the plan, as drafted, did not give effective authority to the Foundation to permit it to carry out its public obligations, as required in its charter.

2 It should be noted that the University of Manitoba Board of Governors had a positive recommendation from the Faculty of Medicine in favour of the establishment of the Manitoba Institute for the Advancement of Medical Education and Research before they gave their support.

Dean Mathers called a special meeting of the Faculty in order to obtain their opinion and reaction to the proposal. The meeting was well-attended, and Dr. Thorlakson was asked to "state his case" and reply to any questions that were put to him.

There was a free and prolonged discussion, and very direct questions were put to Dr. Thorlakson with respect to his motives and objectives in promoting the Institute. Finally an open vote was taken, which gave Dr. Mathers the approval which he needed to make a recommendation to the Board of Governors of the University. As a result, the Board supported the Institute, and the Dean of Medicine, and the President and the Chairman of the University Board became ex-officio members of the Institute Board.

3 Quoted in the *New England Journal of Medicine* (March 5, 1981), p. 601.

4 Signatories to the Petition to incorporate The Manitoba Institute for Medical Education and Research were as follows: Harry C. Ashdown; Dr. Lennox G. Bell; H.A. Bergman; Dr. A.T. Cameron; Dr. Bruce Chown; Dorothy Cocking; Dr. C.R. Gilmour; Cecil S. Gunn; Joseph Harris; G.F. Jonasson; Grace M. Lawson; H.W. Manning; Dr. Harry D. Morse; W.A. Murphy; J.A. MacAulay; Dr. P.A. McDonald; Dr. Neil John Maclean; Wesley McCurdy; J.D. Perrin; R.G. Persse; Mrs. James A. Richardson; C.S. Riley; O.W. Struthers; Esther Snider; H.E. Sellers; Victor Sifton; Dr. C.B. Stewart; Dr. P.H.T. Thorlakson; Donald A. Thompson; Mr. Justice A.K. Dysart; Dr. Sidney E. Smith; Dr. A.T. Mathers; and Dr. Thorlakson signed a second time in his capacity as Chairman of the Research Committee of the Faculty of Medicine.

5 The $60,000 advanced under the first mortgage consisted of $30,000 from Mrs. James A. Richardson and $30,000 from Mr. C.S. Gunn. The balance of the land and building cost, advanced without interest, was provided by the following:

G.F. Jonasson		$10,000.00
J.A. MacAulay		$ 4,000.00
Dr. Thorlakson:		
Land at cost	$13,800.00	
Cash	$19,750.00	
		$33,550.00
		$47,550.00

6 The first cash contributors to the Institute were members of the Winnipeg Clinic (as reported at the first meeting of the members of the Manitoba Institute for the Advancement of Medical Education and Research on June 22, 1943): Dr. Neil John McLean, $1,000; Dr. P.H.T. Thorlakson, $1,000; Dr. H.D. Morse, $1,000; Dr. C.B. Stewart, $1,000; Dr. Lennox Bell, $500; Dr. C.R. Gilmour, $500; Dr. K.R. Trueman $500; Mr. C.S. Gunn (not a member of the Clinic), $500.

7 Charles F. Code was born in Winnipeg in 1910, the grandson of Mr. and Mrs. E.L. Drewry, a distinguished pioneer family of this city. He graduated from the University of Manitoba in 1934 with the degrees of Doctor of Medicine and Bachelor of Science. He was a brilliant student, and immediately after graduation was selected to be Fellow in Physiology and Medicine at the Mayo Graduate School of Medicine in Rochester, Minnesota. He spent 1936–37 as a lecturer in Physiology at University College, London, working with Sir Charles Lovatt Evans, and with Sir Henry H. Dale at the National Institute for Medical Research in Hampstead.

He returned to Rochester, and in the ensuing years held positions of ever-widening responsibility in the Mayo Graduate School of Medicine, the University of Minnesota, the Mayo Foundation, and the Mayo Medical School. He obtained his Ph.D. from the University of Minnesota in 1940. From 1940 to 1975 he was Consultant in Physiology, Mayo Clinic and Mayo Foundation, and subsequently Professor of Physiology, Chairman of the Department, and Director of Medical Education and Research in the Mayo organization. From 1957 to 1964 he was a member of the Board of Governors of the Mayo Clinic and the Mayo Foundation.

In 1975 Dr. Code became Associate Chief of Staff and Senior Research Scientist, and Associate Director of the Centre for Ulcer Research and Education, at the Veteran's Administration Wadsworth Hospital Centre in Los Angeles.

8 The Board of Directors of the Institute had appointed an advisory committee to review and recommend the action to be taken on all applications for assistance. Membership of the Advisory Committee: H.P. Armes, Dean of Arts and Science at the University of Manitoba; Dean Mathers, of the Faculty of Medicine; Dr. A.T. Cameron, Chairman of the Research Committee of the Faculty; Dr. F.G. McGuinness, Chairman of the Postgraduate Committee of the Faculty; Dr. H.D. Morse; Dr. Bruce Chown; and Dr. H. Rice.

9 Other physicians (i.e., in addition to Dr. Hudson of Hamiota and Dr. Johnston of Thompson) who received a General Practitioner Postgraduate Award were: Dr. Robert E. Helgason, Glenboro (1957); Dr. Stephen S. Toni, Altona (1958); Dr. Joseph Leicester, The Pas (1959); Dr. Kjartan L. Johnson, Gladstone (1960); Dr. H.W. Clinton North, Carman (1961); Dr. James M. McMahon, Lynn Lake (1962); Dr. Carleton M. Thomas, Portage la Prairie (1964); Dr. Richard Giesbrecht, Beausejour (1965).

CHAPTER 10

1 By current standards the scholarships and grants made by the Institute to individuals in these times were not large. But they provided an opportunity for undergraduate students and others to gain experience, knowledge, and intellectual rewards through carrying out short-term research projects, or undertaking brief studies of special value to them, which were not eligible for support under the policies of the major funding bodies.

Perhaps of even more importance in the long run, the Institute awards were usually made at times when youth and enthusiasm were combined in a scientific voyage of discovery; and though the objectives may have been limited and the voyage short, the venture was made possible at a critical time in the life of the recipient, when small investments could yield large returns in later achievement.

2 The members of the Board of Directors of the Winnipeg Clinic Research Institute at this time were: Mr. Joseph Harris, President; Dr. L.G. Bell and Dr. C.B. Stewart, Vice-Presidents; together with Mr. H.W. Manning, Mr. W.A. Murphy, Mrs. James A. Richardson, President H.H. Saunderson (University of Manitoba), Mr. H.E. Sellers, Mr. C. Gordon Smith, Dr. P.H.T. Thorlakson, and Mr. J.E. Woods. The Honorary Treasurer was Mr. John A. MacAulay; and the Honorary Secretary was Dr. Thomas A. Lebbetter.

3 Members of the Winnipeg Clinic who were invited by universities in Canada to occupy full-time positions: Dr. Lennox G. Bell, Dean of the Faculty of Medicine, and Professor of Medicine, University of Manitoba; Dr. E.G. Brownell, Associate Professor of Medicine, and Head, Section of General Medicine, University of Manitoba; Dr. Louis Cherniack, Assistant Professor of Medicine, Respiratory Centre, University of Manitoba; Dr. J.C. Martin del Campo, Assistant Professor, Department of Neurology, University of Manitoba; Dr. K.C. Finkel, Associate Professor of Pediatrics, McMaster University, Hamilton, Ontario; Dr. J.P. Gemmell, Professor of Medicine, University of Manitoba; Dr. B.J. Grogono, Chief of Orthopedics, Halifax Infirmary, and Assistant Professor of Orthopedics, Dalhousie University, Halifax, Nova Scotia; Dr. J.C. Haworth, Professor of Pediatrics, and Director of Pediatric Research, University of Manitoba; Dr. Walter C. MacKenzie, Professor of Surgery, University of Alberta, Edmonton; Dr. J. Wendell Macleod, Dean of the Faculty of Medicine, University of Saskatchewan, Saskatoon; Dr. A.S. Majury, Department of Obstetrics and Gynecology, Health Sciences Centre, Winnipeg and Associate Professor of Obstetrics and Gynecology, University of Manitoba; Dr. J.K. Martin, Professor and Head, Department of Pediatrics, University of Alberta, Edmonton; Dr. T.M. Roulston, Professor and Head, Department of Obstetrics and Gynecology, University of Manitoba.

4 At the Annual Meeting of the members of the Manitoba Institute for the Advancement of Medical Education and Research on April 23, 1951, Dr. Thorlakson had reported that a gift of $20,000 in securities had been received by the Institute from Miss Agnes B. Dougall in memory of her sister, Elizabeth Dougall.

CHAPTER 12

1 In later years, when he was one of Manitoba's outstanding surgeons, Dr. Neil John Maclean used to recall that his first rela-

tion to the Medical College occurred when in 1883, as a sixteen-year-old office boy for Dr. J.R. Jones, he was sent on his bicycle to collect the signatures of prospective sponsoring physicians and surgeons for the Medical School, on a petition urging the provision of training facilities in Winnipeg.

The sponsors were: Dr. R.J. Blanchard, Dr. R.G. Brett, Dr. T. Fafard, Dr. A.H. Ferguson, Dr. R.B. Ferguson, Dr. J.W. Good, Dr. J.R. Jones, Dr. J. Kerr, Dr. A. McDiarmid, Dr. J. Patterson, Dr. W.R.D. Sutherland, Dr. J.W. Whiteford and Dr. D.H. Wilson. (Dr. R.J. Blanchard's grandson became Professor and Head, Department of Surgery, University of Manitoba, in 1985.)

2 At that time the University of Manitoba was an examining and degree-granting institution only. The teaching units were five independent colleges: St. Boniface College, St. John's College, Manitoba College, Wesley College and the Medical College.

3 It is of interest to note that the architect was the father of Dr. F.T. Cadham, after whom the Provincial Laboratory – "the Cadham Lab" – was named; and the grandfather of Dr. Roper Cadham, longtime Medical Health Officer of the City of Winnipeg.

4 From "Historical Sketch" in the Faculty of Medicine calendar, 1952–53.

5 Ross Mitchell, "Maternity Hospitals in Greater Winnipeg," *Manitoba Medical Review* (May, 1946), p. 274.

6 Harry Medovy, *A Vision Fulfilled* (Winnipeg: Peguis Publishers Limited, 1979), p. 85.

CHAPTER 14

1 Dr. Rice's project almost failed of completion for want of funds. Meeting Dr. Rice one day in the coffee room, Dr. Thorlakson asked him how the construction of his new machine was progressing. Dr. Rice said that work on it had temporarily stopped because he lacked funds. "How much do you need to complete the job?" asked Dr. Thorlakson. "Eight hundred dollars," Dr. Rice replied. When Dr. Thorlakson went back to his office, his first action was to send a cheque for $800 to Dean A.T. Mathers at the Medical College to enable Dr. Rice to finish building the encephalograph and put it into service at the Winnipeg General Hospital.

The effect of this timely assistance was described in a letter from Dr. Rice to Dr. Harry Medovy (in his capacity as Archivist for the Winnipeg Clinic) in August, 1981. The letter reads in part as follows:

> . . . I well recall the occasion when the EEG grant was made. I think it was in 1940, and followed a Faculty Council meeting at which I described to

Dr. Thorlakson the merits of the electroencephalograph as it was being developed in such places as the Montreal Neurological Institute under Penfield's encouragement. I mentioned to Thor that I felt, with my interest in electronics and my hobby of mechanical devices, I could assemble the circuitry and make the pen recorders for such a machine.

The next morning [after my coffee room meeting with Thor] I had a call from Dr. A.T. Mathers, then Dean of Medicine, to say that a cheque for $800 had been given to him to be made available to me in the construction of an EEG.

I was astonished at this "gift." It was a tremendous demonstration of the direct and forthright manner in which Thor would make a decision and act on it; and it was a new experience to me, who was used to waiting months, and filling reams of applications, for decisions on grants to be made by such bodies as the National Research Council. . . .

In some ways this grant was a turning point in my career, for it opened the door to my interest in clinical physiology. It was this interest that expanded later into active clinical physiology in Edmonton, in connection not only with the EEG and neurological disorders, but also in connection with respiratory problems dramatically shown during the polio epidemic and the use of the iron lung; and also in the diagnosis of cardiac disease and its surgical treatment. All involved applied or clinical physiology, electronics, mechanics, physics, optics and related sciences with which I was familiar.

Within the then-established academic organization there was no means of combining clinical and physiological pursuits in any serious manner. That is why I had to give up my established academic position and get into a hospital. So I finished my active career by being known as a biomedical engineer, and something of a pioneer in these fields.

Thus the ultimate denouement of my EEG experience.

2 Thousands of patients and visitors to the Winnipeg General Hospital and the Manitoba Cancer Relief and Research Foundation will have noticed a bronze plaque, located near the first-floor entrance on the east side of the Hospital, which reads as follows:

ANNE FORLONG
In whose memory a
Radiotherapy Department
was first erected on this
site in the year 1937.

Dr. Thorlakson has recorded how the Forlong Memorial Unit for the treatment of cancer patients came into being:

Mrs. Grace Anne (MacDonald) Forlong was referred to me in 1935 by Dr. H.M. Murdoff for a surgical opinion regarding a persistent lower abdominal complaint. Physical examination revealed a mass which proved at operation to be an advanced malignant growth.

At that period of time, the 400,000-volt x-ray therapy unit had been developed but was not available in many North American medical centres. From Dr. Currie McMillan, the senior radiologist and radiotherapist on the staff of the Winnipeg General Hospital, we learned that the University of Minnesota had installed such a high-powered radiation unit in the University Hospital.

I contacted the radiotherapist for an appointment and tentative admission to the hospital for our patient. Mrs. Forlong asked me to accompany her and her husband to Minneapolis. During my brief stay in Minneapolis, I was able to obtain an insight into some of the rigid requirements for housing such a unit: the need to provide adequate protection for the patient, professional staff and others in the Department with thick cement walls and floors and heavy lead screening, which were much more costly than the machine itself.

During my brief stay in Minneapolis, Mr. Forlong asked why this new form of treatment was not available in Winnipeg. My answer was that no one had offered to purchase this expensive x-ray machine for the Winnipeg General Hospital.

Some months after Mrs. Forlong's death in 1936, I called on Mr. Forlong at his home on a Saturday afternoon. At that interview, I asked Mr. Forlong if he might consider financing the establishment of a special radiotherapy unit attached to the Winnipeg General Hospital in memory of his wife. I well remember emphasizing a therapy unit as a memorial but I soon discovered that my explanation had not been understood. However, at the time, he accepted my suggestion which, in essence, was that "a memorial, when completed, would cost in the neighbourhood of $50,000."

Naturally, I was pleased by his immediate acceptance of my proposal. As it was late in the afternoon, I decided not to inform Dr. George Stephens, the Superintendent of the Winnipeg General Hospital, of this turn of events until Monday. However, John Forlong, having made a decision and a commitment, called Dr. Stephens that evening. His first question was the cost of the 400,000-volt radiation unit. Dr. Stephens told him that to the best of his knowledge at the time that it would be $13,500.

Later that evening, I received a call from Mr. Forlong to check on the wide difference between the quotation from Dr. Stephens and my earlier figure. Everything was cleared up when I explained that I had proposed "a special memorial radiotherapy unit" of which the $13,500 machine was only one part. I then explained that if the hospital accepted the gift of the machine they would then have to build, at considerable cost, a building with thick cement walls together with adequate thick lead insulation to protect the personnel working in the unit, and that great care would be taken to direct the radiation to only the site of the malignant tumour and that other parts of the patient would also require careful screening.

The upshot was that an emergency meeting of the Executive Committee of the Board of Directors of the Winnipeg General Hospital was held. Mr. W.L. Parrish was Chairman at the time and Mr. Forlong and I were in attendance. The final cost of the completed unit, built outside the walls of the hospital on the east side, was $60,000.

This donation by Mr. Forlong in memory of his wife was the beginning of the present large building occupied by the Manitoba Cancer Treatment and Research Foundation.

My contact with Mr. Forlong, however, did not end there; we would meet casually from time to time. He had a magnificent yacht on Lake of the Woods, named the Grace Anne, which he offered to sell to me for $7,000 when he moved to Florida in 1940. If I sold it to someone else for a higher price, the additional sum would be donated to medical research. In retrospect, I fully realize that this was a very generous offer, but I was in no position to accept it. The yacht is still plying the channels and the broad expanse of the Lake of the Woods.

While spending a holiday in Florida in March 1958, I saw Mr. Forlong for the last time in company with Mr. Harry Sellers, in a hospital in St. Petersburg, shortly before his death.

3 It should be said here that later the Bronfman family did contribute very substantially to the cultural resources of Winnipeg by undertaking in 1967 a major share of the cost of building and equipping the Planetarium in the Centennial Centre.

Approval was given for this donation at a meeting of the directors of the Bronfman Family Charitable Foundation held at the Fort Garry Hotel in Winnipeg. Samuel Bronfman's son Charles was the chairman on this occasion.

Dr. Thorlakson was one of the guests invited to attend a reception following this meeting. He recalls that Charles Bronfman was telling a group of guests that it took only about three minutes to get approval of the directors for this support for the Planetarium; upon which his father observed wryly, "Charles hasn't shown yet that he can make a dollar, but he can sure get rid of it in a hell of a hurry!"

4 Letter from Dr. Harvey Agnew, Executive Secretary, Canadian Hospital Council, July 10, 1945.

5 The doctors at the meeting of September 10, 1944, voted unanimous approval for presentation of the Medical Centre Plan to the City Council. They constituted an important segment of the medical staff of the Winnipeg General Hospital. Attending and approving the plan, were: W.C. Aikenhead; F.G. Allison; I.H. Beckman; Brian D. Best; A.R. Birt; Elinore Black; Robert Black; C.W. Burns; W.E. Campbell; H. Coppinger; A.E. Deacon; M.L. Hollenberg; E.S. James; H.W. Kitchen; J.M. Lederman; M.R. MacCharles; A.T. Mathers; J.M. McEachern; R.A. McPherson; J.D. McQueen; Daniel Nicholson; D.W. Penner; T.A. Pincock; James Rennie; D.L. Scott; P.H.T. Thorlakson; K.R. Trueman; E.J. Washington; C. Wallox; J.A. Waugh; and O.S. Waugh.

CHAPTER 16

1 The Committee, named by the Honourable Ivan Schultz, consisted of Dr. F.W. Jackson, Deputy Minister of Health, Dean A.T. Math-

ers, Acting University President H.P. Armes, and Dr. T.A. Pincock, the Provincial Psychiatrist.

CHAPTER 18

1 D.G. Mckenzie was Chief Commissioner, the Board of Grain Commissions for Canada. The Board's Head Office was in Winnipeg. He was a member of the Board of Governors, University of Manitoba, 1944–45.
2 Mr. T.P. Green and Mr. O'Malley were both senior editorial writers on the staff of the *Winnipeg Tribune*.
3 Mr. Justice C. Rhodes Smith was at that time Member of the Legislative Assembly representing Winnipeg Centre, first elected in 1941, and re-elected in 1945 and 1949. He was appointed Minister of Labour in the Garson cabinet on February 15, 1945, and in December 1948 was named Minister of Education by the new Premier, Hon. D.L. Campbell. He was appointed to the Bench in 1963 and became Chief Justice of Manitoba in 1967.
4 *Winnipeg Tribune*, March 30, 1945.
5 The only amendments were the addition of the word "research" to the preamble, and the provision for St. Boniface Hospital and St. Boniface Council representatives.
6 Section 7 of the Act of Incorporation, Manitoba Medical Centre.
7 Ibid., Section 11.
8 Ibid., Section 12.

CHAPTER 19

1 Donald M. Cox was a competent, well-trained, experienced hospital administrator, and a Fellow of the American College of Hospital Administrators. Some years later he moved to British Columbia to head their Hospital Insurance Plan.
2 However, in place of the meeting of October 19, the government decided to appoint two new committees, one of which would study the arrangements for medical education; and the other, consisting of members of the Legislature, would study hospital requirements in Manitoba. The Committee on Medical Education consisted of The Honourable Ivan Schultz, Dr. F.W. Jackson, Dean A.T. Mathers, Dr. Bruce Chown, Mr. Steele (an official of Manitoba Pool Elevators), and Mr. Crawford. This committee visited several medical education centres in the United States, but if they formulated a report it cannot be located, and no recommendations seem to have resulted from their enquiry. The Committee on Hospital Requirements was never appointed.

CHAPTER 20

1 Mr. G.L. Pickering was appointed by the provincial government to plan and direct the organization of the Manitoba Hospital Services Insurance Plan. This required the enrolment of every resident of the Province; design of a system to collect premiums, which were in effect during the early years of the Plan; and determination of a funding method for hospitals providing the services. He and the staff assisting him performed a remarkable feat in completing this immense task in the few months allotted to them, enabling the program to become effective on July 1, 1958.

2 Dr. George Johnson, who served in the Royal Canadian Navy in World War II, graduated in medicine after the War and practised at Gimli for ten years. His medical skills were overlaid with a warm-hearted, compassionate devotion to the needs of his patients, whatever their means or status, in the tradition of the highest ideals of his profession. Highly respected and popular in the district, he was persuaded to run for public office in the Provincial election of 1958, won his seat, and in June, 1958, was appointed Minister of Health and Public Welfare in the newly formed Roblin government.

3 In a study of Saskatchewan experience, where government-funded hospital care had been in place for some time, it was found that in the absence of alternative care facilities about five percent of the patients admitted to general hospitals required more than thirty days of hospital care. This relatively small proportion of patients accounted for about thirty-one percent of all the patient-days in general hospitals, although these facilities were designed and equipped to provide short-term acute care.

4 Clearwater Lake Hospital at The Pas and Assiniboine Hospital at Brandon were operated by the Sanatorium Board of Manitoba for the federal government, which owned or leased the property. They were used by the Board for the treatment of Indians and Eskimos suffering from tuberculosis, under a contract entered into with the federal government at the end of World War II. The Federal authorities concurred in the Board's action in converting the facilities for patients requiring extended treatment because the program to control tuberculosis among Indians and Eskimos had been highly successful, and the needs could be accommodated at Ninette and at St. Boniface Sanatorium in St. Vital.

5 The Manitoba Rehabilitation Hospital, including the D.A. Stewart Centre, was built at a cost of about $4.5 million. It had a total of 222 beds, and accommodation for the treatment of 200 out-patients daily. Average construction cost was nineteen to twenty dollars a

square foot. It represented a pioneering effort in this hitherto neglected field, and professionals interested in rehabilitation care came from many parts of Canada and the United States to see the facilities and study the programs of treatment.

6 It is of interest to note that in a formal proposal I.M. Pei stated that the nature of the medical facilities and their general relationship ought to be settled by the members of the Medical Centre; and with this policy matter settled, they would prepare a medical-centre development plan for $24,000, in four and a half months. Jack Meltzer offered to do a development program, including that of the medical facilities, for a fee of $52,000, in twelve to eighteen months.

7 It was customary that in the Faculty of Medicine the department heads in the several specialties were also appointed by the General Hospital as its corresponding department heads. It was also a requirement that the University have representatives on the Hospital board and its Executive Committee. On policy and planning matters the views of "the University" and "the Hospital" tended to be closely related.

8 The announcement of the development that was to become the Health Sciences Centre appeared in the Winnipeg Free Press of October 31, 1967, with the following lead: "Details of a $97 million plan to expand Manitoba's Medical Education and Research programs to make the province the leading medical centre in North America were unveiled by Premier Duff Roblin on Tuesday" (i.e., October 30, 1967).

CHAPTER 22

1 The importance attached to the work of this committee was attested by the calibre of its members, appointed by Dean Mathers: Dr. J.D. Adamson, Dr. J.D. McEachern, Dr. F.W. Jackson, Dr. Fred G. McGuinness, Dr. C.E. Corrigan, Dr. Lennox Bell, and Dr. P.H.T. Thorlakson, Chairman.

2 In 1934 the only medical college west of Winnipeg was at the University of Saskatchewan, which offered the first two years of training toward a medical degree. These students went to other Universities to complete their professional education.

3 In 1975 a plan was introduced under which every medical student, during his fourth clinical clerkship, has the opportunity to work under the guidance of cooperating private physicians in their office practice, giving them the experience to which Dr. Thorlakson referred.

CHAPTER 24

1 The Flexner study was funded by the Carnegie Foundation for the Advancement of Teaching. Abraham Flexner (M.A., Harvard) was a staff member of the Foundation from 1908 to 1912. During this time he was the author of two famous reports: in 1910, *Medical Education in the United States and Canada*, which revolutionized medical education in North America; and, in 1912, *Medical Education in Europe*. His brother Simon was a noted pathologist and director of laboratories for the Rockefeller Institute of Medical Research. The Flexner comments on his visit to the Manitoba Medical College in May, 1909 are of historical interest:

> Instruction in chemistry, bacteriology, histology and pathology is competently given in the University of Manitoba. Other branches are carried on by the medical faculty. The equipment is adequate for routine instruction, new, and steadily increasing. There is a beautifully kept collection of several hundred wet specimens. Appearances indicate a conscientious and intelligent employment of such resources as the school has had.
>
> Clinical Facilities: The excellent Winnipeg General Hospital of 400 beds adjoins the school. The school faculty is practically the staff of the free wards. The relation between the school and the hospital is admirable. Students work freely on the wards, clinical laboratory, operating rooms, obstetrical ward, etc.

2 The principles of Faculty organization suggested in this paper were largely adopted in later years, including the appointment of a full-time dean assisted by two associate deans and a director of post-graduate studies; and students regularly review professorial performance and course organization and content.

3 Chaired initially by Dr. William Boyd, followed in turn by Dr. Daniel Nicholson and Dr. Donald Penner.

CHAPTER 25

1 Dr. C. Edwin Corrigan graduated in medicine from the University of Manitoba in 1925. After a short period of practice at Lampman, Saskatchewan, he went overseas for training in surgery and obtained his FRCS (Eng.) in 1930. He returned to Winnipeg and in 1931 began the practice of general surgery at St. Boniface General Hospital. His first University appointment came in 1931. In 1939 he was appointed Chief of Surgery at St. Boniface, but within a year took leave of absence to serve in the Royal Canadian Medical Corps in World War II. He had a distinguished military service,

was awarded the DSO, and achieved the rank of lieutenant colonel. At the end of the War he resumed the position of Chief of Surgery at St. Boniface, and was appointed to the equivalent post at Deer Lodge Hospital. Dr. Corrigan was honoured by appointment to senior offices in a number of medical and surgical organizations. He retired as an associate professor of surgery at the University of Manitoba in 1962. Throughout his life he served his profession, his university and his country with distinction. He died at Deer Lodge Hospital on July 14, 1979.

2 The Medical Faculty Council Excutive for 1945–46 consisted of: Dr. A.W. Trueman, President of the University of Manitoba; Dr. A.T. Mathers, Dean of the Faculty of Medicine; Dr. J.D. Adamson, Professor of Medicine and Head of the Department of Medicine at Winnipeg General Hospital; Dr. O.S. Waugh, Professor of Surgery and Head of the Department of Surgery at Winnipeg General Hospital. There were also four representatives of the Faculty Council at large: Dr. J.D. McQueen, Dr. M.R. MacCharles, Dr. P.H.T. Thorlakson, and Dr. Digby Wheeler. There were also two representatives of the pre-clinical years, Dr. A.T. Cameron and Dr. Ian MacLaren Thompson.

CHAPTER 26

1 The descriptive terms were used by Dr. Mathers' successor as Dean of the Faculty of Medicine, Dr. L.G. Bell, in "An Appreciation," which appeared in the *Canadian Medical Association Journal* (February 6, 1960).

2 The four teaching hospitals at that time were: Winnipeg General Hospital; St. Boniface General Hospital; Deer Lodge Hospital; and The Children's Hospital of Winnipeg.

3 P.H.T. Thorlakson, "Trends in Medical Practice," *Manitoba Medical Review* (September, 1944), pp. 243–246.

4 One example occurred a year after the Report was prepared. In November, 1947, Dr. Thorlakson was invited to be the guest speaker at the Annual Meeting of the North Pacific Surgical Association in Victoria. Dr. Henry N. Harkins, then Professor of Surgery at the University of Washington in Seattle, and Dr. Livingstone, Professor of Surgery at the University of Oregon, both of whom were members of the Association and were attending the meeting, arranged to discuss with Dr. Thorlakson some of the teaching and organizational problems with which they were struggling. At the conclusion of their long and interesting interview, Dr. Thorlakson told them that he had prepared a report which addressed many of the problems they had raised and on a strictly confidential basis he

would supply them with copies. On January 5, 1948, Dr. Harkins responded with a comprehensive analysis:

Dear Dr. Thorlakson:

Your prospectus arrived, and I have read it from cover to cover. I am certain that many of the problems that have faced the Department of Surgery of the University of Manitoba in the past will face our own department in the future, and I have received many helpful suggestions from your very thorough analysis of your problems.

I am treating this as a confidential report as you requested and, except for the Dean of the Medical School and a few of the higher men in my own department, will not allow it to be read further.

There are a number of conclusions that you have reached that struck a very responsive chord in me. I might list a few of these in order.

1. A new course in the fundamentals of surgical technique: I am heartily in agreement with this and even though the Medical School that I attended (Rush) did not have such a course, I fully intend to have one here. The reasoning that you used for giving such a course and its importance in the training of general practitioners as well as specialists seems to me to be quite logical.

2. Re-organization of the surgical staff, Winnipeg General Hospital: This is one element in the organization of a Surgical Service with which I am in hearty accord. In the various places that I have worked, both in the Midwest and in the East, I notice that the Eastern portion of the United States is distinctly more backward than is the Midwest in adopting this plan. At the University of Chicago where all cases are used for teaching, the plan works out very well, and I am sure that the private patients get better care. Certainly in a public institution there is every reason to use the private patients for teaching as long as it will improve their care, which I am sure it always does. One other item that might be mentioned is that certainly there will be occasional private patients who will not want to be seen by students, but the same occasionally applies to public patients as well. The organization of a vertical service is one that has interested me for some ten years, and again I might cite my own experience in working in teaching institutions: those in which there has been the vertical organization of the service seem to me to have better teaching, better care of the patients and to avoid assembly-line type of medical care.

3. Combining of patients with one type of illness in one geographic section of the hospital: The combining of neurologic and neurosurgical patients, even though one group is medical and the other surgical, as you have outlined on Page 40, seems to be very logical. The further suggestion that the patient's condition be considered, rather than whether he is public, semi-private or private also is logical. I have always despaired of the way many hospitals are organized whereby for one service, to see ten pa-

tients some five to eight different wards have to be visited with a great loss of time. Furthermore, for any purposes of clinical research, such as special metabolic studies, if patients with one condition are put on one ward, whether they be private or public, it permits those studies to be carried out more efficiently by the nurses.

4. Intermittent versus continuous ward assignments: I am heartily in agreement with your ideas as expressed in favor of the continuous ward assignments.

5. Use of consultants assigned to wards and to ward rounds rather than merely being called in to see special patients: This seems to me to be one of the most helpful suggestions that I have seen in some time and certainly it is one that I intend to bring up in planning our own departmental organization. I also hope that the Medical Department and other departments here will consider the plan as well. I have even thought of having anatomists, physiologists and the like participate in rounds as well as clinicians.

6. The quotation, "All progress in the prevention and control of disease is based primarily on research," is one that I am sure I would like to use in the future. The same applies to the quotation on the bottom of Page 76: "The finest hospital building staffed with third rate personnel becomes a third rate hospital."

7. Adequate clinical facilities: The importance of these cannot be overemphasized, and I am glad to see the arguments for them so succinctly expressed. . . .

9. Idea of keeping leaders in the province or state: This also seems to me to be an especially interesting viewpoint and represents a different approach to the problem than any I had previously considered. . . .

I have heard a great deal about getting numbers of men to stay in general practice in different states or communities, but I have never before seen in print an expression of a method of keeping outstanding leaders in a state or community. . . .

10. Bringing of anatomy and physiology teaching to the clinical level: The idea expressed in the statement, "Freer access to patients for the teaching of anatomy and physiology would be advantageous," seems to me to be very important.

11. Importance of departmental heads visiting other clinics: I heartily agree with you that it is of great importance to visit other schools and the fact that you have visited every other medical school in Canada as well as many in the United States indicates to me that you have a very good approach to the whole problem of organization. I am hoping to pattern after this as much as I can. . . .

After commenting favourably on the remaining subjects in the report, Dr. Harkins concluded his appraisal:

I want to tell you again how much I appreciated reading this report, and I have given all the items in it considerable thought. I have been so stimulated by reading it and look forward to seeing you and discussing some of these problems first hand some time in the future. I am sure that one who is just starting out to organize a department as I am here can get many ideas from one who, like yourself, has had experience in meeting these problems over some time.

With best regards.

Very sincerely yours,

Henry N. Harkins, M.D.

CHAPTER 27

1 The report of the sub-committee of the Executive Committee of the Medical Staff of the Winnipeg General Hospital, appointed to consider "A Plan to establish a subsidized Cancer Diagnostic Clinic at St. Boniface Hospital and Winnipeg General Hospital for cancer subjects from rural Manitoba" had been submitted on May 20, 1949. Dr. Thorlakson's suggestions were offered in the hope of gaining some modification of the initial stand. The following quotation from the sub-committee's report indicates their position:

Your committee has given careful consideration to the plan brought forward by the Cancer Relief and Research Institute for the establishment of subsidized cancer diagnostic clinics at the two principal teaching hospitals. They have arrived at certain general conclusions which might well apply to any plan directed towards the improvement of cancer diagnosis in the Province, and have then applied these criteria to the specific plan under consideration. It is therefore their considered opinion that:

1. Before accepting any new plan for the diagnosis of cancer it must be clear that it possesses definite advantages over existing arrangements either in their present form or after reasonable modification.

2. As one of the primary objectives in cancer diagnosis is its early detection, attention should be focussed on that level of screening where the patient first comes into contact with the medical profession. Whereas a central point of reference is an essential feature of such an organization it is equally important not to remove from the individual medical practitioner his responsibility for the early diagnosis of cancer. Emphasis must be placed upon improving the knowledge and awareness of cancer of all physicians in private practice.

3. The diagnosis of cancer cannot be separated from the problem of diagnosis in general. For example, the middle-aged patient who has abdominal symptoms may be suffering from any one of many diseases, including cancer.

4. Anticipating the problems of medical care under an over-all governmental plan for social security, the physicians and surgeons of Manitoba, at considerable cost in time and money, have developed a plan for medical care which is believed to be in the best interests of the patient as well as of the profession. The Manitoba Medical Service, after several years of voluntary participation, has met with the general approval of the public and the profession; a fact which indicates the soundness of the principles upon which the plan was founded. It is felt that the medical profession of Manitoba should see to it that any ventures into the field of socialized medicine, without exception, should be effected through the structure of the Manitoba Medical Service and only where it can be conclusively shown that such action is not in the interests of both parties should arrangements outside the sphere of the Manitoba Medical Service be accepted.

5. Any partial or total plan for socialized medicine must conform to the twelve principles of social security adopted by the World Medical Association in Geneva in 1948.

With specific reference to the plan submitted by the Cancer Relief and Research Institute your committee have found the plan unacceptable for the following reasons:

1. It is felt that there are adequate facilities for the diagnosis of cancer in Manitoba. Moreover, tumor clinics are now functioning at both hospitals where any doctor may send patients for free diagnosis and treatment recommendations.

2. Concentrating facilities and skilled personnel into a few centres will provide the satisfactory diagnostic handling of patients who appear at the clinics. It is believed, however, that these same patients are at the present time reaching the identical physicians and surgeons who would see them under the proposed plan. The plan fails to emphasize the importance of early diagnosis in the field, and does not provide adequate means of improving the quality of the work at that level.

3. The proposed plan separates the diagnosis of cancer from the general problem of diagnosis, which is the responsibility of private practice.

4. It constitutes a step in socialized medicine outside of the sphere of the Manitoba Medical Service, and in so doing contravenes the principle of private practice. . . . It is the opinion of your Committee that the basic principles involved in the proposed plan are essentially similar to those in-

> volved in the plan to establish a diagnostic centre in the Winnipeg General Hospital for the Stonewall area. At that time ... it was the unanimous opinion of the Executive and the Honorary Attending Staff that such a plan was not in the interests of either the patient or the medical profession....
>
> Your Committee realizes that it is probably exceeding its terms of reference in making alternative suggestions, but feels that to offer only adverse criticism of the plan submitted might indicate unwillingness on their part to recognize any deficiencies in the present arrangements for cancer diagnosis. The truth is quite the contrary and your Committee feels that the medical profession both collectively and individually who, after all, are primarily responsible for the care of cancer in this Province should be only too willing to accept advice and financial assistance when offered in good faith....

The paper concluded with a brief statement of basic principles which the Committee felt should be observed.

2 Both the Honourable Ivan Schultz and Mr. I.B. Griffiths were members of the Board of the Cancer Relief and Research Institute. Mr. Griffiths had been Minister of Health and Public Welfare from 1935 to 1940, after which he retired from the Legislature as member for Russell Constituency and was appointed Commissioner of the Manitoba Farm Loans Board.

CHAPTER 28

1 The Commonwealth Fund, with headquarters at 1 East 75th Street, New York, is one of the great philanthropic foundations in the United States which has supported efforts to improve the health services in North America. In recent years, it has devoted its primary funding to encouragement of the publication of significant and scholarly books in medicine and health; and to experimental and developmental activities devoted to the improvement of medical education, including projects relative to the role of University Medical Centres in strengthening the health-care system.

2 Ivan Schultz, "Surveys and Health Insurance," *Canadian Journal of Public Health* (Vol. 36, no. 2, February, 1945).

3 Paper presented at the annual meeting of the Canadian Medical Association, Montreal, June, 1945.

4 See pages 221–222 for a copy of this resolution.

CHAPTER 29

1 The first Board of Directors of the Manitoba Medical Services, Inc., appointed by the Manitoba Medical Association, consisted of Dr.

M.R. MacCharles, Chairman; Dr. H.D. Kitchen; Dr. Ross Mitchell; Dr. J.S. McInnes; Dr. Claude McRae; Dr. Hugh Cameron; Dr. Brian Best; and Dr. Clifford Abbott. The non-medical members of the Board were: John B. Richardson; Robert McKay; Frederick W. Ross; Milton D. Grant; Gerald F. Pearson; Donald H. Murdock; and Donovan Swailes. Dr. E.S. Moorhead was the first Executive Director.

CHAPTER 30

1 Quoted by Dr. Thorlakson in the preface of his Brief to the Royal Commission on Health Services.
2 The commemorative plaque presented by the Icelandic community in Canada to mark Canada's centenary can be seen in the National Library, Ottawa, on the south wall just inside the entrance to its building on Wellington Street.
3 Dr. Peart was extremely helpful in many other ways. During World War II he had served in the Royal Canadian Army Medical Corps as hygiene officer in Canada and Europe. Later, among other experiences, he had served from 1948 to 1953 as Chief of the Division of Epidemiology in the Department of National Health and Welfare. In addition, he was on the Executive of the World Medical Association, and became its president in 1970. Consequently, he was able to advise Dr. Thorlakson in considerable detail about the international marshalling of medical interest in the Congress.
4 Elected first to the Manitoba Legislature in 1969, Mr. Sherman was re-elected in 1973 and 1977; and he was appointed Minister of Health and Social Development on October 24, 1977, in the government of Premier Sterling Lyon.
5 Under the general direction of Dr. Thorlakson, the President and General Manager of the Congress, eighty-five people serving on eleven committees took an active part in the organization of the First International Congress of Group Medicine. Other than two from the United States, two from Ottawa, two from Oshawa and one from Edmonton, all were from Winnipeg. The committees and their respective chairmen were: Budget Committee, Mr. A.T. Burstow; Citizen's Committee, Mr. Perry S. Bower; Dean's Advisory Committee, Dr. T.W. Fyles; Exhibits Committee, Dr. B. Derbach; Finance Committee, Mr. M. Neaman; Ladies' Committee, Mrs. P.H.T. Thorlakson, Honorary Chairman, Mrs. J.M. Gillis, Chairman; Program and Facilities Committee, Dr. R.E. Beamish; Public Relations Committee, Dr. C. Hollenberg; Reception and Hospitality Committee, Dr. K.R. Trueman; Social Events Committee, Dr. T.K. Thorlakson; Transportation Committee, Dr. I.M.

Grant. The Housing Bureau was operated by Mr. S. Petrow, Director of Sales for the Fort Garry Hotel; and the Executive Secretary was Mrs. Dora Sorell.

6 Vice-Presidents of the First International Congress on Group Medicine were appointed as follows: Dr. Omar Barreneche, Uruguay; Dr. Jacques Beaupere, France; Dr. Chr. F. Borchgrevink, Norway; Dr. J.C. Cameron, United Kingdom; Dr. Julian D. Czapski, Brazil; Dr. Gustave Gingras, Canada; Dr. M.O. Kent-Hughes, Australia; Dr. K.H. Metzner, Federal Republic of Germany; Dr. Alton Ochsner, United States of America; Dr. J.F. Patino, Colombia; Dr. Antonio Spinelli, Italy; Dr. Taro Takemi, Japan; Dr. P.R. Trivedi, India.

7 Dr. R.E. Beamish is a prominent Winnipeg heart specialist, a Vice-President of the Great-West Life Assurance Company, holding high office in many other national and international organizations. One day, as he was in conversation with Dr. Thorlakson, the question of his place of birth arose. "Well," said Dr. Beamish, "I was born at Shoal Lake, Manitoba." "Why," exclaimed Dr. Thorlakson, "that must have been about the time I was practising there. I may have delivered you!" "Is that so?" responded Dr. Beamish. "I must say, I thought your face looked familiar the first time I met you here in Winnipeg!"

CHAPTER 31

1 Published in full in the Icelandic weekly newspaper, *Lögberg-Heimskringla* (January 10, 1974); and in the English-language section of the monthly journal of the Ukrainian Women's Association of Canada, *Promin* (Vol. 5, no. 4, April, 1964).

2 The Reverend Dr. Marteinsson had two children: a son who graduated in medicine and practised for many years in British Columbia; and one daughter who is the wife of Dr. A.L. Paine, for some thirty years the Medical Superintendent of Manitoba Sanatorium at Ninette. Mrs. Paine is a registered nurse. Dr. and Mrs. Paine, now retired, were not only deeply respected for their professional dedication and skill; they are affectionately remembered by countless hundreds of former tuberculosis patients for their warm hospitality and friendship.

3 The Organizing Committee, known after initial plans were formulated as the Foundation Committee, consisted of: Dr. Thorlakson, Chairman; Judge W.J. Lindal; Mr. Grettir L. Johannson, Consul General of Iceland in Winnipeg; Dr. L.A. Sigurdson; and Mr. Arni G. Eggertson, Q.C. Before the fund-raising campaign began, the following organizations had agreed to act as sponsors: The

Icelandic National League; The Icelandic Canadian Club; The Jon Sigurdson Chapter, Imperial Order of the Daughters of the Empire; The Icelandic Good Templars Society of Winnipeg; The Icelandic Celebration Committee; the two Icelandic newspapers, *Lögberg* and *Heimskringla;* and representatives of the Icelandic churches.

4 *Lögberg,* May 7, 1953.

5 *The Winnipeg Tribune,* May 1, 1953.

6 The late Dr. D.A. Stewart, M.D., LL.D., the first Medical Superintendent of the Manitoba Sanatorium at Ninette, used the expression "The Home of the Happy Sunset" in a tribute he wrote to the Betel Home after a visit there in 1933.

CHAPTER 32

1 The Manitoba Conference on Education Planning Committee consisted of Mr. Justice Tritschler, Chairman; Brigadier General N.E. Rodger, Vice-Chairman; Mr. John Gordon; Dr. W.C. Lorimer; Mr. R.F.T. Thompson; Mr. George Brisbin; Mr. Frank Spencer; Mr. R.O.A. Hunter; and Mr. E.L. Arnett, Secretary to the Committee.

2 Dr. Thorlakson's introduction was commendably concise:

> DR. WILDER PENFIELD
> It is now my great pleasure to introduce our guest speaker, Dr. Wilder Penfield of Montreal. Dr. Penfield is an internationally famous neurosurgeon; a medical scientist who has made a substantial contribution to our knowledge of the normal physiology and the diseases of the brain; an author of several scientific books dealing with his specialty; an author of the well-known book entitled *No Other Gods* [Toronto: Little, Brown, 1954] depicting in fiction the life stories of the biblical characters Abraham and Sarah.
>
> Dr. Penfield was created a Companion of St. Michael and St. George in 1943 by His Majesty, the late King George VI. In 1953, Queen Elizabeth conferred upon him the Order of Merit.
>
> Our guest speaker has been the recipient of many honorary degrees from universities in North America and in Europe. In May 1955, the University of Manitoba gave recognition to his outstanding contribution to medical science by conferring upon him at its annual convocation the degree of Doctor of Science, *honoris causa.*
>
> He will speak to us on "Education Seen in Long Perspective."

3 Dr. Hugh Ross, well-known Winnipeg pathologist and long associated with the Victoria General Hospital, was at the time of the Manitoba Conference on Education a member of the Pathology Department at Winnipeg General Hospital.

CHAPTER 33

1 For a definitive history of the founding colleges of the University of Winnipeg and the events leading up to the chartering of the University on July 1, 1967, the reader is referred to the book on these subjects by Professor A.G. Bedford, *The University of Winnipeg: A History of the Founding Colleges* (University of Toronto Press, 1976). Dr. Bedford is a graduate of the United College, which was later incorporated into the University of Winnipeg. For many years he has been an esteemed member of its Department of English. He has written an account of Dr. Thorlakson's experience as Chancellor, which is now one of the valued documents in the Thorlakson papers.

In *The Saga of Dr. Thor,* attention has been focussed to some extent on the more informal duties of the Chancellor, which in fact had particular importance at a time when many University campuses were being disrupted by waves of student unrest. The warm and friendly, and at the same time dignified, way in which Dr. Thorlakson carried out the many official duties of the Chancellor, his sincere interest in the University, and his willingness to meet with students or Faculty on appropriate occasions, brought him into a closer relationship with the members of the University than is normally the case.

2 R.H.G. Bonnycastle was a quiet, unassuming, amiable, conscientious and fair-minded man, strong and effective in each of the widely varying vocations to which he devoted himself. He inherited the pioneering spirit that brought his parents from Ontario to Binscarth, Manitoba, in the early 1880s. He was educated at St. John's College, Winnipeg; Trinity College, Toronto; and Oxford University, which he attended as a Rhodes Scholar. He graduated in law, and became a member of the Honourable Society of Lincoln's Inn. He toured Europe for three years as a member of the same Oxford ice-hockey team that included Lester B. Pearson, who later became the Prime Minister of Canada, and Edward Pitblado, the well-known Winnipeg lawyer. He returned to Winnipeg in 1924, and after a year in a legal firm he joined the Hudson's Bay Company, becoming their chief trader, responsible for the direction of all their Arctic and other northern operations. He travelled regularly to all the HBC trading posts by air, boat and dog team. On an 11,000-mile inspection trip in 1931, he and his staff aboard the S.S. Baychimo were trapped in 50-foot-thick ice west of Pt. Barrow, Alaska. Rescuers of the passengers and crew came by plane from Nome. In 1937, Mr. Bonnycastle represented the Company in a trip

down the Mackenzie River as far as Aklavik by Lord Tweedsmuir, then Governor-General of Canada.

Mr. Bonnycastle left the HBC after nearly a quarter century of service to manage his own business. In 1960 he was appointed the first chairman of the newly created Metropolitan Government of Greater Winnipeg. After six successful years in this office he resigned to return to the direction of his business interests. He gave generously of his time to a number of community enterprises, including the Sanatorium Board of Manitoba, and St. John's Ravenscourt School.

3 The dinner for the class of '69 was held on March 14, 1969.

4 It is of interest to note that Dr. Thorlakson has three first cousins on his mother's side of the family who for many years have been deeply involved in post-secondary education in Norway: Professor Erik Waaler, world-renowned pathologist and research worker, faculty member of the University of Bergen, for five years (1957 to 1962) Rector of that university, and for one year interim Rector of the University of Oslo; his brother, Professor Rolf Waaler, an Engineer by profession, and longtime Rector of the School of Commerce in Bergen; and his elder brother, Professor Georg Waaler, a doctor of medicine, for many years Professor of Forensic Medicine at the University of Oslo. All three men were recently honoured by being appointed Knights First Class of the Order of St. Olav (Norway).

APPENDIX 5

1 Dr. Thorlakson wishes to record his appreciation for the advice and information provided by Dr. O.H. Warwick during the preparation of this part of the paper on research, relating to cancer. Dr. Warwick graduated in Medicine from McGill University in 1940, subsequently obtaining the FACP; FRCP (Lond.); and FRCP (Can.). He is Professor of Medicine at the University of Western Ontario and has been for many years associated with the London Clinic of the Ontario Cancer Treatment and Research Foundation at the Victoria Hospital, London, Ontario.

Index